Clinical Dermatology

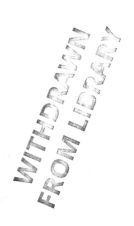

For my mother Alison and for Julie, Hiwot and Girma; Foz, Jack and Isabella; Daniel and Samuel.

Clinical Dermatology

Richard B. Weller MD, FRCP (Edin)

Senior Lecturer
Department of Dermatology
University of Edinburgh
Edinburgh, UK

Hamish J.A. Hunter BSc (Hons), MBChB, MRCP (UK) (Derm)

Clinical Research Fellow in Dermatology
University of Manchester
Manchester, UK

Margaret W. Mann MD, FAAD

Assistant Professor of Dermatology
Director of Aesthetic Dermatology
Associate Director of Dermatologic Surgery
University Hospitals / Case Western School of Medicine
Cleveland, OH, USA

FIFTH EDITION

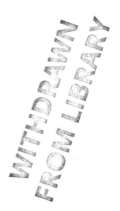

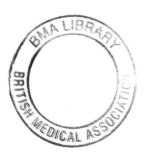

WILEY Blackwell

This edition first published 2015 © 2015 by John Wiley & Sons Ltd.

Registered office: John Wiley & Sons, Ltd, The Atrium, Southern Gate, Chichester,
West Sussex, PO19 8SQ, UK

Editorial offices: 9600 Garsington Road, Oxford, OX4 2DQ, UK
The Atrium, Southern Gate, Chichester, West Sussex, PO19 8SQ, UK
111 River Street, Hoboken, NJ 07030-5774, USA

For details of our global editorial offices, for customer services and for information about how
to apply for permission to reuse the copyright material in this book please see our website at
www.wiley.com/wiley-blackwell

The right of the authors to be identified as the authors of this work has been asserted in
accordance with the UK Copyright, Designs and Patents Act 1988.

Library of Congress Cataloging-in-Publication Data

Weller, Richard P. J. B., author.
   Clinical dermatology / Richard B. Weller, Hamish J.A. Hunter, Margaret W. Mann. – Fifth
edition.
      p. ; cm.
   Preceded by Clinical dermatology / Richard P.J.B. Weller … [et al.]. 4th ed. 2008.
   Includes bibliographical references and index.
   ISBN 978-0-470-65952-6 (pbk.)
   I. Hunter, Hamish J.A., author.   II. Mann, Margaret W., author.   III. Title.
   [DNLM: 1. Skin Diseases–diagnosis.   2. Skin Diseases–therapy.   WR 140]
   RL71
   616.5–dc23
                                                                              2014032478

A catalogue record for this book is available from the British Library.

Wiley also publishes its books in a variety of electronic formats. Some content that appears in
print may not be available in electronic books.

Set in 9.25/11.5pt Minion by Aptara Inc., New Delhi, India
Printed and bound in Singapore by Markono Print Media Pte Ltd

1   2015

Contents

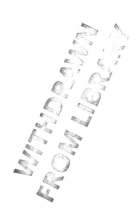

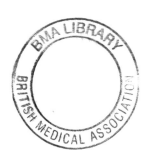

Preface to the Fifth Edition

Clinical Dermatology is now quarter of a century old, and this fifth edition is the first not to include any of the original authors. Hamish Hunter is one of the two British authors and has an interest in inflammatory dermatoses and the brain–skin axis. Margaret Mann has joined the team as our American author bringing particular expertise in dermatologic surgery and cosmetic dermatology. While the authors may have changed, we hope that the book retains its original feel as an approachable and useful text to the practicing clinician, but underpinned by the science behind the disease. As always we have striven to make the text enjoyable and useful to a wide audience, whether medical students, family doctors or neophyte dermatologists.

Dermatology as a speciality has grown enormously since the first edition. The constant improvements in our understanding of skin disease and developments in the treatments are both exciting and, it must be admitted, sometimes a little daunting for the editors! Traditional medical dermatology has been joined by surgical and cosmetic dermatology; an evolution we have tried to reflect by enhancing these sections of our book. The biologics revolution, now well embedded in our practice, has been a gratifying example of how a basic science understanding has led to real improvements in therapy for our patients; truly 'bench to bedside'. We hope that the arrival of BRAF inhibitors for melanoma may be a sign of similar improvements in care for our melanoma patients. Every chapter has benefited from being revised and updated and together they reflect changes in a vigorous and scientifically grounded speciality.

We hope you enjoy the latest edition of our book. All medical textbooks are a snapshot of the state of the art when written, but we trust that you will find this book useful for at least the next five years!

Richard Weller, Edinburgh
Margaret Mann, Cleveland
Hamish Hunter, Manchester

Acknowledgements

Many people have helped in the production of this book. First of course we must thank John Hunter, the late John Savin and Mark Dahl who wrote the first edition a quarter of a century ago and have been responsible for each subsequent edition until now. We are immensely grateful that they have entrusted their text to us, and hope that we have lived up to the standard that they set.

Martin Sugden, latterly Oliver Walter and Jennifer Seward have chivvied and supported us through the delayed gestation of our manuscript. We are also grateful to our friends and colleagues who have generously provided illustrations and feedback. Many of the clinical photographs come from the collections of the Department of Dermatology at the Royal Infirmary of Edinburgh, and we wish to thank all those who presented them. Dr Kelly Nelson of Duke University kindly supplied all the dermoscopic pictures in Chapter 28. Drs Nelson and Meg Gerstenblith of Case Western University provided invaluable feedback on the dermoscopy chapter and Dr Amr Gohar of Cairo on the acne chapter.

Introduction

Our overall aim in this book has been to make dermatology easy to understand by the many busy doctors who glimpsed it only briefly, if at all, during their medical training. All too often the subject has been squeezed out of its proper place in the undergraduate curriculum, leaving growing numbers who quail before the skin and its reputed 2000 conditions, each with its own diverse presentations. They can see the eruptions clearly enough, but cannot describe or identify them. There are no machines to help them; although our new Chapter 28 on dermoscopy should help in this respect. Even official 'clinical guidelines' for treatment are no use if a diagnosis has not been made. Their patients quickly sense weakness and lose faith. We hope that this book will give them confidence in their ability to make the right diagnosis and then to prescribe safe and effective treatments.

An understanding of the anatomy, physiology and immunology of the skin (Chapter 2) is the bedrock on which all diagnostic efforts must be based. Remembering Osler's aphorism that 'we miss more by not seeing than by not knowing', the identification and description of primary skin lesions and the patterns these have taken up on the skin surface follows (Chapter 3) and will lead to a sensible working diagnosis. After this has been achieved, investigations can be directed along sensible lines (Chapter 3) until a firm diagnosis is reached. Then, and only then, will the correct line of treatment snap into place.

General rules for the choice of topical treatments are dealt with in Chapter 26, while more specific information on topical and systemic drugs are covered in the chapters on individual conditions. Correct choices here will be repaid by good results. Patients may be quick to complain if they are not doing well: equally they are delighted if their eruptions can be seen to melt rapidly away. Many of them are now joining in the quest for cosmetic perfection that is already well advanced in the United States and rapidly becoming equally fashionable in the United Kingdom. Family doctors who are asked about this topic can

find their answers in our chapter on cosmetic dermatology (Chapter 22).

We do not pretend that all of the problems in the classification of skin diseases have been solved in this book. Far from it: some will remain as long as their causes are still unknown, but we make no apology for trying to keep our terminology as simple as possible. Many doctors are put off by the cumbersome Latin names left behind by earlier pseudo-botanical classifications. Names like *painful*

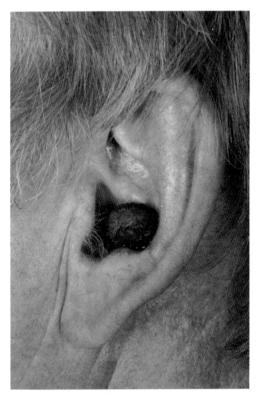

Describe the primary lesion. What is your diagnosis? Turn over the page to find the answer.

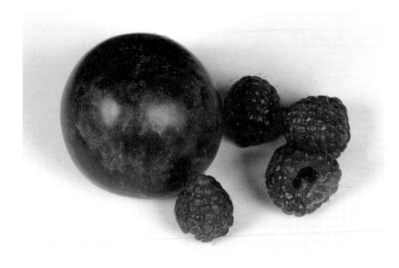

A raspberry! 'See and then reason and compare and control, but see first.' (W. Osler)

nodule of the ear or *ear corn* must now be allowed to take over from more traditional ones such as *chondrodermatitis nodularis helicis chronica*.

As well as simplifying the terminology, we have concentrated mainly on common conditions, which make up the bulk of dermatology in developed countries, although we do mention some others, which may be rare, but which illustrate important general principles. We have also tried to cut out as many synonyms and eponyms as possible. We have included some further reading at the end of each chapter for those wanting more information and, for the connoisseur, the names of some reference books at the end of this section.

We have, wherever possible, grouped together conditions that have the same cause, for example fungal infections (Chapter 16) and drug reactions (Chapter 25). Failing this, some chapters are based on a shared physiology, for example disorders of keratinization (Chapter 4) or on a shared anatomy, fer example disorders of hair and nails (Chapter 13), of blood vessels (Chapter 11) or of the sweat glands (Chapter 12). In some chapters we have, reluctantly, been forced to group together conditions that share physical characteristics, for example the bullous diseases (Chapter 9) and the papulosquamous disorders (Chapter 6): but this is unsound, and brings together some strange bedfellows. Modern research will surely soon reallocate their positions in the dormitory of dermatology. Finally, we must mention, sooner rather than later, electronic communication and the help that it can offer both patients and doctors. Websites are proliferating almost as rapidly as the epidermal cells in psoriasis; this section deserves its own heading.

Dermatology on the internet

Websites come and go, but we hope that the ones we suggest here will last at least as long as this book. The best are packed with useful information: others are less trustworthy. We rely heavily on those of the British Association of Dermatologists (www.bad.org.uk) and the American Academy of Dermatology (www.aad.org) for current guidelines on how to manage a variety of individual skin conditions. They also provide excellent patient information leaflets, and the addresses of patient support groups.

Two other favourite sites are those of the New Zealand Dermatological Society (http://dermnetnz.org) which provides both patient information and a useful pictorial quiz for the budding dermatologist, and Dermatology Information System (www.dermis.net), an online dermatology atlas produced in a collaboration between several European dermatology organisations.

For medical searches, the two main engines we use are the long-standing PubMed (www.pubmed.gov), which ranks publications by date, and the newer Google Scholar (http://scholar.google.com) which attempts to sort them by relevance. We watch the debate on open access to medical journals with interest. The Public Library of Science (www.plos.org) publishes an ever increasing number of dermatology papers, and a growing number of journals are allowing free access to their content 12 months after publication. The full text of over half of the world's 200 most cited journals is now available on a website (http://highwire.stanford.edu).

Further reading

Burgdorf WHC, Plewig G, Wolff HH, Landthaler M. (eds) (2008) *Braun-Falco's Dermatology*, 3rd edition. Springer Verlag, Berlin & Heidelberg.

Burns DA, Breathnach SM, Cox N, Griffiths CEM. (eds). (2010) *Rook's Textbook of Dermatology*, 8th edn. Wiley-Blackwell, Oxford.

Goldsmith LA, Katz SI, Gilchrest BA, Paller AS, Leffell DJ, Wolff K. (eds) (2012) *Fitzpatrick's Dermatology in General Medicine*, 8th edition. McGraw Hill, New York.

Irvine AD, Hoeger PH, Yan AC. (eds) (2011) *Harper's Textbook of Pediatric Dermatology*, 3rd edition. Wiley-Blackwell, Oxford.

Lebwohl MG, Heymann WR, Berth-Jones J, Coulson I. (2014) *Treatment of Skin Diseases: Comprehensive Therapeutic Strategies*, 4th edition. Elsevier Saunders, Philadelphia.

Shelley WB, Shelley DE. (2001) *Advanced Dermatologic Therapy II*, 2nd edition. Elsevier Saunders, Philadelphia.

1 Skin Disease in Perspective

This chapter presents an overview of the causes, prevalence and impact of skin disease.

The many roles of the skin

The skin is the largest organ in the body. It is the boundary between ourselves and the world around us, and its primary role is that of a barrier, preventing the entry of noxious chemicals and infectious organisms, and the exit of water and other chemicals. It is a sort of 'space suit', nicely evolved to house all the other organs and chemicals in our body.

Skin has other roles too. It is an important sense organ, and controls heat and water loss. It reflects internal changes (see Chapter 21) and reacts to external ones. It can sweat, grow hair, erect its hairs, change colour, smell, grow nails, secrete sebum, synthesize vitamin D and release nitric oxide. When confronted with insults from outside, it usually adapts easily and returns to a normal state, but sometimes it fails to do so and a skin disorder appears. Some of the internal and external factors that are important causes of skin disease are shown in Figure 1.1. Often several will be operating at the same time. Just as often, however, no obvious cause for a skin abnormality can be found, and here lies much of the difficulty of dermatology. When a cause is obvious, for example when the washing of dishes leads to an irritant hand dermatitis, or when episodes of severe sunburn are followed by the development of a melanoma, education and prevention are just as important as treatment.

The prevalence and cost of skin disorders

Skin diseases are very common. Probably everyone has experienced a skin disorder, such as sunburn, irritation, dry skin, acne, warts or pigment changes. The most common skin disorders in the United Kingdom are given in Table 1.1. People in other countries and in other environments may also develop skin diseases peculiar to their surroundings, or common skin diseases at different rates. For example, people living in tropical areas develop infectious diseases, such as leishmaniasis, not seen in more temperate climates. Different age groups experience different skin conditions. In the United States, for example, diseases of the sebaceous glands (mainly acne) peak at the age of about 18 years and then decline, while the prevalence of skin tumours steadily mounts with age (Figure 1.2).

The idea that 'common things occur commonly' is well known to surgeons as an aid to diagnosis. It is equally true of dermatology – an immense subject embracing more than 2000 conditions. In the United Kingdom some 70% of a dermatologist's work is caused by only nine types of skin disorder (Table 1.1). Latest figures suggest that approximately one-quarter of the population of England and Wales, some 13 million people, will have a skin condition for which they will seek medical advice over a 12-month period. In the United States approximately one-third of the population has a skin disorder at any given time.

The most recent estimate of the annual cost of skin disease in the United States was $39.3 billion dollars ($29.1 billion dollars in direct medical costs and $10.2 billion in lost productivity costs). Table 1.2 shows a breakdown of the top five most costly skin conditions seen in the United States.

In the United Kingdom, skin disorders are the most common reason for a patient to consult their general practitioner with a new problem; on average each general practitioner conducts over 600 consultations per year related to skin disorders. These figures are likely to be an under-estimation of the problem given the complexities of the classification of skin conditions. However, this is only the tip of an iceberg of skin disease, the sunken part

Clinical Dermatology, Fifth Edition. Richard B. Weller, Hamish J.A. Hunter and Margaret W. Mann.
© 2015 John Wiley & Sons, Ltd. Published 2015 by John Wiley & Sons, Ltd.

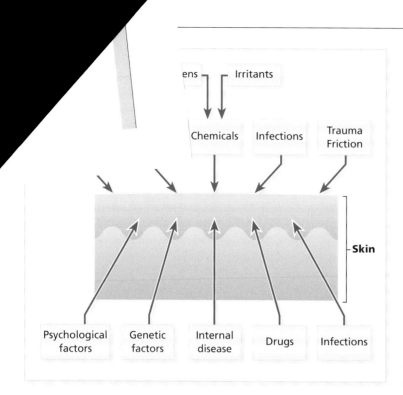

Figure 1.1 Internal and external factors causing skin diseases.

of which consists of problems that never get to doctors, being dealt with or ignored in the community.

How large is this problem? No one quite knows, as those who are not keen to see their doctors seldom star in the medical literature. People tend to be shy about skin diseases, and many of them settle spontaneously, often before patients seek help. The Proprietary Association of Great Britain (PAGB) conducted a survey in 2005 in which 1500 members of the general public were asked questions about their everyday health in the preceding 12 months. Of these, 818 (54%) respondents had experienced a skin condition, of which 69% 'self cared' for their condition and only 14% sought professional advice, usually from their general practitioner or practice nurse.

Table 1.1 The most common categories of skin disorder in the United Kingdom.

Skin cancer
Acne
Atopic eczema
Psoriasis
Viral warts
Other infective skin disorders
Benign tumours and vascular lesions
Leg ulcers
Contact dermatitis and other eczemas

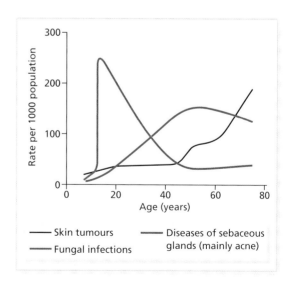

Figure 1.2 The age-dependent prevalence of some skin conditions.

Table 1.2 Most costly skin conditions in the United States (2004).

Condition	Direct medical cost ($billions)
Skin ulcers/wounds	9.7
Acne	2.5
Herpes simplex/zoster	1.7
Cutaneous fungal infection	1.7
Contact dermatitis	1.6

Adapted from Bickers *et al.* (2006). Reproduced with permission of Elsevier.

Figure 1.3 summarizes what happens to those with skin problems in the United Kingdom.

Psoriasis is a common chronic inflammatory condition of the skin which affects aproximately 1.5% of the population. Figure 1.4 demonstrates how the 'iceberg' analogy can be applied to UK psoriasis patients. In the course of a single year most of those with psoriasis see no doctor, and only a few will see a dermatologist. Some may have fallen victim to fraudulent practices, such as 'herbal' preparations laced with steroids, and baseless advice on 'allergies'.

Several population-based studies have confirmed that this is the case with other skin diseases too. In another UK study, 14% of adults and 19% of children had used a skin medication during the previous 2 weeks; only one-tenth of these were prescribed by doctors. In a study of several

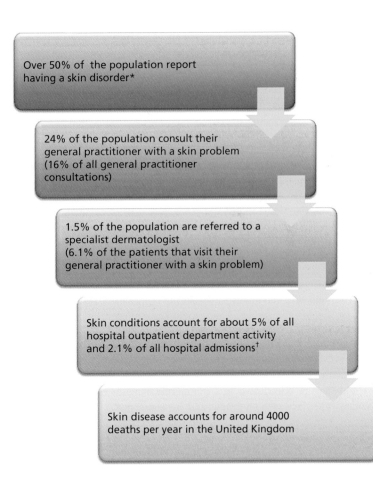

Over 50% of the population report having a skin disorder*

24% of the population consult their general practitioner with a skin problem (16% of all general practitioner consultations)

1.5% of the population are referred to a specialist dermatologist (6.1% of the patients that visit their general practitioner with a skin problem)

Skin conditions account for about 5% of all hospital outpatient department activity and 2.1% of all hospital admissions[†]

Skin disease accounts for around 4000 deaths per year in the United Kingdom

Figure 1.3 Skin problems in the United Kingdom and how they are dealt with in 1 year. Patients in the United States usually refer themselves to dermatologists. (Adapted from Schofield *et al.* (2009) Skin conditions in the UK: a healthcare needs assessment. Metro Commercial Printing Ltd, Watford.)

*Between one-third and two-thirds of the population self-treat their condition.
[†]A significant proportion of these are day case admissions.

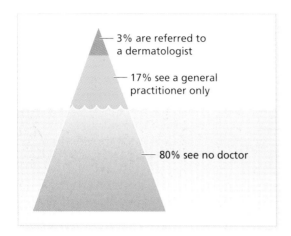

Figure 1.4 The 'iceberg' of psoriasis in the United Kingdom during a single year.

— 3% are referred to a dermatologist

— 17% see a general practitioner only

— 80% see no doctor

Table 1.3 Factors influencing the prevalence of skin diseases in a community.

High level of	High incidence of
Ultraviolet radiation	Skin malignancy in Caucasoids
Heat and humidity	Fungal and bacterial infections
Industrialization	Contact dermatitis
Underdevelopment	Infestations
	Bacterial and fungal infections

tons of unused medicinal preparations, 7% by weight had been manufactured for topical use on the skin.

In 2007, £413.9 million was spent in the United Kingdom on over-the-counter (non-prescribed) treatments for skin disorders, 18% of all over-the-counter sales. Preparations used to treat skin disease can be found in about half of all homes in the United Kingdom; the ratio of non-prescribed to prescribed remedies is about 6 : 1. Skin treatments come second only to painkillers in the list of non-prescription medicines.

No one who has worked in any branch of medicine can doubt the importance of diseases of the skin. A neurologist, for example, will know all about the Sturge–Weber syndrome (p. 302), a gastroenterologist about the Peutz–Jeghers syndrome (p. 275) and a cardiologist about the LEOPARD syndrome (p. 275); yet paradoxically, even in their own wards, they will see far more of other, more common skin conditions, such as drug eruptions, asteatotic eczema and scabies. They should know about these too. In primary care, skin problems are even more important, and the prevalence of some common skin conditions, such as skin cancer and atopic eczema, is undoubtedly rising.

The pattern of skin disease in a community depends on many other factors, both genetic and environmental; some are listed in Table 1.3. In developing countries, for example, overcrowding and poor sanitation play a major part. Skin disorders there are common, particularly in the young, and are dominated by infections and infestations – the so-called 'dermatoses of poverty' – amplified by the presence of HIV infection.

The impact of skin disorders

Much of this book is taken up with ways in which skin diseases can do harm. Most fit into the five D's shown in Figure 1.5; others are more subtle. Topical treatment, for example, can seem illogical to those who think that their skin disease is emotional in origin; it has been shown recently that psoriatics with great disability comply especially poorly with topical treatment.

In addition, the problems created by skin disease do not necessarily tally with the extent and severity of the eruption as judged by an outside observer. In all branches of medicine, quality-of-life studies have come to the fore. They give a different, patient-based, view of the skin condition, and provide an objective, validated and reproduceable outcome measure. They have many applications, ranging from the monitoring of a response to treatment, to the justification of clinical expenditure. There are specialty specific questionnaires such as the Dermatology Life Quality Index (DLQI) and disease-specific questionnaires such as the Cardiff Acne Disability Score.

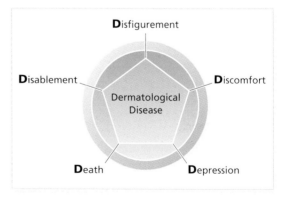

Disfigurement

Disablement

Discomfort

Dermatological Disease

Death

Depression

Figure 1.5 The five D's of dermatological disease.

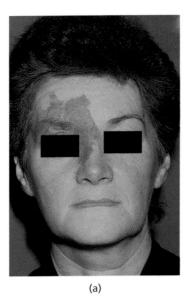 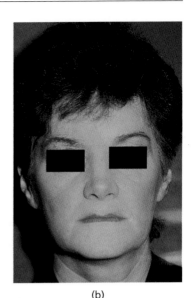

(a)   (b)

Figure 1.6 (a) This patient has a port-wine stain. (b) Her life is transformed by her clever use of modern camouflage cosmetics, which take her less than a minute to apply.

Questionnaires have been designed to compare the impact of skin diseases with those of other conditions; patients with bad psoriasis, for example, have at least as great a disability as those with angina and some cancers. Given the high cost of some of the newer dermatological treatments, the biological drugs for example, quality of life questionnaires are becoming commonplace in the office or clinic.

Disfigurement

The possible reactions to disfiguring skin disease are described in Chapter 23. They range from a leper complex (e.g. some patients with psoriasis, p. 52), to embarrassment (e.g. port-wine stains, Figure 1.6, or androgenetic alopecia in both men and women, p. 175). Disorders of body image can lead those who have no skin disease to think that they have, and even to commit suicide in this mistaken belief (dermatological non-disease, p. 335).

Discomfort

Some people prefer pain to itch; skin diseases can provide both. Itchy skin disorders include eczema (p. 76), lichen planus (p. 69), scabies (p. 253) and dermatitis herpetiformis (p. 119). Pain is marked in shingles (p. 231), pyoderma gangrenosum (p. 321) and glomus tumours (p. 187).

Disability

Skin conditions are capable of ruining the quality of anyone's life and each carries its own set of problems. At the most obvious level, dermatitis of the hands can quickly destroy a manual worker's earning capacity, as many hairdressers, nurses, cooks and mechanics know to their cost. In the United States, skin diseases account for almost half of all cases of occupational illness and cause more than 50 million days to be lost from work each year; in 2004, days lost as a result of contact dermatitis alone accounted for an annual cost of $294.6 million dollars.

Disability and disfigurement can blend in a more subtle way, so that, for example, in times of unemployment people with acne find it hard to get jobs. People with psoriasis in the United States, already plagued by tactless hairdressers and messy treatments, have been shown to lose thousands of dollars in earnings by virtue of time taken off work. Even trivial psoriasis, if it is on the fingertips of a blind person can have a huge effect by making it impossible to read Braille.

Depression

The physical, sensory and functional problems listed above often lead to depression and anxiety, even in the most stable people. Depression also seems to modulate the perception of itching, which becomes much worse. Feelings of stigmatization and rejection are common in patients with chronic skin diseases: latest figures suggest that 17–32% of patients with psoriasis will report depression, 22% have symptoms of anxiety and up to 10% of patients with psoriasis that they think is bad have had suicidal thoughts. The risk of suicide in patients with severe acne is discussed on p. 163.

Table 1.4 The consequences of skin failure.

Function	Skin failure	Treatment
Temperature control	Cannot sweat when too hot; cannot vasoconstrict when too cold. Hence temperature swings dangerously up and down.	Controlled environmental temperature
Barrier function	Raw skin surfaces lose much fluid and electrolytes.	Monitor and replace
	Heavy protein loss.	High protein diet
	Bacterial pathogens multiply on damaged skin.	Antibiotic
		Bathing/wet compresses
Cutaneous blood flow	Shunt through skin may lead to high output cardiac failure in those with poor cardiac reserve.	Aggressively treat skin
		Support vital signs
Others	Erythroderma may lead to malabsorption.	Usually none needed
	Hair and nail loss later.	Regrow spontaneously
	Nursing problems handling patients particularly with toxic epidermal necrolysis (p. 121) and pemphigus (p. 113).	Nurse as for burns

Death

Deaths from skin disease are fortunately rare, but they do occur (e.g. in pemphigus, toxic epidermal necrolysis and cutaneous malignancies). In 2005 there were nearly 4000 deaths from skin disease in the United Kingdom, of which 1817 were attributable to malignant melanoma. In addition, the stresses generated by a chronic skin disorder such as psoriasis predispose to heavy smoking and drinking, which carry their own risks.

In this context, the concept of skin failure is an important one. It may occur when any inflammatory skin disease becomes so widespread that it prevents normal functioning of the skin, with the results listed in Table 1.4. Its causes include erythroderma (p. 74), toxic epidermal necrolysis (p. 121), severe erythema multiforme (p. 105), pustular psoriasis (p. 57), and pemphigus (p. 113).

Learning points

1 'Prevalence' and 'incidence' are not the same thing. Learn the difference and join a small select band.
   • The *prevalence* of a disease is the proportion of a defined population affected by it at a particular point in time.
   • The *incidence* rate is the proportion of a defined population developing the disease within a specified period of time.
2 Quality of life studies have revealed that many skin diseases that seem trivial to a doctor can still wreck a patient's life.
3 Remember that many patients, by the time they see you, will have tried numerous home remedies.

Further reading

Bickers DR, Lim HW, Margolis D, *et al.* (2006) The burden of skin disease: 2004. *Journal of the American Academy of Dermatology* **55**, 490–500.

David SE, Ahmed Z, Salek MS, Finlay A. (2005) Does enough quality of life-related discussion occur during dermatology outpatient consultations? *British Journal of Dermatology* **153**, 997–1000.

Finlay AY. (1997) Quality of life measurement in dermatology: a practical guide. *British Journal of Dermatology* **136**, 305–314.

Grob JJ, Stern RS, Mackie RM, Weinstock WA, eds. (1997) *Epidemiology, Causes and Prevention of Skin Diseases.* Blackwell Science, Oxford.

Savin JA. (2003) Psychosocial aspects. In Van De Kerkhof P, ed. *Textbook of Psoriasis*, 2nd edition. Blackwell Science, Oxford: 43–54.

Schofield JK, Grindlay D, Williams HC. (2009) *Skin conditions in the UK: a healthcare needs assessment.* Metro Commercial Printing Ltd, Watford.

2   The Function and Structure of the Skin

The skin is the interface between humans and their environment. It weighs an average of 4 kg and covers an area of 2 m². It acts as a barrier, protecting the body from harsh external conditions and preventing the loss of important body constituents, especially water. A death from destruction of skin, as in a burn, or in toxic epidermal necrolysis (p. 121), and the misery of unpleasant acne, remind us of its many important functions, which range from the vital to the cosmetic (Table 2.1).

The skin has three layers. The outer one is the *epidermis*, which is firmly attached to, and supported by connective tissue in the underlying *dermis*. Beneath the dermis is loose connective tissue, the *subcutis* or *hypo-dermis*, which usually contains abundant fat (Figure 2.1).

Epidermis

The epidermis consists of many layers of closely packed cells, the most superficial of which are flattened and filled with keratins; it is therefore a stratified squamous epithelium. It adheres to the dermis at the basement membrane where downward projections (*epidermal ridges* or *pegs*) interlock with upward projections of the dermis (*dermal papillae*) (Figure 2.1).

The epidermis contains no blood vessels. It varies in thickness from less than 0.1 mm on the eyelids to nearly 1 mm on the palms and soles. As dead surface squames are shed (accounting for some of the dust in our houses), the thickness is kept constant by cells dividing in the deepest (*basal*) layer. A generated cell moves, to the surface, passing through the *prickle* and *granular cell layers* before dying in the *horny layer*. The journey from the basal layer to the surface (epidermal turnover or transit time) takes about 30 days. During this time the appearance and function of the cell changes in a process known as terminal differentiation. A vertical section through the epidermis summarizes the life history of a single epidermal cell (Figure 2.2).

The *basal layer*, the deepest layer, rests on a basement membrane, which attaches it to the dermis. It is a single layer of columnar cells, whose basal surfaces sprout many fine processes and hemidesmosomes, anchoring them to the *lamina densa* of the basement membrane.

In normal skin some 30% of basal cells are preparing for division (growth fraction). Following mitosis, a cell enters the G_1 phase, synthesizes RNA and protein, and grows in size (Figure 2.3). Later, when the cell is triggered to divide, DNA is synthesized (S phase) and chromosomal DNA is replicated. A short post-synthetic (G_2) phase of further growth occurs before mitosis (M). DNA synthesis continues through the S and G_2 phases, but not during mitosis. The G_1 phase is then repeated, and one of the daughter cells moves into the suprabasal layer. It then differentiates (Figure 2.2), having lost the capacity to divide, and synthesizes keratins. Some basal cells remain inactive in a so-called G_0 phase but may re-enter the cycle and resume proliferation. Stem cells reside amongst the interfollicular basal cells, the base of sebaceous glands, and amongst the cells of the external root sheath at the bulge in the hair follicle at the level of attachment of the arrector pili muscle. These cells divide infrequently, but can generate new proliferative cells in the epidermis and hair follicle in response to damage.

Keratinocytes

The *spinous* or *prickle cell* layer (Figure 2.4) is composed of *keratinocytes*. These differentiating cells, which synthesize keratins, are larger than basal cells. Keratinocytes are firmly attached to each other by small interlocking

Clinical Dermatology, Fifth Edition. Richard B. Weller, Hamish J.A. Hunter and Margaret W. Mann.
© 2015 John Wiley & Sons, Ltd. Published 2015 by John Wiley & Sons, Ltd.

Table 2.1 Functions of the skin.

Function	Structure/cell involved
Protection against:	
chemicals, particles	Horny layer
ultraviolet radiation	Melanocytes
antigens, haptens	Langerhans cells
microbes	Langerhans cells
Preservation of a balanced internal environment	Horny layer
Prevents loss of water, electrolytes and macromolecules	Horny layer
Shock absorber	Dermis and subcutaneous fat
Strong, yet elastic and compliant	
Temperature regulation	Blood vessels
	Eccrine sweat glands
Insulation	Subcutaneous fat
Sensation	Specialized nerve endings
Lubrication	Sebaceous glands
Protection and prising	Nails
Calorie reserve	Subcutaneous fat
Vitamin D synthesis	Keratinocytes
Body odour/pheromones	Apocrine sweat glands
Psychosocial, display	Skin, lips, hair and nails

cytoplasmic processes, by abundant desmosomes, and by other cadherins separated by an intercellular layer of glycoproteins and lipoproteins. Under the light microscope, the desmosomes look like 'prickles'. They are specialized attachment plaques that physically bind adjacent keratinocytes to one another and connect keratin intermediate filaments within keratinocytes to the cell membrane. Desmosomes are composed of transmembranous desmoglein–desmocollin pairs, which bind to the tonofilaments via desmoplakins, plakoglobin and plakophilin-1. There are four types of desmoglein found in the epidermis. Desmoglein (Dsg) 1 is expressed in the upper epidermis while Dsg 3 is mostly expressed in the basal epidermis. Desmoglein 1 is expressed at lower levels in the mucosal epithelium than Dsg 3. Autoantibodies to the desmogleins are found in pemphigus (p. 113), when they are responsible for the detachment of keratinocytes from one another and so for intraepidermal blister formation. Cytoplasmic continuity between keratinocytes occurs at

gap junctions, specialized areas on opposing cell walls. Tonofilaments are small fibres running from the cytoplasm to the desmosomes. They are more numerous in cells of the spinous layer than of the basal layer, and are packed into bundles called *tonofibrils*. Many *lamellar granules* (otherwise known as membrane-coating granules, Odland bodies or keratinosomes), derived from the Golgi apparatus, appear in the superficial keratinocytes of this layer. They contain polysaccharides, hydrolytic enzymes, and stacks of lipid lamellae composed of phospholipids, cholesterol and glucosylceramides. Their contents are discharged into the intercellular space of the granular cell layer to become precursors of the lipids in the intercellular space of the horny layer (see *Barrier function* below).

Cellular differentiation continues in the granular layer, which normally consists of two or three layers of cells that are flatter than those in the spinous layer, and have more tonofibrils. As the name of the layer implies, these cells contain large irregular basophilic granules of *keratohyalin,* which merge with tonofibrils. These keratohyalin granules contain proteins, including involucrin, loricrin and profilaggrin, which is cleaved into filaggrin by specific phosphatases as the granular cells move into the horny layer.

As keratinocytes migrate out through the outermost layers, their keratohyalin granules break up and their contents are dispersed throughout the cytoplasm. Filaggrin peptides aggregate the keratin cytoskeleton, collapsing it, and thus converting the granular cells to flattened squames. These make up the thick and tough peripheral protein coating of the *horny envelope.* Its structural proteins include loricrin and involucrin, the latter binding to ceramides in the surrounding intercellular space under the influence of transglutaminase. Filaggrin, involucrin and loricrin can all be detected histochemically and are useful as markers of epidermal differentiation.

The *horny layer* (stratum corneum) is made of piled-up layers of flattened dead cells (corneocytes) – the bricks – separated by lipids – the mortar – in the intercellular space. Together these provide an effective barrier to water loss and to invasion by infectious agents and toxic chemicals. The corneocyte cytoplasm is packed with keratin filaments, embedded in a matrix and enclosed by an envelope derived from the keratohyalin granules. This envelope, along with the aggregated keratins that it encloses, gives the corneocyte its toughness, allowing the skin to withstand all sorts of chemical and mechanical insults. Horny cells normally have no nuclei or intracytoplasmic

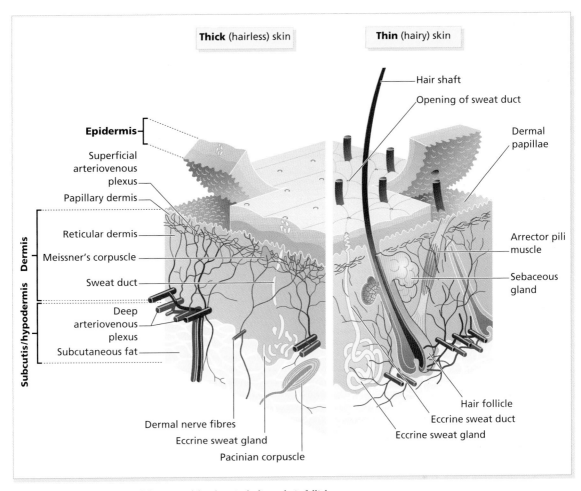

Thick (hairless) skin

Thin (hairy) skin

- Hair shaft
- Opening of sweat duct
- Dermal papillae

Epidermis

Superficial arteriovenous plexus

Papillary dermis

Reticular dermis

Meissner's corpuscle

Sweat duct

- Arrector pili muscle
- Sebaceous gland

Deep arteriovenous plexus

Subcutaneous fat

Dermis

Subcutis/hypodermis

- Hair follicle
- Eccrine sweat duct
- Eccrine sweat gland

Dermal nerve fibres

Eccrine sweat gland

Pacinian corpuscle

Figure 2.1 Three-dimensional diagram of the skin, including a hair follicle.

organelles, these having been destroyed by hydrolytic and degrading enzymes found in lamellar granules and the lysosomes of granular cells.

Keratinization

All cells have an internal skeleton made up of micro-filaments (7 nm diameter; actin), microtubules (20–35 nm diameter; tubulin), and intermediate filaments (10 nm diameter). Keratins (from the Greek *keras* meaning 'horn') are the main intermediate filaments in epithelial cells and are comparable to vimentin in mesenchymal cells, neurofilaments in neurons, and desmin in muscle cells. Keratins are not just a biochemical curiosity, as mutations in their genes cause a number of skin diseases including simple epidermolysis bullosa (p. 123) and bullous ichthyosiform erythroderma (p. 47).

The keratins are a family of more than 30 proteins, each produced by different genes. These separate into two gene families: one responsible for basic and the other for acidic keratins. The keratin polypeptide has a central helical portion with a non-helical N-terminal head and C-terminal tail. Individual keratins exist in pairs so that their double filament always consists of one acidic and one basic keratin polypeptide. The intertwining of adjacent filaments forms larger fibrils.

Different keratins are found at different levels of the epidermis depending on the stage of differentiation and disease; normal basal cells make keratins 5 and 14, but terminally differentiated suprabasal cells make keratins 1 and 10 (Figure 2.2). Keratins 6 and 16 become prominent in hyperproliferative states such as psoriasis.

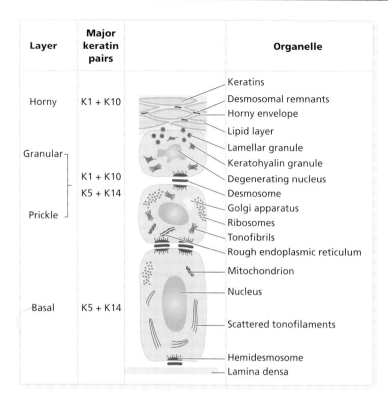

Layer	Major keratin pairs	Organelle
Horny	K1 + K10	Keratins
		Desmosomal remnants
		Horny envelope
		Lipid layer
Granular		Lamellar granule
	K1 + K10	Keratohyalin granule
	K5 + K14	Degenerating nucleus
Prickle		Desmosome
		Golgi apparatus
		Ribosomes
		Tonofibrils
		Rough endoplasmic reticulum
		Mitochondrion
		Nucleus
Basal	K5 + K14	Scattered tonofilaments
		Hemidesmosome
		Lamina densa

Figure 2.2 Changes during keratinization.

During differentiation, the keratin fibrils in the cells of the horny layer align and aggregate, under the influence of filaggrin. Cysteine, found in keratins of the horny layer, allows cross-linking of fibrils to give the epidermis strength to withstand injury.

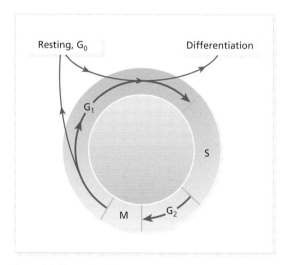

Figure 2.3 The cell cycle.

Cell cohesion and desquamation

Firm cohesion in the spinous layer is ensured by 'stick and grip' mechanisms. A glycoprotein intercellular substance acts as a cement, sticking the cells together, and the intertwining of the small cytoplasmic processes of the prickle cells, together with their desmosomal attachments, accounts for the grip. The cytoskeleton of tonofibrils also maintains the cell shape rigidly.

The typical 'basket weave' appearance of the horny layer in routine histological sections is artefactual and deceptive. In fact, cells deep in the horny layer stick tightly together and only those at the surface flake off; this is in part caused by the activity of cholesterol sulfatase. This enzyme is deficient in X-linked recessive ichthyosis (p. 46), in which poor shedding leads to the piling up of corneocytes in the horny layer. Desquamation is normally responsible for the removal of harmful exogenous substances from the skin surface. The cells lost are replaced by newly formed corneocytes; regeneration and turnover of the horny layer is therefore continuous.

The epidermal barrier

The horny layer prevents the loss of interstitial fluid from within, and acts as a barrier to the penetration of

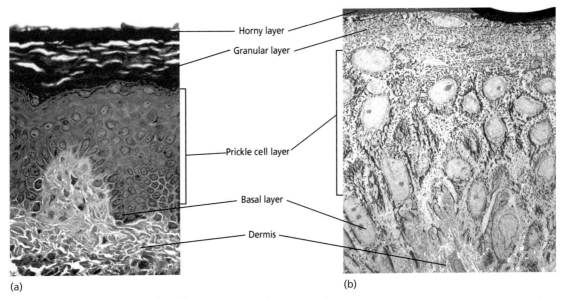

Horny layer
Granular layer
Prickle cell layer
Basal layer
Dermis

(a)   (b)

Figure 2.4 Layers of the epidermis. (a) Light microscopy and (b) electron micrograph.

potentially harmful substances from outside. Solvent extraction of the epidermis leads to an increased permeability to water, and it has been known for years that essential fatty acid deficiency causes poor cutaneous barrier function. These facts implicate ceramides, cholesterol, free fatty acids (from lamellar granules; p. 10) and smaller quantities of other lipids, in cutaneous barrier formation. Natural moisturising factor (NMF), predominantly made up of amino acids and their metabolites, also helps maintain the properties of the stratum corneum. Barrier function is impaired when the horny layer is removed – experimentally, by successive strippings with adhesive tape, or clinically, by injury or skin disease. It is also decreased by excessive hydration or dehydration of the horny layer and by detergents.

The relative impermeability of the stratum corneum and 'moving staircase' effect of continually shedding the outer corneocytes provides a passive barrier to infective organisms. In addition to this, protection is given by the various antimicrobial peptides (AMPs) found on epithelial surfaces. The two major families of AMPs are the defensins and the cathelicidins which have a broad range of antimicrobial activity and form the first line of immune defence of the body.

The speed at which a substance penetrates through the epidermis is directly proportional to its concentration difference across the barrier layer, and inversely proportional to the thickness of the horny layer. A rise in skin temperature aids penetration. A normal horny layer is slightly permeable to water, but relatively impermeable to ions such as sodium and potassium. Some other substances (e.g. glucose and urea) also penetrate poorly, whereas some aliphatic alcohols pass through easily. The penetration of a solute dissolved in an organic liquid depends mainly on the qualities of the solvent.

Epidermopoiesis and its regulation

Both the thickness of the normal epidermis, and the number of cells in it, remain constant, as cell loss at the surface is balanced by cell production in the basal layer. Locally produced cytokines, transcription factors and integrins stimulate or inhibit epidermal proliferation and differentiation, interacting in complex ways to ensure homeostasis (Table 2.2).

Table 2.2 Regulators of epidermopoiesis.

Designation	Function
P63	Probable stem cell marker. Encourages stem cell proliferation
β1 integrin	Drives stem cell proliferation
TGF-α	
C-myc	
TGF-β	Inhibits stem cell proliferation
Notch signalling	Controls epidermal differentiation
PPARα	

Vitamin D synthesis

The steroid 7-dehydrocholesterol, found in keratinocytes, is converted by sunlight to cholecalciferol. The vitamin becomes active after 25-hydroxylation in the kidney. Kidney disease and lack of sun, particularly in dark-skinned peoples, can both cause vitamin D deficiency and rickets. Low vitamin D levels have been linked to a wide range of diseases including multiple sclerosis, cardiovascular disease, hypertension and solid organ tumours. However, results of vitamin D supplementation trials have been variable. Vitamin D may merely be a marker for sun exposure, with other sun-related factors such as cutaneous nitric oxide leading to health improvements. Alternatively, the direction of association may be the other way, with unhealthy patients unable to spend as much time outside and thus prone to low sun exposure and vitamin D levels.

Other cells in the epidermis

Keratinocytes make up about 85% of cells in the epidermis, but three other types of cell are also found there: melanocytes, Langerhans cells and Merkel cells (Figure 2.5).

Melanocytes

Melanocytes are the only cells that can synthesize melanin. They migrate from the neural crest into the basal layer of the ectoderm where, in human embryos, they are seen as early as 8 weeks' gestation. They are also found in hair bulbs, the retina and pia arachnoid. Each dendritic

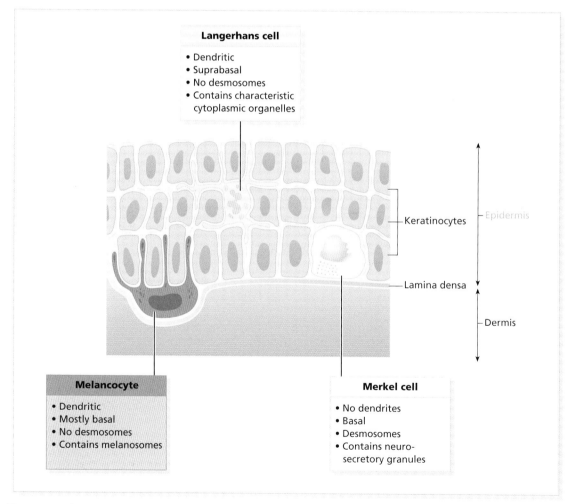

Langerhans cell
- Dendritic
- Suprabasal
- No desmosomes
- Contains characteristic cytoplasmic organelles

Keratinocytes

Epidermis

Lamina densa

Dermis

Melanocyte
- Dendritic
- Mostly basal
- No desmosomes
- Contains melanosomes

Merkel cell
- No dendrites
- Basal
- Desmosomes
- Contains neuro-secretory granules

Figure 2.5 Melanocyte, Langerhans cell and Merkel cell.

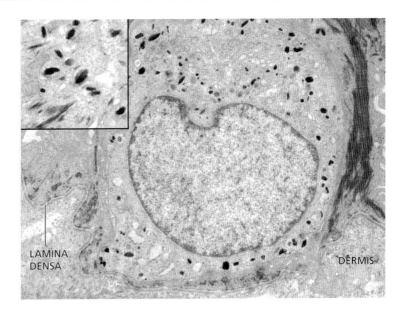

LAMINA
DENSA

DERMIS

Figure 2.6 Melanocyte (electron micrograph), with melanosomes (inset).

melanocyte associates with a number of keratinocytes, forming an epidermal melanin unit (Figure 2.5). The dendritic processes of melanocytes wind between the epidermal cells and end as discs in contact with them. Their cytoplasm contains discrete organelles, the *melanosomes*, containing varying amounts of the pigment melanin (Figure 2.6). This is 'injected' into surrounding keratinocytes to provide them with pigmentation to help protect the skin against damaging ultraviolet radiation.

Melanogenesis is described at the beginning of Chapter 19 on disorders of pigmentation.

Langerhans cells

The Langerhans cell is a dendritic cell (Figures 2.5 and 2.7) like the melanocyte. It also lacks desmosomes and tonofibrils, but has a lobulated nucleus. The specific granules within the cell look like a tennis racket when seen in two dimensions in an electron micrograph (Figure 2.8), or like a sycamore seed when reconstructed in three dimensions. They are plate-like, with a rounded bleb protruding from the surface.

Langerhans cells come from a mobile pool of precursors originating in the bone marrow. There are approximately 800 Langerhans cells per mm^2 in human skin and their dendritic processes fan out to form a striking network seen best in epidermal sheets (Figure 2.7). Langerhans cells are alone among epidermal cells in possessing surface receptors for C3b and the Fc portions of IgG and IgE, and in bearing major histocompatibility complex

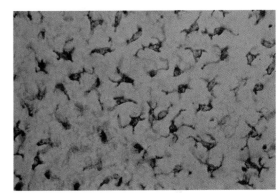

Figure 2.7 Adenosine triphosphase-positive Langerhans cells in an epidermal sheet. The network provides a reticulo-epithelial trap for contact allergens.

(MHC) Class II antigens (HLA-DR, -DP and -DQ). They are best thought of as highly specialized macrophages.

Langerhans cells have a key role in many immune reactions. They take up exogenous antigen, process it and present it to T lymphocytes either in the skin or in the local lymph nodes (p. 26). They probably play a part in immunosurveillance for viral and tumour antigens. Topical or systemic glucocorticoids reduce the density of epidermal Langerhans cells as does ultraviolet radiation.

Merkel cells

Merkel cells are found in normal epidermis (Figure 2.5) and act as transducers for fine touch. They are

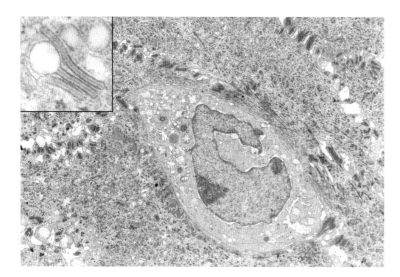

Figure 2.8 Langerhans cell (electron micrograph), with characteristic granule (inset).

non-dendritic cells, lying in or near the basal layer, and are of the same size as keratinocytes. They are concentrated in localized thickenings of the epidermis near hair follicles (hair discs), and contain membrane-bound spherical granules, 80–100 nm in diameter, which have a core of varying density, separated from the membrane by a clear halo. Sparse desmosomes connect these cells to neighbouring keratinocytes. Fine unmyelinated nerve endings are often associated with Merkel cells, which express immunoreactivity for various neuropeptides.

Epidermal appendages

The skin appendages are derived from epithelial germs during embryogenesis and, except for the nails, lie in the dermis. They include hair, nails, and sweat and sebaceous glands. They are described, along with the diseases that affect them, in Chapters 12 and 13, respectively.

Dermo-epidermal junction

The basement membrane lies at the interface between the epidermis and dermis. With light microscopy it can be highlighted using a periodic acid–Schiff (PAS) stain, because of its abundance of neutral mucopolysaccharides. Electron microscopy (Figure 2.9) shows that the *lamina densa* (rich in type IV collagen) is separated from the basal cells by an electron-lucent area, the *lamina lucida*. *Hemidesmosomes* span the basal plasma membrane of basal keratinocytes and structurally bind the epidermis to the dermis. They are complex structures made up of bullous pemphigoid antigens 1 (a 230-kDa plakin) and 2 (180 kDa collagen XVII), plectin and α6 β4 integrin. Anti-

bodies to BP antigens 1 and 2 are found in pemphigoid (p. 117), a subcutaneous blistering condition. The intracellular component of the hemidesmosome binds to the intermediate filament network within keratinocytes.

Fine *anchoring filaments,* largely composed of laminin-332, cross the lamina lucida and connect the lamina densa to the plasma membrane of the basal cells by interacting with the α6 β4 integrin component of the hemidesmosome. *Anchoring fibrils* (of type VII collagen), dermal microfibril bundles and single small collagen fibres (types I and III), extend from the papillary dermis to the deep part of the lamina densa.

Laminins, large non-collagen glycoproteins produced by keratinocytes, aided by nidogen, promote adhesion between the basal cells above the lamina lucida and type IV collagen, the main constituent of the lamina densa, below it. Laminin 332 is the most important member of this family, which also includes laminins 311 and 511. Laminins bind to cells by interactions with cellular integrins.

The structures within the dermo-epidermal junction provide mechanical support, encouraging the adhesion, growth, differentiation and migration of the overlying basal cells, and also act as a semipermeable filter that regulates the transfer of nutrients and cells from dermis to epidermis.

Dermis

The dermis lies between the epidermis and the subcutaneous fat. It supports the epidermis structurally and nutritionally. Its thickness varies, being greatest in the palms

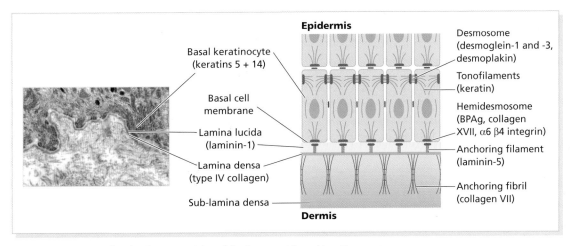

Epidermis

Basal keratinocyte
(keratins 5 + 14)

Basal cell
membrane

Lamina lucida
(laminin-1)

Lamina densa
(type IV collagen)

Sub-lamina densa

Desmosome
(desmoglein-1 and -3,
desmoplakin)

Tonofilaments
(keratin)

Hemidesmosome
(BPAg, collagen
XVII, α6 β4 integrin)

Anchoring filament
(laminin-5)

Anchoring fibril
(collagen VII)

Dermis

Figure 2.9 Structure and molecular composition of the dermo-epidermal junction.

and soles and least in the eyelids and penis. In old age, the dermis thins and loses its elasticity.

The dermis interdigitates with the epidermis (Figure 2.1) so that upward projections of the dermis, the dermal papillae, interlock with downward ridges of the epidermis, the rete pegs. This interdigitation is responsible for the ridges seen most readily on the fingertips (as fingerprints). It is important in the adhesion between epidermis and dermis as it increases the area of contact between them.

Like all connective tissues the dermis has three components: cells, fibres and amorphous ground substance.

Cells of the dermis

The main cells of the dermis are fibroblasts, but there are also small numbers of resident and transitory mononuclear phagocytes, lymphocytes, dermal dendritic cells and mast cells. Other blood cells (e.g. polymorphs) are seen during inflammation. The main functions of the resident dermal cells are listed in Table 2.3 and their role in immunological reactions is discussed later in this chapter.

Fibres of the dermis

The dermis is largely made up of interwoven fibres, principally of collagen, packed in bundles. Those in the papillary dermis are finer than those in the deeper reticular dermis. When the skin is stretched, collagen, with its high tensile strength, prevents tearing, and the elastic fibres, intermingled with the collagen, later return it to the unstretched state.

Collagen makes up 70–80% of the dry weight of the dermis. Its fibres are composed of thinner fibrils, which are in turn made up of microfibrils built from individual collagen molecules. These molecules consist of three polypeptide chains (molecular weight 150 kDa) forming a triple helix with a non-helical segment at both ends. The alignment of the chains is stabilized by covalent cross-links involving lysine and hydroxylysine. Collagen is an unusual protein as it contains a high proportion of proline and hydroxyproline and many glycine residues; the spacing of glycine as every third amino acid is a prerequisite for the formation of a triple helix. Defects in the enzymes needed for collagen synthesis are

Table 2.3 Functions of some resident dermal cells.

Fibroblast	Synthesis of collagen, reticulin, elastin, fibronectin, glycosaminoglycans, collagenase
Mononuclear phagocyte	Mobile: phagocytose and destroy bacteria
	Secrete cytokines
Lymphocyte	Immunosurveillance
Langerhans cell and dermal dendritic cell	In transit between local lymph node and epidermis
	Antigen presentation
Mast cell	Stimulated by antigens, complement components, and other substances to release many inflammatory mediators including histamine, heparin, prostaglandins, leukotrienes, tryptase and chemotactic factors for eosinophils and neutrophils
Merkel cell	Act as transducers for fine touch

Table 2.4 Distribution of some types of collagen.

Collagen type	Tissue distribution
I	Most connective tissues including tendon and bone
	Accounts for approximately 85% of skin collagen
II	Cartilage
III	Accounts for about 15% of skin collagen
	Blood vessels
IV	Skin (lamina densa) and basement membranes of other tissues
V	Ubiquitous, including placenta
VII	Skin (anchoring fibrils)
	Fetal membranes

responsible for some skin diseases, including Ehlers–Danlos syndrome (see Chapter 21), and conditions involving other systems, including lathyrism (fragility of skin and other connective tissues) and osteogenesis imperfecta (fragility of bones).

There are many, genetically distinct, collagen proteins, all with triple helical molecules, and all rich in hydroxyproline and hydroxylysine. The distribution of some of them is summarized in Table 2.4.

Reticulin fibres are fine collagen fibres, seen in fetal skin and around the blood vessels and appendages of adult skin.

Elastic fibres account for about 2% of the dry weight of adult dermis. They have two distinct protein components: an amorphous elastin core and a surrounding elastic tissue microfibrillar component. Elastin (molecular weight 72 kDa) is made up of polypeptides (rich in glycine, desmosine and valine) linked to the microfibrillar component through their desmosine residues. Abnormalities in the elastic tissue cause cutis laxa (sagging inelastic skin) and pseudoxanthoma elasticum (see Chapter 21).

Ground substance of the dermis

The amorphous ground substance of the dermis consists largely of two glycosaminoglycans (hyaluronic acid and dermatan sulfate) with smaller amounts of heparan sulfate and chondroitin sulfate. The glycosaminoglycans are complexed to core protein and exist as proteoglycans.

The ground substance has several important functions:
• it binds water, allowing nutrients, hormones and waste products to pass through the dermis;
• it acts as a lubricant between the collagen and elastic fibre networks during skin movement; and

• it provides bulk, allowing the dermis to act as a shock absorber.

Muscles

Both smooth and striated muscle are found in the skin. The smooth arrector pili muscles (see Figure 13.1) are used by animals to raise their fur and so protect them from the cold. They are vestigial in humans, but may help to express sebum. Smooth muscle is also responsible for 'goose pimples' (bumps) from cold, nipple erection and the raising of the scrotum by the dartos muscle. Striated fibres (e.g. the platysma) and some of the muscles of facial expression, are also found in the dermis.

Blood vessels

Although the skin consumes little oxygen, its abundant blood supply regulates body temperature. The blood vessels lie in two main horizontal layers (Figure 2.10). The deep plexus is just above the subcutaneous fat, and its arterioles supply the sweat glands and hair papillae. The superficial plexus is in the papillary dermis and arterioles from it become capillary loops in the dermal papillae. An arteriole arising in the deep dermis supplies an inverted cone of tissue, with its base at the epidermis.

The blood vessels in the skin are important in thermoregulation. Under sympathetic nervous control, arteriovenous anastamoses at the level of the deep plexus can shunt blood to the venous plexus at the expense of the capillary loops, thereby reducing surface heat loss by convection.

Cutaneous lymphatics

Afferent lymphatics begin as blind-ended capillaries in the dermal papilla and pass to a superficial lymphatic plexus in the papillary dermis. There are also two deeper horizontal plexuses, and collecting lymphatics from the deeper one run with the veins in the superficial fascia.

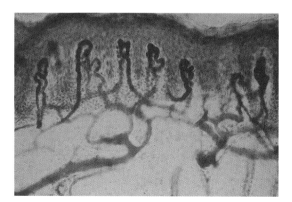

Figure 2.10 Blood vessels of the skin (carmine stain).

Nerves

The skin is liberally supplied with an estimated 1 million nerve fibres. Most are found in the face and extremities. Their cell bodies lie in the dorsal root ganglia. Both myelinated and non-myelinated fibres exist, with the latter making up an increasing proportion peripherally. Most free sensory nerves end in the dermis; however, a few non-myelinated nerve endings penetrate into the epidermis. Some of these are associated with Merkel cells (p. 13). Free nerve endings detect the potentially damaging stimuli of heat and pain (nociceptors), while specialized end organs in the dermis, Pacinian and Meissner corpuscles, register deformation of the skin caused by pressure (mechanoreceptors) as well as vibration and touch. Autonomic nerves supply the blood vessels, sweat glands and arrector pili muscles.

Itching is an important feature of many skin diseases. It follows the stimulation of fine free nerve endings lying close to the dermo-epidermal junction. Areas with a high density of such endings (itch spots) are especially sensitive to itch-provoking stimuli. Impulses from these free endings pass centrally in two ways: quickly along myelinated A fibres, and more slowly along non-myelinated C fibres. As a result, itch has two components: a quick localized pricking sensation followed by a slow burning diffuse itching.

Many stimuli can induce itching (electrical, chemical and mechanical). In itchy skin diseases, pruritogenic chemicals such as histamine and proteolytic enzymes are liberated close to the dermo-epidermal junction. The detailed pharmacology of individual diseases is still poorly understood but prostaglandins potentiate chemically induced itching in inflammatory skin diseases.

Learning points

1 More diseases are now being classified by abnormalities of function and structure rather than by their appearance.
2 Today's patients are inquisitive and knowledgeable. If you understand the structure and function of the skin, your explanations to them will be easier and more convincing.

The skin immune system

The skin acts as a barrier to prevent injury of underlying tissues and to prevent infections from entering the body. Simply put, it keeps the inside in and the outside out. The horny layer is a physical barrier that minimizes the loss of fluid and electrolytes, and also stops the penetration of harmful substances and traumas (p. 7). It is a dry mechanical barrier from which contaminating organisms and chemicals are continually being removed by washing and desquamation. Only when these breach the horny layer do the cellular components, described below, come into play.

The skin is involved in so many immunological reactions, seen regularly in the clinic (e.g. urticaria, allergic contact dermatitis, psoriasis, vasculitis), that a special mention has to be made of the peripheral arm of the immune system based in the skin – the skin immune system (SIS). The coordinated actions of the innate and acquired immune systems are mediated by cells such as macrophages, dendritic cells and T cells, and by effector proteins such as cytokines and antibodies. Although it is beyond the scope of this book to cover general immunology, this section outlines some of the intricate ways in which the skin defends itself and the body, and how antigens are recognized by specialized skin cells, such as the Langerhans cells. It also reviews the ways in which antibodies, lymphocytes, macrophages and polymorphs elicit inflammation in skin.

Cellular components of the skin immune system

Keratinocytes (p. 7)

The prime role of keratinocytes is to make the protective horny layer (p. 7) and to support the outermost epithelium of the body, but they also have important immunological functions in their own right and act as a link between the innate and acquired immune systems. Keratinocytes synthesize and release the cationic antimicrobial peptides cathelicidin and β-defensin. They can recognize pattern-associated molecular patterns (PAMPs) on bacteria by the toll-like receptors (TLRs) that they carry on their surface and in the cytosol. Activation of these leads to interferon release and a T-helper 1 (Th1) immune response. Proinflammatory pathways are activated after TLR ligation via an organized cluster of proteins known as the inflammosome in the keratinocyte cytosol. Keratinocytes produce chemokines that attract cells of the immune system to the skin, and large numbers of cytokines that can activate and guide an immune response. Their release of IL-1 after injury initiates various immune and inflammatory cascades (Figure 2.11). γ-interferon induces the expression of MHC Class II molecule on keratinocytes enabling them to act as non-professional antigen-presenting cells. Keratinocytes play a central part in healing after epidermal injury by self-regulating epidermal proliferation and differentiation (Figure 2.11).

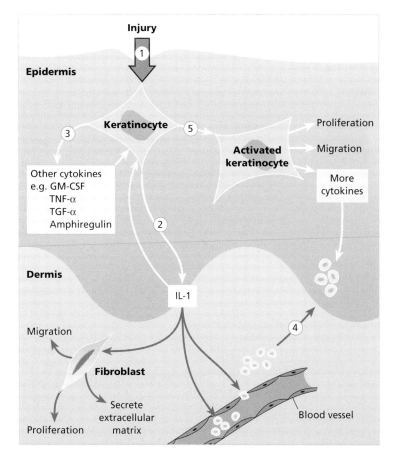

Figure 2.11 The keratinocyte and wound healing. The injured keratinocyte turns on wound healing responses. When a keratinocyte is injured (1), it releases interleukin-1 (IL-1) (2). IL-1 activates endothelial cells causing them to express selectins that slow down lymphocytes passing over them. Once lymphocytes stop on the endothelial cells lining the vessels, IL-1 acts as a chemotactic factor to draw lymphocytes into the epidermis (4). At the same time, IL-1 activates keratinocytes by binding to their IL-1 receptors. Activated keratinocytes produce other cytokines (3). Among these is tumour necrosis factor α (TNF-α) which additionally activates keratinocytes and keeps them in an activated state (5). Activation of keratinocytes causes them to proliferate, migrate and secrete additional cytokines. GM-CSF, granulocyte–macrophage colony-stimulating factor; TGF, transforming growth factor.

Langerhans cells (p. 13)

These dendritic cells come from the bone marrow and move into the epidermis and mucous membranes. Their dendrites intercalate between keratinocytes and their peripheral location in the body makes them an early sentinel in defence against infection. They can be identified in tissue sections by demonstrating their characteristic surface marker langerin, and also express MHC Class II molecules, CD1a antigen, and carry Birbeck granules. The function of Langerhans cells is an area of active research, but it is clear that they are key players in the induction of T-cell responses. Following antigen uptake and activation, they migrate to the draining lymph nodes and can induce either immunity or tolerance to an antigen, depending on the circumstances in which it is presented.

Dermal dendritic cells

Several subsets of dendritic cells are found within the dermis, particularly just below the basement membrane. They are identified by the different surface markers they carry, and their roles are gradually being elucidated. Different subsets are seen in inflamed and uninflamed skin, and activated dermal dendritic cells can secrete cytokines. Dermal dendritic cells can migrate to lymph nodes and stimulate T-cell proliferation, but they are probably more specifically involved in regulating the humoral antibody-mediated immune response.

T lymphocytes

Like T cells elsewhere, these develop and acquire their antigen receptors (T-cell receptors, TCR) in the thymus. They differentiate into subpopulations, recognizable by their different surface molecules (CD meaning cluster of differentiation markers), which are functionally distinct. T lymphocytes that express CD4 on their surfaces work to induce immune reactions and elicit inflammation. T cells that express CD8 are cytotoxic and can lyse infected, grafted and cancerous cells. A subset of these, the CD8 skin resident memory T cells, remain permanently in the skin and can rapidly amplify a reaction to an infectious challenge without circulating to the regional lymph nodes. CD4 (helper) cells are subdivided into Th1 cells that produce interleukin-2 (IL-2; T-cell growth factor) and γ-interferon. Th2 cells produce other interleukins such as IL-4, IL-5, IL-9 and IL-13. A third subset of CD4 cells has been described, called (somewhat confusingly) Th17 cells. IL-23 directs these to release IL-17 and IL-22. The amounts of IL-12 and IL-4 secreted by antigen-processing cells seem important in determining exactly which path of differentiation is followed.

Th1 cells induce cell-mediated immune reactions in the skin – for example, allergic contact dermatitis and delayed hypersensitivity reactions – and are involved in elicitation reactions as well. Th2 cells help B cells produce antibody. Th17 cells are involved in the clearance of infectious agents, and also mediate autoimmune inflammation and psoriasis. Th cells recognize antigen in association with MHC Class II molecules (Figures 2.12 and 2.13) and, when triggered by antigen, release cytokines that attract and activate other inflammatory cells (see Figure 2.18).

Some skin diseases display a predominantly Th1 response (e.g. tuberculoid leprosy), others a mainly Th2 response (e.g. atopic dermatitis) and others a Th17 response (psoriasis).

T-cytotoxic (Tc) cells

These lymphocytes are capable of destroying allogeneic and virally infected cells, which they recognize by the MHC Class I molecules on their surface. They express CD8.

T-regulatory (Treg) cells

This subset of T cells are strongly immunosuppressive and are characterized by the expression of the transcription factor Foxp3. Tregs are found in the skin and the circulation and help balance inflammatory responses. Ultraviolet radiation induces Tregs in the skin, and both the

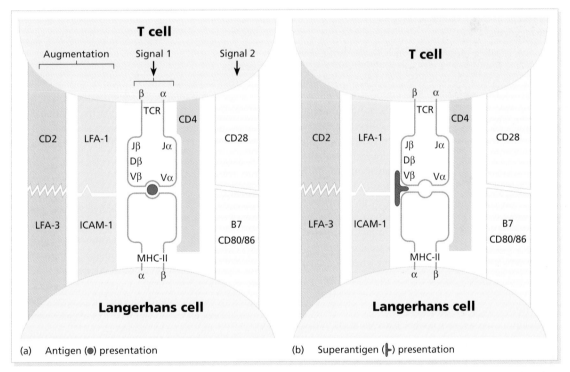

Figure 2.12 T-lymphocyte activation by (a) antigen and (b) superantigen. When antigen has been processed it is presented on the surface of the Langerhans cell in association with major histocompatibility complex (MHC) Class II. The complex formation that takes place between the antigen, MHC Class II and T-cell receptor (TCR) provides signal 1, which is enhanced by the coupling of CD4 with the MHC molecule. A second signal for T-cell activation is provided by the interaction between the co-stimulatory molecules CD28 (T cell) and B7 (Langerhans cell). CD2/LFA-3 and LFA-1/ICAM-1 adhesion augment the response to signals 1 and 2. Superantigen interacts with the TCR Vβ and MHC Class II without processing, binding outside the normal antigen binding site. Activated T cells secrete many cytokines, including IL-1, IL-8 and γ-interferon, which promote inflammation (Figure 2.13).

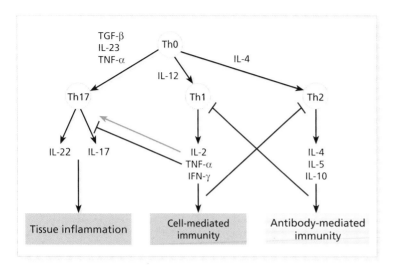

Figure 2.13 Characteristics of Th1, Th2 and Th17 responses.

sensitization and elicitation phases of the contact hypersensitivity response are moderated by these cells.

T-cell receptor and T-cell gene receptor rearrangements

Most T-cell receptors are composed of an α and a β chain, each with a variable (antigen binding) and a constant domain, which are associated with the CD3 cell surface molecules (Figure 2.12). The amino acid sequence of the variable portion determines its antigen-binding specificity – different sequences bind different antigens. To provide diversity and the ability to bind almost any antigen, the genes coding for the amino acid sequence undergo rearrangent. Antigenic stimulation results in expansion of appropriate clones carrying TCR capable of binding to the antigen. Most responses are polyclonal. On the other hand, malignant transformation is associated with proliferation of a unique clone. In fact, an analysis of the degree of clonality of rearrangements of the gene for the receptor can be used to determine whether a T-cell infiltrate in skin is likely to be malignant or reactive.

Other (non-T, non-B) lymphocytes

Some lymphocytes express neither CD4 nor CD8. These leucocytes have some properties of T lymphocytes and some properties of myelomonocytic cells. Most have receptors for FcIgG. This subpopulation contains natural killer (NK) and killer (K) cells.

Natural killer cells

These are large granular leucocytes that can kill virally infected cells, or tumour cells that have not previously been sensitized with antibody. They develop in the bone marrow, but have no antigen-specific receptors, reacting instead with self antigens. They especially kill tumour and virally infected cells. These cells can sometimes recognize glycolipid antigens using CD1 surface molecules that do not require presentation by antigen-presenting cells.

Killer cells

These are cytotoxic T cells, NK cells, or monocytic leucocytes that can kill target cells sensitized with antibody. In antibody-mediated cellular cytotoxicity, antibody binds to antigen on the surface of the target cell: the K cell binds to the antibody at its other (Fc) end by its Fc receptor and the target cell is then lysed.

Mast cells

These are present in most connective tissues, predominantly around blood vessels. Their numerous granules contain inflammatory mediators (see Figure 8.1). In rodents – and probably in humans – there are two distinct populations of mast cells, connective tissue and mucosal, which differ in their staining properties, content of inflammatory mediators and proteolytic enzymes. Skin mast cells play a central part in the pathogenesis of urticaria (p. 99) and also influence the development of contact allergic responses to haptens.

Molecular components of the skin immune system

Antigens

Antigens are molecules that are recognized by the immune system thereby provoking an immune reaction, usually in the form of a humoral or cell-mediated immune response. The immune system can usually identify its own molecules so that it does not direct a reaction against them. If it does, autoimmune reactions occur. Otherwise, the skin immune system readily responds to non-self antigens, such as chemicals, proteins, allografted cells and infectious agents. The process of recognizing antigens and developing immunity is called induction or sensitization.

Superantigens

Some bacterial toxins (e.g. those released by *Staphylococcus aureus*) are prototypic superantigens. They align with MHC Class II molecules of antigen-presenting cells outside their antigen-presentation groove and, without any cellular processing, may directly induce massive T-cell proliferation and cytokine production leading to disorders such as the toxic shock syndrome (p. 217). Streptococcal toxins act as superantigens to activate T cells in the pathogenesis of guttate psoriasis.

Antibodies (immunoglobulins)

Antibodies are immunoglobulins that react with antigens.
• Immunoglobulin G (IgG) is responsible for long-lasting humoral immunity. It can cross the placenta, and binds complement to activate the classic complement pathway. IgG can coat neutrophils and macrophages (by their FcIgG receptors), and acts as an opsonin by cross-bridging antigen. IgG can also sensitize target cells for destruction by K cells.
• IgM is the largest immunoglobulin molecule. It is the first antibody to appear after immunization or infection. Like IgG, it can fix complement but unlike IgG it cannot cross the placenta.
• IgA is the most common immunoglobulin in secretions. It acts as a protective paint in the gastrointestinal and respiratory tracts. It does not bind complement but can activate it via the alternative pathway.
• IgE binds to Fc receptors on mast cells and basophils, where it sensitizes them to release inflammatory mediators in type I immediate hypersensitivity reactions (Figure 2.14).

Cytokines

Cytokines are small proteins secreted by cells such as lymphocytes and macrophages, and also by keratinocytes. They regulate the amplitude and duration of inflammation by acting locally on nearby cells (paracrine action), on those cells that secreted them (autocrine) and occasionally on distant target cells (endocrine) via the circulation. The term cytokine covers interleukins, interferons, colony-stimulating factors, cytotoxins and growth factors. Interleukins are produced predominantly by leucocytes, have a known amino acid sequence and are active in inflammation or immunity.

There are many cytokines, and each may act on more than one type of cell, causing many different effects. Cytokines frequently have overlapping actions. In any inflammatory reaction some cytokines are acting synergistically while others will antagonize these effects. This network of potent chemicals, each acting alone and in concert, moves the inflammatory response along in a controlled way. Cytokines bind to high affinity (but not usually specific) cell surface receptors, and elicit a biological response by regulating the transcription of genes in the target cell via signal transduction pathways involving, for example, the Janus protein tyrosine kinase or calcium influx systems. The biological response is a balance between the production of the cytokine, the expression of its receptors on the target cells and the presence of inhibitors.

Adhesion molecules

Cellular adhesion molecules (CAMs) are surface glycoproteins that are expressed on many different types of cell; they are involved in cell–cell and cell–matrix adhesion and interactions. CAMs are fundamental in the interaction of lymphocytes with antigen-presenting cells (Figure 2.12), keratinocytes and endothelial cells, and are important in lymphocyte trafficking in the skin during inflammation (Figure 2.11). CAMs have been classified into four families: cadherins, immunoglobulin superfamily, integrins and selectins. E-cadherins are found on the surface of keratinocytes between the desmosomes. γ-Interferon causes upregulation of Fas on epidermal lymphocytes. Interaction of these with Fas ligand on keratinocytes causes e-cadherins to 'disappear', leading to intercellular edema (spongiosis) between desmosomes.

CAMs of special relevance in the skin are listed in Table 2.5.

Histocompatibility antigens

Like other cells, those in the skin express surface antigens directed by genes. The human leucocyte antigen (HLA) region lies within the major histocompatability locus (MHC) on chromosome 6. In particular, HLA-A, -B and -C antigens (the Class I antigens) are expressed on all nucleated cells including keratinocytes, Langerhans cells and cells of the dermis. HLA-DR, -DP, -DQ and -DZ antigens (the Class II antigens) are expressed only on some cells (e.g. Langerhans cells and B cells). They are usually not found on keratinocytes except during certain

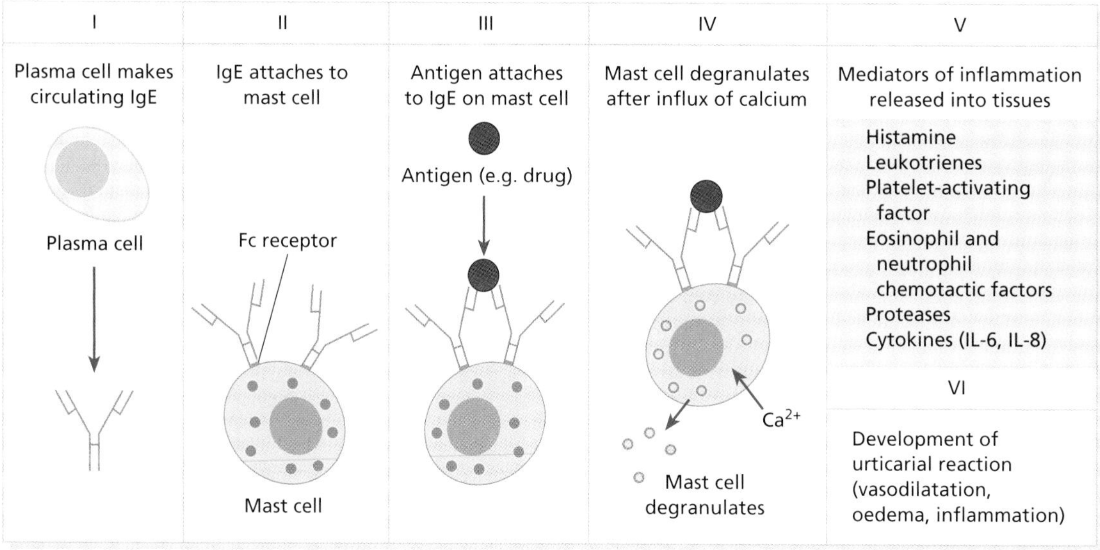

I	II	III	IV	V
Plasma cell makes circulating IgE	IgE attaches to mast cell	Antigen attaches to IgE on mast cell	Mast cell degranulates after influx of calcium	Mediators of inflammation released into tissues

Histamine
Leukotrienes
Platelet-activating factor
Eosinophil and neutrophil chemotactic factors
Proteases
Cytokines (IL-6, IL-8)

VI

Development of urticarial reaction (vasodilatation, oedema, inflammation)

Plasma cell

Fc receptor

Antigen (e.g. drug)

Mast cell

Ca²⁺

Mast cell degranulates

Figure 2.14 Urticaria: an immediate (type I) hypersensitivity reaction.

reactions (e.g. allergic contact dermatitis) or diseases (e.g. lichen planus). Helper T cells recognize antigens only in the presence of cells bearing Class II antigens. Class II antigens are also important for certain cell–cell interac-

tions. On the other hand, Class I antigens mark target cells for cell-mediated cytotoxic reactions, such as the rejection of skin allografts and the destruction of cells infected by viruses.

Table 2.5 Cellular adhesion molecules important in the skin.

Family	Nature	Example	Site	Ligand
Cadherins	Glycoproteins Adherence dependent on calcium	Desmoglein	Desmosomes in epidermis	Other cadherins
Immunoglobulin	Numerous molecules that are structurally similar to immunoglobulins	ICAM-1	Endothelial cells Keratinocytes Langerhans cells	LFA-1
		CD2	T lymphocytes Some NK cells	LFA-3
		VCAM-1 (β1-VLA)	Endothelial cells	VLA-4
Integrins	Surface proteins comprising two non-covalently bound α and β chains	LFA-1	T lymphocyte T lymphocyte	VCAM ICAM-1
		Mac-1	Macrophages Monocytes Granulocytes	C3b component of complement
Selectins	Adhesion molecules with lectin-like domain which binds carbohydrate	E selectin	Endothelial cells	CD15

CD, Cluster of differentiation antigen; ICAM, Intercellular adhesion molecule; LFA, leucocyte function antigen; Mac, macrophage activation; VCAM, vascular cell adhesion molecule; VLA, very late activation proteins.

Types of immune reactions in the skin

Innate immune system

The epidermal barrier is the major defence against infection in human skin. When it is breached, cells in the dermis and epidermis can telegraph the danger and engage the innate immunity and inflammatory systems. Innate immunity allows reaction to infectious agents and noxious chemicals, without the need to activate specific lymphocytes or use antibodies. This is fortunate. If an infected person had to wait for immunity to develop, the onset of the reaction might take a week or two, and by then the infection might be widespread or lethal.

For example, defensins in the epidermis inhibit bacterial replication there. Complement can be activated by many infectious agents via the alternative pathway without the need for antigen–antibody interaction. Complement activation generates C5a, which attracts neutrophils, and C3b and C5b, which opsonize the agents so they can be more readily engulfed and killed by the phagocytes when these arrive. Chemicals such as detergents can activate keratinocytes to produce cytokines leading to epidermal proliferation and eventual shedding of the toxic agent. After infection or stimulation, certain cells can non-specifically secrete chemokines that bring inflammatory cells to the area. The main effector cells of the innate immune system are neutrophils, monocytes and macrophages.

The antigen-presenting cells have a role in both innate and acquired immunity. They can recognize certain patterns of molecules or chemicals common to many infectious agents. The lipo-polysaccharide of Gram-negative bacteria is an example of such a pathogen-associated molecular pattern. The receptors for these reside on cell membranes and are genetically derived.

Toll-like receptors provide the innate immune system with a certain specificity. These are transmembrane proteins, which also recognize patterns, and different toll receptors recognize different patterns and chemicals. For example, toll-like receptor 2 recognizes lipoproteins, while toll-like receptor 3 recognizes double-stranded RNA. Toll-like receptors also upregulate the expression of co-stimulatory molecules that allow appropriate recognition and response of the adaptive immune system.

Adaptive immune system

Adaptive immunity is not only more specific, but is also long-lasting. It generates cells that can persist in a relatively dormant state. These are ready to react quickly and powerfully when they encounter their antigen again – even years later.

Specific immune responses allow a targeted and amplified inflammatory response. To induce such a response, an antigen must be processed by an antigen-presenting cell such as a Langerhans or dermal dendritic cell, and it must be presented to a T cell, with unique receptor molecules on its surface, that can bind the antigen presented to it. To elicit an inflammatory response, this antigen processing, presenting and binding process is repeated but, this time, with the purpose of bringing in inflammatory, phagocytic and cytotoxic cells to control the inflammation within the arena.

It is still helpful, if rather artificial, to separate these elicited specific immune responses into four main types using the original classification of Coombs and Gell. All of these types cause reactions in the skin.

Type I: Immediate hypersensitivity reactions

These are characterized by vasodilatation and an outpouring of fluid from blood vessels. Such reactions can be mimicked by drugs or toxins, which act directly, but immunological reactions are mediated by antibodies, and are manifestations of allergy. IgE and IgG4 antibodies, produced by plasma cells in organs other than the skin, attach themselves to mast cells in the dermis. These contain inflammatory mediators, both in granules and in their cytoplasm. The IgE antibody is attached to the mast cell by its Fc end, so that the antigen combining site dangles from the mast cell like a hand on an arm (Figure 2.14). When specific antigen combines with the hand parts of the immunoglobulin (the antigen-binding site or Fab end), the mast cell liberates its mediators into the surrounding tissue. Of these mediators, histamine (from the granules) and leukotrienes (from the cell membrane) induce vasodilatation, and endothelial cells retract allowing transudation into the extravascular space. The vasodilatation causes a pink colour, and the transudation causes swelling. Urticaria and angioedema (p. 99) are examples of immediate hypersensitivity reactions occurring in the skin.

Antigen may be delivered to the skin from the outside (e.g. in a bee sting). This will induce a swelling in everyone by a direct pharmacological action. However, some people, with IgE antibodies against antigens in the venom, swell even more at the site of the sting as the result of a specific immunological reaction. If they are extremely sensitive, they may develop wheezing, wheals and anaphylactic shock (see Figure 25.5) because of a massive release of histamine into the circulation.

Antigens can also reach mast cells from inside the body. Those who are allergic to shellfish, for example, may develop urticaria within seconds, minutes or hours of eating one. Antigenic material, absorbed from the gut, passes to tissue mast cells via the circulation, and elicits an urticarial reaction after binding to specific IgE on mast cells in the skin.

Type II: Humoral cytotoxic reactions

In the main, these involve IgG and IgM antibodies, which, like IgE, are produced by plasma cells and are present in the interstitial fluid of the skin. When they meet an antigen, they fix and activate complement through a series of enzymatic reactions that generate mediator and cytotoxic proteins. If bacteria enter the skin, IgG and IgM antibodies bind to antigens on them. Complement is activated through the classic pathway, and a number of mediators are generated. Amongst these are the chemotactic factor, C5a, which attracts polymorphs to the area of bacterial invasion, and the opsonin, C3b, which coats the bacteria so that they can be ingested and killed by polymorphs

when these arrive (Figure 2.15). Under certain circumstances, activation of complement can kill cells or organisms directly by the *membrane attack complex* (C5b6789) in the terminal complement pathway. Complement can also be activated by bacteria directly through the alternative pathway; antibody is not required. The bacterial cell wall causes more C3b to be produced by the alternative pathway factors B, D and P (properdin). Aggregated IgA can also activate the alternative pathway.

Activation of either pathway produces C3b, the pivotal component of the complement system. Through the amplification loop, a single reaction can flood the area with C3b, C5a and other amplification loop and terminal pathway components. Complement is the mediator of humoral reactions.

Humoral cytotoxic reactions are typical of defence against infectious agents such as bacteria. However, they are also involved in certain autoimmune diseases such as pemphigoid (see Chapter 9).

Occasionally, antibodies bind to the surface of a cell and activate it without causing its death or activating

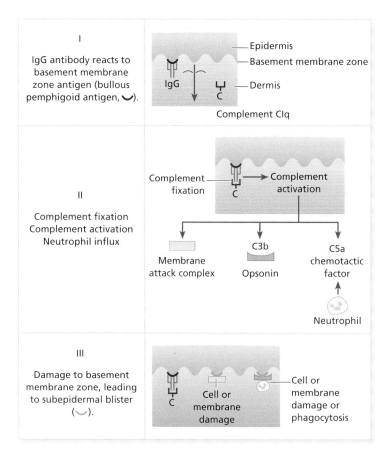

I	Epidermis
IgG antibody reacts to basement membrane zone antigen (bullous pemphigoid antigen, ⌣).	Basement membrane zone
	IgG C Dermis
	Complement C1q

II	Complement fixation → Complement activation
Complement fixation Complement activation Neutrophil influx	C
	Membrane attack complex C3b Opsonin C5a chemotactic factor
	Neutrophil

| III | |
| Damage to basement membrane zone, leading to subepidermal blister (⌣). | Cell or membrane damage   Cell or membrane damage or phagocytosis |

Figure 2.15 Bullous pemphigoid: a humoral cytotoxic (type II) reaction against a basement membrane zone antigen.

complement. Instead, the cell is stimulated to produce a hormone-like substance that may mediate disease. Pemphigus (see Chapter 9) is a blistering disease of skin in which this type of reaction may be important.

Type III: Immune complex-mediated reactions

Antigen may combine with antibodies near vital tissues so that the ensuing inflammatory response damages them. When an antigen arrives in the dermis, for example after a bite or an injection, it may combine with appropriate antibodies on the walls of blood vessels. Complement is activated, and polymorphonuclear leucocytes are brought to the area (an Arthus reaction). Degranulation of poly-

morphs liberates lysosomal enzymes that damage the vessel walls.

Antigen–antibody complexes can also be formed in the circulation, move to the small vessels in the skin and lodge there (Figure 2.16). Complement will then be activated and inflammatory cells will injure the vessels as in the Arthus reaction. This causes oedema and the extravasation of red blood cells (e.g. the palpable purpura that characterizes vasculitis; see Chapter 8).

Type IV: Cell-mediated immune reactions

As the name implies, these are mediated by lymphocytes rather than by antibodies. Cell-mediated immune

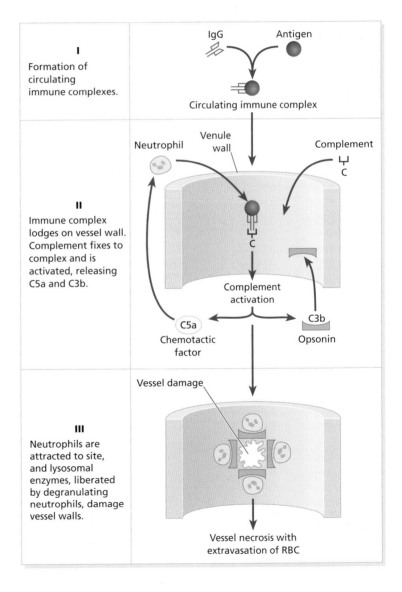

Figure 2.16 Immune complex-mediated vasculitis (type III reaction).

reactions are important in granulomas, delayed hyper-sensitivity reactions and allergic contact dermatitis. They probably also play a part in some photosensitive disorders, in protecting against cancer and in mediating delayed reactions to insect bites.

During the elicitation phase, most protein and chemical antigens entering the skin are processed by antigen-presenting cells such as macrophages and Langerhans cells (Figure 2.17) and then interact with sensitized lymphocytes. The lymphocytes are stimulated to enlarge, divide and to secrete cytokines that can injure tissues directly and kill cells or microbes.

Allergic contact dermatitis

Induction (sensitization) phase (Figure 2.17)

When the epidermal barrier is breached, the immune system provides the second line of defence. Antigens – either in isolation (e.g. nickel), or bound as haptens to self-proteins – activate the innate immune system via Toll-like receptors or the inflammosome in keratinocytes. Cytokines such as IL-1β, IL-18 or TNF are released by activated keratinocytes, and this helps steer the response of the skin resident dendritic cells. Among the keratinocytes are Langerhans cells, highly specialized intraepidermal macrophages with tentacles that intertwine amongst the keratinocytes, providing a net (Figure 2.7) to 'catch' antigens falling down on them from the surface, such as chemicals or the antigens of microbes or tumours. Dermal dendritic cells perform a similar role below the basement membrane. During the initial induction phase, the antigen is trapped by these dendritic cells then leave the skin and migrates to the regional lymph node. The Langerhans cells must retract their dendrites and 'swim upstream' from the prickle cell layer of the epidermis towards the basement membrane, against the 'flow' of keratinocytes generated by the epidermal basal cells. Entering the lymphatic system, the dendritic cells

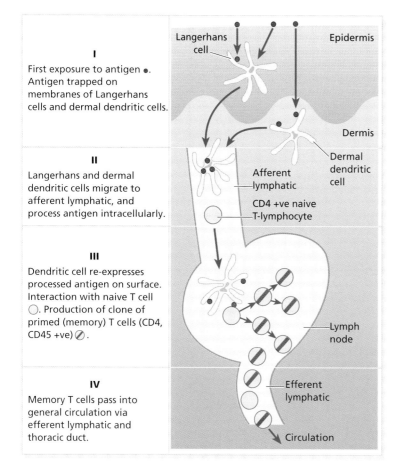

Figure 2.17 Induction phase of allergic contact dermatitis (type IV) reaction.

process the antigens they are carrying and by the time they reach the regional lymph re-express them on their surface in conjunction with MHC Class II molecules. In the node, the dendritic cells mingles with crowds of lymphocytes, and are quite likely to find a T cell with just the right T-cell receptor to bind its now processed antigen. Helper (CD4$^+$) T lymphocytes recognize antigen only in the presence of cells bearing MHC Class II antigens, such as Langerhans cells and dermal dendritic cells. The interactions between surface molecules on a CD4$^+$ T cell and a Langerhans cell are shown in Figure 2.12. To activate, the T lymphocyte must also bind itself tightly to certain *accessory molecules*, also called co-stimulatory molecules. If these are not engaged, then the immune response does not occur.

When a T cell interacts with an antigen-presenting cell carrying an antigen to which it can react, the T lymphocyte divides many times. This continuing division depends upon the persistence of antigen (and the antigen-presenting cells that contain it) and the T-cell growth factor IL-2. Eventually, a whole cadre of memory T cells is available to return to the skin to attack the antigen that stimulated their proliferation.

CD4$^+$, CD45$^+$ memory T lymphocytes then leave the node and circulate via lymphatic vessels, the thoracic duct and blood. They return to the skin aided by *homing molecules* (cutaneous lymphocyte antigen, CLA) on their surfaces that guide their trip so that they preferentially enter the dermis. In the absence of antigen, they merely pass through it, and again enter the lymphatic vessels to return and recirculate. These cells are sentinel cells (Figure 2.18), alert for their own special antigens. They accumulate in the skin if the host again encounters the antigen that initially stimulated their production. This

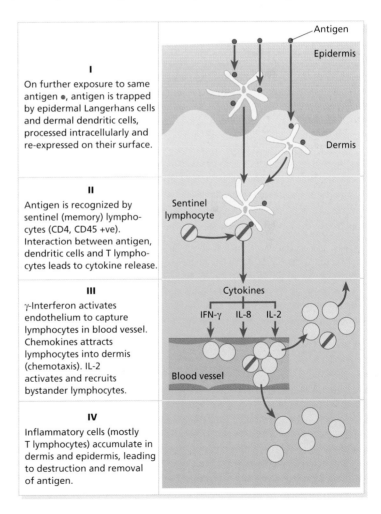

I

On further exposure to same antigen •, antigen is trapped by epidermal Langerhans cells and dermal dendritic cells, processed intracellularly and re-expressed on their surface.

II

Antigen is recognized by sentinel (memory) lymphocytes (CD4, CD45 +ve). Interaction between antigen, dendritic cells and T lymphocytes leads to cytokine release.

III

γ-Interferon activates endothelium to capture lymphocytes in blood vessel. Chemokines attracts lymphocytes into dermis (chemotaxis). IL-2 activates and recruits bystander lymphocytes.

IV

Inflammatory cells (mostly T lymphocytes) accumulate in dermis and epidermis, leading to destruction and removal of antigen.

Figure 2.18 Elicitation phase of allergic contact dermatitis (type IV) reaction.

preferential circulation of lymphocytes into the skin is a special part of the skin immune system and reflects a selective advantage for the body to circulate lymphocytes that react to skin and skin surface-derived antigens.

Elicitation (challenge) phase (Figure 2.18)

When a T lymphocyte again encounters the antigen to which it is sensitized, it is ready to react. If the antigen is extracellular, as on an invading bacterium, toxin or chemical allergen, the CD4$^+$ T-helper cells do the work. The sequence of antigen processing by the skin dendritic cells in the elicitation reaction is similar to the sequence of antigen processing during the induction phase, described above, that leads to the induction of immunity. The antigens get trapped by epidermal Langerhans cells or dermal dendritic cells, which process them intracellularly before re-expressing the modified antigenic determinant on their surfaces. In the elicitation reaction, the Langerhans cells find appropriate T lymphocytes in the dermis, because these are trafficking through the dermis. In the elicitiation phase, most antigen presentation occurs there. The antigen is presented to CD4$^+$ T cells, which are activated and produce cytokines that cause lymphocytes, polymorphonuclear leucocytes and monocytes in blood vessels to slow as they pass through the dermal blood vessels, to stop and emigrate into the dermis causing inflammation (Figure 2.18). Helper or cytotoxic lymphocytes help to stem the infection or eliminate antigen, and polymorphonuclear leucocytes engulf antigens and destroy them. The traffic of inflammatory cells in the epidermis and dermis is determined not only by cytokines produced by lymphocytes, but also by cytokines produced by injured keratinocytes (Figure 2.11). For example, keratinocyte-derived cytokines can activate Langerhans cells and T cells, and IL-8, produced by keratinocytes, is a potent chemotactic factor for lymphocytes and polymorphs, and brings these up into the epidermis.

Response to intracellular antigens

Antigens coming from inside a cell, such as intracellular fungi or viruses and tumour antigens, are presented to cytotoxic T cells (CD8$^+$) by the MHC Class I molecule. Presentation in this manner makes the infected cell liable to destruction by cytotoxic T lymphocytes or K cells. NK cells can also kill such cells, even though they have not been sensitized with antibody.

Granulomas

Granulomas form when cell-mediated immunity fails to eliminate antigen. Foreign body granulomas occur because material remains undigested. Immunological granulomas require the persistence of antigen, but the response is augmented by a cell-mediated immune reaction. Lymphokines, released by lymphocytes sensitized to the antigen, cause macrophages to differentiate into epithelioid cells and giant cells. These secrete other cytokines, which influence inflammatory events. Immunological granulomas of the skin are characterized by Langhans giant cells (not to be confused with Langerhans cells; p. 13), epithelioid cells and a surrounding mantle of lymphocytes.

Granulomatous reactions also occur when organisms cannot be destroyed (e.g. in tuberculosis, leprosy, leishmaniasis), or when a chemical cannot be eliminated (e.g. zirconium or beryllium). Similar reactions are seen in some persisting inflammations of undetermined cause (e.g. rosacea, granuloma annulare, sarcoidosis and certain forms of panniculitis).

Learning points

1 Many skin disorders are good examples of an immune reaction at work. The more you know about the mechanisms, the more interesting the rashes become.
2 However, the immune system may not be the only culprit. If *Treponema pallidum* had not been discovered, syphilis might still be listed as an autoimmune disorder.
3 Because skin protects against infections, it has its own unique immune system to cope quickly with infectious agents breaching its barrier.

Further reading

Asadullah K, Sterry W, Volk HD. (2002) Analysis of cytokine expression in dermatology. *Archives of Dermatology* **138**, 1189–1196.

Blanpain C, Fuchs E. (2009) Epidermal homeostasis: a balancing act of stem cells in the skin. *Nature Reviews Molecular Cell Biology* **10**, 207–217.

Boehncke WH. (2005) *Lymphocyte Homing to Skin: Immunology, Immunopathology, and Therapeutic Perspectives.* CRC Press, Boca Raton.

Chaplin DD. (2006) Overview of the human immune response. *Journal of Allergy and Clinical Immunology* **117**, s430–s435.

Freinkel RK, Woodley DT. (2001) *The Biology of the Skin.* Parthenon, London.

Honda T, Miyachi Y, Kabashima K. (2011) Regulatory T cells in cutaneous immune responses. *Journal of Dermatological Science* **63**, 75–82.

Kang SSW, Sauls LS, Gaspari AA. (2006) Toll-like receptors: Applications to dermatologic disease. *Journal of the American Academy of Dermatology* **54**, 951–983.

Kaplan DH, Igyarto BZ, Gaspari AA. (2012) Early immune events in the induction of allergic contact dermatitis. *Nature Reviews Immunology* **12**, 114–124.

Nestle FO, Di Meglio P, Qin JZ, Nickoloff BJ. (2009) Skin immune sentinels in health and disease. *Nature Reviews Immunology* **9**, 679–691.

Yokoyama WM. (2005) Natual killer cell immune responses. *Immunology Reviews* **32**, 317–326.

3 Diagnosis of Skin Disorders

The key to successful treatment is an accurate diagnosis. You can look up treatments, but you cannot look up diagnoses. Without a proper diagnosis, you will be asking 'What's a good treatment for scaling feet?' instead of 'What's good for tinea pedis?' Would you ever ask yourself 'What's a good treatment for chest pain?' Luckily, dermatology differs from other specialties as its diseases can easily be seen. Keen eyes and a magnifying glass are all that are needed for a complete examination of the skin. Sometimes it is best to examine the patient briefly before obtaining a full history: a quick look will often prompt the right questions. However, a careful history is important in every case, as is the intelligent use of the laboratory.

History

The key points to be covered in the history are listed in Table 3.1 and should include descriptions of the events surrounding the onset of the skin lesions, of the progression of individual lesions and of the disease in general, including any responses to treatment. Many patients try a few salves before seeing a physician. Some try all the medications in their medicine cabinets, many of which can aggravate the problem. A careful enquiry into drugs taken for other conditions is often useful. Ask also about previous skin disorders, occupation, hobbies and disorders in the family.

Examination

To examine the skin properly, the lighting must be uniform and bright. Daylight is best. The patient should usually undress so that the whole skin can be examined, although sometimes this is neither desirable (e.g. hand warts) nor possible. Do not be put off this too easily by the elderly, the stubborn, the shy or the surroundings. The presence of a chaperone, ideally a nurse, is often sen-

sible, and is essential if examination of the genitalia is necessary. Sometimes, make-up must be washed off or wigs removed. It is often important to remove adherent crust overlying the primary lesion to see and determine the underlying sign. There is nothing more embarrassing than missing the right diagnosis because an important sign has been hidden.

Distribution

A dermatological diagnosis is based both on the distribution of lesions and on their morphology and configuration. For example, an area of seborrhoeic dermatitis may look very like an area of atopic dermatitis; but the key to diagnosis lies in the location. Seborrhoeic dermatitis affects the scalp, forehead, eyebrows, nasolabial folds and central chest; atopic dermatitis typically affects the antecubital and popliteal fossae. Figure 3.1 shows the typical distribution of some common skin conditions.

See if the skin disease is localized, universal or symmetrical. Symmetry implies a systemic origin, whereas unilaterality or asymmetry implies an external cause. Depending on the disease suggested by the morphology, you may want to check special areas, like the feet in a patient with hand eczema, or the gluteal cleft in a patient who might have psoriasis. Examine as much of the skin as possible. Look in the mouth and remember to check the hair and the nails (see Chapter 13). Note negative as well as positive findings; for example, the way the shielded areas are spared in a photosensitive dermatitis (see Figure 18.7). Always keep your eyes open for incidental skin cancers which the patient may have ignored.

Morphology

After the distribution has been noted, next define the morphology of the primary lesions. Many skin diseases have a characteristic morphology, but scratching, ulceration and other events can change this. The rule is to find an early or 'primary' lesion and to inspect it closely. What

Clinical Dermatology, Fifth Edition. Richard B. Weller, Hamish J.A. Hunter and Margaret W. Mann.
© 2015 John Wiley & Sons, Ltd. Published 2015 by John Wiley & Sons, Ltd.

Table 3.1 Outline of dermatological history.

History of present skin condition
Duration
Site at onset, details of spread
Itch
Burning
Pain
Wet, dry, blisters, pustules
Exacerbating factors
Relationship of rash to work and holidays

Drugs used to treat present skin condition and clinical response
Topical
Systemic
Physician prescribed
Patient initiated

General health at present
Ask about fever, weight loss and night sweats

Past history of skin disorders
Past general medical history
Enquire specifically about asthma and hay fever
    (atopy)

Drugs prescribed for other disorders (including those taken before onset of skin disorder)
Any known drug allergies?
Family history of skin disorders
If positive, the disorder or the tendency to have it may
    be inherited. Sometimes, family members may be
    exposed to a common infectious agent or scabies or
    to a injurious chemical

Family history of other medical disorders
Social and occupational history
Alcohol intake
Smoking history
Hobbies
History of sun exposure:
    Skin type (p. 260)
    Outdoor work/hobbies
    Travel abroad
    Sunbed usage
    History of sunburn
Recent foreign travel

Table 3.2 Terminology of primary lesions.

	Small (<0.5 cm)	Large (>0.5 cm)
Elevated solid lesion	Papule	Nodule (>0.5 cm in both width and depth)
		Plaque >2 cm in width but without substantial depth)
Flat area of altered colour or texture	Macule	Large macule (patch)
Fluid-filled blister	Vesicle	Bulla
Pus-filled lesion	Pustule	Abscess Furuncle/ carbuncle
Extravasation of blood into skin	Petechia (pinhead size)	Ecchymosis
	Purpura (up to 2 mm in diameter)	Haematoma
Accumulation of dermal oedema	Wheal (can be any size)	Angioedema

There are many reasons why you should describe skin diseases properly.
• Skin disorders are often grouped by their morphology. Once the morphology is clear, a differential diagnosis comes easily to mind.
• If you have to describe a condition accurately, you will have to look at it carefully.
• You can paint a verbal picture if you have to refer the patient for another opinion.
• You will sound like a physician and not a homoeopath.
• You will be able to understand the terminology of this book.

Terminology of lesions (Figure 3.2)

Primary lesions
The size in many of the definitions given below (e.g. papule, nodule, macule, patch) is arbitrary and it is often helpful to record the actual measurement.
A *papule* is a small solid elevation of skin, less than 0.5 cm
    in diameter.
A *plaque* is an elevated area of skin greater than 2 cm in
    diameter but without substantial depth.

is its shape? What is its size? What is its colour? What are its margins like? What are the surface characteristics? What does it feel like?

Most types of primary lesion have one name if small, and a different one if large. The scheme is summarized in Table 3.2.

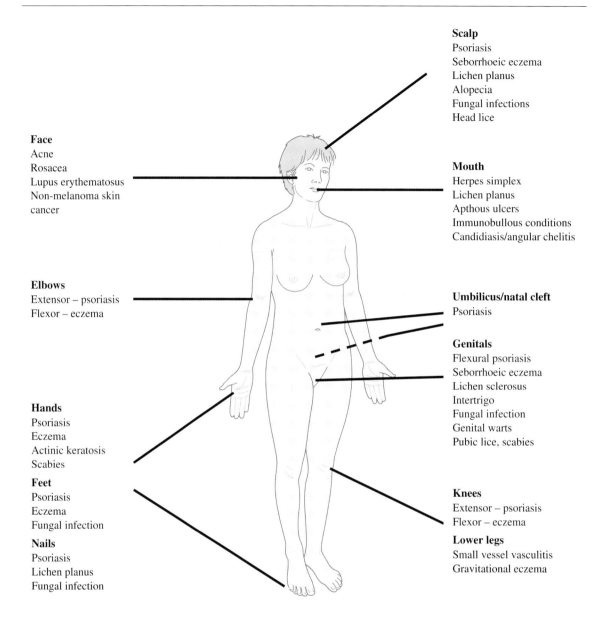

Scalp
Psoriasis
Seborrhoeic eczema
Lichen planus
Alopecia
Fungal infections
Head lice

Face
Acne
Rosacea
Lupus erythematosus
Non-melanoma skin
cancer

Mouth
Herpes simplex
Lichen planus
Apthous ulcers
Immunobullous conditions
Candidiasis/angular chelitis

Elbows
Extensor – psoriasis
Flexor – eczema

Umbilicus/natal cleft
Psoriasis

Genitals
Flexural psoriasis
Seborrhoeic eczema
Lichen sclerosus
Intertrigo
Fungal infection
Genital warts
Pubic lice, scabies

Hands
Psoriasis
Eczema
Actinic keratosis
Scabies

Feet
Psoriasis
Eczema
Fungal infection

Knees
Extensor – psoriasis
Flexor – eczema

Lower legs
Small vessel vasculitis
Gravitational eczema

Nails
Psoriasis
Lichen planus
Fungal infection

Rashes with an unusual distribution may give a clue to the diagnosis:

- Photo-exposed sites (e.g. lupus erythematosus, polymorphic light eruption)
- Sites of trauma, the Köbner phenomenon (e.g. psoriasis, lichen planus)
- Possible contact allergy (e.g. nickel earrings, leather or rubber shoes)

Figure 3.1 The typical distribution of some common skin conditions.

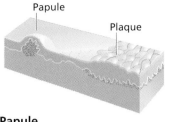

Papule
Small solid elevation of skin
<0.5 cm in diameter

Plaque
Elevated area of skin
>2 cm in diameter
Without substantial depth

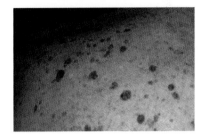

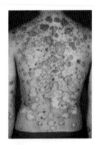

Seborrhoeic keratoses
Multiple pale to mid brown
'stuck on' warty papules

Psoriasis
Extensive, sharply demarcated,
plaques covered by large silver
polygonal scales

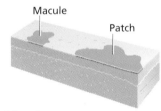

Macule
Small flat area
<0.5 cm in diameter

Patch
A large macule
>0.5 cm in diameter

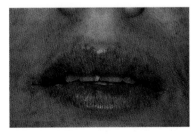

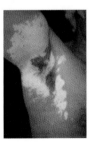

Peutz–Jeghers syndrome
Multiple brown macules of the
lips and perioral skin

Vitiligo
Localized, well-defined,
depigmented patch of the right axilla

Figure 3.2 Terminology of skin lesions.

Exophytic nodule

Endophytic nodule

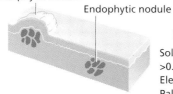

Nodule

Solid mass in the skin
>0.5 cm in width and depth
Elevated – exophytic
Palpated – endophytic

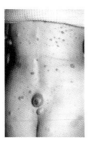

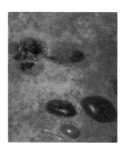

Neurofibromatosis

Multiple exophytic ulcerated and
non-ulcerated nodules, associated
with pale brown café au lait patches

Lipomas

Multiple endophytic rubbery nodules

Vesicles

Bulla

Vesicle
Fluid-filled blister
<0.5 cm in diameter

Bulla
Fluid-filled blister
>0.5 cm in diameter

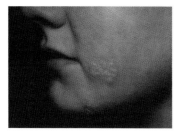

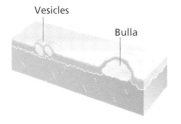

Herpes simplex

Grouped, yellow vesicles with
secondary crusting of the lower
group

Bullous pemphigoid

Large, tense, yellow or haemorrhagic
bullae often on a pink, urticated base

Figure 3.2 (*Continued*)

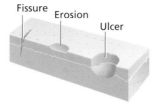

Fissure
Slit in the skin

Erosion
Complete or partial loss of the
epidermis (heals with no scarring)

Ulcer
Loss of entire epidermis and at
least part of the dermis (heals with
scarring)

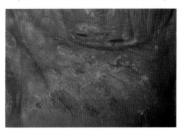

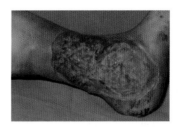

Chronic hand eczema

Palmar inflammation with
lichenification, hyperkeratosis and
fissuring

Venous leg ulcer

A large sloughy ulcer overlying the
medial malleolus with surrounding
evidence of vascular stasis

Figure 3.2 (*Continued*)

A *macule* is a small flat area, less than 0.5 cm in diameter, of altered colour or texture.

A *patch* is a large macule.

A *vesicle* is a circumscribed elevation of skin, less than 0.5 cm in diameter, and containing fluid.

A *bulla* is a circumscribed elevation of skin over 0.5 cm in diameter and containing fluid.

A *pustule* is a visible accumulation of pus in the skin.

An *abscess* is a localized collection of pus in a cavity, more than 1 cm in diameter. Abscesses are usually nodules, and the term 'purulent bulla' is sometimes used to describe a pus-filled blister that is situated on top of the skin rather than within it.

A *furuncle* or 'boil' is an infection of a single hair follicle and surrounding tissue.

A *carbuncle* is an infection of a group of hair follicles and surrounding tissue.

Folliculitis is inflammation of one or more hair follicles.

A *wheal* is an elevated white compressible evanescent area produced by dermal oedema. It is often surrounded by a red axon-mediated flare. Although usually less than 2 cm in diameter, some wheals are huge.

Angioedema is a diffuse swelling caused by oedema extending to the subcutaneous tissue.

A *nodule* is a solid mass in the skin, usually greater than 0.5 cm in diameter, in both width and depth, which can be seen to be elevated (exophytic) or can be palpated (endophytic).

A *tumour* is harder to define as the term is based more correctly on microscopic pathology than on clinical morphology. We keep it here as a convenient term to describe an enlargement of the tissues by normal or pathological material or cells that form a mass, usually more than 1 cm in diameter. Because the word 'tumour' can scare patients, tumours may courteously be called 'large nodules', especially if they are not malignant.

A *papilloma* is a nipple-like projection from the skin.

Petechiae are pinhead-sized macules of blood in the skin.

The term *purpura* describes a larger macule or papule of blood in the skin. Such blood-filled lesions do not blanch if a glass lens is pushed against them (see below under *Diascopy*)

An *ecchymosis (bruise)* is a larger extravasation of blood into the skin and deeper structures.

A *haematoma* is a swelling from gross bleeding.

A *burrow* is a linear or curvilinear papule, with some scaling, caused by a scabies mite.

A *comedo* is a plug of greasy keratin wedged in a dilated pilosebaceous orifice. Open comedones are *blackheads*. The follicle opening of a closed comedo is nearly covered over by skin so that it looks like a pinhead-sized, ivory-coloured papule.

Erythema is redness caused by vascular dilatation.

Telangiectasia is the visible dilatation of small cutaneous blood vessels.

Poikiloderma is a combination of atrophy, reticulate hyperpigmentation and telangiectasia.

Horn is a keratin projection that is taller than it is broad.

Erthyroderma is a generalized redness involving 90% or more of the skin, which may be scaling (exfoliative erythroderma) or smooth.

Secondary lesions

These evolve from primary lesions.

A *scale* is a flake arising from the horny layer. Scales may be seen on the surface of many primary lesions (e.g. macules, patches, nodules, plaques).

A *keratosis* is a horn-like thickening of the stratum corneum.

A *crust* may look like a scale, but is composed of dried blood or tissue fluid.

An *ulcer* is an area of skin from which the whole of the epidermis and at least the upper part of the dermis has been lost. Ulcers may extend into subcutaneous fat, and heal with scarring.

An *erosion* is an area of skin denuded by a complete or partial loss of only the epidermis. Erosions heal without scarring.

An *excoriation* is an ulcer or erosion produced by scratching.

A *fissure* is a slit in the skin.

A *sinus* is a cavity or channel that permits the escape of pus or fluid.

A *scar* is a result of healing, where normal structures are permanently replaced by fibrous tissue.

Atrophy is a thinning of skin caused by diminution of the epidermis, dermis or subcutaneous fat. When the epidermis is atrophic it may crinkle like cigarette paper, appear thin and translucent, and lose normal surface markings. Blood vessels may be easy to see in both epidermal and dermal atrophy.

Lichenification is an area of thickened skin with increased markings.

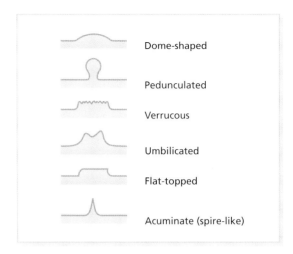

Figure 3.3 Surface contours of papules.

A *stria* (stretch mark) is a streak-like linear atrophic pink, purple or white lesion of the skin caused by changes in the connective tissue.

Pigmentation, either more (hyper) or less (hypo) than surrounding skin, can develop after lesions heal.

Having identified the lesions as primary or secondary, adjectives can be used to describe them in terms of their other features.

• Colour (e.g. salmon-pink, lilac, violet).
• Sharpness of edge (e.g. well-defined, ill-defined).
• Surface contour (e.g. dome-shaped, umbilicated, spire-like; Figure 3.3).
• Geometric shape (e.g. nummular, oval, irregular, like the coast of Maine).
• Texture (e.g. rough, silky, smooth, hard).
• Smell (e.g. foul-smelling).
• Temperature (e.g. hot, warm).

Dermatologists also use a few special adjectives which warrant definition.

• *Nummular* means round or coin-like.
• *Annular* means ring-like.
• *Circinate* means circular.
• *Arcuate* means curved.
• *Discoid* means disc-like.
• *Gyrate* means wave-like.
• *Retiform* and *reticulate* mean net-like.
• *Targetoid* means target-like or 'bull's eye'.
• *Polycyclic* means formed from coalescing circles, or incomplete rings.

To describe a skin lesion, use the term for the primary lesion as the noun, and the adjectives mentioned above to

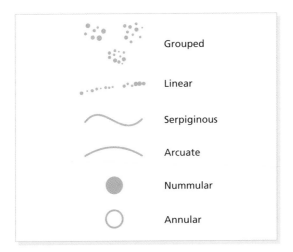

Figure 3.4 Configuration of lesions.

define it. For example, the lesions of psoriasis may appear as 'salmon-pink sharply demarcated nummular plaques covered by large silver polygonal scales'. This principle is illustrated in Figure 3.2. Try not to use the term 'erythema' as it means a shade of red and therefore is less specific than for example 'fire engine red'.

Try also not to use the terms 'lesion' or 'area'. Why say 'papular lesion' when you can say papule? It is almost as bad as the ubiquitous term 'skin rash'. By the way, there are very few diseases that are truly 'maculopapular'. The term is best avoided except to describe some drug eruptions and viral exanthems. Even then, the terms 'scarlatiniform' (like scarlet fever – punctate, slightly elevated papules) or 'morbilliform' (like measles – a net-like, blotchy, slightly elevated, pink exanthem) are more helpful.

Configuration

After unravelling the primary and secondary lesions, look for arrangements and configurations that can be, for example, discrete, confluent, grouped, annular, arcuate, segmental or dermatomal (Figure 3.4). Note that while individual lesions may be annular, several individual lesions may arrange themselves into an annular or polycyclic configurations. Other adjectives discussed under the morphology of individual lesions can apply to their groupings too. The Köbner or isomorphic phenomenon is the induction of skin lesions by, and at the site of, trauma such as scratch marks or operative incisions.

Special tools and techniques

A *magnifying lens* is a helpful aid to diagnosis because subtle changes in the skin become more apparent when enlarged. One attached to spectacles will leave your hand free.

A *Wood's light*, emitting long wavelength ultraviolet radiation, will help with the examination of some skin conditions. Fluorescence is seen in some fungal infections (see Chapter 16), erythrasma (p. 214) and pseudomonas infections. Some subtle disorders of pigmentation can be seen more clearly under Wood's light, (e.g. the pale patches of tuberous sclerosis, low-grade vitiligo and pityriasis versicolor, and the darker café au lait patches of neurofibromatosis). The urine in Porphyria cutanea tarda (p. 317) often fluoresces coral pink, even without solvent extraction of the porphyrins (see Figure 21.10).

Diascopy is the name given to the technique in which a glass slide or clear plastic spoon is pressed on vascular lesions to blanch them and verify that their redness is caused by vasodilatation and to unmask their underlying colour. Diascopy is also used to confirm the presence of extravasated blood in the dermis (i.e. petechia and purpura, the appearance of which do not change on pressure). This technique may also be helpful in the diagnosis of granulomatous conditions (e.g. sarcoid; p. 313) where pressure reveals a colour reminiscent of apple jelly.

Dermatoscopy (also known as dermoscopy, epiluminescence microscopy, skin surface microscopy) is a non-invasive technique, now commonplace in the clinic or office setting. It has many potential uses: not least as an aide in the diagnosis of pigmented lesions (benign and malignant); the visualization of scabies mites in their burrows; and in deciding if alopecia is scarring or non-scarring. Dermatoscopy is covered in depth in Chapter 28. Figure 3.5 demonstrates the dermatoscopic appearance of a malignant melanoma.

Photography, mostly digital nowadays, helps to record the baseline appearance of a lesion or rash, so that change can be assessed objectively at later visits. Small changes in pigmented lesions can be detected by analysing sequential digital images stored in computerized systems.

Assessment

Next, try to put the disease into a general class; the titles of the chapters in this book are representative. Once classified, a differential diagnosis is usually forthcoming. Each

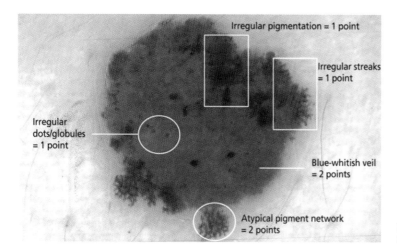

Irregular pigmentation = 1 point

Irregular streaks = 1 point

Irregular dots/globules = 1 point

Blue-whitish veil = 2 points

Atypical pigment network = 2 points

Figure 3.5 Dermatoscopic appearance of a malignant melanoma.

diagnosis can then be considered on its merits, and laboratory tests may be used to confirm or refute diagnoses in the differential list. At this stage you must make a working diagnosis or formulate a plan to do so!

Learning points

1 As Osler said: 'See and then reason and compare and control, but see first.'
2 A correct diagnosis is the key to correct treatment.
3 The term 'skin rash' is as bad as 'gastric stomach'.
4 Avoid using too many long Latin descriptive names as a cloak for ignorance.
5 The history is especially important when the diagnosis is difficult.
6 Undress the patients and use a lens, even if it only gives you more time to think.
7 A modern dermatologist without a dermatoscope is like a cardiologist without a stethoscope.
8 Remember the old adage that if you do not look in the mouth you will put your foot in it.

Side-room and office tests

A number of tests are commonly carried out in the practice office.

Potassium hydroxide preparations for fungal infections

If a fungal infection is suspected, scales or plucked hairs can be dissolved in an aqueous solution of 20% potassium hydroxide (KOH) containing 40% dimethyl sulfoxide (DMSO). The scale from the edge of a scaling lesion is

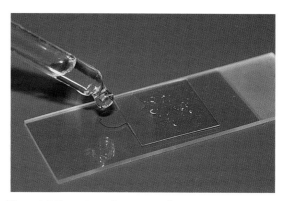

Figure 3.6 Preparing a skin scraping for microscopy by adding potassium hydroxide (KOH) from a pipette.

vigorously scraped on to a glass slide with a No. 15 scalpel blade or the edge of a second glass slide. Other samples can include nail clippings, the roofs of blisters, hair pluckings and the contents of pustules when a candidal infection is suspected. A drop or two of the KOH solution is run under the coverslip (Figure 3.6). After 5–10 minutes the mount is examined under a microscope with the condenser lens lowered to increase contrast. Nail clippings take longer to clear – up to a couple of hours. With experience, fungal and candidal hyphae can be readily detected (Figure 3.7). No heat is required if DMSO is included in the KOH solution.

Bacterial swabs

If a wound or rash is smelly, weeping, crusting or has a yellow (*Staphylococcus aureus*) or green (*Pseudomonas*) discoloration it may be worth while taking swabs for

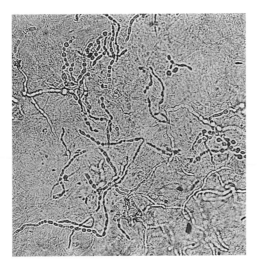

Figure 3.7 Fungal hyphae in a KOH preparation. The polygonal shadows in the background are horny layer cells.

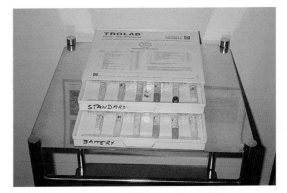

Figure 3.8 Patch testing equipment. Syringes contain commercially prepared antigens, to be applied in aluminium cups.

bacterial culture and sensitivity. These may identify a pathogenic organism, which should respond to appropriate antibiotic therapy. Often an antibiotic is given empirically on clinical suspicion, but if the condition is slow to respond swabs taken before the start of treatment will confirm the pathogen and its antibiotic sensitivity. There is a growing consensus that the empirical prescription of antibiotics for colonizing non-pathogenic bacteria may be fuelling bacterial resistance, so antibiotics should only be given for clinically significant infection.

Detection of a scabies mite

Burrows in an itchy patient are diagnostic of scabies. Retrieving a mite from the skin will confirm the diagnosis and convince a sceptical patient of the infestation. The burrow should be examined under a magnifying glass or dermatoscope; the acarus is seen as a tiny black or gray dot at the most recent, least scaly end (see Figure 17.5). It can be removed by a sterile needle and placed on a slide within a marked circle. Alternatively, if mites are not seen, possible burrows can be vigorously scraped with a No. 15 scalpel blade, moistened with liquid paraffin or vegetable oil, and the scrapings transferred to a slide. Patients never argue the toss when confronted by a magnified mobile mite.

Cytology (Tzanck smear)

Cytology can aid the diagnosis of viral infections such as herpes simplex and zoster, and of bullous diseases such as

pemphigus. A blister roof is removed and the cells from the base of the blister are scraped off with a No. 10 or 15 surgical blade. These cells are smeared on to a microscope slide, air-dried and fixed with methanol. They are then stained with Giemsa, toluidine blue or Wright's stain. Acantholytic cells (see Chapter 9) are seen in pemphigus and multinucleate giant cells are diagnostic of herpes simplex or varicella zoster infections (see Chapter 16). Practice is needed to get good preparations. The technique has fallen out of favour as histology, virological culture, polymerase chain reaction (PCR) and electron microscopy have become more accessible.

Patch tests

Patch tests are invaluable in detecting the allergens responsible for allergic contact dermatitis (see Chapter 7). A patch test involves applying a chemical to the skin and then watching for dermatitis to develop 48–96 hours later.

Either suspected individual antigens, or a battery of antigens that are common culprits, can be tested. Standard dilutions of the common antigens in appropriate bases are available commercially (Figure 3.8). The test materials are applied to the back under aluminium discs or patches; the occlusion encourages penetration of the allergen. The patches are left in place for 48 hours and then, after careful marking, are removed. The sites are inspected 10 minutes later, again 2 days later, and sometimes even later if doubtful reactions require further assessment. The test detects type IV delayed hypersensitivity reactions (see Chapter 2). The readings are scored according to the reaction seen:
NT Not tested.
−No reaction.
±Doubtful reaction (minimal erythema).

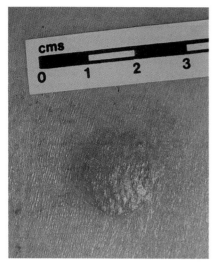

Figure 3.9 A strong positive reaction to a rubber additive.

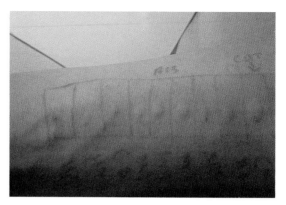

Figure 3.10 Prick testing: many positive results in an atopic individual.

+Weak positive reaction (erythema and maybe papules).

++ Strong reaction (palpable erythema and/or vesicles; Figure 3.9).

+++ Extreme reaction (intense palpable erythema, coalescing vesicles and/or bullae).

IR Irritant reaction (variable, but often sharply circumscribed, with a glazed appearance and increased skin markings).

A positive patch test does not prove that the allergen in question has caused the current episode of contact dermatitis; the results must be interpreted in the light of the history and possible previous exposure to the allergen.

Patch testing requires attention to detail in applying the patches properly and skill and experience in interpreting the results. The concentration of allergen must be sufficient to penetrate the thick skin of the back and yet not so high as to create a false positive irritation reaction.

Prick testing

Prick testing is much less helpful in dermatology. It detects immediate (type I) hypersensitivity (see Chapter 2) and patients should not have taken systemic antihistamines for at least 48 hours before the test. Commercially prepared diluted antigens and a control are placed as single drops on marked areas of the forearm. The skin is gently pricked through the drops using separate sterile fine (e.g. size 25 gauge, or smaller) needles. The prick should not cause bleeding. The drops are then removed with a tissue wipe. After 10 minutes the sites are inspected and the diameter of any wheal measured and recorded. A result

is considered positive if the test antigen causes a wheal of 4 mm or greater (Figure 3.10) and the control elicits a negligible reaction. Like patch testing, prick testing should not be undertaken by those without formal training in the procedure. Although the risk of anaphylaxis is small, resuscitation facilities including epinephrine and oxygen (p. 354) must be available. The relevance of positive results to the cause of the condition under investigation – usually urticaria or atopic dermatitis – is often debatable. Positive results should correlate with specific immunoglobulin E (IgE) levels to inhaled or ingested allergens, meaured either by a radio-allergosorbent test (RAST; p. 80) or its more specific modern replacement, the fluorescence enzyme labelled test (ImmunoCAP). These tests, carried out on patient's blood, although more expensive, pose no risk of anaphylaxis and take up less of the patient's time in the clinic. They are now used more often than prick tests. If total IgE levels are very high (often in atopic individuals), interpretation of the relevance of specific IgE levels to a particular allergen may be difficult.

Skin biopsy

Biopsy (from the Greek *bios* meaning 'life' and *opsis* 'sight') of skin lesions is useful to establish or confirm a clinical diagnosis. A piece of tissue is removed surgically for histological examination and, sometimes, for other tests (e.g. culture for organisms). When used selectively, a skin biopsy can solve the most perplexing problem but, conversely, will be unhelpful in conditions without a specific histology (e.g. most drug eruptions, pityriasis rosea, reactive erythemas).

Skin biopsies may be *incisional*, when just part of a lesion is removed for laboratory examination, or *excisional*, when the whole lesion is cut out. Excisional

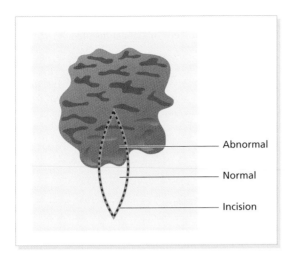

Abnormal

Normal

Incision

Figure 3.11 Incision biopsy. This should include adjacent normal skin.

biopsy is preferable for most small lesions (up to 0.5 cm diameter) but incisional biopsy is chosen when the partial removal of a larger lesion is adequate for diagnosis, and complete removal might leave an unnecessary and unsightly scar. Ideally, an incisional biopsy should include a piece of the surrounding normal skin (Figure 3.11), although this may not be possible if a small punch is used.

The main steps in skin biopsy:

1 Obtain written and informed consent from the patient before starting the procedure;

2 Administration of local anaesthesia; and

3 Removal of all (excision) or part (incision) of the lesion and repair of the defect made by a scalpel or punch.

Local anaesthetic

Lidocaine 1–2% is used. Sometimes, epinephrine 1 : 200 000 is added. This causes vasoconstriction, reduced clearance of the local anaesthetic and prolongation of the local anaesthetic effect. Plain lidocaine should be used on the fingers, toes and the penis as the prolonged vasoconstriction produced by epinephrine can be dangerous here. Epinephrine is also best avoided in diabetics with small vessel disease, in those with a history of heart disease (including dysrhythmias), in patients taking non-selective α-blockers and tricyclic antidepressants (because of potential interactions) and in uncontrolled hyperthyroidism. There are exceptions to these general rules and, undoubtedly, the total dose of local anaesthetic and/or epinephrine is important. Nevertheless, the rules should not be broken unless the

surgeon is quite sure that the procedure that he or she is about to embark on is safe.

It is wise to avoid local anaesthesia during early pregnancy and to delay non-urgent procedures until after the first trimester.

As B follows A in the alphabet, get into the habit of checking the precise concentration of the lidocaine ± added epinephrine on the label *before* withdrawing it into the syringe and then, *before* injecting it, confirm that the patient has not had any previous allergic reactions to local anaesthetic.

Infiltration of the local anaesthetic into the skin under and around the area to be biopsied is the most widely used method. If the local anaesthetic is injected into the subcutaneous fat, it will be relatively pain-free, will produce a diffuse swelling of the skin and will take several minutes to induce anaesthesia. Intradermal injections are painful and produce a discrete wheal associated with rapid anaesthesia. The application of EMLA cream (eutectic mixture of local anaesthesia) to the operation site 2 hours before giving a local anaesthetic to children helps to numb the initial prick.

Scalpel biopsy

This provides more tissue than a punch biopsy. It can be used routinely, but is especially useful for biopsying disorders of the subcutaneous fat, for obtaining specimens with both normal and abnormal skin for comparison (Fig. 3.11) and for removing small lesions in toto (excision biopsy; p. 368). After selecting the lesion for biopsy, an elliptical piece of skin is excised. The specimen should include the subcutaneous fat. Removing the specimen with forceps may cause crush artefact, which can be avoided by lifting the specimen with either a Gillies hook or a syringe needle. The wound is then sutured; firm compression for 5 minutes stops oozing. Non-absorbable 3/0 sutures are used for biopsies on the legs and back, 5/0 for the face and 4/0 for elsewhere. Stitches are usually removed from the face in 4–7 days, from the anterior trunk and arms in 7–10 days and from the back and legs in 10–14 days.

Some guidelines for skin biopsies are listed in Table 3.3.

Punch biopsy

The skin is sampled with a small (3–4 mm diameter) tissue punch. Lidocaine 1% is injected intradermally first, and a cylinder of skin is incised with the punch by rotating it back and forth (Figure 3.12). Skin is lifted up carefully with a needle or forceps and the base is cut off at the level of subcutaneous fat. The defect is cauterized or repaired

Table 3.3 Guidelines for skin biopsies.

Sample a fresh lesion.
Obtain your specimen from near the edge of the lesion.
Avoid sites where a scar would be conspicuous.
Avoid the upper trunk or jaw line where keloids are most
    likely to form.
Avoid the legs, where healing is slow.
Avoid lesions over bony prominences, where infection is
    more likely.
Use the scalpel technique for scalp disorders and diseases
    of the subcutaneous fat or vessels.
Do not crush the tissue.
Place in appropriate fixative,* usually 10% formalin for
    routine histology.
If two lesions are sampled, be sure they do not get mixed
    up or mislabelled. Label specimen containers before the
    biopsy is placed in them.
Make sure that the patient's name, age and sex are clearly
    indicated on the pathology form.
Provide the pathologist with a legible summary of the
    history (including laboratory numbers of previous
    relevant biopsies), the site of the biopsy and a
    differential diagnosis.
Discuss the results with the pathologist.

*Specimens for immunofluorescence should be
immediately frozen or placed in special transport
medium. Transport of specimens for microbiology
should be discussed with the laboratory.
Preservative-free lidocaine may be indicated to keep
the local anaesthesia from killing organisms during the
process of biopsy.

with a single suture. The biopsy specimen must not be
crushed with the forceps or critical histological patterns
may be distorted.

The tissue can be sent to the pathologist with a summary of the history, a differential diagnosis and the
patient's age. Close liaison with the pathologist is essential, because the diagnosis may only become apparent
with knowledge of both the clinical and histological
features.

Laboratory tests

The laboratory is vital for the accurate diagnosis of
many skin disorders. Tests include various assays of
blood, serum and urine, bacterial, fungal, and viral culture from skin and other specimens, immunofluorescent
and immunohistologic examinations (Figures 3.13 and
3.14), radiography, ultrasonography and other methods
of image intensification. Specific details are discussed as
each disease is presented.

Conclusions

Clinical dermatology is a visual specialty. You must see
the disease, and understand what you are seeing. Look
closely and thoroughly. Take time. Examine the whole
body. Locate primary lesions and check configuration and
distribution. Ask appropriate questions, especially if the
diagnosis is difficult. Classify the disorder and list the differential diagnoses. Use the history, examination and laboratory tests to make a diagnosis if this cannot be made

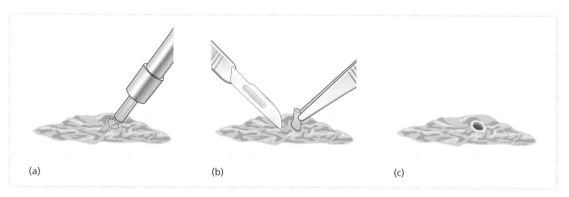

(a)   (b)   (c)

Figure 3.12 Steps in taking a punch biopsy.

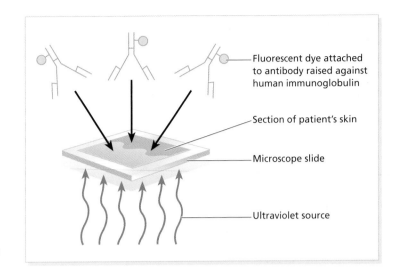

Figure 3.13 Direct immunofluorescence detects antibodies in a patient's skin. Here immunoglobulin G (IgG) antibodies are detected by staining with a fluorescent dye attached to antihuman IgG.

by clinical features alone. Then treat. Refer the patient to a dermatologist if:

- You cannot make a diagnosis;
- The disorder does not respond to treatment;
- The disorder is unusual or severe; or
- You are just not sure.

Learning points

1 A biopsy is the refuge of a bankrupt mind when dealing with conditions that do not have a specific histology. Here, a return to the history and examination is more likely to reveal diagnostic clues than a pathologist.

2 If you do not remember the three essential checks before injecting local anaesthetic then read p. 41 again.

Further reading

Cox NH, Lawrence CM. (1998) *Diagnostic Problems in Dermatology*. Mosby Wolfe, Edinburgh.

General Medical Council Publications (2006) Supplementary report, Maintaining Boundaries. http://www.gmc-uk.org/guidance/good_medical_practice.asp (accessed 11 July 2014).

Graham-Brown R, Bourke J. (2006) *Mosby's Color Atlas and Text of Dermatology*, 2nd edn. Mosby, London.

Lawrence CM, Cox NM. (2001) *Physical Signs in Dermatology*, 2nd edn. Mosby, Edinburgh.

Mutasim DF, Adams BB. (2001) Immuno-fluorescence in dermatology. *Journal of the American Academy of Dermatology* **45**, 803–822.

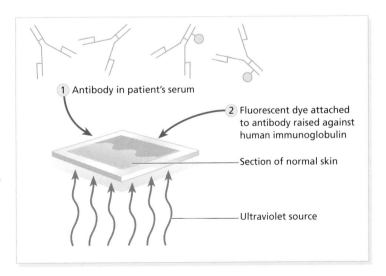

Figure 3.14 Indirect immunofluorescence detects antibodies in a patient's serum. There are two steps. (1) Antibodies in this serum are made to bind to antigens in a section of normal skin. (2) Antibody raised against human immunoglobulin, conjugated with a fluorescent dye can then be used to stain these bound antibodies (as in the direct immunofluorescence test).

Savin JA, Hunter JAA, Hepburn NC. (1997) *Skin Signs in Clinical Medicine: Diagnosis in Colour.* Mosby Wolfe, London.

Shelley WB, Shelley ED. (1992) *Advanced Dermatologic Diagnosis.* W.B. Saunders, Philadelphia, PA.

Shelley WB, Shelley ED. (2006) *Consultations in Dermatology. Studies of Orphan and Unique Patients.* Cambridge University Press, New York.

Stolz W, *et al.* (2011) *Color Atlas of Dermatoscopy*, 3rd edn. Blackwell Science, Oxford.

Walsh A, Walsh S. (2011) Local anaesthesia and the dermatologist. *Clinical and Experimental Dermatology* **36**, 337–343.

4 Disorders of Keratinization

The complex but orderly processes of keratinization, and of cell cohesion and proliferation within the epidermis, have been described in Chapter 2. As they proceed, the living keratinocytes of the deeper epidermis change into the dead corneocytes of the horny layer, where they are stuck together by intercellular lipids. They are then shed in such a way that the surface of the normal skin does not seem scaly to the naked eye. Shedding balances production, so that the thickness of the horny layer does not alter. However, if keratinization or cell cohesion is abnormal, the horny layer may become thick or the skin surface may become dry and scaly; this impairs barrier function, which if severe can lead to excessive water loss, dehydration and, in extreme cases, death. Such changes can be localized or generalized.

In this chapter we describe a variety of skin disorders that have as their basis a disorder of keratinization. The term Mendelian disorders of cornification (MEDOC) has recently been used to classify these conditions. During the last few years the molecular mechanisms underlying many of these have become clearer, including abnormal genetic coding for keratins, the enzymes involved in cell cohesion in the horny layer and the molecules that are critical in the signalling pathway governing cell cohesion in the spinous layer.

The ichthyoses

The word *ichthyosis* comes from the Greek word for a fish. It is applied to disorders that share, as their main feature, a dry rough skin with marked scaling but no inflammation. Strictly speaking, the scales lack the regular overlapping pattern of fish scales, but the term is usefully descriptive and too well entrenched to be discarded. Much information on icthyoses is coming to light from national patient registers, both in the United Kingdom and the United States. In 2009, experts in the field of ichthyosis met to agree on an international consensus classification (see *Further reading*). This supersedes older nomenclature and as such has been adopted in this chapter.

The genetics underlying the ichthyoses is complex; to date there are 36 forms of inherited ichthyosis, including conditions primarily affecting the skin, and rarer 'syndromic' associations involving other organs. Over 25 genes have now been implicated, with multiple mutations on each gene. Recent research has focused on the molecular pathways by which the genetic defects produce the ichthyosiform phenotype. This chapter reviews the more commonly encountered ichthyoses and provides suggestions for further reading on the rarer forms.

Common ichthyoses

Ichthyosis vulgaris

Cause
Inherited as an autosomal semidominant disorder, this condition is common, affecting about 1 in 250 people in the United Kingdom. Mutations in the filaggrin gene lead to a loss or reduction of profilaggrin, the major component of the keratohyalin granule. Profilaggrin is cleaved to filaggrin, which in turn is responsible for aggregating keratin filaments in the cornified cell envelope. The breakdown of filaggrin results in the formation of filaggrin degradation products, which reduce transepidermal water loss. The reduction in keratohyalin granules gives icthyosis vulgaris its characteristic histology; a paucity or absence of the granular layer of the epidermis. Mutant alleles of the filaggrin gene have a frequency of 4% in European populations, which accounts for it being such a common disorder. Heterozygotes have milder disease than compound heterozygotes and homozygotes.

Presentation
The dryness is usually mild and symptoms are few. The scales are small and branny, being most obvious on the

Clinical Dermatology, Fifth Edition. Richard B. Weller, Hamish J.A. Hunter and Margaret W. Mann.
© 2015 John Wiley & Sons, Ltd. Published 2015 by John Wiley & Sons, Ltd.

limbs and least obvious in the major flexures. The skin creases of the palm may be accentuated. Keratosis pilaris (p. 48) is often present on the limbs.

Clinical course

The skin changes are not usually present at birth but develop over the first few years of life. Some patients improve in adult life, particularly during warm weather, but the condition seldom clears completely.

Complications

The already dry skin chaps in winter and is easily irritated by degreasing agents. This should be taken into account in the choice of a career. Ichthyosis of this type is apt to appear in a stubborn combination with atopic eczema, as mutations in the filaggrin gene are strong predisposing factors for atopic eczema (p. 88).

Differential diagnosis

It can usually be distinguished from less common types of ichthyosis on the basis of the pattern of inheritance and the type and distribution of the scaling. Mild variants may be difficult to differentiate from the xerosis of atopic eczema, which is not surprising given their common genetic basis.

Investigations

None are usually needed.

Treatment

This is palliative. The dryness can be helped by the regular use of emollients, which are best applied after a shower or bath. Emulsifying ointment, soft white paraffin, E45 and Unguentum Merck are all quite suitable (Formulary 1, p. 397) and the selection depends on the patient's preference. Many find proprietary bath oils and creams containing humectants such as glycerin, urea or lactic acid helpful (Formulary 1, p. 397).

Recessive X-linked ichthyosis

Cause

This less common type of ichthyosis is inherited as an X-linked recessive trait and therefore, in its complete form, is seen only in males, although some female carriers show mild scaling. The condition affects about 1 in 6000 males in the United Kingdom and is associated with a deficiency of the enzyme steroid sulfatase, which hydrolyses cholesterol sulfate. The responsible gene has been localized to the end of the short arm of the X chromosome, at Xp 22.3 (see Chapter 24).

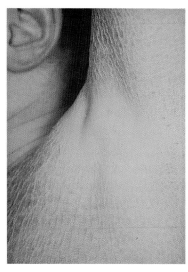

Figure 4.1 Ichthyosis: large rather dark scales suggest recessive X-linked ichthyosis.

Presentation and course

In contrast to the delayed onset of the dominantly inherited ichthyosis vulgaris, scaling appears early, often soon after birth, and always by the first birthday. The scales are larger and browner (Figure 4.1), involve the neck, and to a lesser extent the popliteal and antecubital areas, as well as the skin generally. The palms and soles are normal. There is no association with atopy or keratosis pilaris. The condition persists throughout life.

Complications

Affected babies may be born after a prolonged labour. Corneal opacities may appear in adult life. Kallmann's syndrome (hypogonadotrophic hypogonadism and anosmia) is caused by the deletion of a part of the X chromosome that includes the gene for X-linked recessive ichthyosis, which is therefore one of its features. Neurological defects may also occur in this contiguous gene disorder.

Differential diagnosis

This is as for ichthyosis vulgaris. It is helpful to remember that only males are affected. Bear Kallmann's syndrome in mind if there are other congenital abnormalities.

Investigations

None are usually needed. Steroid sulfatase gene deletions can be identified by fluorescence *in situ* hybridization (FISH; see Chapter 24). Electron microscopy shows retained corneodesmosomes within the stratum corneum (see Chapter 2).

Treatment

Oral aromatic retinoids are probably best avoided. Topical measures are as for ichthyosis vulgaris.

Autosomal recessive congenital ichthyoses

There are three major types of autosomal recessive congenital ichthyosis: lamellar ichthyosis, congenital ichthyosiform erythroderma and harlequin ichthyosis. The term 'collodion baby', often associated with these conditions, is a description and not a diagnosis. The bizarre skin changes are seen at birth. At first the stratum corneum is smooth and shiny, and the skin looks as though it has been covered with cellophane or collodion. Its tightness may cause ectropion and feeding difficulties. The shiny outer surface is shed within a few days leaving behind red scaly skin. This is most often a result of congenital ichthyosiform erythroderma, less commonly lamellar ichthyosis, and is very severe in harlequin ichthyosis. Collodion babies may have problems with temperature regulation and high water loss through the skin in the early days of life, best dealt with by the use of a high humidity incubator. Regular application of a greasy emollient also limits fluid loss and makes the skin supple.

Lamellar ichthyosis and congenital ichthyosiform erythroderma

These rare conditions have often been confused in the past, because they look so similar and probably form a spectrum of disease. Both may be inherited as an autosomal recessive trait, and in both the skin changes at birth are those of a collodion baby. Later, the two conditions can be distinguished by the finer scaling and more obvious redness of congenital ichthyosiform erythroderma and the plate-like scales of lamellar ichthyosis. Both last for life and are sufficiently disfiguring for the long-term use of acitretin to be justifiable (Formulary 2, p. 421). Mutations in the transglutaminase-1 gene on chromosome 14q11.2 were the first to be implicated; since then a further five genes have been identified and recent studies suggest that more are yet to be discovered. Transglutaminase-1 is the major cross-linking enzyme in the stratum corneum. Lamellar ichthyosis shows genetic heterogeneity (see Chapter 24); the most severe type is caused by mutations in this gene.

Acral peeling skin syndrome is a milder disorder resulting from mutations in the transglutaminase-5 gene. Here, persistent sunburn-like peeling is limited to the hands and feet. Other minor variants include bathing suit ichthyosis (lamellar ichthyosis confined to axillae, trunk, and scalp) and self-healing collodion baby, which, as its name suggests, almost completely resolves by 3 months of age.

Harlequin fetus

This much rarer condition results from null mutations in the *ABCA12* gene on chromosome 2q35 (a member of the ABC transporter superfamily). It normally has a role in forming the skin lipid barrier. Affected babies are often preterm and covered with an armour-like collodion membrane, which when shed reveals thick fissured hyperkeratosis. Ectropion and eclabium (outward turning of the lips) are extreme and most affected infants die, although early intervention with oral retinoids has improved mortality rates. Needless to say, these babies are best cared for on a neonatal intensive care unit by a multidisciplinary team, including an experienced paediatric dermatologist. Infants that do survive develop a very severe hyperkeratotic erythroderma. Missense mutations in the *ABCA12* gene may have milder repercussions, resulting in lamellar ichthyosis.

Keratinopathic ichthyoses

These conditions have been grouped together under this heading as they all result from mutations in keratin genes.

Epidermolytic ichthyosis (previously called bullous ichthyosiform erythroderma)

This rare condition is inherited as an autosomal dominant disorder. Shortly after birth the baby's skin becomes generally red and shows numerous blisters. The redness fades over a few months, and the tendency to blister also lessens, but during childhood a gross brownish warty hyperkeratosis appears, sometimes in a roughly linear or annular form and usually worst in the flexures. The diseased skin often becomes secondarily infected and painful, and develops a foul odour. For many patients this is as socially disabling as the skin disease. The histology is distinctive: a thickened granular cell layer contains large granules, and clefts may be seen in the upper epidermis. The condition is caused by mutations in the genes (on chromosomes

12q13 and 17q21) controlling the production of keratins 1 and 10. A few patients with localized areas of hyperkeratosis with the same histological features have gonadal mosaicism, and so their children are at risk of developing the generalized form of the disorder.

Treatment is symptomatic. Antibacterial washes and masking fragrances are helpful. Antibiotics may be needed from time to time but should not be used for prolonged periods. Acitretin (Formulary 2, p. 421) has helped in severe cases. Superficial epidermolytic ichthyosis is a milder autosomal dominant keratinopathic ichthyosis resulting from defects in the keratin 2 gene.

Other ichthyosiform disorders

Sometimes, ichthyotic skin changes are a minor part of a multisystem disease, but such associations are very rare. *Refsum's syndrome*, an autosomal recessive trait, is caused by deficiency of a single enzyme concerned in the breakdown of phytanic acid, which then accumulates in the tissues. The other features (retinal degeneration, peripheral neuropathy and ataxia) overshadow the minor dryness of the skin.

Rud's syndrome is an ichthyosiform erythroderma in association with mental retardation and epilepsy. In *Netherton's syndrome*, brittle hairs, with a so-called bamboo deformity, are present as well as a curious gyrate and erythematous hyperkeratotic eruption (ichthyosis linearis circumflexa). Other conditions are identified by confusing acronyms: MEDNIK syndrome stands for Mental retardation, Enteropathy, Deafness Neuropathy, Ichthyosis and Keratoderma; the KID syndrome consists of Keratitis, Ichthyosis and Deafness.

Acquired ichthyosis

It is unusual for ichthyosis to appear for the first time in adult life but, if it does, an underlying disease should be suspected. The most frequent is Hodgkin's disease. Other recorded causes include other lymphomas, leprosy, sarcoidosis, malabsorption or a poor diet. The skin may also appear dry in hypothyroidism.

Other disorders of keratinization

Keratosis pilaris

Cause

This common condition affecting up to 50% of the adolescent population is inherited as an autosomal dominant trait; it is possibly caused by mutations in a gene lying on the short arm of chromosome 18. Heterozygote carriers of an abnormal profilaggrin gene often have keratosis pilaris. The abnormality lies in the keratinization of hair follicles, which become filled with horny plugs.

Presentation and course

The changes begin in childhood and tend to become less obvious in adult life. In the most common type, the greyish horny follicular plugs, sometimes with red areolae, are confined to the outer aspects of the thighs and upper arms, where the skin feels rough. Less often the plugs affect the sides of the face; perifollicular erythema and loss of eyebrow hairs may then occur. There is an association with ichthyosis vulgaris.

Complications

Involvement of the cheeks may lead to an ugly pitted scarring. Rarely, the follicles in the eyebrows may be damaged with subsequent loss of hair.

Differential diagnosis

A rather similar pattern of widespread follicular keratosis (phrynoderma) can occur in severe vitamin deficiency. The lack is probably not just of vitamin A, as was once thought, but of several vitamins.

Investigations

None are needed.

Treatment

Treatment is not usually needed, although keratolytics such as salicylic acid or urea in a cream base may smooth the skin temporarily (Formulary 1, p. 397). Ultraviolet radiation also provides temporary benefit. A move to a more humid climate is helpful.

Keratosis follicularis (Darier's disease)

Cause

This rare condition is inherited as an autosomal dominant trait. Fertility tends to be low and many cases represent new mutations. The abnormal gene, *ATP2A2* on chromosome 12q24.1 encodes for SERCA2, a calcium pump that keeps a high concentration of calcium in the endoplasmic reticulum.

Presentation

The first signs usually appear in the mid-teens, sometimes after overexposure to sunlight. The characteristic lesions

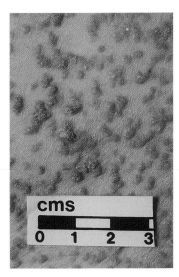

Figure 4.2 The typical yellow–brown greasy papules of Darier's disease.

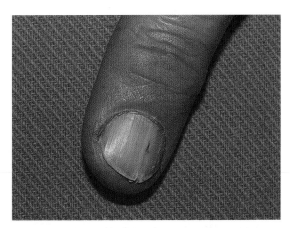

Figure 4.4 The nail in Darier's disease. One or more longitudinal pale or pink stripes run over the lunule to the free margin where they end in a triangular nick.

are small pink or brownish papules with a greasy scale (Figure 4.2). These coalesce into warty plaques in a seborrhoeic distribution (Figure 4.3). Early lesions are often seen on the sternal and interscapular areas, and behind the ears. The severity of the condition varies greatly from person to person: sometimes the skin is widely affected. The abnormalities remain for life, often causing much embarrassment and discomfort.

Other changes include lesions looking like plane warts on the backs of the hands, punctate keratoses or pits on the palms and soles, cobblestone-like irregularities of the mucous membranes in the mouth, and a distinctive nail

dystrophy. White or pinkish lines or ridges run longitudinally to the free edge of the nail where they end in triangular nicks (Figure 4.4).

Complications

Some patients are stunted. In some families, Darier's disease runs with bipolar mood disorder. Personality disorders, including antisocial behaviour, are seen more often than would be expected by chance. In one recent study, over half of patients with Darier's disease were diagnosed with a major psychiatric condition at some point in their life. An impairment of delayed hypersensitivity may be the basis for a tendency to develop widespread herpes simplex and bacterial infections. Bacterial overgrowth is responsible for the unpleasant smell of some severely affected patients.

Differential diagnosis

The distribution of the lesions may be similar to that of seborrhoeic eczema, but this lacks the warty papules of Darier's disease. The distribution differs from that of acanthosis nigricans (mainly flexural) and of keratosis pilaris (favours the outer upper arms and thighs). Other forms of folliculitis and Grover's disease can also cause confusion.

Investigations

The diagnosis should be confirmed by a skin biopsy, which will show characteristic clefts in the epidermis, and dyskeratotic cells.

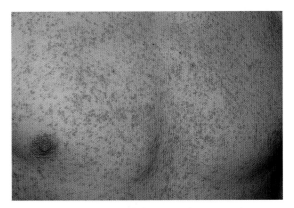

Figure 4.3 Extensive Darier's disease, in this case made worse by sun exposure.

Treatment

Severe and disabling disease can be dramatically alleviated by long-term acitretin (Formulary 2, p. 421). Ablative lasers have shown some promise in the treatment of more severe cases. Varied strengths of topical 5-fluorouracil may be beneficial. Milder cases need only topical keratolytics, such as salicylic acid, and the control of local infection (Formulary 1, p. 401).

Keratoderma of the palms and soles

Inherited types

Many genodermatoses share keratoderma of the palms and soles as their main feature; they are not described in detail here. The clinical patterns and modes of inheritance vary from family to family. Punctate, striate, diffuse and mutilating varieties have been documented, sometimes in association with metabolic disorders such as tyrosinaemia, or with changes elsewhere. The punctate type is caused by mutations in the keratin 16 gene on chromosome 17q12-q21; the epidermolytic type by mutations in the gene for keratin 9, found only on palms and soles.

The most common pattern is a diffuse one, known also as tylosis (Figure 4.5), which is inherited as an autosomal dominant trait linked to changes in chromosome region 12q11-q13, which harbours the type 11 keratin gene cluster. In a few families these changes have been associated with carcinoma of the oesophagus, but in most families this is not the case.

Treatment tends to be unsatisfactory, but keratolytics such as salicylic acid and urea can be used in higher concentrations on the palms and soles than elsewhere (Formulary 1, p. 401). Systemic retinoids may be helpful in some cases.

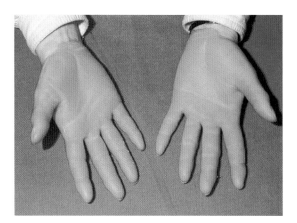

Figure 4.5 Tylosis.

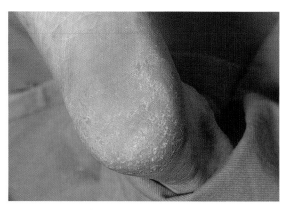

Figure 4.6 Keratoderma climactericum – thickly keratotic skin, especially around the heels. Painful fissures are a problem.

Acquired types

It is not uncommon for healthy people to have a few inconspicuous punctate keratoses on their palms, and it is no longer thought that these relate to internal malignancy, although palmar keratoses caused by arsenic may have this association. Black patients are prone to keratotic papules along their palmar creases.

Keratoderma of the palms and soles may be part of the picture of some generalized skin diseases such as pityriasis rubra pilaris (p. 72) and lichen planus (p. 69).

A distinctive pattern (keratoderma climactericum) is sometimes seen in overweight middle-aged women at about the time of the menopause. It is most marked around the borders of the heels where painful fissures form and interfere with walking (Figure 4.6). Regular paring and the use of keratolytic ointments are often more helpful than attempts at hormone replacement. Many improve with applications of 40% urea in cream or ointment bases. Acitretin in low doses may be worth a trial, especially when the disorder interferes with walking. The condition tends to settle over a few years.

Knuckle pads

Cause

Sometimes these are familial; usually they are not. Trauma seems not to be important.

Presentation

Fibromatous and hyperkeratotic areas appear on the backs of many finger joints, usually beginning in late childhood and persisting thereafter. There may be an association with Dupuytren's contracture.

Differential diagnosis

Occupational callosities (e.g. in carpet layers), granuloma annulare and viral warts should be considered.

Investigations

A biopsy may be helpful in the few cases of genuine clinical difficulty.

Treatment

None, including surgery, is satisfactory.

Callosities and corns

Both are responses to pressure. A *callosity* is a more diffuse type of thickening of the keratin layer, which seems to be a protective response to widely applied repeated friction or pressure. Callosities are often occupational (e.g. they are seen on the hands of manual workers). Usually painless, they need no therapy.

Corns have a central core of hard keratin, which can hurt if forced inwards. They appear where there is high local pressure, often between bony prominences and shoes. Favourite areas include the under surface of the toe joints, and the soles under prominent metatarsals. *Soft corns* arise in the third or fourth toe clefts when the toes are squeezed together by tight shoes; such corns are often macerated and may present as eroded nodules causing diagnostic confusion.

The main differential is from hyperkeratotic warts, but these will show tiny bleeding points when pared down, or pinpoint blood vessels when examined with a dermatoscope, whereas a corn has only its hard compacted avascular core surrounded by a more diffuse thickening of opalescent keratin.

The correct treatment for corns is to eliminate the pressure that caused them, but patients may be slow to accept this. While regular paring reduces the symptoms temporarily, well-fitting shoes are essential. Corns under the metatarsals can be helped by soft spongy soles or orthotic shoe inserts but sometimes orthopaedic surgery is required to alter weight distribution. Especial care is needed with corns on ischaemic or diabetic feet, which are at greater risk of infection and ulceration.

Learning points

- The ichthyosis nomenclature is constantly changing and is likely to further evolve with the discovery of more genotype–phenotype correlations. Simply spelling ichthyosis correctly will differentiate you from many.
- Keratosis pilaris is extremely common and often relatively resistant to therapy; a significant proportion of cases will improve with age.
- Acquired ichthyosis or palmoplantar keratoderma in adult life should prompt a thorough search for an underlying malignancy.

Further reading

Cooper SM, Burge SM. (2003) Darier's disease: epidemiology, pathophysiology and management. *American Journal of Clinical Dermatology* **4**, 97–105.

Dunnill MG. (1998) The molecular basis of inherited disorders of keratinization. *Hospital Medicine* **59**, 17–22.

Gordon-Smith K, Jones LA, Burge SM, Munro CS, Tavadia S, Craddock N. (2010) The neuropsychiatric phenotype in Darier disease. *British Journal of Dermatology* **163**, 515–522.

Hernandez-Martin A, Gonzalez-Sarmiento R, De Unamuno P. (1999) X-linked ichthyosis: an update. *British Journal of Dermatology* **141**, 617–627.

Hwang S, Schwartz RA. (2008) Keratosis pilaris: a common follicular hyperkeratosis. *Cutis* **82**, 177–180.

Patel S, Zirwas M, English JC. (2007) Acquired palmoplantar keratoderma. *American Journal of Clinical Dermatology* **8**, 1–11.

Ratnavel RC, Griffiths WAD. (1997) The inherited palmoplantar keratodermas. *British Journal of Dermatology* **137**, 485–490.

Rugg EL, Leigh IM. (2004) The keratins and their disorders. *American Journal of Medical Genetics Clinical Seminar of Medical Genetics* **131C**, 4–11.

Shwayder T. (2004) Disorders of keratinisation. *American Journal of Clinical Dermatology* **5**, 17–29.

Vinzenz O, Tadini G, Akiyama M, *et al.* (2010) Revised nomenclature and classification of inherited ichthyoses: results of the first ichthyosis consensus conference in Sorèze 2009. *Journal of the American Academy of Dermatology* **63**, 607–641.

5 Psoriasis

Psoriasis is an immunologically mediated chronic inflammatory skin disease, characterized by well-defined salmon-pink plaques bearing large adherent silvery centrally attached scales. One to three per cent of most populations have psoriasis, which is most prevalent in European and North American white people. It can start at any age but is rare under 10 years, and appears most often between 15 and 40 years. Its course is unpredictable but is usually chronic with exacerbations and remissions.

Cause and pathogenesis

Our understanding of the causes of psoriasis has greatly improved in the last 10 years and this has resulted in the development of a range of valuable new treatments, particularly for more severe disease. Psoriasis is also now seen as an inflammatory disease affecting more than just the skin. Psoriatic arthritis has long been recognized, but studies now show that moderate and severe psoriasis is also associated with an increased risk of cardiovascular disease.

There are two key abnormalities in a psoriatic plaque: hyperproliferation of keratinocytes; and an inflammatory cell infiltrate in which neutrophils, tumour necrosis factor and T lymphocytes predominate. Both of these abnormalities can induce the other, leading to a vicious cycle of keratinocyte proliferation and inflammatory reaction; but it is still not clear which is the primary defect. Perhaps the genetic abnormality leads first to keratinocyte hyperproliferation that, in turn, produces a defective skin barrier (p. 10) allowing the penetration by, or unmasking of, hidden antigens to which an immune response is mounted. Alternatively, the psoriatic plaque might reflect a genetically determined reaction to different types of trauma (e.g. physical wounds, environmental irritants and drugs) in which the healing response is exaggerated and uncontrolled.

Genetics

Psoriasis is undoubtedly a genetic condition, but does not follow a simple Mendelian pattern of inheritance. The mode of inheritance is genetically complex, implying a polygenic inheritance. A child with one affected parent has a 14% chance of developing the disease, and this rises to 41% if both parents are affected. Genomic imprinting (p. 343) may explain why psoriatic fathers are more likely to pass on the disease to their children than are psoriatic mothers. If non-psoriatic parents have a child with psoriasis, the risk for subsequent children is about 10%. The disorder is concordant in around 70% of monozygotic (identical) twins but in only 20% of dizygotic ones.

There are two peaks of onset of psoriasis. Type I has onset in the second and third decade and a more common family history of psoriasis. Type II has onset in late adulthood in patients without obvious family history. Early onset psoriasis shows a genetic linkage (p. 342) with a psoriasis susceptibility locus (PSOR-1) located on 6p21 within the major histocompatibility complex Class I (MHC-I) region. The HLA-Cw6 allele at this site, which affects immune function, particularly confers a risk of developing psoriasis; 10% of Cw6+ individuals will develop the disease. Corneodesmosin, a protein that is overexpressed in the differentiating outer epidermis of psoriatic skin, is also coded for by a gene here. So too is the coiled-coil alpha helical rod protein-1, which may be involved in regulation of keratinoctye proliferation. Variants of both of these genes are associated with type I psoriasis, but their close proximity to the Cw6 allele, and thus linkage disequilibrium, makes it difficult to conclusively show that they are independent risk factors. The hereditary element and the HLA associations are much weaker in late-onset psoriasis.

While PSORS-1 is the most important locus in psoriasis, accounting for up to 50% of genetic susceptibility to the disease, at least 11 other loci (PSORS-2 to 12) have been identified. Variants in the genes for interleukin

Clinical Dermatology, Fifth Edition. Richard B. Weller, Hamish J.A. Hunter and Margaret W. Mann.
© 2015 John Wiley & Sons, Ltd. Published 2015 by John Wiley & Sons, Ltd.

23 receptor and interleukin 12B are the most interesting of these with the recent development of effective biological treatments targeted at the p40 subunit common to both cytokines. At present perhaps it is best to consider psoriasis as a multifactorial disease with a complex genetic trait. An individual's predisposition to it is determined by a large number of genes, each of which has only a low penetrance. Clinical expression of the disease may result from environmental stimuli including antigen exposure. Different forms of psoriasis may well be caused by different underlying gene variants.

Epidermal cell kinetics

The epidermis of psoriasis makes itself too fast. Keratinocytes proliferate out of control, and an excessive number of germinative cells enter the cell cycle. This 'out of control' proliferation is rather like a car going too fast because the accelerator is stuck, which cannot be stopped by putting a foot on the brake. The growth fraction (p. 7) of epidermal basal cells is increased sevenfold compared with normal skin. This epidermal hyperproliferation accounts for many of the metabolic abnormalities associated with psoriasis. It is not confined to obvious plaques: similar but less marked changes occur in the apparently normal skin of psoriatic patients as well.

The exact mechanism underlying this increased epidermal proliferation is uncertain, but the skin behaves as though it were trying to repair a wound.

Angiogenesis

Endothelial cells, and thus blood vessels, proliferate in the superficial dermis in response to vascular endothelial growth factor (VEGF) which is overproduced in psoriatic epidermis.

Inflammation

Psoriasis differs from the ichthyoses (p. 45) in its accumulation of inflammatory cells. The importance of T lymphocytes is shown by their presence early in the development of psoriatic plaques and the response of the disease to treatments such as ciclosporin. When nonlesional psoriatic skin is grafted on to severe combined immunodeficient mice, plaques develop more readily following injection of autologous T cells from a psoriatic patient. Defective regulation of the innate immune system is also involved in the development of psoriasis. Psoriatic keratinocytes contain high levels of the antimicrobial peptides LL-37 (cathelicidin), β defensin and psoriasin (S100A7), which may account for the surprisingly low incidence of bacterial skin infection in psori-

atic patients. Cathelicidin forms complexes with DNA, and these complexes activate plasmacytoid dendritic cells via Toll-like receptors. Dendritic cells link the innate and adaptive immune systems. Plasmacytoid dendritic cells are overexpressed in early psoriatic plaques and on activation produce α-interferon which stimulates myeloid dendritic cells to move to the local draining lymph nodes. Here, the myeloid dendritic cells drive naïve T cells to proliferate and differentiate. Release of interleukin-12 (p. 19) causes differentiation to type 1 helper cells (Th1), and interleukin-23 differentiation to type 17 helper cells (Th17). These T cells are drawn from the circulation back to the psoriatic dermis by the interaction of $\alpha_1\beta_1$ integrin on the T cells with collagen IV at the basement membrane. Once in the dermis, Th1 cells release γ-interferon and TNF-α, and Th17 cells release interleukin-17 and 22. Dendritic cells themselves release further TNF-α and also inducible nitric oxide synthase. This rich cocktail of cytokines acts on keratinocytes, making them proliferate and produce antimicrobial peptides and various chemokines. Neutrophils are drawn to the epidermis by these chemokines, particularly IL-8, producing the characteristic pustules of severe psoriasis.

Precipitating factors

1 Trauma – if the psoriasis is active, lesions can appear in skin damaged by scratches or surgical wounds (the Köbner phenomenon; Figure 5.1).
2 Infection – tonsillitis caused by β-haemolytic streptococci often triggers guttate psoriasis. Bacterial exotoxins produced by *Staphylococcus aureus* and certain streptococci can act as superantigens (p. 21) and promote

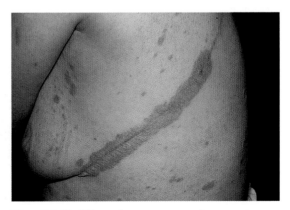

Figure 5.1 The Köbner phenomenon seen after a recent thoracotomy operation.

polyclonal T-cell proliferation. AIDS depresses cell-mediated immunity, so one might expect HIV infection to ameliorate psoriasis. Actually, HIV infection often worsens psoriasis, or precipitates explosive forms. The reason for this remains unclear, but may be a result of a reduction in regulatory T cells late in HIV allowing for unchecked inflammation, or because of the the relatively high proportion of CD8 T cells found in HIV infected patients.

3 Hormonal – psoriasis frequently improves in pregnancy only to relapse postpartum. Hypocalcaemia secondary to hypoparathyroidism is a rare precipitating cause.

4 Sunlight – improves most psoriatics but 10% become worse.

5 Drugs – antimalarials, β-blockers, IFN-α and lithium may worsen psoriasis. Psoriasis may 'rebound' after withdrawal of treatment with systemic steroids or potent topical steroids. The case against non-steroidal anti-inflammatory drugs (NSAIDs) remains unproven.

6 Cigarette smoking and alcohol – psoriasis is more common in smokers and ex-smokers but cause and effect relationships are uncertain. Alcohol consumption is associated with psoriasis, and may affect treatment options.

7 Emotion – emotional upsets seem to cause some exacerbations, and psoriasis itself has an adverse effect on patients' self-esteem.

8 Paradoxically, patients with rheumatoid arthritis treated with anti-TNFα agents may develop psoriasis, probably because of a reduction in the suppressive effect of TNFα on α-interferon.

Histology (Figure 5.2)

The main changes are the following.
1 Parakeratosis (nuclei retained in the horny layer).

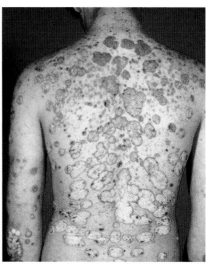

Figure 5.3 Psoriasis: extensive plaque psoriasis.

2 Irregular thickening of the epidermis over the rete ridges, but thinning over dermal papillae. Bleeding may occur when scale is scratched off (Auspitz sign).
3 Epidermal polymorphonuclear leucocyte infiltrates and microabscesses (described originally by Munro).
4 Dilated and tortuous capillary loops in the dermal papillae.
5 T-lymphocyte infiltrate in upper dermis.

Presentation
Common patterns are as follows.

Plaque pattern
This is the most common type. Lesions are well demarcated and range from a few millimetres to many centimetres in diameter (Figure 5.3). The lesions are pink or red

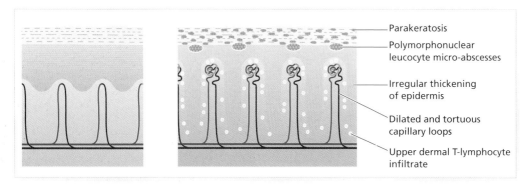

Figure 5.2 Histology of psoriasis (right) compared with normal skin (left).

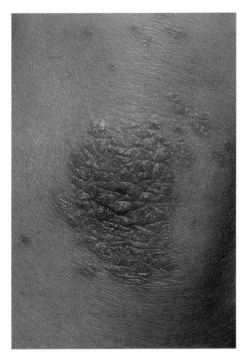

Figure 5.4 Psoriasis favours the extensor aspects of the knees and elbows.

with large centrally adherent silvery-white built-up polygonal scales. Symmetrical sites on the elbows, knees, lower back and scalp are sites of predilection (Figure 5.4).

Guttate pattern

This is usually seen in children and adolescents and may be the first sign of the disease, often triggered by streptococcal tonsillitis. The word guttate means 'drop-shaped'. Numerous small round red macules come up suddenly on the trunk and soon become scaly (Figure 5.5). The rash often clears in a few months but plaque psoriasis may develop later.

Scalp

The scalp is often involved. Areas of scaling are interspersed with normal skin; their lumpiness is sometimes more easily felt than seen (Figure 5.6). Frequently, the psoriasis overflows just beyond the scalp margin. Significant hair loss is rare.

Nails

Involvement of the nails is common, with 'thimble pitting' (Figure 5.7), onycholysis (separation of the nail from the

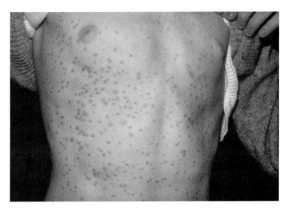

Figure 5.5 Guttate psoriasis.

nail bed; Figure 5.8) and sometimes subungual hyperkeratosis.

Flexures

Psoriasis of the submammary, axillary and anogenital folds is not scaly although the glistening sharply demarcated red plaques (Figure 5.9), often with fissuring in the depth of the fold, are still readily recognizable. Flexural psoriasis is most common in women and in the elderly, and is more common among HIV-infected individuals than uninfected ones. Many patients with plaque psoriasis harbour inverse psoriasis in their gluteal folds. Sometimes, when the diagnosis is in doubt, it pays to check for this and for relatively scaleless red papules on the penis.

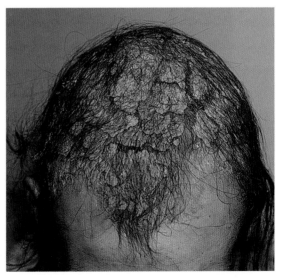

Figure 5.6 Untreated severe and extensive scalp psoriasis.

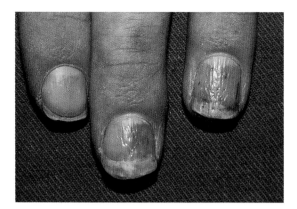

Figure 5.7 Thimble-like pitting of nails with onycholysis.

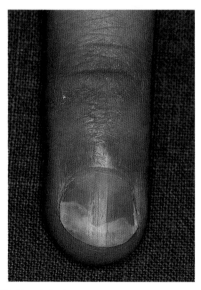

Figure 5.8 Onycholysis.

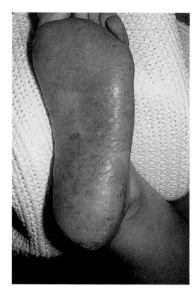

Figure 5.10 Pustular psoriasis of the sole.

Palms and soles

Palmar psoriasis may be hard to recognize, as its lesions are often poorly demarcated and barely erythematous. The fingers may develop painful fissures. At other times lesions are inflamed and studded with 1–2 mm pustules (palmoplantar pustulosis) (Figures 5.10 and 5.11). Psoriasis of the palms and soles may be disabling.

Less common patterns

Napkin psoriasis

A psoriasiform spread outside the napkin (nappy/diaper) area may give the first clue to a psoriatic tendency in an

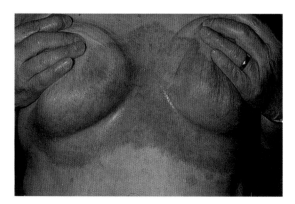

Figure 5.9 Sharply defined glistening erythematous patches of flexural psoriasis.

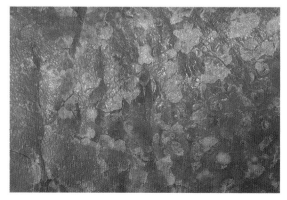

Figure 5.11 A closer view of pustules on the sole.

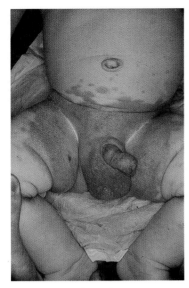

Figure 5.12 An irritant napkin rash now turning into napkin psoriasis.

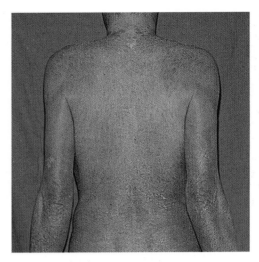

Figure 5.13 Erythrodermic psoriasis.

infant (Figure 5.12). Usually, it clears quickly but there is an increased risk of ordinary psoriasis developing in later life.

Generalized pustular psoriasis

This is a rare but serious condition, with fever and recurrent episodes of pustulation within areas of erythema.

Erythrodermic psoriasis

This is also rare and can be sparked off by the irritant effect of tar or dithranol, by a drug eruption or by the withdrawal of potent topical or systemic steroids. The skin becomes universally and uniformly red with variable scaling (Figure 5.13). Malaise is accompanied by shivering and the skin feels hot and uncomfortable.

Complications

Psoriatic arthropathy

Arthritis occurs in about 5–10% of psoriatic patients. Several patterns are recognized. Distal arthritis involves the terminal interphalangeal joints of the toes and fingers, especially those with marked nail changes (Figure 5.14). Other patterns include involvement of a single large joint; one that mimics rheumatoid arthritis and may become mutilating (Figure 5.15); and one where the brunt is borne by the sacro-iliac joints and spine. Tests for rheumatoid

factor are negative and nodules are absent. In patients with spondylitis and sacroiliitis there is a strong correlation with the presence of HLA-B27. Other patients develop painful inflammation where tendons meet bones (enthetitis).

Psoriasis and systemic disease

Perhaps unexpectedly for a condition causing such widespread inflammation of the skin, patients with psoriasis have a lower incidence of bacterial skin infections than people with healthy skin. This is in marked contrast

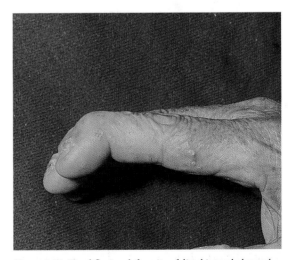

Figure 5.14 Fixed flexion deformity of distal interphalangeal joints following arthropathy.

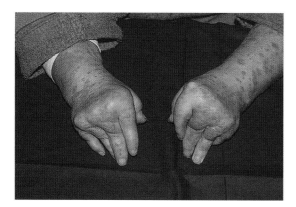

Figure 5.15 Rheumatoid-like changes associated with severe psoriasis of hands.

to the very frequent episodes of impetigo that complicate eczema. High quantities of antimicrobial peptides such as β-defensin and cathelicidin are found in psoriatic epidermis, and these important elements of the innate immune defences probably account for this. Psoriatic patients have an increased risk of developing cardiovascular disease, a complication that is most marked in younger people with severe disease. Patients with psoriasis have a relatively high prevalence of the metabolic syndrome, with obesity and impaired glucose tolerance, but the increased risk of heart disease exists even after allowing for this, and may be caused by the background degree of inflammation in the disease.

Differential diagnosis

Discoid eczema (p. 93)
Lesions are less well defined and may be exudative or crusted, lack thick scales and may be extremely itchy. Lesions do not favour scalp, extensor aspects of elbows and knees but rather the trunk and proximal parts of the extremities.

Seborrhoeic eczema (p. 92)
Scalp involvement is more diffuse and less lumpy. Intervening areas of normal scalp skin are unusual. Plaques are not so sharply marginated.

Flexural plaques are also less well defined and more exudative. There may be signs of seborrhoeic eczema elsewhere, such as in the eyebrows, nasolabial folds or on the chest.

Pityriasis rosea (p. 68)
This may be confused with guttate psoriasis but the lesions, which are oval rather than round, tend to run along rib lines. Scaling is of collarette type and a herald plaque may precede the rash. Lesions are mostly confined to the upper trunk.

Secondary syphilis (p. 219)
There is usually a history of a primary chancre. The scaly lesions are brownish and characteristically the palms and soles are involved. Oral changes, patchy alopecia, condylomata lata and lymphadenopathy complete the picture.

Cutaneous T-cell lymphoma (p. 307)
The lesions, which tend to persist, are not in typical locations and are often annular, arcuate, kidney-shaped or show bizarre outlines. Atrophy or poikiloderma may be present and individual lesions may vary in their thickness. About half of patients report that somebody wrongly diagnosed psoriasis, so tread carefully here. Erythrodermic psoriasis mimics the erythroderma of Sézary's syndrome.

Tinea unguium (p. 240)
The distal subungual form is often confused with nail psoriasis but is more asymmetrical and there may be obvious tinea of neighbouring skin. Uninvolved nails are common. Pitting is not seen and nails tend to be crumbly and discoloured at their free edge.

Investigations

1 Biopsy is seldom necessary. Usually, the diagnosis of common plaque psoriasis is obvious from clinical appearance. Treated psoriasis and variant forms may pose diagnostic problems, made worse because atypical clinical forms are also frequently atypical histologically.
2 Throat swabbing for β-haemolytic streptococci is needed in guttate psoriasis.
3 Skin scrapings and nail clippings may be required to exclude tinea.
4 Radiology and tests for rheumatoid factor are helpful in assessing arthritis.

Treatment

The need for this depends both on the patient's own perception of his or her disability, and on the doctor's objective assessment of how severe the skin disease is. The two do not always tally. The cosmetic disfigurement and psychological disability may be severe. Who is worse and needs treatment more – a woman with localized plaque psoriasis who will not go out and who becomes reclusive, or a man with generalized psoriasis who would rather wear shorts than cover up his many more plaques?

The effect of psoriasis on the quality of life as perceived by the patient can be scored with such measures as the Dermatology Life Quality Instrument (DLQI). The questionnaire asks questions such as 'Over the past week, how itchy, painful or stinging has your psoriasis been?' and 'Over the past week, how embarrassed or self-conscious have you been?' The questionnaire tallies three points for 'very much', two points for 'a lot', one point for 'some', and zero points for 'not at all'. Scores for the 10 questions are summed. A DLQI of 10 or more implies severe disease.

Meanwhile, the severity of psoriasis can be scored on the Psoriasis Area and Severity Index (PASI), which quantifies the scaliness, erythema, thickness and extent. Although the maximum score is 72, most dermatologists would interpret a PASI of 12 as severe disease. While very useful and reproducible for clinical research studies, the PASI is cumbersome for routine use in the clinic. However, it is important in the assessment of patients before starting treatment with biological agents. To ensure consistency in the use of these expensive and powerful new drugs, and to assess response in an impartial way, the UK guidelines require PASI scores to measured before treatment and while it is underway.

General measures

Explanations and reassurances must be geared to the patient's or the parent's intelligence. Information leaflets help to reinforce verbal advice. The doctor as well as the patient should keep the disease in perspective, and treatment must never be allowed to be more troublesome than the disease itself. The disease is not contagious. In the end, the treatment is one that is chosen by patient and doctor together after an informed and frank discussion of treatment options, including risks, mess, costs, compliance and comorbidities.

At present there is no cure for psoriasis; all treatments are suppressive and aimed at either inducing a remission or making the condition more tolerable. However, spontaneous remissions will occur in 50% of patients. Treatment for patients with chronic stable plaque psoriasis is relatively simple and may be safely administered by the family practitioner. However, systemic treatment for severe psoriasis should be monitored by a dermatologist. No treatment, at present, alters the overall course of the disease.

Physical and mental rest help to back up the specific management of acute episodes. Concomitant anxiety and depression should be treated on their own merits (see Table 5.1 for appropriate treatments).

Main types of treatment

These can be divided into four main categories: topical, ultraviolet radiation, systemic and biological. Broad recommendations are listed in Table 5.1, but most physicians will have their own favourites. In many ways it is better to become familiar with a few remedies than dabble with many. The management of patients with psoriasis is an art as well as a science and few other skin conditions benefit so much from patience and experience – of both patients and doctors.

Local treatments

Vitamin D analogues

Calcipotriol (calcipotriene), calcitriol and tacalcitol are analogues of chlolecalciferol, which do not cause hypercalcaemia and calciuria when used topically in the recommended dosage. They can be used for mild to moderate psoriasis affecting less than 40% of the skin. Vitamin D analogues work by influencing vitamin D receptors in keratinocytes, reducing epidermal proliferation and restoring a normal horny layer and are the mainstay of long-term topical treatment of chronic plaque psoriasis.

Patients like calcipotriol because it is odourless, colourless and does not stain. It seldom clears plaques of psoriasis completely, but does reduce their scaling and thickness. Local and usually transient irritation may occur with the recommended twice-daily application and for this reason it may not suit treatment for psoriasis of the face. One way of lessening this irritation is to combine the use of calcipotriol with a topical corticosteroid. This can either be achieved by applying the calcipotriol in the evening and the steroid in the morning (see *Topical corticosteroids*), or more conveniently by using a combined calcipotriol – betamethasone preparation. Up to 15 g/day or 100 g/week calcipotriol may be used, but the manufacturer's recommendations should be consulted when it is used in children under 6 years old. Calcitriol appears less irritant than calcipotriol. Tacalcitol ointment is applied sparingly once daily at bedtime, the maximum amount being 10 g/day. As with calcipotriol, irritation – often transient – may occur. The drug should not be used for longer than a year at

Table 5.1 Treatment options in psoriasis.

Type of psoriasis	Treatment of choice	Alternative treatments
Stable plaque	Vitamin D analogue (long term)	Tazarotene
	Local corticosteroid (short term)	Dithranol
	Corticosteroid–calcipotriol combination (short term)	Coal tar
	Narrowband UVB phototherapy	
Extensive stable plaque (>30% surface area) recalcitrant to local therapy	Narrowband UVB	Methotrexate
	PUVA	Ciclosporin
	PUVA + acitretin	Acitretin
		Fumarates
		Biological agents
Widespread small plaque	UVB	Vitamin D analogue
		Coal tar
		Systemic therapies
Guttate	Systemic antibiotic	Weak tar preparation
	Emollients while erupting; then UVB	Mild local steroids
Facial	Mild to moderately potent local corticosteroid	Tacrolimus
		Calcitriol
Flexural	Mild to moderately potent local steroid tacrolimus	Coal tar
	Vitamin D analogue (caution: may irritate. Calcitriol less irritant than calcipotriol)	
Pustular psoriasis of hands and feet	Moderately potent or potent local steroid	Acitretin
	Local retinoid	Topical PUVA
Acute erythrodermic, unstable or generalized pustular	Inpatient treatment with ichthammol paste	Gentle phototherapy (UVB), acitretin
	Local steroid may be used initially with or without wet compresses	Methotrexate, ciclosporin
		Biological agents

a time and is not yet recommended for children under 12 years.

Topical corticosteroids

Practice varies from centre to centre and from country to country. Patients like topical corticosteroids because they are clean and reduce scaling and redness. Potent topical corticosteroids are of similar efficacy to vitamin D analogues, but should not be used long term because of the risk of skin thinning. They are thus best used for short-term, or intermittent, treatment of psoriasis.

In our view such usage is safe, but only under proper supervision by doctors well aware of problems such as dermal atrophy, tachyphylaxis, early relapses, the occasional precipitation of unstable psoriasis (Figure 5.16) and, rarely, in extensive cases, of adrenal suppression caused by systemic absorption. A commitment by the prescriber to keep the patient under regular clinical review is especially important if more than 50 g/week of a moderately potent topical corticosteroid preparation is being

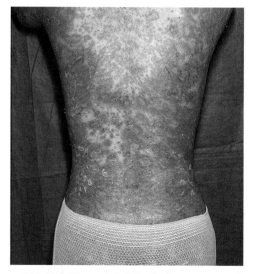

Figure 5.16 Unstable psoriasis following long-term use of a potent topical steroid.

used. A combined calcipotriol–corticosteroid preparations is more effective than either agent alone.

The regular use of topical corticosteroids is less controversial under the following circumstances.

1 In 'limited choice' areas such as the face, ears, genitals and flexures where tar and dithranol are seldom tolerated. Mild or moderately potent steroid preparations can be used here for 2–4 weeks.

2 For patients who cannot use vitamin D analogues, tar or dithranol because of allergic or irritant reactions (moderately potent preparations, except for 'no choice' areas where mildly potent ones should be used if possible).

3 For unresponsive psoriasis on the scalp, palms and soles (moderately potent, potent and very potent – but only in the short term – preparations).

4 For patients with minor localized psoriasis (moderately potent or potent preparations).

Local retinoids

Tazarotene is a topically active retinoid. It has a selective affinity for retinoic acid receptors (RARs) and, when bound to these, improves psoriasis by reducing keratinocyte proliferation, normalizing the disturbed differentiation and lessening the infiltrate of dermal inflammatory cells. It is recommended for chronic stable plaque psoriasis on the trunk and limbs covering up to 20% of the body. It is applied sparingly once a day, in the evening, and can be used for courses of up to 12 weeks. It works slowly and seldom clears psoriasis but reduces the induration, scaling and redness of plaques. It is available as either a 0.05% or 0.1% gel. Like the vitamin D analogues, its main adverse effect is irritation. If this occurs, the strength should be reduced to 0.05%; if irritation persists, applications should be cut to alternate days and a combination treatment with a local steroid considered.

In the United States, tazarotene is licenced for children aged 12 years and over; in Europe it is currently licenced only for adults over 18 years old. The drug should not be used in pregnancy or during lactation. Females of childbearing age should use adequate contraception during therapy.

Dithranol (anthralin)

Dithranol is rarely used in the United States nowadays but remains popular in the United Kingdom. Like coal tar it inhibits DNA synthesis, but some of its benefits may be brought about by the formation of free radicals of oxygen.

Dithranol is more tricky to use than coal tar. It has to be applied carefully, to the plaques only; often it needs to be covered with gauze dressings to prevent movement on to uninvolved skin and clothing, which it stains a rather indelible purple colour. Dithranol also stains normal skin, but the purple–brown discoloration peels off after a few days. It also stains bathtubs, which need to be scrubbed down. It is irritant, so treatment should start with a weak (0.1%) preparation, thereafter the strength can be stepped up at weekly intervals. Dithranol stronger than 1% is seldom necessary. Irritation of the surrounding skin can be lessened by the application of a protective bland paste (e.g. zinc paste). One popular regimen is to apply dithranol daily for 5 days in the week; after 1 month many patients will be clear.

Short contact therapy, in which dithranol is applied for no longer than 30 minutes, is also effective. Initially, a test patch of psoriasis is treated with a 0.1% dithranol cream, left on for 20 minutes and then washed off. If there is no undue reaction, the application can be extended the next day and, if tolerated, can be left on for 30 minutes. After the cream is washed off, a bland application such as soft white paraffin or emulsifying ointment is applied. Depending on response, the strength of the dithranol can be increased from 0.1% to 2% over 2–3 weeks. Suitable preparations are listed in Formulary 1 (p. 406).

Dithranol is too irritant to apply to the face, the inner thighs, genital region or skin folds. Special care must be taken to avoid contact with the eyes. It can be used to treat resistant plaques in the scalp, but stains pale-coloured hair.

Coal tar preparations

Crude coal tar and its distillation products have been used to treat psoriasis for many years. Their precise mode of action is uncertain but tar does inhibit DNA synthesis and photosensitizes the skin.

Many preparations are available but it is wise to become familiar with a few. The less refined tars are smelly, messy and stain clothes, but are more effective than the cleaner refined preparations. Tar emulsions can also be added to the bath. Suitable preparations are listed in Formulary 1 (p. 407). Despite its reputation as a carcinogen, no increase in skin cancer has been found in patients treated for long periods with tar preparations.

Salicylic acid

This is a common constituent of psoriasis remedies sold without prescriptions, usually at 2% concentrations. Dermatologists often use 3–6% concentrations. Salicylic acid debrides scales that contain chemotactic factors, enhances the penetration of other topical therapies and may have anti-inflammatory effects.

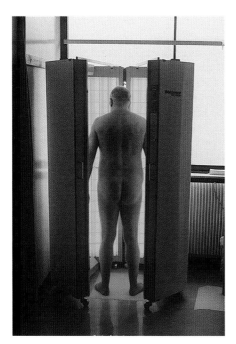

Figure 5.17 Ultraviolet radiation therapy.

Calcineurin inhibitors (topical immunomodulators)

Both tacrolimus and pimecrolimus are useful where chronic treatment of psoriasis on the face, genitals or intertriginous areas is needed.

Ultraviolet radiation

Most patients improve with natural sunlight and should be encouraged to sunbathe. During the winter, courses of artificial ultraviolet radiation (UVB), as an outpatient or at home, may help (Figure 5.17). Both broadband UVB and narrowband UVB can be used. Narrowband UVB uses intense ultraviolet radiation at wavelength 311 nm. This wavelength of ultraviolet radiation is especially effective for clearing psoriasis while minimizing exposure to potentially carcinogenic wavelengths less than 300 nm.

Treatments should be given by an expert, twice to three times weekly for 8 weeks or until the skin clears. Goggles should be worn. The initial dose is calculated either by establishing the skin type (p. 260) or by determining the minimal dose of UVB that causes erythema in a test patch 24 hours after radiation. The initial small dose is increased incrementally after each exposure providing it is well tolerated. The number of treatments and doses employed should be recorded. The main risk of UVB therapies in the short term is acute phototoxicity (sunburn-like reac-

tion) and, in the long term, the induction of photodamage and skin cancer.

Special situations

Scalp psoriasis

This is often recalcitrant. Oily preparations containing 3–6% salicylic acid are useful for treating scaling of the scalp (Formulary 1, p. 407). They should be rubbed into the scalp three times a week and washed out with a tar shampoo 4–6 hours later. If progress is slow, they can be left on for one or two nights before shampooing. Once the scale has been removed, intermittent potent topical corticosteroids can be used, either alone, or in combination with a vitamin D analogue such as calcipotriol.

Guttate psoriasis

A course of penicillin V or erythromycin is indicated for any associated streptococcal throat infection. Bland local treatment is often enough as the natural trend is towards remission. Suitable preparations include emulsifying ointment and zinc and ichthammol cream. Tar–steroid preparations are reasonable alternatives. A course of ultraviolet therapy (UVB) may be helpful after the eruptive phase is over.

Eruptive/unstable psoriasis

Bland treatment is needed and rest is important. Tar, dithranol and ultraviolet therapy are best avoided. Suitable preparations include oilated baths, mild or moderately potent topical steroids, emulsifying ointment, and zinc and ichthammol cream. Refer these patients to dermatologists.

Systemic treatment

A systemic approach should be considered for extensive psoriasis (more than 20% of the body surface) that fails to improve with prolonged courses of tar or dithranol, and for patients whose quality of life is low. As the potential adverse effects are sometimes great, local measures should be given a good trial first. The most commonly used systemic treatments are photochemotherapy with psoralen and ultraviolet A (PUVA) treatment, retinoids, methotrexate, ciclosporin, fumaric acid (fumarate), hydroxyurea (hydroxycarbamide) and an array of biological agents.

Photochemotherapy (PUVA)

In this ingenious therapy, a drug is photo-activated in the skin by ultraviolet radiation. An oral dose of

8-methoxypsoralen (8-MOP) or 5-methoxypsoralen (5-MOP) is followed by exposure to long-wave ultraviolet radiation (UVA: 320–400 nm). The psoralen reaches the skin and, in the presence of UVA, forms photo-adducts with DNA pyrimidine bases and cross-links between complementary DNA strands; this inhibits DNA synthesis and epidermal cell division.

The 8-MOP (crystalline formulation 0.6–0.8 mg/kg body weight or liquid formulation 0.3–0.4 mg/kg) or 5-MOP (1.2–1.6 mg/kg) is taken 1–2 h before exposure to a bank of UVA tubes mounted in a cabinet similar to that seen in Figure 5.17. Psoralens may also be administered in bath water for those unable to tolerate the oral regimen. The initial exposure is calculated either by determining the patient's minimal phototoxic dose (the least dose of UVA that after ingestion of 8-MOP produces a barely perceptible erythema 72 hours after testing) or by assessing skin colour and ability to tan. Treatment is given two or three times a week with increasing doses of UVA, depending on erythema production and the therapeutic response. Protective goggles are worn during radiation and UVA opaque plastic glasses must be used after taking the tablets and for 24 hours after each treatment (p. 259). All phototherapy equipment should be serviced and calibrated regularly by trained personnel. An accurate record of each patient's cumulative dosage and number of treatments should be kept.

Clearance takes 5–10 weeks.

Adverse effects. Painful erythema is the most common adverse effect but the risk of this can be minimized by careful dosimetry. One-quarter of patients itch during and immediately after radiation; fewer feel nauseated after taking 8-MOP. 5-MOP, not available in the United States, is worth trying if these effects become intolerable. Long-term adverse effects include premature ageing of the skin (with mottled pigmentation, scattered lentigines, wrinkles and atrophy), cutaneous malignancies (usually after a cumulative dose greater than 1000 J or after more than 250 treatments) and, theoretically at least, cataract formation. The use of UVA blocking glasses (p. 259) for 24 hours after each treatment should protect against the latter. The long-term adverse effects relate to the total amount of UVA received over the years; this must be recorded and kept as low as possible, without denying treatment when it is clearly needed. As far as possible, PUVA therapy is avoided in younger patients. In most centres there is a move to replacing PUVA with narrowband UVB as the major form of phototherapy.

Retinoids

Acitretin (10–25 mg/day; Formulary 2, p. 420) is an analogue of vitamin A, and is one of the few drugs helpful in pustular psoriasis. It is also used to thin down thick hyperkeratotic plaques. Minor adverse effects are frequent and dose-related. They include dry lips, mouth, vagina and eyes, peeling of the skin, pruritus and unpleasant paronychia. All settle on stopping or reducing the dosage of the drug, but the use of emollients and artificial tears is often recommended. Hair thinning or loss is common. Occasionally, all hair is lost when acetretin is used as monotherapy at higher doses of 0.5–1 mg/kg/day. Hair regrows when treatment is stopped, but meanwhile patients generally hate their baldness.

Acitretin can be used for long periods, but regular blood tests are needed to exclude abnormal liver function and the elevation of serum lipids (mainly triglycerides but also cholesterol). Yearly X-rays should detect bone spurs and ossification of ligaments, especially the paraspinal ones (disseminated interstitial skeletal hyperostosis (DISH) syndrome). Monitor, too, for depression, although a causal relationship between retinoids and depression has not been proved. Children, and those with persistently abnormal liver function tests or hyperlipidaemia, should not be treated.

The most important adverse effect is teratogenicity, so acitretin should not normally be prescribed to women of childbearing age. If, for unavoidable clinical reasons, it is still the drug of choice, effective oral contraceptive measures must be taken and, in view of the long half-life of its metabolite, these should continue for 2 years after treatment has ceased. Blood donation should be avoided for a similar period.

Retinoids and PUVA act synergistically and are often used together in the so-called Re-PUVA regimen. This clears plaque psoriasis quicker than PUVA alone, and needs a smaller cumulative dose of UVA. The standard precautions for both PUVA and retinoid treatment should, of course, still be observed. Low doses of acitretin are often used in combination with other topical therapies for palmoplantar psoriasis.

Methotrexate

Methotrexate, at the doses used for the treatment of psoriasis, inhibits proliferating lymphoid cells by its effects on purine biosynthesis. These effects are caused by inhibition of both dihydrofolate reductase, and 5-aminoimidazole-4-carboxamide ribonucleotide (AICAR) transferase. AICAR accumulation reduces adenosine deaminase activity causing adenosine to accumulate in

T cells and inhibit their effects. Folate supplementation may reduce methotrexate toxicity, but does not appear to greatly reduce its therapeutic effectiveness.

After an initial trial dose of 2.5 mg, in an adult of average weight, the drug is given orally once a week and the dose increased gradually to a maintenance dose of 7.5–20 mg/week. This often controls even aggressive psoriasis. The drug is eliminated largely by the kidneys and so the dose must be reduced if renal function is poor. Aspirin and sulfonamides displace the drug from binding with plasma albumin, and furosemide (frusemide) decreases its renal clearance: note must therefore be taken of concurrent drug therapy (Formulary 2, p. 419) and the dose reduced accordingly. Minor and temporary adverse effects, such as nausea and malaise, are common in the 48 hours after administration. The most serious drawback to this treatment is hepatic fibrosis, the risk of which is greatly increased in those who drink alcohol. Unfortunately, routine liver function tests and scans cannot predict this reliably, and a liver biopsy to exclude active liver disease has hitherto been advised for those with risk factors, and repeated after every cumulative dose of 1.5–2 g, especially in less than perfectly healthy drinking adults. Liver biopsy is now being replaced by serial assays of serum procollagen III aminopeptide (PIIINP), which appears to be an adequately sensitive marker for hepatic fibrosis. Blood checks to exclude marrow suppression, and to monitor renal and liver function, should also be performed – weekly at the start of treatment, with the interval being slowly increased to monthly or every third month depending on when stable maintenance therapy is established.

The drug is teratogenic and should not be given to females in their reproductive years. Oligospermia has been noted in men and fertility may be lowered; however, a child fathered by a man on methotrexate can be expected to be normal. Folic acid, 5 mg/day, taken on days when the patient does not have methotrexate, can lessen nausea and reduce marrow suppression. Methotrexate should not be taken at the same time as retinoids or ciclosporin.

Ciclosporin

Ciclosporin inhibits cell-mediated immune reactions. It blocks resting lymphocytes in the G_0 or early G_1 phase of the cell cycle and inhibits lymphokine release, especially that of IL-2.

Ciclosporin is effective in severe psoriasis, but patients needing it should be under the care of specialists. Most prefer to use the drug only for short periods to stabilize disease or to buy time while other therapies are started.

The initial daily dose is 3–4 mg/kg/day and not more than 5 mg/kg/day. With improvement, the dose can often be reduced but the adverse effects of long-term treatment include hypertension, kidney damage and persistent viral warts with a risk of skin cancer. Blood pressure and renal function should be assessed carefully before starting treatment. The serum creatinine should be measured two or three times before starting therapy to be sure of the baseline and then every other week for the first 3 months of therapy. Thereafter, if the results are stable, the frequency of testing will depend on the dosage (monthly for >2.5 mg/kg/day or every other month for <2.5 mg/kg/day). The dosage should be reduced if the serum creatinine concentration rises to 30% above the baseline level on two occasions within 2 weeks. If these changes do not reverse themselves when the dosage has been reduced for 1 month, then the drug should be stopped.

Hypertension is a common adverse effect of ciclosporin: nearly 50% of patients develop a systolic blood pressure over 160 mmHg and/or a diastolic blood pressure over 95 mmHg. Usually, these rises are mild or moderate, and respond to concomitant treatment with a calcium channel blocker, such as nifedipine. If this cannot be tolerated, an angiotensin-converting enzyme inhibitor should be used under specialist supervision. Diuretics, which may themselves worsen renal function, and β-blockers, which may themselves worsen psoriasis, should probably be avoided. Ciclosporin interacts with a number of drugs (Formulary 2, p. 418). It is also advisable to watch levels of cholesterol, triglycerides, potassium and magnesium, and advise patients that they will become hirsute and that they may develop gingival hyperplasia. Treatment with ciclosporin should not continue for longer than 1 year without careful assessment and close monitoring.

Fumaric acid esters

Fumaric acid esters, although unlicensed, have been effective in some patients with treatment resistant psoriasis, but with a high incidence of gastrointestinal upset and flushing. These generally settle with time and in those who can tolerate the drug efficacy appears similar to methotrexate.

Other systemic drugs

Antimetabolites such as mycophenolate mofetil, 6-thioguanine, azathioprine and hydroxyurea help psoriasis, but less than methotrexate; they tend to damage the marrow rather than the liver. Regular blood monitoring is again essential. Sulfasalazine occasionally helps psoriasis.

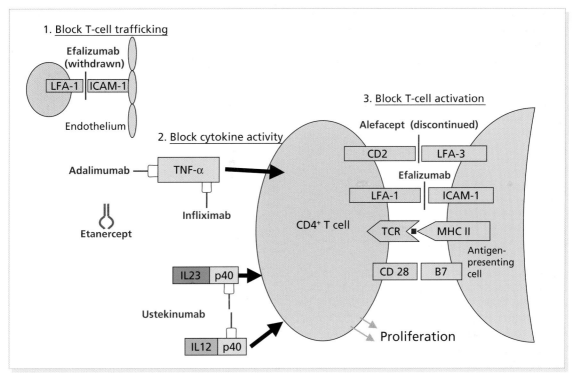

Figure 5.18 Therapeutic targets of biological treatments.

Biological agents

The immunologically based pathogenesis of psoriasis presents many targets for therapeutic exploitation and the development of synthesized monoclonal antibodies that bind key molecules (Figure 5.18) has been a major advance in the treatment. Clinical experience is growing with these agents, and their effectiveness in treating moderate and severe psoriasis means that hospital admission can now often be avoided, but they are very expensive. Efalizumab, a humanized murine IgG that binds to CD11a and one of the early biological agents, has been withdrawn because of the development of progressive multifocal leukoencephalopathy in three patients on the drug. In the United Kingdom, all patients being treated with biological agents must be under the supervision of a dermatologist, and are entered on to a centrally held register so that such rare but serious adverse effects can be rapidly identified.

Etanercept is a fusion protein of IgG and the extracellular TNFα receptor, so that it effectively mops up free TNFα, preventing its action. Infliximab is a chimeric antibody against TNFα that binds both soluble and bound

TNFα. Adalimumab is a recombinant IgG monoclonal antibody against TNFα with similar action.

Ustekinumab is a fully human recombinant antibody to the shared p40 subunit of IL12 and IL23.

Alefacept (not licensed for use in the United Kingdom) does not bind TNFα. It is a fusion protein of human LFA-3 and IgG that inhibits T-cell activation by blocking the action of accessory molecules needed for lymphocyte activation (p. 19).

Both dermatologists and patients often ponder when to use biological treatments, and then which agent to use. As with other therapies, the choice depends upon type of psoriasis, comorbidities (including arthritis), insurance coverage, cost, efficacy, mode of administration and safety. In the United Kingdom, guidelines have been produced by the British Association of Dermatologists (BAD) and also by the National Institute for Health and Clinical Excellence (NICE). Patients must have severe psoriasis and have failed, or been intolerant of standard systemic therapy and phototherapy for biological therapy to be considered (Table 5.2). The TNFα blocking agents are generally recommended as the first line biological

Table 5.2 Elements suggesting the need for treatment with biological agents.

PASI score more than 10
DLQI score more than 10
Globally severe disease
Life-threatening psoriasis
Unstable psoriasis
Unresponsive to other therapies
Intolerant to other therapies
Would otherwise need hospitalization
Significant comorbidities
Associated significant psoriatic arthritis

DLQI, Dermatology Life Quality Instrument; PASI, Psoriasis Area and Severity Index.

treatments, with etanercept and adalimumab being favoured in stable chronic plaque psoriasis. If a first anti-TNFα agent is ineffective, an alternative anti-TNFα, or ustekinumab (a second line agent) can be used. For unstable and general pustular psoriasis, infliximab has the advantage of rapid onset of action and disease control. In the United States, many dermatologists first choose etanercept, because of its good safety profile, relative efficacy and relative ease of administration (it can be injected at home by the patient). There are worries about opportunistic infections and about precipitating multiple sclerosis, congestive heart failure, lupus-like syndromes and lymphomas. It can be used in children.

Infliximab probably works fastest of all the biological agents, but requires intravenous infusions. Alefacept requires weekly counts of CD4 lymphocytes, because it can cause lymphopenias. It is given in courses.

Reactivation of tuberculosis is a concern with all of the anti-TNF agents and also probably ustekinumab, so patients should be screened for the disease before and then be assessed during treatment. Live vaccines cannot be used during biological therapy as they have reduced effectiveness. TNF antagonists are contraindicated in those with a history of demyelinating disease. While there is no firm evidence that biological treatments increase the incidence of malignancy, they are probably best avoided in those with active cancer. Entering all patients treated with biological agents into treatment registers will ultimately produce definitive data as to these risks.

All the biological agents are expensive. Payers could buy a car each year for the money they will spend. However, the treatments are very effective and relatively safe.

They minimize costs of laboratory test monitoring, physician visits, phototherapies, and costs associated with long-term adverse effects of other choices such as liver disease (methotrexate), renal disease (ciclosporin) and heart disease (hyperlipidaemias from retinoids).

Combination therapy

If psoriasis is resistant to one treatment, a combination of treatments used together may be the answer. Combination treatments can even prevent adverse effects by allowing less of each drug to be used. Common combinations include topical vitamin D analogues with either local steroids or UVB, dithranol following a tar bath, and UVB (Ingram regimen) and coal tar following a tar bath and UVB (Goeckerman regimen). Combination therapy with biological agents is possible, but experience is limited.

Rotational therapy may also minimize the toxicity of some treatments – an example would be PUVA, methotrexate, acitretin and ciclosporin, each used separately for a while before moving on to the next treatment.

Learning points

1 Discuss a treatment plan with the patient. Consider disability, cost, time, mess and risk of systemic therapy to general health.
2 The treatment must not be worse than the disease.
3 Do not aggravate eruptive psoriasis.
4 Never use systemic steroids.
5 Avoid the long-term use of potent or very potent topical corticosteroids.
6 Never promise a permanent cure, but be encouraging.
7 Great advances have been made over the last 20 years in the treatment of severe psoriasis, but patients taking modern systemic agents require careful monitoring.

Further reading

British Association of Dermatologists and Primary Care Dermatology Society. (2009) Recommendations for the initial management of psoriasis 29. www.eGuidelines.co.uk (accessed 1 June 2014).

Elder JT, Bruce AT, Gudjonsson JE, et al. (2010) Molecular dissection of psoriasis: integrating genetics and biology. *Journal of Investigative Dermatology* **130**, 1213–1226.

Lapolla W, Yentzer BA, Bagel J, Halvorson CR, Feldman SR. (2011) A review of phototherapy protocols for psoriasis treatment. *Journal of the American Academy of Dermatology* **64**, 936–949.

Nestle FO, Kaplan DH, Barker J. (2009) Psoriasis. *New England Journal of Medicine* **361**, 496–509.

Scottish Intercollegiate Guidelines Network (SIGN). (2010) Diagnosis and management of psoriasis and psoriatic arthri-tis in adults. SIGN, Edinburgh. (SIGN publication no. 121). www.sign.ac.uk (accessed 1 June 2014).

Smith CH, Anstey AV, Barker JN, *et al.* (2009) British Association of Dermatologists guidelines for use of biological inter-ventions for psoriasis 2009. *British Journal of Dermatology* **161**, 987–1019.

6 Other Papulosquamous Disorders

Psoriasis is not the only skin disease that is sharply marginated and scaly. Table 6.1 lists some of the most common ones. Eczema can also be raised and scaly, but is usually poorly marginated with fissures, crusts or lichenification and signs of epidermal disruption such as weeping, and yellow scaling (see Chapter 7). Psoriasis is discussed in Chapter 5.

Pityriasis rosea

Cause
Pityriasis rosea is caused by reactivation of either human herpes virus 7 or human herpes virus 8. The disease may occur in clusters, both geographical and temporal, and seems not to be contagious.

Presentation
Pityriasis rosea is common. It mainly affects children and young adults, and second attacks are rare. Most patients develop one plaque (the 'herald' or 'mother' plaque) before the others (Figure 6.1). It is larger (2–5 cm in diameter) than later lesions, and is rounder, redder and more scaly. After several days many smaller plaques appear, mainly on the trunk, but some also on the neck and extremities. About half of the patients complain of itching. An individual plaque is oval, salmon pink and shows a delicate scaling, adherent peripherally as a collarette. The configuration of such plaques is often characteristic. Their longitudinal axes run down and out from the spine in a 'fir tree' pattern (Figure 6.2), along the lines of the ribs. Purpuric lesions are rare.

Course
The herald plaque precedes the generalized eruption by several days. Subsequent lesions enlarge over the first week or two. Many patients have systemic symptoms such as aching and tiredness. The eruption lasts between 2 and 10 weeks and then resolves spontaneously, sometimes leaving hyperpigmented patches that fade more slowly.

Differential diagnosis
Although herald plaques are often mistaken for ringworm (tinea corporis), the two disorders most likely to be misdiagnosed early in the general eruption are guttate psoriasis and secondary syphilis. Tinea corporis and pityriasis versicolor can be distinguished by the microscopical examination of scales (p. 37), and secondary syphilis by its other features (mouth lesions, palmar lesions, condyloma lata, lymphadenopathy, alopecia) and by serology. Gold and captopril are the drugs most likely to cause a pityriasis rosea-like drug reaction, but barbiturates, penicillamine, some antibiotics, tyrosine kinase inhibitors and other drugs can also do so. These drug-induced rashes show an interface dermatitis and eosinophils on histology. A transient pityriasis rosea like rash has been reported after a number of vaccinations.

Investigations
Because secondary syphilis can mimic pityriasis rosea so closely, testing for syphilis is usually wise.

Treatment
No treatment is curative, and active treatment is seldom needed for this self-limiting disease. Symptomatic agents such as calamine lotion may help the itching. So far, treatment with antiviral agents has not been helpful.

> **Learning points**
> 1 Check serology for syphilis if in doubt about the diagnosis.
> 2 Revise the diagnosis if the rash lasts for longer than 3 months.

Clinical Dermatology, Fifth Edition. Richard B. Weller, Hamish J.A. Hunter and Margaret W. Mann.
© 2015 John Wiley & Sons, Ltd. Published 2015 by John Wiley & Sons, Ltd.

Table 6.1 Some important papulosquamous diseases.

Psoriasis
Pityriasis rosea
Lichen planus
Pityriasis rubra pilaris
Parapsoriasis
Mycosis fungoides (cutaneous T-cell lymphoma)
Pityriasis lichenoides
Discoid lupus erythematosus
Subacute cutaneous lupus erythematosus
Tinea corporis
Pityriasis versicolor
Nummular eczema
Seborrhoeic dermatitis
Secondary syphilis
Drug eruptions
Extramammary Paget's disease
Squamous cell carcinoma *in situ*

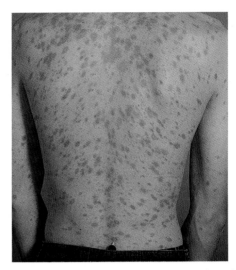

Figure 6.2 An extensive pityriasis rosea showing a 'fir tree' distribution on the back.

Lichen planus

Cause

The precise cause of lichen planus is unknown, but the disease seems to be mediated immunologically. Activated

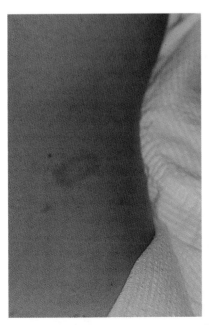

Figure 6.1 The herald plaque of pityriasis rosea is usually on the trunk and is larger than the other lesions. Its annular configuration is shown well here.

T lymphocytes are recruited to the dermo-epidermal junction where CD8$^+$ cytotoxic and to a lesser extent CD4$^+$ T cells predominate in the lichenoid infiltrate. T helper 1 (Th1) cytokines are overexpressed together with the pro-apoptotic molecules fas and Bcl-2. The resultant basal keratinocyte apoptosis is characteristic of lichen planus. Similar basal keratinocyte apoptosis also occurs in subacute cutaneous lupus erythematosus and erythema multiforme, but elevated intercellular adhesion molecule 1 (ICAM-1) expression is specific to lichen planus. Chronic graft versus host disease can cause an eruption rather like lichen planus in which histoincompatibility causes lymphocytes to attack the epidermis. There may be a genetic susceptibility to idiopathic lichen planus although an abnormal gene has not yet been identified. Rarely, familial cases are reported. Lichen planus is also associated with autoimmune disorders, such as alopecia areata, vitiligo and ulcerative colitis, more commonly than would be expected by chance. Contact with mercury compounds or amalgam in dental fillings seems to be an important cause of oral lichen planus, especially if there is no concomitant cutaneous lichen planus. Only about one-third of these patients have a positive patch test response to mercury, so this may be an irritant rather than allergic reaction. Drugs too can cause lichen planus (see *Differential diagnosis*). Some patients with lichen planus also have a hepatitis C infection, although this association is rarely seen in northern Europe. Lichen planus itself is not infectious.

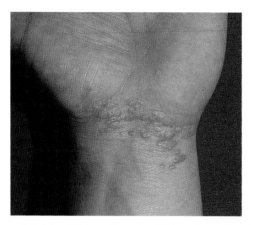

Figure 6.3 Shiny flat-topped papules of lichen planus. Note the Wickham's striae.

Table 6.2 Variants of lichen planus.

Annular
Atrophic
Bullous
Follicular
Hypertrophic (Figure 6.6)
Ulcerative

Presentation

Typical lesions are violaceous or lilac-coloured, intensely itchy, flat-topped papules that usually arise on the extremities, particularly on the volar aspects of the wrists and legs (Figure 6.3). A close look is needed to see a white streaky pattern on the surface of these papules (Wickham's striae). White asymptomatic lacy lines, dots, and occasionally small white plaques, are also found in the mouth, particularly inside the cheeks, in about 50% of patients (Figure 6.4), and oral lesions may be the sole manifestation of the disease. The genital skin may be similarly affected (see Figure 13.37). Variants of the classic pattern are rare and often difficult to diagnose (Table 6.2). Curiously, although the skin plaques are usually itchy, patients rub rather than scratch, so that excoriations are uncommon. As in psoriasis, the Köbner phenomenon may occur

(Figure 6.5). The nails are usually normal, but in about 10% of patients show changes ranging from fine longitudinal grooves to destruction of the entire nail fold and bed (see Figure 13.26). Scalp lesions can cause a patchy scarring alopecia.

Course

Individual lesions may last for many months and the eruption as a whole tends to last about 1 year. However, the hypertrophic variant of the disease, with thick warty lesions usually around the ankles (Figure 6.6), often lasts for many years. As lesions resolve, they become darker, flatter and leave discrete brown or grey macules. About one in six patients will have a recurrence.

Complications

Nail and hair loss can be permanent. The ulcerative form of lichen planus in the mouth may lead to squamous cell carcinoma. Ulceration, usually over bony prominences, may be disabling, especially if it is on the soles. Any association with liver disease may be caused by a coexisting hepatitis C infection (see *Cause*).

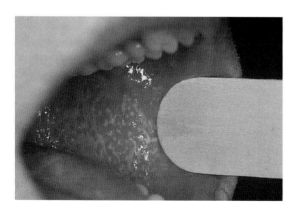

Figure 6.4 Lichen planus: classic white lacy network lying on the buccal mucosa.

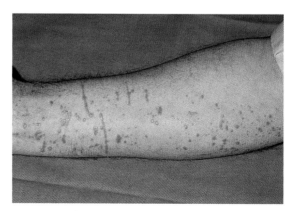

Figure 6.5 Lichen planus: striking Köbner effect on the forearm.

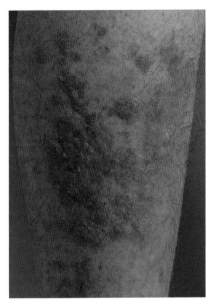

Figure 6.6 The thickened purplish lesions characteristic of hypertrophic lichen planus on the shins.

Differential diagnosis

Lichen planus should be differentiated from the other papulosquamous diseases listed in Table 6.1. Lichenoid drug reactions can mimic lichen planus closely. Gold and other heavy metals have often been implicated. Other drug causes include antimalarials, β-blockers, non-steroidal anti-inflammatory drugs, para-aminobenzoic acid, thiazide diuretics and penicillamine. Contact with chemicals used to develop colour photographic film can also produce similar lesions. It may be hard to tell lichen planus from generalized discoid lupus erythematosus if only a few large lesions are present, or if the eruption is on the palms, soles or scalp. Wickham's striae or oral lesions favour the diagnosis of lichen planus. Oral candidiasis (pp. 189, 243) can also cause confusion.

Investigations

The diagnosis is usually obvious clinically. The histology is characteristic (Figure 6.7), so a biopsy will confirm the diagnosis if necessary.

Treatment

Treatment can be difficult. If drugs are suspected as the cause, they should be stopped and unrelated ones substituted. Potent topical steroids will sometimes relieve symptoms and flatten the plaques. Systemic steroid courses work too, but are recommended only in special situations (e.g. unusually extensive involvement, nail destruction or painful and erosive oral lichen planus). Treatment with photochemotherapy with psoralen and ultraviolet A (PUVA; p. 373) or with narrowband UVB (p. 373) may reduce pruritus and help to clear up the skin lesions. Oral ciclosporin (Formulary 2, p. 418) or acitretin (Formulary 2, p. 420) have also helped some patients with stubborn lichen planus. Antihistamines may blunt the itch. Mucous membrane lesions, both oral and genital, are usually asymptomatic and do not require treatment; if they do, then applications of a corticosteroid or calcineurin inhibitor such as tacrolimus in a gel base may be helpful.

Learning points

1 A good diagnostic tip is to look for light reflected from shiny papules.
2 Always look in the mouth.
3 If you can recognize lichen planus, you have pulled ahead of 75% of your colleagues.

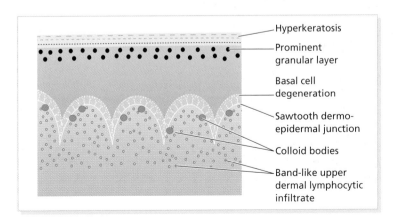

Figure 6.7 Histology of lichen planus.

Pityriasis rubra pilaris

This heading describes a group of uncommon skin disorders characterized by fine scaling (pityriasis), redness (rubra) and involvement of hair follicles (pilaris). It is unclear if the different presentations of this combination of signs are separate conditions or variants of one disease. The prevalence of pityriasis rubra pilaris, including all types, is very low at around 1 in 5000 of the population in the United Kingdom.

Cause

No cause has been identified for any type. There is epidermal hyperproliferation in lesional skin and the epidermal turnover time (p. 7) is decreased, but not to the extent seen in psoriasis. A defect in vitamin A metabolism was once suggested but has been disproved. The rare familial type has an autosomal dominant inheritance.

Presentation

The most common acquired type begins in adult life with erythema and scaling of the face and scalp. Later, the disease spreads to the trunk and limbs (termed cephalocaudal spread) and red or orange plaques grow quickly and merge, so that patients with pityriasis rubra pilaris are often erythrodermic. Peri-follicular papules and keratinous follicular plugs develop at this stage. Small islands of skin may be 'spared' from this general erythema, but even here the follicles may be red and plugged with keratin (Figure 6.8). Equally striking may be the relative sparing of the peri-areolar and axillary skin. The generalized plaques, although otherwise rather like psoriasis,

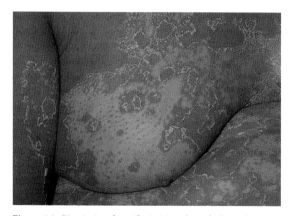

Figure 6.8 Pityriasis rubra pilaris. Note the red plugged follicles, seen even in the 'spared' areas.

may also show follicular plugging. The palms and soles become thickened, smooth and yellow. Fissures are common there. The nails also thicken, because of an accumulation of keratin under them without pitting of the nail plate (cf. psoriasis), appearing as 'half and half' nails (p. 315). The scalp becomes covered with fine bran-like scales in contrast to the larger scales of psoriasis and the greasier ones of seborrhoeic dermatitis. The ability to sweat is often impaired. Pityriasis rubra pilaris in childhood is similar to the adult disease, but tends to start on the lower part of the body. Onset is usually between 5 and 10 years of age and it develops slowly in the familial form, and more rapidly in the acquired. A circumscribed juvenile type affects the palms and soles, and fronts of the knees and backs of the elbows in younger children.

Course

The most common acquired form generally resolves within 3 years, but may recur. Even when the plaques have gone, the skin may retain a rough scaly texture with persistent small scattered follicular plugs. Acquired generalized childhood pityriasis rubra pilaris has a better prognosis and usually resolves within a couple of years. The familial type, developing in childhood, persists throughout life. The juvenile circumscribed type usually clears in the teens.

Complications

There are usually few complications although ectropion may be a problem. Accompanying arthritis, as seen in psoriasis, is not a feature. Erythroderma (see *Erythroderma/exfoliative dermatitis*) causes the patients to tolerate cold poorly.

Differential diagnosis

Psoriasis is the disorder closest in appearance to pityriasis rubra pilaris, but lacks its slightly orange tinge. The thickening of the palms and soles, the follicular erythema in islands of uninvolved skin, and follicular plugging within the plaques, especially over the knuckles, are other features, besides those mentioned already, that help to separate them.

Investigations

A biopsy may help to distinguish psoriasis from pityriasis rubra pilaris. There are no polymorphonuclear leucocyte micro-abscesses of Munro, less parakeratosis and broader rete pegs in pityriasis rubra pilaris. Even so, the two disorders share many histological features.

Treatment

Most patients require copious topical treatment and many prefer this to systemic treatment. Emollients (Formulary 1, p. 397) and keratolytics (Formulary 1, p. 401) for the palms and soles are the mainstay of this. About 50% of patients respond slowly to systemic retinoids such as acitretin (in adults, 25–50 mg/day for 6–8 months; p. 420). Oral methotrexate in low doses, taken once a week, may also help a similar percentage (p. 419). In contrast to psoriasis, phototherapy does not help much unless given concomitantly with orally administered retinoids. A growing number of reports show benefit from the tumour necrosis factor α (TNFα) inhibitors infliximab, etanercept and adalimumab, but comparative clinical trials have not yet been performed. Systemic steroids are not indicated.

Parapsoriasis and premycotic eruption

Parapsoriasis is a contentious term, which many would like to drop. We still find it useful clinically for lesions that look a little like psoriasis but which scale subtly rather than grossly, and which persist despite antipsoriasis treatment. It is worth trying to distinguish a benign type of parapsoriasis from a *premycotic* type, which is a forerunner of cutaneous T-cell lymphoma (mycosis fungoides) (Figure 6.9), although they can look alike early in their development. Clonality of infiltrating lymphocytes suggest that these lesions are mycosis fungoides right from the start. Many prefer to call this form of parapsoriasis *patch stage cutaneous T-cell lymphoma*, particularly if there is lymphocyte clonality in the patches and plaques (p. 307).

Cause

The cause is otherwise unknown.

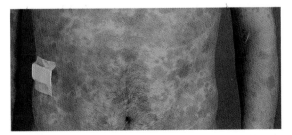

Figure 6.9 A bizarre eruption: its persistence and variable colour suggested a prelymphomatous eruption. Biopsy confirmed this.

Table 6.3 Distinguishing features of parapsoriasis and premycotic/prelymphomatous eruptions.

Parapsoriasis (benign type)	Premycotic/prelymphomatous eruptions
Smaller plaques	Larger
Yellowish	Not yellow – pink, slightly violet, or brown
Sometimes finger-shaped lesions	Asymmetrical with bizarre outline running around the trunk
No atrophy	Atrophy ± poikiloderma
Responds to UVB	Responds better to PUVA
Remains benign although rarely	May progress to a cutaneous T-cell lymphoma clears

Presentation

Pink scaly well-marginated plaques appear, typically on the buttocks, breasts, abdomen or flexural skin. Often they are large and irregularly shaped, and develop asymmetrically. The clinical features that distinguish the small-plaque (benign) and large-plaque (premycotic/prelymphomatous) types are given in Table 6.3. Perhaps the most important point is the presence of poikiloderma (atrophy, telangiectasia and reticulate pigmentation) in the latter type. Both conditions are stubborn in their response to topical treatment, although often responding temporarily to phototherapy. Itching is variable.

Complications

Patients with suspected premycotic/prelymphomatous eruptions should be followed up carefully, even though a cutaneous T-cell lymphoma may not develop for years. If poikiloderma or induration develops, the diagnosis of a cutaneous T-cell lymphoma becomes likely.

Differential diagnosis

This includes psoriasis, tinea and nummular (discoid) eczema. In contrast to psoriasis and pityriasis rosea, the lesions of parapsoriasis, characteristically, are asymmetrical. Topical steroids can cause atrophy and confusion.

Investigations

Several biopsies should be taken if a premycotic eruption is suspected, if possible from thick or atrophic untreated areas. These may suggest an early cutaneous T-cell lymphoma, with bizarre mononuclear cells both in the dermis and in microscopic abscesses within the epidermis. T-cell receptor gene rearrangement studies (p. 20) can determine clonality of the T cells within the lymphoid infiltrate, and in combination with immunophenotyping helps to differentiate benign parapsoriasis from premycotic/prelymphomatous eruptions. Staging studies rarely disclose lymphoma of nodes or internal organs at this stage, but it may be worth feeling for lymphadenopathy and hepatosplenolomegaly. In the same spirit, some experts advocate baseline tomography, chest roentgenography, blood counts and determinations of lactic dehydrogenase levels.

Treatment
Treatment is symptomatic and does not appear to slow down or prevent the frequency of development of any subsequent cutaneous T-cell lymphoma. Usually, moderately potent steroids or ultraviolet radiation bring some resolution, although topical steroids should be used cautiously where there is atrophic skin.

Pityriasis lichenoides

Pityriasis lichenoides is uncommon. It can be precipitated by infection which may precipitate proliferation and skin recruitment of cytotoxic CD8$^+$ T cells. It occurs in two forms (both Latin mouthfuls) at each end of a spectrum that, more often than not, includes patients with overlapping features.
• **Pityriasis lichenoides et varioliformis acuta.** This acute type is characterized by crops of papules that become necrotic and leave scars like those of chickenpox. They rarely affect the face and the rash, which lasts much longer than chickenpox, is usually scattered on the trunk and limbs.
• **Pityriasis lichenoides chronica.** The numerous small circular scaly macules and papules of the chronic type are easy to confuse with guttate psoriasis (p. 55). However, their scaling is distinctive in that single silver-grey scales (mica scales) surmount the lesions. The rash usually grumbles on for months or, rarely, years.

Treatment
Long-term antibiotics (tetracycline or erythromycin) have their advocates and UVB radiation can reduce

the number of lesions. Spontaneous resolution occurs eventually.

Other papulosquamous diseases

Discoid lupus erythematosus is typically papulosquamous; it is discussed with subacute cutaneous lupus erythematosus in Chapter 10. Fungus infections are nummular and scaly and can appear papulosquamous or eczematous; they are dealt with in Chapter 16. Seborrhoeic and nummular discoid eczema are discussed in Chapter 7. Secondary syphilis is discussed in Chapter 16.

Erythroderma/exfoliative dermatitis

Sometimes the whole skin becomes red and scaly (see Figure 5.13). The disorders that can cause this are listed in Table 6.4. The best clue to the underlying cause is a history of a previous skin disease. Sometimes, the histology is helpful but often it is non-specific. *Erythroderma* is the term used when the skin is red with little or no scaling, while the term *exfoliative dermatitis* is preferred if scaling predominates. In dark skin the presence of pigment may mask the erythema, giving a purplish hue.

Most patients have lymphadenopathy, and many have hepatomegaly as well. If the condition becomes chronic, tightness of the facial skin leads to ectropion, scalp and body hair may be lost, and the nails become thickened and may be shed too. Temperature regulation is impaired and heat loss through the skin usually makes the patient feel cold and shiver. Oedema, high output cardiac failure, tachycardia, anaemia, failure to sweat and

Table 6.4 Some causes of erythroderma/exfoliative dermatitis.

Psoriasis
Pityriasis rubra pilaris
Ichthyosiform erythroderma
Pemphigus erythematosus
Contact, atopic, or seborrhoeic eczema
Reiter's syndrome
Lymphoma (including the Sézary syndrome)
Drug eruptions
Crusted (Norwegian) scabies

dehydration can occur. Treatment is that of the underlying condition.

Learning points

The dangers of erythroderma are the following.
1 Poor temperature regulation.
2 High-output cardiac failure.
3 Protein deficiency.

Further reading

Chuh AA, Dofitas BL, Comisel GG, *et al.* (2007) Interventions for pityriasis rosea. *Cochrane Database of Systematic Reviews* **2**, CD005068.

Drago F, Broccolo F, Rebora A. (2009) Pityriasis rosea: an update with a critical appraisal of its possible herpesviral etiology. *Journal of the American Academy of Dermatology* **61**, 303–318.

Klein A, Landthaler M, Karrer S. (2010) Pityriasis rubra pilaris: a review of diagnosis and treatment. *American Journal of Clinical Dermatology* **11**, 157–170.

Le Cleach L, Chosidow O. (2012) Clinical practice. Lichen planus. *New England Journal of Medicine* **366**, 723–732.

Lehman JS, Tollefson MM, Gibson LE. (2009) Lichen planus. *International Journal of Dermatology* **48**, 682–694.

Lodi G, Carrozzo M, Furness S, Thongprasom K. (2012) Interventions for treating oral lichen planus: a systematic review. *British Journal of Dermatology* **166**, 938–947.

Sarveswari KN, Yesudian P. (2009) The conundrum of parapsoriasis versus patch stage of mycosis fungoides. *Indian Journal of Dermatology, Venereology and Leprology* **75**, 229–235.

Scarisbrick JJ. (2006) Staging and management of cutaneous T cell lymphoma. *Clinical and Experimental Dermatology* **31**, 181–186.

7 Eczema and Dermatitis

The disorders grouped under this heading are the most common skin conditions seen by family doctors, and make up some 20% of all new patients referred to our clinics.

The eczemas are a disparate group of diseases, but unified by the presence of itch and in the acute stages, of oedema (spongiosis) in the epidermis. In early disease the stratum corneum remains intact, so the eczema appears as a red smooth oedematous plaque. With worsening disease the oedema becomes more severe, tense blisters appear on the plaques, or they may weep plasma. If less severe or if the eczema becomes chronic, scaling and epithelial disruption occurs, giving chronic eczemas a characteristic appearance. All these are phases of the reaction pattern are known as *eczema*.

Terminology

The word eczema comes from the Greek for 'boiling' – a reference to the tiny vesicles (bubbles) that are often seen in the early acute stages of the disorder, but less often in its later chronic stages. Dermatitis means inflammation of the skin and is therefore, strictly speaking, a broader term than eczema – which is just one of several possible types of skin inflammation.

To further complicate matters, the classification of eczemas is a messy legacy from a time when little was known about the subject. Some are given names based on etiology, for example irritant contact dermatitis, and venous eczema. Others are based on the appearance of lesions (e.g. discoid eczema and hyperkeratotic eczema), while still others are classified by site (e.g. flexural eczema and hand eczema) or age (e.g. infantile eczema and senile eczema). These classifications invite overlap. However, until the causes of all eczemas are clear, both students and dermatologists are stuck with the time-honoured, yet muddled, nomenclature (Table 7.1) that we use here.

A rational subdivision of dermatitis into exogenous (or contact) and endogenous (or constitutional) types has recently been formalized by the World Allergy Organization into the classification shown in Table 7.2 although this is not widely used.

> **Learning point**
>
> 'When I use a word it means just what I choose it to mean' said Humpty Dumpty. Choose to make the words eczema and dermatitis mean the same to you.

Pathogenesis

Inflammation is the hallmark of all eczemas. The skin is a large and complex organ and exposed to all the existential hazards of the environment. Unsuprisingly, there has evolved a sophisticated array of innate and acquired immune defences. Different challenges will produce different responses and types of eczema, described in more detail below. Common to all eczemas is an interaction between precipitating factors, keratinocytes and T lymphocyes. In allergic contact dermatitis (ACD) an initial exposure to an allergen, involves antigen-processing Langerhans and dermal dendritic cells carrying the antigen to the regional lymph nodes and presenting it to naïve T cells. On subsequent exposure, $CD8^+$ cytotoxic T cells are activated and release Th1 cytokines including γ-interferon (IFN-γ). These T cells express Fas ligand on their surface and release the cytotoxins perforin and granzyme-B. Simultaneously, and stimulated by IFN-γ exposure, keratinocytes express Fas, major histocompatibility complex Class II (MHC-II) molecules and intercellular adhesion molecule 1 (ICAM-1) on their surface. This potent combination of factors leads to keratinocyte apoptosis, spongiosis and further chemokine

Clinical Dermatology, Fifth Edition. Richard B. Weller, Hamish J.A. Hunter and Margaret W. Mann.
© 2015 John Wiley & Sons, Ltd. Published 2015 by John Wiley & Sons, Ltd.

Table 7.1 Eczema: a working classification.

Mainly caused by exogenous (contact) factors	Irritant
	Allergic
	Photodermatitis (see Chapter 18)
Other types of eczema	Atopic
	Seborrhoeic
	Discoid (nummular)
	Pompholyx
	Gravitational (venous, stasis)
	Asteatotic
	Neurodermatitis
	Juvenile plantar dermatosis
	Napkin (diaper) dermatitis

release which perpetuates the infiltration of inflammatory cells. In atopic eczema, skin barrier defects (p. 10) probably allow enhanced allergen penetrations. In contrast to ACD, CD4+ helper T cells predominate, displaying a Th2 profile of cytokine release in acute lesions, but progressing to Th2 with time. Ultimately, similar histological changes are seen in the skin of atopic patients as in allergic and irritant eczemas.

Histology

The clinical appearance of the different stages of eczema mirrors their histology. In the acute stage, oedema in the epidermis (spongiosis) progresses to the formation of intraepidermal vesicles, which may coalesce into larger blisters or rupture. The chronic stages of eczema show less spongiosis and vesication but more thickening of the prickle cell layer (acanthosis) and horny layers (hyperker-

Table 7.2 Dermatitis: World Allergy Organization classification.

Eczema
  Atopic
  Non-atopic
Contact dermatitis
  Allergic
  Non-allergic (irritant)
Other types of dermatitis
  e.g. nummular, photosensitive, seborrhoeic

atosis and parakeratosis). These changes are accompanied by a variable degree of vasodilatation and infiltration with lymphocytes.

Clinical appearance

The different types of eczema have their own distinguishing marks, and these will be dealt with later; most share certain general features, which it is convenient to consider here. The absence of a sharp margin is a particularly important feature that separates eczema from most papulosquamous eruptions. Other distinguishing features are epithelial disruption (Figure 7.1) shown by coalescing vesicles, bullae and oedematous papules on pink plaques, and a tendency for intense itching.

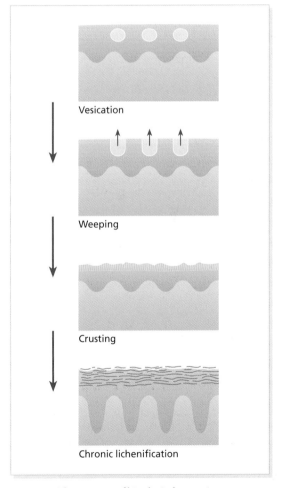

Vesication

Weeping

Crusting

Chronic lichenification

Figure 7.1 The sequence of histological events in eczema.

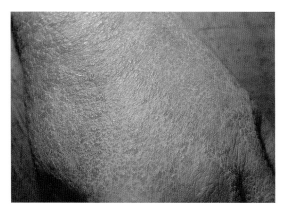

Figure 7.2 Acute vesicular contact eczema of the hand.

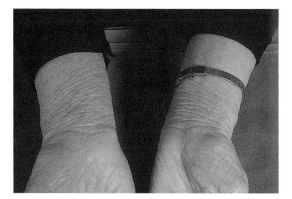

Figure 7.4 Lichenification of the wrists – note also the increased skin markings on the palms (atopic palms).

Acute eczema

Acute eczema (Figures 7.2 and 7.3) is recognized by:
- Weeping and crusting;
- Blistering – usually with vesicles but, in fierce cases, with large blisters;
- Redness, papules and swelling – usually with an ill-defined border; and
- Scaling.

Chronic eczema

Chronic eczema may show all of the above changes but is, in general:
- Less vesicular and exudative;
- More scaly, pigmented and thickened;
- More likely to show lichenification (Figures 7.4 and 7.5) – a dry leathery thickened state, with increased skin markings, secondary to repeated scratching or rubbing; and
- More likely to fissure.

Complications

Heavy bacterial colonization is common in all types of eczema but overt infection is most troublesome in the seborrhoeic, nummular and atopic types. Local superimposed allergic reactions to medicaments can provoke dissemination, especially in gravitational eczema.

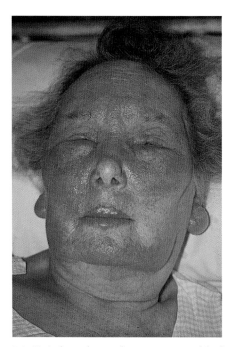

Figure 7.3 Vesicular and crusted contact eczema of the face (cosmetic allergy).

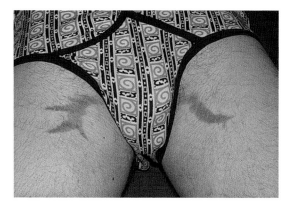

Figure 7.5 Stretch marks following the use of too potent topical steroids to the groin.

All severe forms of eczema have a huge effect on the quality of life. An itchy sleepless child can wreck family life. Eczema can interfere with work, sporting activities and sex lives. Jobs can be lost through it.

Differential diagnosis

This falls into two halves. First, eczema has to be separated from other skin conditions that look like it. Table 7.3 plots a way through this maze. Always remember that eczemas are scaly, with poorly defined margins. They also exhibit features of epidermal disruption such as weeping, crust, excoriation, fissures and yellow scale (due to plasma coating the scale). Papulosquamous dermatoses, such as psoriasis or lichen planus are sharply defined and show no signs of epidermal disruption.

Occasionally a biopsy is helpful in confirming a diagnosis of eczema, but it will not determine the cause or type. Once the diagnosis of eczema becomes solid, look for clinical pointers towards an external cause. This determines both the need for investigations and the best line of treatment. Sometimes an eruption will follow one of the well-known patterns of eczema, such as the way atopic

Table 7.3 Is the rash eczematous?

Atypical physical signs? Could be eczema but consider other erythematosquamous eruptions. ↓				
Sharply marginated, strong colour, very scaly? Points of elbows and knees involved? ↓No	Yes →	Likely to be psoriasis (see Chapter 5)	→	Can be confused with seborrhoeic eczema and neurodermatitis on the scalp, with seborrhoeic eczema in the flexures and discoid eczema on the limbs. Look for confirmatory nail and joint changes. Ask about family history.
Itchy social contacts? Face spared? Burrows found? Genitals and nipples affected? ↓No	Yes →	This is scabies (p. 253)	→	Ensure all contacts are treated adequately – whether itchy or not.
Mouth lesions? Violaceous tinge? Shiny flat topped papules? ↓No	Yes →	Could be lichen planus (p. 69)	→	Also consider lichenoid drug eruptions.
Annular lesions with active scaly edges? ↓No	Yes →	Probably a fungal infection (see Chapter 16	→	More likely if the rash affects the groin, or is asymmetrical, perhaps affecting the palm of one hand only; and not doing well with topical steroids. Look at scales, cleared with potassium hydroxide, under a microscope or send scrapings to mycology laboratory. Check for contact with animals and for thickened toe nails.
Localized to palms and soles? Obvious pustules? ↓No	Yes →	Probably palmoplantar pustulosis (p. 56)	→	Expect poor response to most topical treatments.
Unusually swollen; on the face? ↓No	Yes →	Consider angioedema (p. 99) or erysipelas (p. 217)	→	Needs rapid treatment with antihistamines or antibiotics.
Consider dermatitis herpetiformis, not the various pityriases (rosea, versicolor and rubra pilaris) and drug eruptions (see Chapter 25).	Yes →			

eczema picks out the skin behind the knees, and a diagnosis can then be made readily enough. Often, however, this is not the case, and the history then becomes especially important.

A contact element is likely if:
• There is obvious contact with known irritants or allergens;
• The eruption clears when the patient goes on holiday, or at the weekends;
• The eczema is asymmetrical, or has a linear or rectilinear configuration; or
• The rash picks out the eyelids, external ear canals, hands and feet, the skin around stasis ulcers, or the peri-anal skin.

Learning point

Time spent thinking about contact factors may well help even those patients with the most blatantly 'constitutional' types of eczema.

Investigations

Each pattern of eczema needs a different line of enquiry.

Exogenous eczema

Exogenous eczemas can be irritant or allergic. They are diagnosed predominantly on the distribution, which suggests contact with a precipitating factor. Irritant eczemas are a result of agents that produce keratinocyte damage without immunological memory. Allergic contact dermatitis is a type IV delayed type hypersensitivity reaction involving sensitization and then elicitation. Thus, the main decision when investigating an exogenous eczema is whether to undertake patch testing (p. 38) to confirm allergic contact dermatitis and to identify the allergens responsible. In patch testing, standardized non-irritating concentrations of common allergens are applied to the normal skin of the back. If the patient is allergic to the allergen, eczema will develop at the site of contact after 48–96 hours. Patch testing with irritants is of no value in any type of eczema, but testing with suitably diluted allergens is essential in suspected allergic contact eczema. The technique is not easy. Its problems include separating irritant from allergic patch test reactions, and picking the right allergens to test. If legal issues depend on the results, testing should be carried out by a dermatologist who will have the standard equipment and a suitable selection of properly standardized allergens (see Figure 3.8). Patch testing can be used to confirm a suspected allergy or, by the use of a battery of common sensitizers, to discover unsuspected allergies, which then have to be assessed in the light of the history and the clinical picture. A visit to the home or workplace may help with this.

Photopatch testing is more specialized and facilities are only available in a few centres. A chemical is applied to the skin for 24 hours and then the site is irradiated with a suberythema dose of ultraviolet irradiation; the patches are inspected for an eczematous reaction 48 hours later.

Other types of eczema

The only indication for patch testing here is when an added contact allergic element is suspected. This is most common in gravitational eczema; neomycin, framycetin, lanolin or preservative allergy can perpetuate the condition and even trigger dissemination. Ironically, rubber gloves, so often used to protect eczematous hands, can themselves sensitize.

The role of prick testing in atopic eczema is discussed on p. 39.

The presence of a raised level of immunoglobulin E (IgE) antibodies is necessary to make a diagnosis of atopic eczema under the new World Allergy Organization criteria (Table 7.2) but this information only rarely affects management and is thus not routinely carried out in our practice. If the patient also has asthma or allergic rhinitis, the test results may be misleading even though they do tend to indicate an atopic state. Total and specific IgE antibodies are measured by a fluorescence enzyme labelled test (ImmunoCAP). Prick and ImmunoCAP testing give similar results but many now prefer the more expensive ImmunoCAP test as it carries no risk of anaphylaxis, is easier to perform and is less time consuming. Although not all children with atopic eczema have elevated IgE levels, those that do are more likely to have eczema persisting into adult life, and are also more likely to develop asthma.

If the eczema is worsening despite treatment, or if there is much crusting, bacterial superinfection may be present. *Staphylococcus aureus* is the most common cause of an infective flare in atopic eczema and background colonisation with *S. aureus* is found in around 90% of patients with atopic eczema. Staphylococcal superantigen enhances Th2 responses and it also releases a number of proteases that damage the skin barrier. Treatment of *S. aureus* induced flares with appropriate antibiotics – usually flucloxacillin or erythromycin – helps bring the disease back under control. Scrapings for microscopical examination (p. 37) and culture for fungus will rule out tinea if there is clinical doubt – as in some cases of discoid eczema.

Finally, malabsorption should be considered in otherwise unexplained widespread pigmented atypical patterns of endogenous eczema.

Treatment

Topical treatment

Topical treatment of eczema relies on two components: emollients and anti-inflammatory agents. The importance of emollients has been underscored by the growing understanding of the relevance of defects in the skin barrier to the aetiology of eczema. Emollients should be used daily and in generous quantities by eczema patients. A good rule of thumb is that 10 times as much emollient should be prescribed (and used!) as corticosteroid. For chronic eczema with dry skin, emollient ointments such as soft white/liquid paraffin mix, or emulsifying ointment should be used. For acute inflammatory eczemas emollient creams such as Aveeno, Diprobase or Oilatum are preferred (Formulary 1, p. 397). Strong soaps should be avoided as they can be irritant and impair the skin barrier. Aqueous cream or emulsifying ointment can be used in their place. Aqueous cream should be avoided as a leave on emollient as it contains the detergent sodium laurel sulfate which damages the skin barrier and can worsen eczema.

The inflammation of eczema needs treatment with topical corticosteroids or calcineurin inhibitors. The potency of corticosteroids is graded as mild, moderate, potent and very potent (Formulary 1, p. 401) and the strength used is determined by age, body site and severity of eczema. The major side effect of corticosteroids is epidermal atrophy (Figure 7.6), but by avoiding use of too potent a steroid for too long this can be avoided. An inadequately strong preparation will not settle the eczema and should equally be avoided. Nothing stronger than 0.5 or 1% hydrocortisone ointment should be used in infancy. In adults, only mild corticosteroids, or moderately potent ones for no more than 1 week should be used for treatment of the face. On the body in adults, moderately potent or potent steroid creams will be needed. The hands and feet have a thick stratum corneum and weaker steroid creams produce little benefit. Very potent steroids should be reserved for use at these sites or for short periods of time on the body when severe eczema is difficult to bring under control. Corticosteroids should be applied once daily to eczema, increasing to twice daily if it fails to improve. The quantities needed for once daily application to different body sites are shown

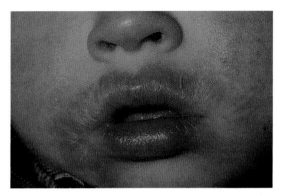

Figure 7.6 Licking the lips as a nervous habit has caused this characteristic pattern of dry fissured irritant eczema.

in Table 26.4 (p. 364). If patients are suffering from more than three or four flares of eczema per year, a good trick is to apply corticosteroids to previously affected body sites on two days of the week during remissions. This reduces the number of flares of eczema and thus overall long-term steroid use and such twice weekly steroid application is unlikely to induce atrophy. Emollients should be used at least twice daily, and this should continue during remissions.

The topical calcineurin inhibitors pimecrolimus and tacrolimus have the advantage of not inducing skin atrophy. Tacrolimus (Formulary 1, p. 403) is a macrolide immunosuppressant produced by a streptomycete. The anti-inflammatory actions of 0.1% tacrolimus are similar to a potent corticosteroid. Pimecrolimus (Formulary 1, p. 403) is another topical immunosuppressant and a derivative of askamycin, but has less anti-inflammatory actions than moderate topical corticosteroids. Tacrolimus is particularly useful in adult patients with facial eczema which is failing to respond do mild or moderate corticosteroids and can also be used in eczema on the body where long-term potent corticosteroids would be needed to maintain control. Pimecrolimus and.03% tacrolimus can be used in children. As with corticosteroids, twice weekly use of tacrolimus during periods of remission extends the time to relapse. Patients should be advised to avoid excessive exposure to sunlight or UV lamps while using tacrolimus.

Systemic treatment

If topical treatment fails to control eczema, systemic treatment or phototherapy may be needed. Short courses of systemic steroids can occasionally be justified in extremely acute and severe eczema, particularly when the cause is known and already eliminated (e.g. allergic contact dermatitis from a plant such as poison ivy). However, prolonged systemic steroid treatment should be avoided in chronic cases, particularly in atopic eczema. Hydroxyzine, doxepin, alimemazine and other antihistamines (Formulary 2, p. 415) may help at night. Systemic antibiotics may be needed in widespread bacterial superinfection. *Staphylococcus aureus* routinely colonizes all weeping eczemas and most dry ones as well. Simply isolating it does not automatically prompt a prescription for an antibiotic, although if the density of organisms is high, usually manifest as extensive crusting, then systemic antibiotics can help.

For longer term systemic management, patients with moderate to severe eczema can benefit from the purine analogue azathioprine (Formulary 2. p. 418). Relatively common polymorphisms in the gene coding for thiopurine methyltransferase (TPMT) lead to low or absent levels of this azathioprine metabolizing enzyme. TPMT levels must thus be checked before starting azathioprine to determine in whom the drug must be avoided because of absent activity, and in whom lower doses should be given because of low activity.

Severe and unresponsive cases may be helped by short courses of ciclosporin under specialist supervision (Formulary 2, p. 418). Short (6-week) courses may induce long-term remission in adults, but in children continuous therapy is usually needed.

For chronic hand eczema that is not responding to potent topical corticosteroids, alitretinoin is the only licensed systemic treatment. It clears hand eczema in almost half of patients, but should be discontinued if there has been no improvement after the first 12 weeks of treatment. Like all systemic retinoids it is highly teratogenic and should be prescribed with great caution in women of childbearing years.

Phototherapy with UVB, or narrowband UVB is effective for widespread eczema. For hand or foot eczema, local PUVA can be given (see Chapter 27).

Acute weeping eczema

This does best with rest and liquid applications. Non-steroidal preparations are helpful and the techniques used will vary with the facilities available and the site of the lesions. In general practice, a simple and convenient way of dealing with weeping eczema of the hands or feet is to use thrice daily 10-minute soaks in a cool 0.65% aluminium acetate solution (Formulary 1, p. 398) – saline or even tap water will do almost as well – each soaking being followed by a smear of a corticosteroid cream and the

application of a non-stick dressing or cotton gloves. One reason for dropping the dilute potassium permanganate solution that was once so popular is because it stains the skin and nails brown.

Wider areas on the trunk respond well to corticosteroid creams. However, traditional remedies such as exposure and frequent applications of calamine lotion, and the use of half-strength magenta paint for the flexures are also effective.

An experienced doctor or nurse can teach patients how to use wet dressings, and supervise this. The aluminium acetate solution, saline or water can be applied on cotton gauze, under a polythene covering, and changed twice daily. Details of wet wrap techniques are given below. Rest at home will help too.

Wet wrap dressings

This is a labour-intensive but highly effective technique, of value in the treatment of troublesome atopic eczema in children. After a bath, a corticosteroid is applied to the skin and then covered with two layers of tubular dressing – the inner layer already soaked in warm water, the outer layer being applied dry. Cotton pyjamas or a T-shirt can be used to cover these, and the dressings can then be left in place for several hours. The corticosteroid may be one that is rapidly metabolized after systemic absorption such as a beclometasone diproprionate ointment diluted to 0.025%. Alternatives include 1% or 2.5% hydrocortisone cream for children and 0.025% or 0.1% triamcinolone cream for adults. The bandages can be washed and reused. The evaporation of fluid from the bandages cools the skin and provides rapid relief of itching. With improvement, the frequency of the dressings can be cut down and a moisturizer can be substituted for the corticosteroid. Parents can be taught the technique by a trained nurse, who must follow up treatment closely. Parents easily learn how to modify the technique to suit the needs of their own child. Side effects seem to be minimal.

Subacute eczema

Steroid lotions or creams are the mainstay of treatment; their strength is determined by the severity of the attack. The yellow crust and yellow scales suggest impetigo, and *Staphylococcus aureus* can be routinely isolated from most lesions. Frank infection, requiring systemic antibiotic treatment is suggested by sudden worsening, cellulitis, pustule formation, weeping and crusting. Flucloxacillin, or erythromycin in the penicillin-allergic patient, is usually a sensible first-line antibiotic, but microbial swabs will confirm antibiotic sensitivity and also whether other bacterial infections with for example Streptococci are complicating the eczema. Bacitracin, fusidic acid, mupirocin or neomycin (Formulary 1, p. 401) can be incorporated into the topical treatment if an infective element is present, but watch out for sensitization to neomycin, especially when treating gravitational eczema.

Chronic eczema

This responds best to steroids in an ointment base, but is also often helped by non-steroid applications such as ichthammol and zinc cream or paste.

Bacterial superinfection may need systemic antibiotics but can often be controlled by the incorporation of antibiotics (e.g. fusidic acid, mupirocin, neomycin or chlortetracycline) or antiseptics (e.g. Vioform) into the steroid formulation. Many proprietary mixtures of this type are available in the United Kingdom. Chronic localized hyperkeratotic eczema of the palms or soles can be helped by salicylic acid (1–6% in emulsifying ointment) or stabilized urea preparations (Formulary 1, p. 401).

Common patterns of eczema

Irritant contact dermatitis

This accounts for more than 80% of all cases of contact dermatitis, and for the vast majority of industrial cases. However, it can also occur in children (e.g. as a reaction to a bubble bath, play dough or lip-licking; Figure 7.6).

Cause

Strong irritants elicit an acute reaction after brief contact and the diagnosis is then usually obvious. Prolonged exposure, sometimes over years, is needed for weak irritants to cause dermatitis, usually of the hands and forearms (Figure 7.7). Water, detergents, chemicals, solvents, cutting oils and abrasive dusts are common culprits. There is a wide range of susceptibility; those with very dry skin are especially vulnerable. Past or present atopic dermatitis doubles the risk of irritant hand eczema developing.

Course

The need to continue at work, or with housework, often stops the skin regaining its normal barrier function. Even under ideal circumstances this may take several months. All too often therefore irritant eczema, probably reversible in the early stages, becomes chronic.

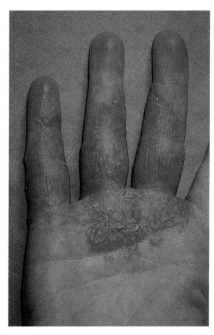

Figure 7.7 Typical chronic hand eczema – irritants have played a part here.

Complications

The condition may lead to loss of work.

Differential diagnosis

It is often hard to differentiate irritant from allergic contact dermatitis, and from atopic eczema of the hands – the more so as atopic patients are especially prone to develop irritant eczema.

Investigations

Patch testing with irritants is not helpful and may be misleading; but patch testing to a battery of common allergens (p. 38) is worthwhile if an allergic element is suspected. Even if the results are negative, patch testing is not a waste of time, and provides a valuable opportunity to educate patients about their condition.

Treatment

Management is based upon avoidance of the irritants responsible for the condition, but often this is not possible and the best that can be achieved is reduced exposure by the use of protective gloves and clothing. The factory doctor or nurse can often advise here. Washing facilities at work should be good. Barrier creams seldom help established cases, and dirty hands should not be cleaned with harsh solvents.

Prevention is better than cure because, once started, irritant eczema can persist long after contact with offending substances has ceased, despite the vigorous use of emollients and topical corticosteroids. Vulnerable people should be advised to avoid jobs that carry an especially heavy exposure to skin irritants (Table 7.5). If the right person can be placed in the right job, fewer trainee hairdressers and mechanics will find out the hard way that their skins are easily irritated. Moderately potent topical corticosteroids and emollients are valuable, but are secondary to the avoidance of irritants and protective measures.

Allergic contact dermatitis

Cause
The mechanism is that of delayed (type IV) hypersensitivity (p. 25). It has the following features.
• Previous contact is needed to induce allergy.
• It is specific to one chemical and its close relatives.
• After allergy has been established, all areas of skin will react to the allergen.
• Sensitization persists indefinitely.
• Desensitization is seldom possible.

Allergens
In an ideal world, allergens would be replaced by less harmful substances, and some attempts are already being made to achieve this. A whole new industry has arisen around the need for predictive patch testing before new substances or cosmetics are let out into the community. Similarly, chrome allergy is less of a problem now in enlightened countries that insist on adding ferrous sulfate to cement to reduce its water-soluble chromate content. However, contact allergens will never be abolished completely and family doctors still need to know about the most common ones and where to find them (Table 7.4). It is not possible to guess which substances are likely to sensitize just by looking at their formulae. In fact, most allergens are relatively simple chemicals that have to bind to protein to become 'complete' antigens. Their ability to sensitize varies – from substances that can do so after a single exposure (e.g. poison ivy), to those that need prolonged exposure (e.g. chrome – bricklayers take an average of 10 years to become allergic to it).

Presentation and clinical course
The original site of the eruption gives a clue to the likely allergen but secondary spread may later obscure this. Easily recognizable patterns exist. Nickel allergy, for example,

gives rise to eczema under jewellery, bra clips and jean studs (Figure 7.8). The lax skin of the eyelids and genitalia is especially likely to become oedematous. Possible allergens are numerous and to spot the less common ones in the environment needs specialist knowledge. Table 7.4 lists some common allergens and their distribution.

Allergic contact dermatitis should be suspected if:
1 Certain areas are involved (e.g. the eyelids, external auditory meati, hands (Figure 7.9) or feet, and around gravitational ulcers);
2 There is known contact with the allergens mentioned in Table 7.4; or
3 The individual's work carries a high risk (e.g. hairdressing, working in a flower shop, or dentistry).

Investigations
Questioning should cover both occupational and domestic exposure to allergens. The indications for patch testing are discussed on p. 38. Techniques are constantly improving and dermatologists will have access to a battery of common allergens, suitably diluted in a bland vehicle. These are applied in aluminium cups held in position on the skin for 2–3 days by tape. Patch testing will often start with a standard series (battery) of allergens whose selection is based on local experience. Table 7.4 shows the battery used by the authors and how it helps with the most common types of contact allergy. This picks up some 80% of reactions. Extra series of relevant allergens will be used for problems such as hand eczema, leg ulcers and suspected cosmetic allergy, and for those in jobs like dentistry or hairdressing, which carry unusual risks. Some allergies are more common than others. In most centres, nickel tops the list, with a positive reaction in some 15% of those tested; fragrance allergy usually comes second. It is important to remember that positive reactions are not necessarily relevant to the patient's current skin problem: some are simply 'immunological scars' left behind by previous unrelated problems.

Treatment
Topical corticosteroids give temporary relief, but far more important is avoidance of the relevant allergen. Reducing exposure is usually not enough: active steps have to be taken to avoid the allergen completely. Job changes are sometimes needed to achieve this. Even then, other factors may come into play; for example, some believe that reactions to nickel can be kept going by nickel in the diet, released from cans or steel saucepans, as changes in diet and cooking utensils may rarely be helpful.

Table 7.4 The allergens in our battery and what they mean.

Allergen	Common sources	Comments
Metals		
The classic metal allergy for men is still to chrome, present in cement. In the past, more women than men have been allergic to nickel but the current fashion for men to have their ears and other parts of their body pierced is changing this.		
Chrome	Cement; chromium plating processes; antirust paints; tattoos (green) and some leathers. Sensitization follows contact with chrome salts rather than chromium metal.	A common problem for building site workers. In Scandinavia, putting iron sulfate into cement has been shown to reduce its allergenicity by making the chrome salts insoluble.
Nickel	Nickel-plated objects, especially cheap jewellery. Remember jean studs.	The best way of becoming sensitive is to pierce your ears. Nickel is being taken out of some good costume jewellery. Stainless steel is relatively safe.
Cobalt	A contaminant of nickel and occurs with it.	Eruption similar to that of nickel allergy. The main allergen for those with metal on metal arthroplasties.
Cosmetics		
Despite attempts to design 'hypoallergenic' cosmetics, allergic reactions are still seen. The most common culprits are fragrances, followed by preservatives, dyes and lanolin.		
Fragrance mix	An infinite variety of cosmetics, sprays and toiletries.	Any perfume will contain many ingredients. This convenient mix picks up some 80% of perfume allergies. Some perfume allergic subjects also react to balsam of Peru, tars or colophony.
Balsam of Peru	Used in some scented cosmetics. Also in some spices and suppositories (e.g. Anusol).	May indicate allergy to perfumes also. Can cross-react with colophony, orange peel, cinnamon and benzyl benzoate.
Paraphenylene diamine (PPD)	Dark dyes for hair and clothing.	Few heed the manufacturer's warning to patch test themselves before dyeing their hair. May cross-react with other chemicals containing the 'para' group (e.g. some local anaesthetics, sulfonamides or para-aminobenzoic acid, in some sunscreens).
Wool alcohols	Anything with lanolin in it.	Common cause of reactions to cosmetics and topical medicaments. The newer purified lanolins cause fewer problems.
Cetosteryl alcohol	Emollient, and base for many cosmetics.	Taking over now as a vehicle from lanolin.
Preservatives and biocides		
No one likes rancid cosmetics, or smelly cutting oils. Biocides are hidden in many materials to stop this sort of thing happening.		
Formaldehyde	Used as a preservative in some shampoos and cosmetics. Also in pathology laboratories and white shoes.	Many pathologists are allergic to it. Quaternium 15 (see below) releases formaldehyde as do some formaldehyde resins.
Parabens-mix	Preservatives in a wide variety of creams and lotions, both medical and cosmetic.	Common cause of allergy in those who react to a number of seemingly unrelated creams.
Chlorocresol	Common preservative.	Cross reacts with chloroxylenol – a popular antiseptic.
Kathon	Preservative in many cosmetics, shampoos, soaps and sunscreens.	Also found in some odd places such as moist toilet papers and washing-up liquids.
Quaternium 15	Preservative in many topical medicaments and cosmetics.	Releases formaldehyde and may cross-react with it.
Imidazolidinyl urea	Common ingredient of moisturizers and cosmetics.	Cosmetic allergy.
Other biocides	In glues, paints, cutting oils, etc.	Responsible for some cases of occupational dermatitis.

Table 7.4 (*Continued*)

Allergen	Common sources	Comments
Medicaments		
These may share allergens, such as preservatives and lanolin, with cosmetics (see above). In addition, the active ingredients can sensitize, especially when applied long term to venous ulcers, pruritus ani, eczema or otitis externa.		
Neomycin	Popular topical antibiotic. Safe in short bursts (e.g. for impetigo or cuts).	Common sensitizer in those with leg ulcers. Simply swapping to another antibiotic may not always help as neomycin cross-reacts with framycetin and gentamycin.
Quinoline mix	Used as an antiseptic in creams, often in combination with a corticosteroid.	Its aliases include Vioform and chinoform.
Ethylenediamine dihydrochloride	Stabilizer in some topical steroid mixtures (e.g. Mycolog and the alleged active ingredient in fat removal creams). A component in aminophylline. A hardener for epoxy resin.	Cross-reacts with some antihistamines (e.g hydroxyzine).
Benzocaine	A local anaesthetic which lurks in some topical applications (e.g. for piles and sunburn).	Dermatologists seldom recommend using these preparations – they have seen too many reactions.
Tixocortol pivalate	Topical steroid.	A marker for allergy to various topical steroids. Hydrocortisone allergy exists. Think of this when steroid applications seem to be making things worse.
Budesonide	Topical steroid.	Testing with both tixocortol pivalate and budesonide will detect 95% of topical steroid allergies.
Rubber		
Rubber itself is often not the problem, but it has to be converted from soft latex (p. 101) to usable rubber by adding vulcanizers to make it harder, accelerators to speed up vulcanization, and antioxidants to stop it perishing in the air. These additives are allergens.		
Mercapto-mix	Chemicals used to harden rubber.	Diagnosis is often obvious: sometimes less so. Remember shoe soles, rubber bands and golf club grips.
Thiuram-mix	Another set of rubber accelerators.	Common culprit in rubber glove allergy.
Black rubber mix	All black heavy-duty rubber (e.g. tyres, rubber boots, squash balls).	These are PPD derivatives, cross-reacting with PPD dyes (see above).
Carba mix	Mainly in rubber gloves.	Patch testing with rubber chemicals occasionally sensitizes patients to them.
Plants		
In the United States, the Rhus family (poison ivy and poison oak) are important allergens. In Europe, *Primula obconica* holds pride of place. Both cause severe reactions with streaky erythema and blistering. The Rhus antigen is such a potent sensitizer that patch testing with it is unwise. Other reaction patterns include a lichenified dermatitis of exposed areas from chrysanthemums, and a fingertip dermatitis from tulip bulbs		
Primin	Allergen in *Primula obconica*.	More reliable than patch testing to *Primula* leaves.
Sesquiterpene lactone mix	Compositae plant allergy.	Picks up chrysanth allergy. Flying pollen affects exposed parts and reactions can look like light sensitivity.
Resins		
Common sensitizers such as epoxy resins can cause trouble both at home, as adhesives, and in industry		
Epoxy resin	Common in 'two-component' adhesive mixtures (e.g. Araldite). Also used in electrical and plastics industries.	'Cured' resin does not sensitize. A few become allergic to the added hardener rather than to the resin itself.
Paratertiary butylphenol formaldehyde resin	Used as an adhesive (e.g. in shoes, wrist watch straps, prostheses, hobbies).	Cross-reacts with formaldehyde. Depigmentation has been recorded.
Colophony	Naturally occurring and found in pine sawdust. Used as an adhesive in sticking plasters bandages. Also found in various varnishes, paper and rosin.	The usual cause of sticking plaster allergy; also, of dermatitis of the hands of violinists who handle rosin.

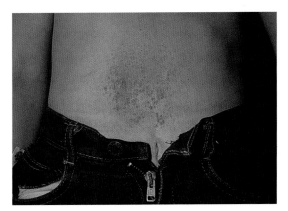

Figure 7.8 Contact eczema caused by allergy to nickel in a jean stud.

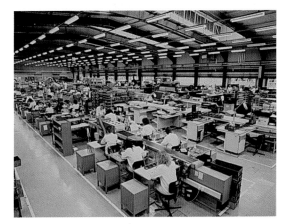

Figure 7.10 Assembly workers in an electronic factory – potential victims of industrial dermatitis. (Dr P.K. Buxton. Reproduced with permission of Dr P.K. Buxton.)

Occupational dermatitis

The size of this problem has been underestimated in the past but, both in the United Kingdom and the United States, dermatitis is the second most common occupational disorder – second only to musculoskeletal injuries. In the United Kingdom, it is most common in younger women (Figure 7.10), and then is often associated with wet work. The incidence in men rises with age, and in older workers it is often caused by contact with cutting oils. Table 7.5 lists the types of work particularly associated with high rates of contact dermatitis in the United Kingdom. The hands are affected in 80–90% of cases. Often several factors (constitutional, irritant and allergic) have combined to cause this, and a change of job does not always lead to a cure, particularly in long-established cases. In one large series, hand dermatitis was most common in caterers, metal workers, hairdressers, health care workers and mechanics.

Atopic eczema

The word atopy comes from the Greek (*a-topos*: 'without a place'). It was introduced by Coca and Cooke in 1923 and refers to the lack of a niche in the medical classifications then in use for the grouping of asthma, hay fever and eczema. Atopy is a state in which an exuberant production of IgE occurs as a response to common environmental allergens. Atopic subjects may, or may not, develop one or more of the atopic diseases such as asthma, hay fever, eczema and food allergies, and the prevalence of atopy is steadily rising.

The prevalence of atopic eczema varies around the world from around 2% in parts of the developing world to 20% in children in western Europe, Australia and the United States. This prevalence has risen over the last

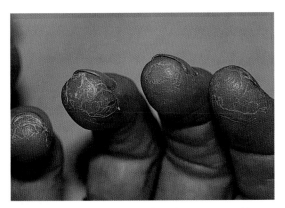

Figure 7.9 Dry fissured eczema of the fingertips caused by handling garlic.

Table 7.5 Occupations with the highest rates of contact dermatitis in the United Kingdom.

Men	Women
Chemical plant workers	Hairdressers
Machine tool setters and operatives	Biological scientists and laboratory workers
Coach and spray painters	Nurses
Metal workers	Catering workers

20 years, but now appears to have stabilized. The reasons for this rise are not yet clear, but cannot be due to a change in the genetic pool in the population. Several environmental factors have been shown to reduce the risk of developing atopic disease. These include having many older siblings, growing up on a farm, having childhood measles and gut infections. The 'hygiene hypothesis' unites these, blaming the early use of antibiotics and a reduced exposure to orofaecal and other infections for preventing normal immunological maturation and shifting the circulating T lymphocytes of children destined to develop allergies from a Th1 to a Th2 response. However, this theory of a simple Th1–Th2 imbalance fails to explain the simultaneous rise in Th1-mediated diseases such as diabetes and inflammatory bowel disease. More recently it has been suggested that failure to develop regulatory T cells, which also develop as part of the response to infection, may explain the rise in incidence of allergic and autoimmune disease.

Inheritance

A strong genetic component is obvious, although affected children can be born to clinically normal parents. The concordance rates for atopic eczema in monozygotic and dizygotic twins are around 80% and 22%, respectively; and atopic diseases tend to run true to type within each family. In some, most of the affected members will have eczema; in others respiratory allergy will predominate. There is also a tendency for atopic diseases to be inherited more often from the mother than the father, and if both parents have atopic eczema, a child has a 75% chance of developing the disease. Environmental factors too are important and, not surprisingly, a simple genetic explanation has not yet been found in all patients.

Many patients are heterozygous or homozygous for a mutation of the filaggrin gene. New insights have come from the finding that a 50% reduction or complete absence of a critical structural protein in the skin due to highly prevalent genetic mutations are a major genetic factor in eczema development. Loss of function mutations in the filaggrin gene cause ichthyosis vulgaris (p. 45) but are also strongly predictive for atopic eczema. In European populations, about 10% of individuals carry mutations that completely deactivate one copy of the filaggrin gene; 1 in 400 make no filaggrin whatsoever. In cohorts of patients with eczema, 18–48% of subjects carry one or more filaggrin-deactivating mutations and these mutations are also strongly linked with eczema-associated asthma and peanut allergy. Filaggrin-associated eczema tends to more severe, more likely to involve irritant hand

eczema and more likely to be complicated by eczema herpeticum than eczema in patients with a wild-type filaggrin gene. Interestingly, Asian patients with eczema show a different spectrum of filaggrin mutations from European patients and this suggests that there has been a selective evolutionary pressure for filaggrin inactivation, which leads to eczema when combined with modern environmental factors. Mutations in the filaggrin gene are the most significant genetic factor yet identified in atopy and points to a skin barrier defect being an early initiating event or even a prerequisite for development of the disease. Th2 cytokines, typical of atopic eczema, will themselves reduce expression of filaggrin and in this way atopic eczema patients with the wild-type filaggrin gene may have reduced filaggrin protein. Filaggrin is involved in the collapse of the cytoskeleton of keratinocytes, leading to there collapse into the squames of the stratum corneum. Filaggrin itself is broken down to form a major constituent of natural moisturizing factor, which fills the interstices between squames, and helps ensure the physical integrity of the stratum corneum.

The inheritance of atopic eczema probably requires genes that predispose to the state of atopy itself, and others that determine whether it is asthma, eczema or hay fever that occurs. Genome-wide scans in different populations have suggested various linkages with atopic eczema but there has been a disappointing lack of overlap between findings in these studies, perhaps because of lack of a consistent phenotype and definition of atopic eczema. Variations in the genes for the Th2 cytokines interleukin 4 (IL-4), IL-13 and the also the IL-4 receptor have been consistently linked with atopic eczema. Similarly, variations in the mast cell chymase gene, which is involved in regulating accumulation of inflammatory cells are also linked. Netherton's syndrome, in which eczema and raised serum IgE predominate, is caused by mutations in the *SPINK5* gene which codes for a serine protease inhibitor involved in epidermal differentiation and also highlights the significance of skin barrier defects in the aetiology of atopic eczema. In genome scans, several areas of overlap have also been reported with psoriasis susceptibility loci.

Presentation and course

Seventy-five per cent of cases of atopic eczema begin before the age of 6 months, and 80–90% before the age of 5 years. It affects at least 3% of infants, but the onset may be delayed until childhood or adult life. Some 60–70% of children with atopic eczema will clear by their early teens, although subsequent relapses are possible. The distribution and character of the lesions vary with age

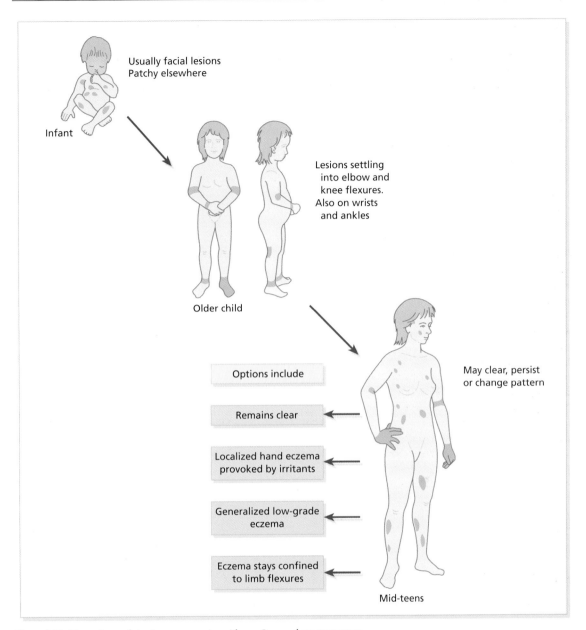

Usually facial lesions
Patchy elsewhere

Infant

Lesions settling
into elbow and
knee flexures.
Also on wrists
and ankles

Older child

Options include

Remains clear

Localized hand eczema
provoked by irritants

Generalized low-grade
eczema

Eczema stays confined
to limb flexures

May clear, persist
or change pattern

Mid-teens

Figure 7.11 The pattern of atopic eczema varies with age. It may clear at any stage.

(Figure 7.11) but a general dryness of the skin may persist throughout life.

• In infancy, atopic eczema tends to be vesicular and weeping. It often starts on the face (Figure 7.12) with a non-specific distribution elsewhere, commonly sparing the napkin (diaper) area.

• In childhood, the eczema becomes leathery, dry and excoriated, affecting mainly the elbow and knee flexures (Figure 7.13), wrists and ankles. A stubborn 'reverse' pattern affecting the extensor aspects of the limbs is also recognized.

• In adults, the distribution is as in childhood with a marked tendency towards lichenification and a more widespread but low-grade involvement of the trunk, face and hands. White dermographism (Figure 7.14) is often striking, but not diagnostic of atopic eczema.

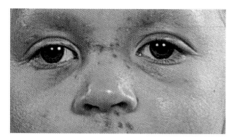

Figure 7.12 Atopic eczema in a child: worse around the eyes due to rubbing. (Dr Olivia Schofield. Reproduced with permission of Dr Olivia Schofield.)

The cardinal feature of atopic eczema is itching; and scratching may account for most of the clinical picture. Affected children may sleep poorly, be hyperactive and sometimes manipulative, using the state of their eczema to get what they want from their parents. Luckily, the condition remits spontaneously before the age of 10 years in at least two-thirds of affected children, although it may come back at times of stress. Eczema and asthma may seesaw, so that while one improves the other may get worse.

Learning points

1 Eczema is like jazz; it is hard to define – but it should be easy to recognize if you bear in mind the physical signs.
2 If it does not itch, it is probably not eczema.

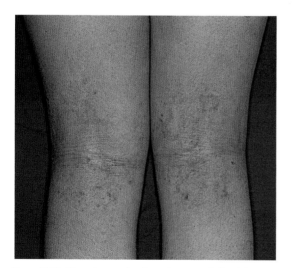

Figure 7.13 Chronic excoriated atopic eczema behind the knees.

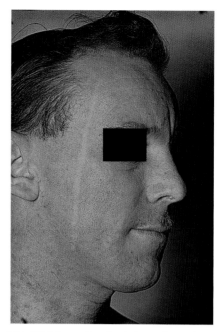

Figure 7.14 Trivial scratching has led to striking white dermographism.

Diagnostic criteria

Diagnostic criteria shown to be accurate in hospital and community settings, and used for epidemiological research worldwide, are shown in Table 7.6.

Complications

Overt bacterial infection is troublesome in many patients with atopic eczema (Figure 7.15). They are also especially

Table 7.6 Diagnostic criteria for atopic eczema.

Must have:
• A chronically itchy skin (or report of scratching or rubbing in a child)
Plus three or more of the following:
• History of itchiness in skin creases such as folds of the elbows, behind the knees, fronts of ankles or around the neck (or the cheeks in children under 4 years)
• History of asthma or hay fever (or history of atopic disease in a first-degree relative in children under 4 years)
• General dry skin in the past year
• Visible flexural eczema (or eczema affecting the cheeks or forehead and outer limbs in children under 4 years)
• Onset in the first 2 years of life (not always diagnostic in children under 4 years)

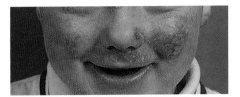

Figure 7.15 Facial eczema in a young boy worsening recently. Crusting on the cheeks and upper lip points to possible bacterial superinfection. (Dr Olivia Schofield. Reproduced with permission of Dr Olivia Schofield.)

prone to viral infections, most dangerously with widespread herpes simplex (eczema herpeticum; Figure 7.16), but also with molluscum contagiosum and warts. Growth hormone levels rise during deep sleep (stages 3 and 4), but these stages may not be reached during the disturbed sleep of children with severe atopic eczema and as a consequence they may grow poorly. The absorption of topical steroids can contribute to this too.

Investigations

Prick testing (see Figure 3.10) demonstrates immediate-type hypersensitivity and is helpful in the investigation of asthma and hay fever. However, the value of prick testing in atopic eczema remains controversial. Often the finding of multiple positive reactions, and a high IgE level, does little more than support a doubtful clinical diagnosis. Treatment of eczema is the same whether atopic (IgE positive) or non-atopic.

Treatment

Management here is complex and should include the following.
• Explanation, reassurance and encouragement. Educating patients and parents has been shown to improve long-term outcome. Many benefit from an introduction to the National Eczema Society in the United Kingdom or the

Table 7.7 Winning ways with emollients.

• Make sure they are applied when the skin is moist
• Prescribe plenty (at least 500 g/week for the whole skin of an adult and 250 g/week for the whole skin of a child) and ensure they are used at least 3–4 times a day
• For maximal effect, combine the use of creams, ointments, bath oils and emollient soap substitutes

National Eczema Association for Science and Education or the Inflammatory Skin Institute in the United States.
• The avoidance of exacerbating factors such as irritants (e.g. woollen clothing next to the skin) and later of careers such as hairdressing and engineering, which would inevitably lead to much exposure to irritants. Also avoid extremes of temperature, and contact with soaps and detergents.
• The regular use of bland emollients (p. 397), either directly to the skin or in the form of oils to be used in the bath. Some of these, such as aqueous cream, can also be used as soap substitutes. A list of suitable preparations is given in Formulary 1 (p. 397). Some rules governing the use of emollients are given in Table 7.7.
• The judicious use of topical steroids or calcineurin inhibitors as for other types of eczema (p. 82; Table 7.8). The strength of corticosteroid used is determined by the patient's age, body site and the severity of the eczema. A technique useful for extensive and troublesome eczema, particularly in children, is that of wet wrap dressings (p. 82). A nurse who is expert in applying such dressings is an asset to any practice (Figure 7.17).
• Those with an associated ichthyosis should generally use ointments rather than creams.
• The scratch–itch cycle can often be interrupted by occlusive bandaging (e.g. with a 1% ichthammol paste bandage). Nails should be kept short.

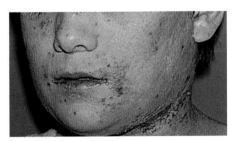

Figure 7.16 Infected facial eczema – herpes simplex was isolated.

Table 7.8 Principles of treatment with topical corticosteroids.

• Use the weakest steroid that controls the eczema effectively
• Review their use regularly: check for local and systemic side effects
• In primary care, avoid using potent and very potent steroids for children with atopic eczema
• Be wary of repeat prescriptions

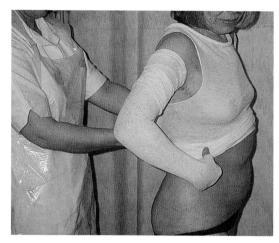

Figure 7.17 Protective tubular gauze dressings being applied over a topical steroid ointment.

• Sedative antihistamines (e.g. alimemazine or hydroxyzine; Formulary 2, p. 415) are of value if sleep is interrupted, but histamine release is not the main cause of the itching, so the newer non-sedative antihistamines help less than might be expected.
• Acute flares are often induced by the surface proliferation of staphylococci, even without frank sepsis. A month's course of a systemic antibiotic (e.g. erythromycin) may then be helpful.
• Allergen avoidance: prick tests confirm that most patients from atopic eczema have immediate hypersensitivity responses to allergens in the faeces of house dust mites. Sometimes, but not always, measures to reduce contact with these allergens help eczema. These measures should include encasing the mattress in a dustproof bag, washing the duvets and pillows every 3 months at a temperature greater than 55°C, and thorough and regular vacuuming in the bedroom, where carpets should preferably be avoided. This approach is time consuming and expensive and rarely replaces the need for conventional treatment based on emollients and topical corticosteroids.
• Do not keep pets to which there is obvious allergy.
• The role of diet in atopic eczema is even more debatable, and treatments based on changing the diet of patients are often disappointing. Similarly, it is not certain that the avoidance of dietary allergens (e.g. cow's milk and eggs) by a pregnant or lactating woman lessens the risk of her baby developing eczema. It may still be wise to breastfeed children at special risk for 6 months.
• Routine inoculations are permissible during quiet phases of the eczema. However, children who are aller-gic to eggs should not be inoculated against measles, influenza and yellow fever.
• Those with active herpes simplex infections should be avoided to cut the risk of developing eczema herpeticum.

> **Learning point**
>
> Do not encourage cranky dieting for atopic eczema: it causes anxiety and seldom if ever does much good.

Seborrhoeic eczema

Presentation and course
The term covers at least three common patterns of eczema, mainly affecting hairy areas, and often showing characteristic greasy yellowish scales. These patterns may merge together (Figure 7.18).
1 A red scaly or exudative eruption of the scalp, ears (Figure 7.19), face (Figure 7.20) and eyebrows. May be associated with chronic blepharitis and otitis externa.
2 Dry scaly petaloid lesions of the presternal (Figure 7.21) and interscapular areas. There may also be extensive follicular papules or pustules on the trunk (seborrhoeic folliculitis or *Malassezia* folliculitis).
3 Intertriginous lesions of the armpits, umbilicus or groins, or under spectacles or hearing aids.

Cause
This condition is not obviously related to seborrhoea. It may run in some families, often affecting those with a tendency to dandruff. The success of treatments directed against yeasts has suggested that overgrowth of the *Malassezia* yeast skin commensals plays an important part in the development of seborrhoeic eczema. This fits well with the fact that seborrhoeic eczema is often an early sign of AIDS, and that it responds to anti-yeast agents such as topical ketoconazole shampoo or cream.

Seborrhoeic eczema may affect infants (Figure 7.22) but is most common in adult males. In infants it clears quickly but in adults its course is unpredictable and may be chronic or recurrent. Some particularly severe cases have occurred in patients with AIDS (p. 235; see Figure 16.35).

Complications
It may be associated with furunculosis. In the intertriginous type, superadded *Candida* infection is common.

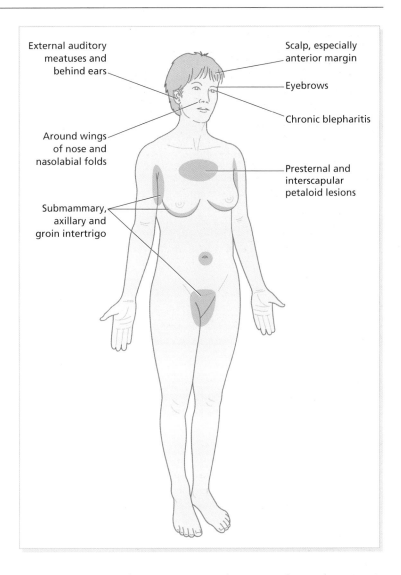

External auditory
meatuses and
behind ears

Scalp, especially
anterior margin

Eyebrows

Chronic blepharitis

Around wings
of nose and
nasolabial folds

Presternal and
interscapular
petaloid lesions

Submammary,
axillary and
groin intertrigo

Figure 7.18 Areas most often affected by
seborrhoeic eczema.

Investigations

None are usually needed, but bear possible HIV infection
and Parkinson's disease in mind.

Treatment

Therapy is suppressive rather than curative and patients
should be told this. Topical imidazoles (Formulary 1,
p. 404) are perhaps the first line of treatment. Two per
cent sulfur and 2% salicylic acid in aqueous cream is often
helpful and avoids the problem of topical steroids. It may
be used on the scalp overnight and removed by a medicated shampoo, which may contain ketoconazole, tar, salicylic acid, sulfur, zinc or selenium sulfide (Formulary 1,
p. 398). A topical lithium preparation may help the facial

rash. For intertriginous lesions a weak steroid – antiseptic
or steroid – antifungal combination (Formulary 1, p. 402)
is often effective. For severe and unresponsive cases a
short course of oral itraconazole may be helpful.

Discoid (nummular) eczema

Cause

No cause has been established but chronic stress is often
present. A reaction to bacterial antigens has been suspected as the lesions often yield staphylococci on culture,
and as steroid – antiseptic or steroid – antibiotic mixtures
do better than either separately.

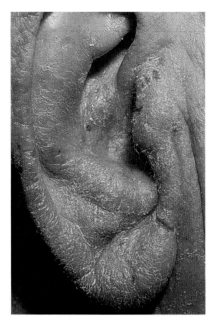

Figure 7.19 Dry scaly seborrhoeic eczema of the ear.

Presentation and course

This common pattern of endogenous eczema classically affects the limbs of middle-aged males. The lesions are multiple, coin-shaped, vesicular or crusted, highly itchy plaques (Figure 7.23), usually less than 5 cm across. The

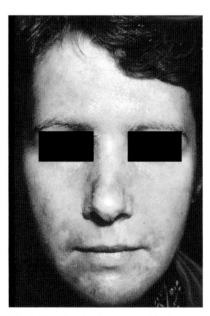

Figure 7.20 Active seborrhoeic eczema of the face.

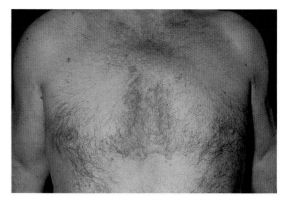

Figure 7.21 Typical presternal patch of seborrhoeic eczema.

condition tends to persist for many months, and recurrences often appear at the site of previous plaques.

Investigations

None are usually needed.

Treatment

With topical steroid – antiseptic or steroid – antibiotic combinations (see *Cause*).

Pompholyx

Cause

The cause is usually unknown, but pompholyx is sometimes provoked by heat or emotional upsets. In subjects allergic to nickel, small amounts of nickel in food may trigger pompholyx. The vesicles are not plugged sweat ducts, and the term dyshidrotic eczema should now be dropped.

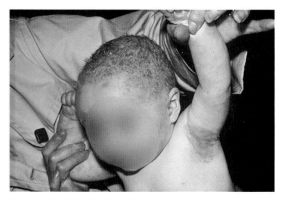

Figure 7.22 Infantile seborrhoeic eczema.

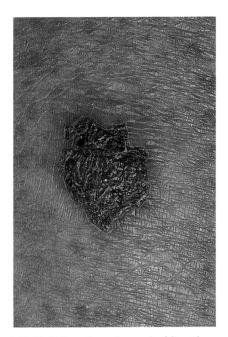

Figure 7.23 Vesicular and weeping patch of discoid eczema.

Presentation and course

In this tiresome and sometimes very unpleasant form of eczema, recurrent bouts of vesicles or larger blisters appear on the palms, fingers (Figure 7.24) and/or the soles of adults. Bouts lasting a few weeks recur at irregular intervals. Secondary infection and lymphangitis are a recurrent problem for some patients.

Investigations

None are usually needed but sometimes a pompholyx-like eruption of the hands can follow acute tinea pedis

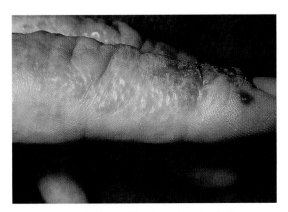

Figure 7.24 Pompholyx vesicles along the side of a finger.

(an ide reaction). If this is suspected, scrapings or blister roofs, not from the hand lesions but from those on the feet, should be sent for mycological examination. Swabs from infected vesicles should be cultured for bacterial pathogens.

Treatment

Treatment is as for acute eczema of the hands and feet (p. 82). Appropriate antibiotics should be given for bacterial infections. Aluminium acetate or potassium permanganate soaks, followed by applications of a very potent corticosteroid cream, are often helpful. If hand eczema fails to respond to potent topical corticosteroids, alitretinoin should be prescribed (p. 421).

Gravitational (stasis) eczema

Cause

Often, but not always, accompanied by obvious venous insufficiency.

Presentation and course

A chronic patchy eczematous condition of the lower legs, sometimes accompanied by varicose veins, oedema and haemosiderin deposition (Figure 7.25). When severe it may spread to the other leg or even become generalized.

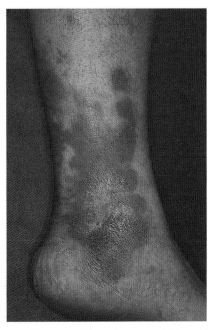

Figure 7.25 Chronic gravitational eczema, perhaps with a superimposed contact dermatitis from a local medication.

Complications

Patients often become sensitized to local antibiotic applications or to the preservatives in medicated bandages. Excoriations may lead to ulcer formation.

Treatment

This should include the elimination of oedema by elevation, pressure bandages or diuretics. A moderately potent topical steroid may be helpful, but stronger ones are best avoided. Bland applications (e.g. Lassar's paste or zinc cream BNF) or medicated bandages (Formulary 1, p. 408) are useful but stasis eczema is liable to persist, despite surgery to the underlying veins.

Asteatotic eczema

Cause

Many who develop asteatotic eczema in old age will always have had a dry skin and a tendency to chap. Other contributory factors include the removal of surface lipids by over-washing, the low humidity of winter and central heating, the use of diuretics and hypothyroidism.

Presentation and course

Often unrecognized, this common and itchy pattern of eczema occurs usually on the legs of elderly patients. Against a background of dry skin, a network of fine red superficial fissures creates a 'crazy paving' appearance (Figure 7.26).

Investigations

None are usually needed. Very extensive cases may be part of malabsorption syndromes, zinc deficiency or internal malignancy.

Treatment

The condition can be cleared by the use of a mild or moderately potent topical steroid in a greasy base, and aqueous cream as a soap substitute for the area. Baths should be restricted until clearance. Thereafter, daily use of unmedicated emollients (Formulary 1, p. 296) usually prevents recurrence.

Localized neurodermatitis (lichen simplex)

Cause

The skin is damaged as a result of repeated rubbing or scratching, as a habit or in response to stress, but there is no underlying skin disorder.

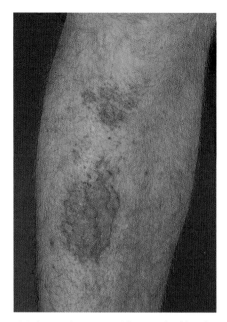

Figure 7.26 Asteatotic eczema with network of fine fissures in the stratum corneum.

Presentation and course

Usually occurs as a single fixed itchy lichenified plaque (Figure 7.27). Favourite areas are the nape of the neck in women, the legs in men and the anogenital area in both sexes. Lesions may resolve with treatment but tend to recur either in the same place or elsewhere.

Investigations

None are usually needed.

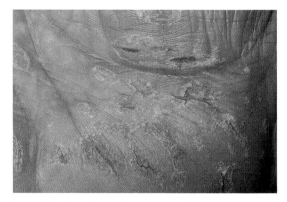

Figure 7.27 It is often hard to tell palmar lichen simplex from hyperkeratotic fissured eczema, as shown here.

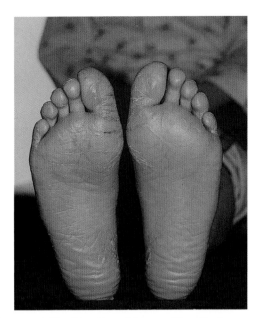

Figure 7.28 The shiny skin and fissures of juvenile plantar dermatosis.

Treatment
Potent topical steroids or occlusive bandaging, where feasible, help to break the scratch–itch cycle. Tranquillizers are often disappointing.

Juvenile plantar dermatosis (Figure 7.28)

Cause
This condition is thought to be related to the impermeability of modern socks and shoe linings with subsequent sweat gland blockage, and so has been called the 'toxic sock syndrome'! Some feel the condition is a manifestation of atopy.

Presentation and course
The skin of the weight-bearing areas of the feet, particularly the forefeet and undersides of the toes, becomes dry and shiny with deep painful fissures that make walking difficult. The toe webs are spared. Onset can be at any time after shoes are first worn, and even if untreated the condition clears in the early teens.

Investigations
Much time has been wasted in patch testing and scraping for fungus.

Treatment
The child should use a commercially available cork insole in all shoes, and stick to cotton or wool socks. An emollient such as emulsifying ointment or 1% ichthammol paste, or an emollient containing lactic acid, is as good as a topical steroid.

Napkin (diaper) dermatitis

Cause
The most common type of napkin eruption is irritant in origin, and is aggravated by the use of waterproof plastic pants. The mixture of faecal enzymes and ammonia produced by urea-splitting bacteria, if allowed to remain in prolonged contact with the skin, leads to a severe reaction. The overgrowth of yeasts is another aggravating factor. The introduction of modern disposable napkins has helped to reduce the number of cases sent to dermatology clinics.

Presentation
The moist, often glazed and sore erythema affects the napkin area generally (Figure 7.29), with the exception of the skin folds, which tend to be spared.

Complications
Superinfection with *Candida albicans* is common, and this may lead to small erythematous papules or vesicopustules appearing around the periphery of the main eruption.

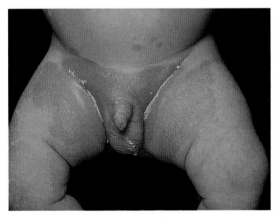

Figure 7.29 Irritant napkin erythema with a hint of sparing of the skin folds.

Differential diagnosis

The sparing of the folds helps to separate this condition from infantile seborrhoeic eczema and candidiasis.

Treatment

It is never easy to keep this area clean and dry, but this is the basis of all treatment. Theoretically, the child should be allowed to be free of napkins as much as possible but this may lead to a messy nightmare. On both sides of the Atlantic, disposable nappies (diapers) have largely replaced washable ones. The superabsorbent type is best and should be changed regularly, especially in the middle of the night. When towelling napkins are used they should be washed thoroughly and changed frequently. The area should be cleaned at each nappy change with aqueous cream and water. Protective ointments (e.g. zinc and castor oil ointment), or silicone protective ointments, are often useful (Formulary 1, p. 399), as are topical imidazole preparations that stop yeast growth. Potent steroids should be avoided but combinations of hydrocortisone with antifungals or antiseptics (Formulary 1, p. 402) are often useful.

Learning points

1 Do not accept 'eczema' as an adequate diagnosis: treatment hinges on establishing its cause and type.
2 Keep fluorinated steroids off the face of adults and off the skin of infants.
3 Monitor repeat prescriptions of topical steroids, keeping an eye on the amount used and their potency.
4 Twice weekly corticosteroids or tacrolimus during eczema remissions reduces the frequency of disease flares.
5 Do not promise that atopic eczema will be clear by any particular age. Guesses are always wrong and the patients lose faith.

Further reading

Brown S, Reynolds NJ. (2006) Atopic and non-atopic eczema. *British Medical Journal* **332**, 584–588.

Brown SJ, McLean WHI. (2009) Eczema genetics: current state of knowledge and future goals. *Journal of Investigative Dermatology* **129**, 543–552.

Cochrane Library. Cochrane reviews: eczema and dermatitis. http://www.thecochranelibrary.com/details/browseReviews/576987/Eczema–dermatitis.html (accessed 17 June 2014).

Flohr C, Johansson SG, Wahlgren CF, Williams H. (2004) How atopic is atopic dermatitis? *Journal of Allergy and Clinical Immunology* **114**,150–158.

Hanifin J, Saurat JH. (2001) Understanding atopic dermatitis pathophysiology and etiology. *Journal of the American Academy of Dermatology* **45** (Suppl), S1.

Irvine AD, McLean WH, Leung DY. (2011) Filaggrin mutations associated with skin and allergic diseases. *New England Journal of Medicine* **365**, 1315–1327.

Kanerva L, Elsner P, Wahlberg JE, Maibach HI. (2000) *Handbook of Occupational Dermatology*. Springer, Berlin.

O'Regan GM, Sandilands A, McLean WH, Irvine AD. (2009) Filaggrin in atopic dermatitis. *Journal of Allergy and Clinical Immunology* **124** (Suppl 2), R2–R6.

Primary Care Dermatology Society and British Association of Dermatologists. (2009) Guidelines for the management of atopic eczema. www.eGuidelines.co.uk (accessed 17 June 2014).

Rietschel R, Fowler JM. (2008) *Fisher's Contact Dermatitis*, 6th edition. McGraw-Hill Medical.

Schmitt J, von Kobyletzki L, Svensson Å, Apfelbacher C. (2011) Efficacy and tolerability of proactive treatment with topical corticosteroids and calcineurin inhibitors for atopic eczema: systematic review and meta-analysis of randomized controlled trials. *British Journal of Dermatology* **164**, 415–428.

8 Reactive Erythemas and Vasculitis

Blood vessels can be affected by a variety of insults, both exogenous and endogenous. When this occurs, the epidermis remains unaffected, but the skin becomes red or pink and often oedematous. This is a reactive erythema. If the blood vessels are damaged more severely – as in vasculitis – purpura or larger areas of haemorrhage mask the erythematous colour.

Urticaria (hives, 'nettle-rash')

Urticaria is a common reaction pattern in which pink, itchy or 'burning' swellings (wheals) can occur anywhere on the body. Individual wheals do not last longer than 24 hours, but new ones may continue to appear for days, months or even years. Traditionally, urticaria is divided into acute and chronic forms, based on the duration of the disease rather than of individual wheals. Urticaria that persists for more than 6 weeks is classified as chronic. More recently, episodic (acute intermittent or recurrent activity) has been added to the classification. Most patients with chronic urticaria, other than those with an obvious physical cause, have what is often known as *ordinary urticaria*. Chronic ordinary urticaria (COU) can be further subdivided depending on the presence (30%) or absence (70%) of histamine-releasing autoantibodies; giving rise to the somewhat cumbersome terms, *autoimmune chronic ordinary urticaria* and *idiopathic chronic ordinary urticaria*, respectively.

Cause

The signs and symptoms of urticaria are caused by mast cell degranulation, with release of multiple vasoactive substances, including histamine (Figure 8.1). The mechanisms underlying this may be different but the end result, increased capillary permeability leading to transient leakage of fluid into the surrounding tissue and development of a wheal, is the same (Figure 8.1). For example, in autoimmune COU circulating antibodies are directed against the high affinity immunoglobulin E receptor (FcIgE) or receptor bound IgE on mast cells whereas the reaction in others in this group may be caused by immediate IgE-mediated hypersensitivity (see Figure 2.14), direct degranulation by a chemical or trauma, or complement activation.

Classification

The various types of urticaria are listed in Table 8.1. They can often be identified by a careful history; laboratory tests are less useful. The duration of the wheals is an important pointer. Contact and physical urticarias, with the exception of delayed pressure urticaria, start shortly after the stimulus and go within an hour. Individual wheals of other forms resolve within 24 hours. If they persist for longer, then urticarial vasculitis should be considered (see *Cutaneous small vessel vasculitis*).

Physical urticarias

Cold urticaria

Patients develop wheals in areas exposed to cold (e.g. on the face when cycling or freezing in a cold wind).

A useful test in the clinic is to reproduce the reaction by holding an ice cube, in a thin plastic bag to avoid wetting, against forearm skin. A few cases are associated with the presence of cryoglobulins, cold agglutinins or cryofibrinogens.

Solar urticaria

Wheals occur within minutes of sun exposure. Some patients with solar urticaria have erythropoietic

Clinical Dermatology, Fifth Edition. Richard B. Weller, Hamish J.A. Hunter and Margaret W. Mann.
© 2015 John Wiley & Sons, Ltd. Published 2015 by John Wiley & Sons, Ltd.

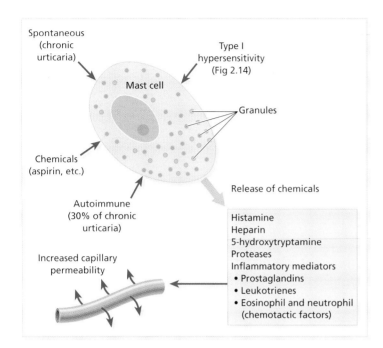

Figure 8.1 Ways in which a mast cell can be degranulated and the ensuing reaction.

protoporphyria (p. 317); most have an IgE-mediated urticarial reaction to sunlight.

Heat urticaria
In this condition wheals arise in areas after contact with hot objects or solutions.

Table 8.1 The main types of urticaria.

Ordinary urticaria
Acute (up to 6 weeks of continuous activity)
Chronic (more than 6 weeks of continuous activity)
    Autoimmune chronic ordinary urticaria
    Idiopathic chronic ordinary urticaria
Episodic (acute intermittent or recurrent activity)

Physical
Cold
Solar
Heat
Cholinergic
Dermographism (immediate pressure urticaria)
Delayed pressure

Hypersensitivity
Autoimmune
Pharmacological
Contact

Cholinergic urticaria
Anxiety, heat, sexual excitement or strenuous exercise elicits this characteristic response. The vessels overreact to acetylcholine liberated from sympathetic nerves in the skin. Transient 2–5 mm follicular macules or papules (Figure 8.2) resemble a blush or viral exanthem. Some patients get blotchy patches on their necks.

Dermographism (Figure 8.3)
This is the most common type of physical urticaria, the skin mast cells releasing extra histamine after rubbing or scratching. The linear wheals are therefore an exaggerated

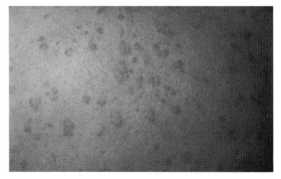

Figure 8.2 Typical small transient wheals of cholinergic urticaria – in this case triggered by exercise.

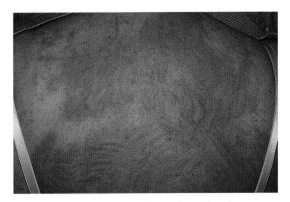

Figure 8.3 Dermographism: a frenzy of scratching by an already dermographic individual led to this dramatic appearance.

triple response of Lewis. They can readily be reproduced by rubbing the skin of the back lightly at different pressures, or by scratching the back with a fingernail or blunt object.

Delayed pressure urticaria

Sustained pressure causes oedema of the underlying skin and subcutaneous tissue 3–6 hours later. The swelling may last up to 48 hours and kinins or prostaglandins rather than histamine probably mediate it. It occurs particularly on the feet after walking, on the hands after clapping and on the buttocks after sitting. It can be disabling for manual labourers.

Other types of urticaria

Hypersensitivity urticaria

This common form of urticaria is caused by hypersensitivity, often an IgE-mediated (type I) immediate hypersensitivity reaction (see Chapter 2). Allergens may be encountered in 10 different ways (the 10 I's listed in Table 8.2).

Autoimmune urticaria

About 30% of patients with COU have an autoimmune disease with IgG antibodies to IgE or to FcIgE receptors on mast cells. Here the autoantibody acts as antigen to trigger mast cell degranulation.

Pharmacological urticaria

This occurs when drugs cause mast cells to release histamine in a non-allergic manner (e.g. opiates such as codeine and morphine, and radiocontrast media).

Table 8.2 The 10 I's of antigen encounter in hypersensitive urticaria.

Ingestion
Inhalation
Instillation
Injection
Insertion
Insect bites
Infestations
Infection
Infusion
Inunction (contact)

Urticaria provoked by aspirin, non-steroidal anti-inflammatory drugs (NSAIDs) and certain food substances may also involve leukotriene release.

Contact urticaria

This may be IgE-mediated or caused by a pharmacological effect. The allergen is delivered to the mast cell from the skin surface rather than from the blood. Wheals occur most often around the mouth. Foods and food additives are the most common culprits but drugs, animal saliva, caterpillars, insect repellents and plants may cause the reaction. Latex allergy has become a significant public health concern although the incidence now appears to be falling.

Latex allergy

Possible skin reactions to the natural rubber latex of the *Hevea brasiliensis* tree include irritant dermatitis, contact allergic dermatitis (see Chapter 7) and type I (immediate hypersensitivity) allergy (see Chapter 2). Reactions associated with the latter include hypersensitivity urticaria (both by contact and by inhalation), hay fever, asthma, anaphylaxis and, rarely, death.

Medical latex gloves became universally popular after precautions were introduced to protect against HIV and hepatitis B infections. The demand for the gloves increased and this led to alterations in their manufacture and to a flood of high allergen gloves on the market. Cornstarch powder in these gloves bound to the latex proteins so that the allergen became airborne when the gloves were put on. Individuals at increased risk of latex allergy include health care workers, those undergoing multiple surgical procedures (e.g. patients with spina bifida) and workers in mechanical, catering and electronic trades.

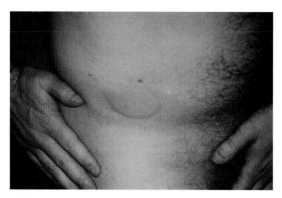

Figure 8.4 A classic wheal.

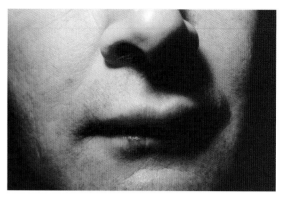

Figure 8.6 Angioedema of the upper lip.

Around 1–6% of the general population is believed to be sensitized to latex.

Latex reactions should be treated on their own merits (see *Urticaria treatment*, p. 104 and Figure 25.5 for anaphylaxis and Chapter 7 for dermatitis). Prevention of latex allergy is equally important. Non-latex (e.g. vinyl) gloves should be worn by those not handling infectious material (e.g. caterers) and, if latex gloves are chosen for those handling infectious material, then powder-free low allergen ones should be used.

Presentation

Most types of urticaria share the sudden appearance of pink itchy wheals, which can come up anywhere on the skin surface (Figures 8.4 and 8.5). Each lasts for less than a day, and most disappear within a few hours. Lesions may enlarge rapidly and some resolve centrally to take up an annular shape. In an acute anaphylactic reaction, wheals

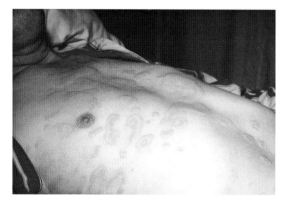

Figure 8.5 Severe and acute urticaria caused by penicillin allergy.

may cover most of the skin surface. In contrast, in chronic urticaria only a few wheals may develop each day.

Angioedema is a variant of urticaria that primarily affects the subcutaneous tissues, so that the swelling is less demarcated and less red than an urticarial wheal. Angioedema most commonly occurs at junctions between skin and mucous membranes (e.g. peri-orbital, peri-oral and genital; Figure 8.6). It may be associated with swelling of the tongue and laryngeal mucosa. It sometimes accompanies chronic urticaria and its causes may be the same. Angioedema without wheals may be the presenting feature of hereditary angioedema (see *Hereditary angioedema*) or more commonly as a result of angiotensin-converting enzyme (ACE) inhibitor consumption (thought to result from the inhibition of kinin degradation).

Course

The course of an urticarial reaction depends on its cause. If the urticaria is allergic, it will continue until the allergen is removed, tolerated or metabolized. Most such patients clear up within a day or two, even if the allergen is not identified. Urticaria may recur if the allergen is met again. At the other end of the scale, only half of patients attending hospital clinics with chronic urticaria and angioedema will be clear 5 years later. Those with urticarial lesions alone do better, half being clear after 6 months.

Complications

Urticaria is normally uncomplicated, although its itch may be enough to interfere with sleep or daily activities and to lead to depression. In acute anaphylactic reactions, oedema of the larynx may lead to asphyxiation, and oedema of the tracheo-bronchial tree to asthma.

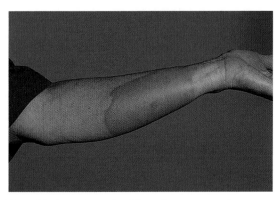

Figure 8.7 A massive urticarial reaction to a wasp sting.

Table 8.3 Endogenous causes of urticaria.

Infection
   Viral (e.g. hepatitis, infectious mononucleosis, HIV
      infection during seroconversion)
   Bacterial
   Mycoplasma
Intestinal parasites
Connective tissue disorders
Hypereosinophilic syndrome (unexplained
   eosinophilia with multiple internal organ
   involvement, especially cardiac)
Hyperthyroidism
Coeliac disease (children and young adults)
Cancer
Lymphomas

Differential diagnosis

There are two aspects to the differential diagnosis of urticaria. The first is to tell urticaria from other eruptions that are not urticaria at all. The second is to define the type of urticaria, according to Table 8.1. Insect bites or stings (Figure 8.7) and infestations commonly elicit urticarial responses, but these may have a central punctum and individual lesions may last longer than 24 hours. Erythema multiforme can mimic an annular urticaria. A form of vasculitis (urticarial vasculitis; p. 109) may resemble urticaria, but individual lesions last for longer than 24 hours, are typically associated with a more burning pain, blanch incompletely and leave bruising in their wake. Some bullous diseases, such as dermatitis herpetiformis, bullous pemphigoid and pemphigoid gestationis, begin as urticarial papules or plaques but, later, bullae make the diagnosis obvious. In these patients, individual lesions last longer than 24 hours, providing an additional tip-off for further investigation (see Chapter 9). On the face, erysipelas can be distinguished from angioedema by its sharp margin, redder colour and accompanying pyrexia. Hereditary angioedema (see *Hereditary angioedema*) must be distinguished from the angioedema accompanying urticaria as their treatments are completely different.

Investigations

The investigations will depend upon the presentation and type of urticaria. Many of the physical urticarias can be reproduced by appropriate physical tests. It is important to remember that antihistamines should be stopped for at least 3 days before these are undertaken.

Almost invariably, more is learned from the history than from the laboratory. The history should include details of the events surrounding the onset of the eruption. A review of systems may uncover evidence of an underlying disease. Careful attention should be paid to drugs, remembering that self-prescribed ones can also cause urticaria. Over-the-counter medications (such as aspirin and herbal remedies) and medications given by other routes (Table 8.2) can produce wheals.

If a patient has ordinary urticaria and its cause is not obvious, investigations are often deferred until it has persisted for a few weeks or months, and are based on the history. If no clues are found in the history, investigations can be confined to a complete blood count and erythrocyte sedimentation rate (ESR). An eosinophilia should lead to consideration of bullous or parasitic disease, and a raised ESR might suggest urticarial vasculitis, or a systemic cause. If the urticaria continues for 2–3 months, the patient may be referred to a dermatologist for further evaluation. In general, the focus of such investigations will be on internal disorders associated with urticaria (Table 8.3) and on external allergens (Table 8.4).

Table 8.4 Exogenous causes of urticaria.

Drugs, both topical and systemic
Preservatives in lotions (especially sorbic acid)
Foods and food additives
Bites
Inhalants
Pollens
Insect venoms
Animal dander

Thyroid function and autoantibody testing may be indicated by the history. Some specialist centres perform autologous serum intradermal injection to test for the presence of histamine-releasing autoantibodies. Patients frequently suspect a food allergy, but this is rarely found in chronic urticaria. Prick tests are unhelpful, although many patients with chronic ordinary urticaria are sure that their problems could be solved by intensive 'allergy tests', and ask repeatedly for them. Fluoroimmunoassays have superseded radioallergosorbent tests (RAST) on blood and are safer than prick or oral challenge testing. Their judicious use may be useful in the investigation of some environmental allergens (latex, nuts, fruit, pollen and animal dander). However, cautious interpretation of the results is required, especially in the presence of a raised total IgE. Even after extensive evaluation and environmental change, the cause cannot always be found; despite this the prognosis for recovery is usually good, a point worth stressing with the patient.

Treatment

The ideal is to find a cause and then to eliminate it. In addition, aspirin – in any form – should be avoided, as should opiates, ACE inhibitors and possibly NSAIDs (in aspirin-sensitive patients). The treatment for each type of urticaria is outlined in Table 8.5. In general, antihistamines are the mainstays of symptomatic treatment although they are not universally effective. First-line therapy usually includes one of the newer non-sedating antihistamines such as cetirizine 10 mg/day or loratadine 10 mg/day, both with half-lives of around 12 hours. Fexofenadine at the higher dose of 180 mg/day may also be useful. If necessary, these can be supplemented with shorter acting antihistamines; for example, hydroxyzine 10–25 mg up to every 6 hours (Formulary 2, p. 415) or acrivastine 8 mg three times daily. Alternatively, they can be combined with a longer acting antihistamine (such as chlorphenamine maleate 12 mg sustained-release tablets every 12 hours) so that peaks and troughs are blunted, and histamine activity is blocked throughout the night. If the eruption is not controlled, the dose of hydroxyzine can often be increased and still tolerated. The sedative effects of the older antihistamines (chlorphenamine, hydroxyzine, alimemazine and promethazine) may be especially helpful for relief of nocturnal symptoms. It should be remembered that all antihistamines can cause sedation so patients should be warned about driving and operating machinery. Response to different H1-blocking antihistamines is variable; therefore patients should be offered an alternative one if the first choice is ineffective. Doses

Table 8.5 Types of urticaria and their management.

Type	Treatment
Cold urticaria	Avoid cold
Protective clothing	
Antihistamines	
Solar urticaria	Avoid sun exposure
Protective clothing	
Sunscreens and sun blocks	
Beta-carotene	
Antihistamines	
Cholinergic urticaria	Avoid heat
Minimize anxiety	Anticholinergics
Avoid excessive exercise	Antihistamines
	Tranquillizers
Dermographism	Avoid trauma
	Antihistamines
Hereditary angioedema	Avoid trauma
	Attenuated androgenic steroids as prophylaxis
	Recombinant C1 esterase inhibitor concentrate for acute exacerbations
	Tracheotomy may be necessary
Hypersensitivity urticarias	Remove cause
	Antihistamines (H1 + H2)
	Sympathomimetics
	Systemic steroids (rarely justified)
	Avoid aspirin-containing drugs

above the manufacturer's guidelines are common practice and may be useful; this clearly requires careful consideration of the risk versus benefit of such treatment. H2-blocking antihistamines (e.g. cimetidine) may add a slight benefit if used in conjunction with an H1 histamine antagonist. Chlorphenamine or diphenhydramine are often used during pregnancy because of their long record of safety, but hydroxyzine, cetirizine, loratadine and mizolastine should be avoided. Sympathomimetic agents can help urticaria, although the effects of epinephrine are short lived. Pseudoephedrine (30 or 60 mg every 4 hours) or terbutaline (2.5 mg every 8 hours) can sometimes be useful adjuncts.

A tapering course of systemic corticosteroids may be used, but only when the cause is known and there are no contraindications, and certainly not as a panacea to control chronic urticaria or urticaria of unknown cause. Low doses of ciclosporin may be used for particularly severe cases. For the treatment of anaphylaxis see p. 357. The British Association of Dermatologists has produced an excellent patient information sheet on urticaria (http://www.bad.org.uk/for-the-public/patient-information-leaflets?l=0).

> **Learning points**
>
> - The treatment of choice is to find the cause and eliminate it.
> - You can learn more about the cause from the history than from tests.
> - Most patients with hives clear up quickly even if the cause is not obvious.
> - Use antihistamines in relatively high doses.
> - Avoid aspirins and systemic steroids in chronic urticaria.
> - Do not promise patients that all will be solved by allergy tests.
> - Take respiratory tract blockage seriously.

Hereditary angioedema

Recurrent attacks of abdominal pain and vomiting, or massive oedema of soft tissues, which may involve the larynx, characterize this autosomal dominant condition. Urticaria does not accompany the tissue swellings. Tooth extraction, cheek biting and other forms of trauma may precipitate an attack. A deficiency of an inhibitor to C1 esterase allows complement consumption to go unchecked so that vasoactive mediators are generated. To confirm the diagnosis, plasma complement C4 levels should be checked and, if low, functional serum C1 esterase inhibitor level measured.

This type of angioedema is controlled with maintenance anabolic steroids, and replacement C1 esterase inhibitor concentrate for acute episodes.

Erythema multiforme

Cause
In erythema multiforme, the patient has usually reacted to an infection (90% of cases), often herpes simplex, or to a drug, but other factors have occasionally been implicated (Table 8.6).

Presentation
The symptoms of an upper respiratory tract infection may precede the eruption. Typically, annular non-scaling

Table 8.6 Causes of erythema multiforme.

Viral infections, especially:
  Herpes simplex
  Hepatitis A, B and C
  Mycoplasma
  Orf
Bacterial infections
Fungal infections
  Coccidioidomycosis
Parasitic infestations
Drugs
Pregnancy
Malignancy, or its treatment with radiotherapy
Idiopathic

plaques appear predominantly on acral sites: the palms, soles, forearms and legs. They may be slightly more purple than the wheals of ordinary urticaria. Individual lesions enlarge but clear centrally. A new lesion may begin at the same site as the original one, so that the two concentric plaques look like a target (Figure 8.8). In erythema multiforme major (Figure 8.9) there is involvement of the mucous membranes (oral, genital, ocular, pharangeal or

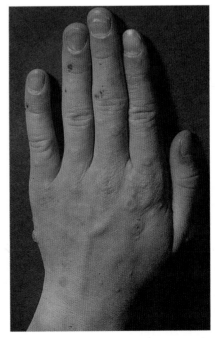

Figure 8.8 Erythema multiforme: bullous and target lesions occurring in a favourite site.

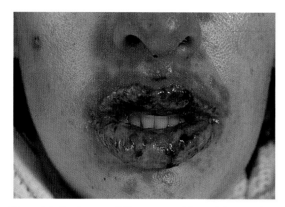

Figure 8.9 Erythema multiforme major. The eyelids were also severely involved.

may be associated with significant mortality. In Stevens–Johnson syndrome, extensive erythematous targetoid macules show an initial preponderance for the trunk. In comparison, the pathognomonic target lesions of erythema multiforme are palpable and favour an acral distribution. It should be noted that this distinction is not always clear-cut. The annular variant of urticaria as described earlier in this chapter should be considered. However, persistence of lesions for longer than 24 hours and the involvement of mucous membranes favour a diagnosis of erythema multiforme. Fixed drug eruptions, Sweet's syndrome (see *Acute febrile neutrophilic dermatosis*) and bullous disorders (see Chapter 9) may enter the differential. Rings of granuloma annulare (p. 312) take weeks or months to develop.

upper respiratory), which may or may not be associated with prodromal symptoms of fever, myalgia and malaise. Some lesions blister. The Stevens–Johnson syndrome is now no longer thought to be a severe form of erythema multiforme but rather part of the toxic epidermal necrolysis (TEN) spectrum of diseases (see Chapter 9).

Course

Crops of new lesions appear for 1–2 weeks, or until the responsible drug or other factor has been eliminated. Individual lesions last several days, and this differentiates them from the more fleeting lesions of an annular urticaria. The site of resolved lesions is marked transiently by grey or brown patches, particularly in pigmented individuals. A recurrent variant of erythema multiforme exists, characterized by repeated attacks; this merges with a rare form in which lesions continue to develop over a prolonged period, even for years. Herpes simplex infection is thought to be the most prevalent precipitant in these cases.

Complications

There are usually no complications. However, severe lesions in the tracheo-bronchial tree of patients with erythema multiforme major can lead to asphyxia, and ulcers of the bulbar conjunctiva to blindness. Corneal ulcers, anterior uveitis and panophthalmitis may also occur. Genital ulcers can cause urinary retention, and phimosis or vaginal stricture after they heal.

Differential diagnosis

Erythema multiforme should be distinguished from Stevens–Johnson syndrome (see Chapter 9) as the latter

Investigations

The histology of erythema multiforme is distinctive. Its main features are epidermal necrosis and dermal changes, consisting of endothelial swelling, a mixed lymphohistiocytic perivascular infiltrate and papillary dermal oedema. The abnormalities may be predominantly epidermal or dermal, or a combination of both; they probably depend on the age of the lesion biopsied.

Most investigations are directed towards identifying a cause. A careful history helps rule out a drug reaction. A PCR test, Tzanck smear (p. 39) or culture of suspicious prodromal vesicles may identify a precipitating herpes simplex infection, which is usually almost healed by the time the erythema multiforme erupts. A chest X-ray and serological tests should identify mycoplasmal pneumonia. A search for other infectious agents, neoplasia, endocrine causes or connective tissue disorder is sometimes necessary, especially when the course is prolonged or recurrent. About 50% of cases have no demonstrable provoking factor.

Treatment

The best treatment for erythema multiforme is to identify and remove its cause. In particular, if drug-induced erythema multiforme is suspected the culprit drug should be discontinued immediately. In mild cases, only symptomatic treatment is needed and this includes the use of antihistamines.

Erythema multiforme major, however, may demand consultation between dermatologists and specialists in other fields such as ophthalmology, urology and infectious diseases, depending on the particular case. Oral mucosal involvement may be treated with topical steroids, and anti-inflammatory or anaesthetic mouth washes. In severe cases where pain impedes swallowing, systemic steroids (prednisolone 40–60 mg/day tapered over 2–4 weeks) may be needed.

Herpes simplex infections should be suspected in recurrent or continuous erythema multiforme of otherwise unknown cause. A 6-month trial of continuous treatment with oral valaciclovir 500 mg once or twice daily or famciclovir 250 mg once or twice daily (Formulary 2, p. 415) may prevent attacks, both of herpes simplex and of the recurrent erythema multiforme that follows it. Treatment can subsequently be tapered according to response.

Learning points

- Look for target lesions and involvement of the palms.
- Herpes simplex infection is the most common provoking factor of recurrent erythema multiforme, but do not forget drugs.

Erythema nodosum

Erythema nodosum is an inflammation of the subcutaneous fat (a panniculitis). It is the prototypical septal panniculitis, with inflammation confined to the fibrous septae running between the fat lobules. It is commonly viewed as a type IV delayed hypersensitivity reaction (see Chapter 2) elicited by various bacterial, viral and fungal infections, malignant disorders, drugs or by a variety of other causes (Table 8.7).

Table 8.7 Causes of erythema nodosum.

Infections
  Bacteria (e.g. streptococci, tuberculosis, brucellosis, leprosy, yersinia)
  Viruses (e.g. hepatitis B, Epstein–Barr virus)
  Mycoplasma
  Rickettsia
  Chlamydia
  Fungi (especially coccidioidomycosis)
Drugs (e.g. sulfonamides, penicillins, oral contraceptive agents)
Systemic disease (e.g. sarcoidosis, ulcerative colitis, Crohn's disease, Behçet's disease)
Pregnancy
Malignancy

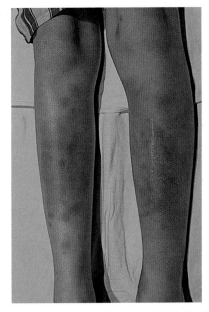

Figure 8.10 Erythema nodosum: large painful dusky plaques on the shins. Always investigate this important reaction pattern (see text).

Presentation

The characteristic lesion is a tender red nodule developing alone or in groups on the legs and forearms or, rarely, on other areas such as the thighs, face, breasts or other areas where there is fat (Figure 8.10). Some patients also have painful joints and fever.

Course

Individual lesions resolve over 2 weeks with new 'crops' appearing for up to 6–8 weeks. In the interim, lesions may enlarge and new ones may occur at other sites. Like other reactive erythemas, erythema nodosum may persist if its cause is not removed. Persisting erythema nodosum is sometimes called nodular vasculitis.

Complications

The nodules may be so tender that walking is difficult. Erythema nodosum leprosum occurs when lepromatous leprosy patients establish cell-mediated immunity to *Mycobacterium leprae*. These patients have severe malaise, arthralgia and fever.

Differential diagnosis

The differential diagnosis of a single tender red nodule is extensive and includes trauma, infection (early cellulitis or abscess) and phlebitis.

When lesions are multiple or bilateral, infection becomes less likely unless the lesions are developing in a sporotrichoid manner (p. 226). Other causes of a nodular panniculitis, which may appear like erythema nodosum, include panniculitis from pancreatitis, cold, trauma, the injection of drugs or other foreign substances, withdrawal from systemic steroids, lupus erythematosus, superficial migratory thrombophlebitis, polyarteritis nodosa and a deficiency of α_1-antitrypsin.

Investigations

Erythema nodosum demands a careful history, physical examination, a chest X-ray, throat culture for streptococcus, a Mantoux test and an antistreptolysin-O (ASO) titre. Serological testing for deep fungal infections such as coccidioidomycosis should be obtained, at least in endemic areas. Pregnancy should be excluded. If the results are normal, and there are no symptoms or physical findings to suggest other causes, extensive investigations can be deferred because the disease will usually resolve.

Treatment

The ideal treatment for erythema nodosum is to identify and eliminate its cause if possible. For example, if culture or an ASO test confirms a streptococcal infection, a suitable antibiotic should be recommended. Bed rest and leg elevation are also an important part of treatment. NSAIDs such as aspirin, indometacin or ibuprofen may be helpful. Systemic steroids are usually not needed. For reasons that are not clear, potassium iodide in a dosage of 400–900 mg/day can help, but should not be used for longer than 6 months.

Acute febrile neutophilic dermatosis (Sweet's syndrome)

Red, indurated, often painful plaques (see Figure 21.2), nodules or tumours erupt suddenly and dramatically, sometimes being associated with fever, malaise, myalgias and ocular signs. Coalescence of areas of more and less acute inflammation may lead to curious irregularities of the surface resembling a mountain range. Neutrophils gather in the dermis and subcutaneous fat to cause this, and peripheral blood counts of these cells are frequently elevated. The ESR is often raised. Involvement of other organs can occur too. Acute myelocytic leukemia is one cause. Other cancers, infections, inflammatory bowel disease, pregnancy, treatments with granulocyte–macrophage colony-stimulating factor (GM-CSF), and

Behçet's disease are among other associated causes. Sometimes a precipitant cannot be found. The differential diagnosis is large, the list of causes is long, the disease may be severe and treatments can be tricky. Refer these patients to a dermatologist.

Vasculitis

Whereas the reactive erythemas are associated with some inflammation around superficial or deep blood vessels, the term vasculitis is reserved for those showing inflammation within the vessel wall, with endothelial cell swelling, necrosis or fibrinoid change. The clinical manifestations depend upon the size of the blood vessel affected.

Cutaneous small vessel vasculitis (involving small vessels) Syn: cutaneous leucocytoclastic angiitis, leucocytoclastic vasculitis, allergic or hypersensitivity vasculitis, anaphylactoid purpura

Cause

Immune complexes may lodge in the walls of blood vessels (principally the postcapillary venules), activate complement and attract polymorphonuclear leucocytes (Figure 8.11). Enzymes released from these can degrade the vessel wall. Antigens in these immune complexes include

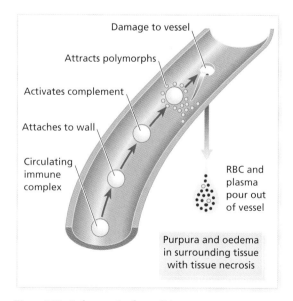

Figure 8.11 Pathogenesis of vasculitis.

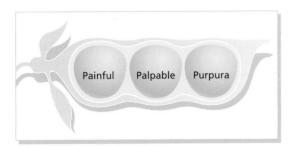

Figure 8.12 The three P's of cutaneous small vessel vasculitis.

drugs, autoantigens, and infectious agents such as viruses and bacteria. In the absence of other signs of systemic disease or malignancy, one should consider whether the onset of the vasculitis is precipitated by a 'drug or bug'.

Presentation

The most common presentation of cutaneous small vessel vasculitis is painful palpable purpura (Figure 8.12). Crops of 3–6 mm purpuric papules arise in dependent areas (the forearms and legs in ambulatory patients, or on the buttocks and flanks in bedridden ones; Figure 8.13). Some have a small, livid or black centre, caused by necrosis of the tissue overlying the affected blood vessel.

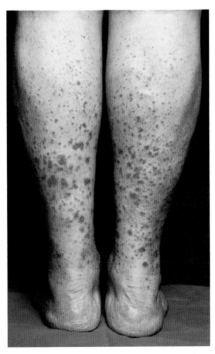

Figure 8.13 The palpable purpuric lesions of cutaneous small vessel vasculitis.

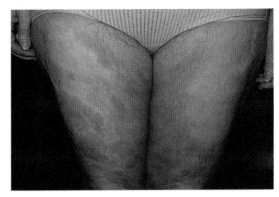

Figure 8.14 Urticarial vasculitis: a combination of urticaria and bruising.

Henoch–Schönlein purpura is a small vessel vasculitis associated with palpable purpura, arthritis, abdominal pain and occasionally nephritis. It typically presents in children following an upper respiratory tract infection.

Urticarial vasculitis (see *Urticaria*) is a small vessel vasculitis characterized by burning urticaria-like lesions (rather than itching found in true urticaria), which last for longer than 24 hours, sometimes leaving bruising and then pigmentation (haemosiderin) at the site of previous lesions (Figure 8.14). There may be foci of purpura in the wheals, low serum complement levels, elevated ESR and sometimes angioedema. General features include malaise and arthralgia.

Course

The course of vasculitis varies with its cause, its extent, the size of blood vessel affected and the involvement of other organs. In cutaneous small vessel vasculitis spontaneous resolution is the norm following removal of the precipitant. However, up to 10% of patients may have repeated episodes. In Henoch–Schönlein purpura the presence of nephritis predicts a worse long-term prognosis.

Complications

The vasculitis may simply be cutaneous; alternatively, it may be systemic and then other organs will be damaged, including the kidney, central nervous system, gastrointestinal tract and lungs.

Differential diagnosis

Cutaneous small vessel vasculitis has to be separated from other causes of purpura (p. 153) such as abnormalities of the clotting system and sepsis (with or without vasculitis). Vasculitic purpuras are raised (palpable).

Occasionally, the vasculitis may look like urticaria if its purpuric element is not marked. Blanching such an urticarial papule with a glass slide (diascopy) may reveal subtle residual purpura.

Investigations

Investigations should be directed toward identifying the cause and detecting internal involvement. Questioning may indicate infections; myalgias, abdominal pain, claudication, mental confusion and mononeuritis may indicate systemic involvement. A physical examination, chest X-ray, ESR and biochemical tests monitoring the function of various organs are indicated. However, the most important test is urine analysis, checking for proteinuria and haematuria, because vasculitis can affect the kidney subtly and so lead to renal insufficiency; in this context the blood pressure should also be checked.

Skin biopsy will confirm the diagnosis of small vessel vasculitis. The finding of circulating immune complexes, or a lowered level of total complement (CH50) or C4, will implicate immune complexes as its cause. Tests for paraproteins, hepatitis viruses, cryoglobulins, rheumatoid factor, antineutrophil cytoplasmic antibody (ANCA) and antinuclear antibodies may also be needed.

Direct immunofluorescence can be used to identify immune complexes in blood vessel walls, but is seldom performed because of false positive and false negative results, as inflammation may destroy the complexes in a true vasculitis and induce non-specific deposition in other diseases. Henoch–Schönlein vasculitis is confirmed if IgA deposits are found in the blood vessels of a patient with the clinical triad of palpable purpura, arthritis and abdominal pain.

Treatment

The treatment of choice is to identify the cause and eliminate it. In addition, antihistamines and bed rest sometimes help. Colchicine 0.6 g twice daily or dapsone 100 g daily may be worth a trial, but require monitoring for side effects (Formulary 2, p. 413). Patients whose vasculitis is damaging the kidneys or other internal organs may need systemic corticosteroids or immunosuppressive agents such as cyclophosphamide. NSAIDs may be useful in treating painful skin lesions and associated arthralgias but should be avoided if there is renal involvement.

Learning point

Cutaneous small vessel vasculitis may involve the kidneys. Be sure to check the urine and blood pressure.

Wegener's granulomatosis (involving small and medium-sized vessels)

In this granulomatous vasculitis of unknown cause, fever, weight loss and fatigue accompany naso-respiratory symptoms such as rhinitis, hearing loss or sinusitis. Only half of the patients have skin lesions, usually symmetrical ulcers or papules on the extremities. Other organs can be affected, including the eye, joints, heart, nerves, lung and kidney. Antineutrophil antibodies (usually C-ANCA with anti-PR3 specificity) are present in most cases and are a useful but non-specific diagnostic marker. Cyclophosphamide is the treatment of choice, used alone or with systemic steroids.

Polyarteritis nodosa (involving medium-sized vessels)

Cause

This necrotizing vasculitis of predominantly medium-sized vessels causes skin nodules, infarctive ulcers and peripheral gangrene. Immune complexes may initiate this vasculitis, and sometimes contain hepatitis B or C virus or antigen. Other known causes are adulterated drugs, B-cell lymphomas and immunotherapy.

Presentation

Tender subcutaneous nodules appear along the line of arteries. The skin over them may ulcerate or develop stellate patches of purpura and necrosis. Splinter haemorrhages and a peculiar net-like vascular pattern (livedo reticularis; p. 141) aid the clinical diagnosis. In approximately 10% of cases the disorder is limited to the skin (cutaneous polyarteritis nodosa); in the remainder there is systemic involvement of the kidneys, gut, heart muscle, nerves, testicles and joints (Figure 8.15). Cutaneous polyarteritis nodosa is associated with streptococcal infection in children. Patients may be febrile, lose weight and feel pain in the muscles, joints or abdomen. Some develop peripheral neuropathy, hypertension and ischaemic heart disease. Renal involvement, with or without hypertension, is common.

Course

Untreated, systemic polyarteritis nodosa becomes chronic. Death, often from renal disease, is common, even in treated patients.

Differential diagnosis

Embolism, panniculitis and infarctions can cause a similar clinical picture. Wegener's granulomatosis, allergic

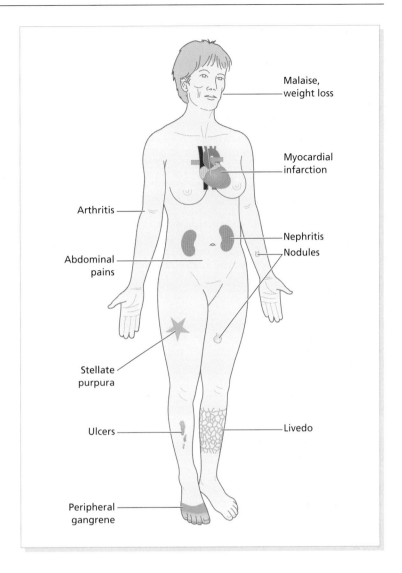

Malaise,
weight loss

Myocardial
infarction

Arthritis

Nephritis

Nodules

Abdominal
pains

Stellate
purpura

Ulcers

Livedo

Peripheral
gangrene

Figure 8.15 Clinical features of
polyarteritis nodosa.

granulomatosis, temporal arteritis, and the vasculitis that accompanies systemic lupus erythematosus and rheumatoid arthritis should be considered. Occasionally, pyoderma gangrenosum can mimic polyarteritis nodosa.

Investigations

The laboratory findings are non-specific. An elevated ESR, neutrophil count and gammaglobulin level are common. Investigations for cryoglobulins, rheumatoid factor, antinuclear antibody, ANCA, hepatitis C antibodies and hepatitis B surface antigen are worthwhile, as are checks for disease in the kidneys, heart, liver and gut. Low levels of complement C4 suggest active disease. The use of

a biopsy to confirm the diagnosis of medium-sized vessel vasculitis is not always easy as the arterial involvement may be segmental, and surgery itself difficult. Histological confirmation is most likely when biopsies are from a fresh lesion. Affected vessels show aneurysmal dilatation or necrosis, fibrinoid changes in their walls and an intense neutrophilic infiltrate around and even in the vessel wall.

Treatment

Systemic steroids and cyclophosphamide improve the chances of survival. Low-dose systemic steroids alone, or methotrexate, are usually sufficient for the purely cutaneous form. Empirical penicillin is often given to children with cutaneous polyarteritis nodosa given the association with streptococcal infection.

Further reading

Carlson JA, Ng BT, Chen KR. (2005) Cutaneous vascultis update: diagnostic criteria, classification, epidemiology, etiology, pathogenegis, evaluation and prognosis. *American Journal of Dermatopathology* **27**, 504–528.

Cousin F, Philips K, Favier B, Bienvenu J, Nicolas JF. (2001) Drug-induced urticaria. *European Journal of Dermatology* **11**, 181–187.

Dibbern DA. (2006) Urticaria: selected highlights and recent advances. *Medical Clinics of North America* **90**, 187–209.

Gilchrist H, Patterson JW. (2010) Erythema nodosum and erythema induratum (nodular vasculitis): diagnosis and management. *Dermatologic Therapy* **23**, 320–327.

Grattan CEH, Humphreys F. (2007) Guidelines for evaluation and management of urticaria in adults and children. *British Journal of Dermatology* **157**, 1116–1123.

Greaves MW. (2005) Antihistamines in dermatology. *Skin Pharmacology and Physiology* **18**, 220–209.

Kaplan AP, Greaves MW. (2005) Angioedema. *Journal of the American Academy of Dermatology* **53**, 373–388.

Russell JP, Gibson LE. (2006) Primary cutaneous small vessel vasculitis: approach to diagnosis and treatment. *International Journal of Dermatology* **45**, 3–13.

Sokumbi O, Wetter DA. (2012) Clinical features, diagnosis and treatment of erythema multiforme: a review for the practicing dermatologist. *International Journal of Dermatology* **51**, 889–902.

Sunderkotter C, Sindrilaru A. (2006) Clinical classification of vasculitis. *European Journal of Dermatology* **16**, 114–124.

Xu LY, Esparza EM, Anadkat MJ, Crone KG, Brasington RD. (2009) Cutaneous manifestations of vasculitis. *Seminars in Arthritis and Rheumatism* **38**, 348–360.

9 Bullous Diseases

Vesicles and bullae are accumulations of fluid within or under the epidermis. They have many causes, and a correct clinical diagnosis must be based on a close study of the physical signs.

The appearance of a blister is determined by the level at which it forms. Subepidermal blisters occur between the dermis and the epidermis. Their roofs are relatively thick and so they tend to be tense and intact. They may contain blood. Intraepidermal blisters appear within the prickle cell layer of the epidermis, and so have thin roofs and rupture easily to leave an oozing denuded surface. This tendency is even more marked with subcorneal blisters, which form just beneath the stratum corneum at the outermost edge of the viable epidermis, and therefore have even thinner roofs.

Sometimes the morphology or distribution of a bullous eruption gives the diagnosis away, as in herpes simplex or zoster. Sometimes the history helps too, as in cold or thermal injury, or in an acute contact dermatitis. When the cause is not obvious, a biopsy should be taken to show the level in the skin at which the blister has arisen. A list of differential diagnoses, based on the level at which blisters form, is given in Figure 9.1.

The bulk of this chapter is taken up by the three most important immunobullous disorders – pemphigus, pemphigoid and dermatitis herpetiformis (Table 9.1) – and by the group of inherited bullous disorders known as epidermolysis bullosa. Our understanding of both groups has advanced in parallel, as several of the skin components targeted by autoantibodies in the acquired immunobullous disorders are the same as those inherited in an abnormal form in epidermolysis bullosa.

Bullous disorders of immunological origin

Many chronic bullous diseases are caused directly or indirectly by antibodies binding to normal tissue antigens. In the pemphigus family, these are cadherins holding keratinocytes of the epidermis together. In the pemphigoid family, antigens are constituents of the dermo-epidermal junction that anchor the epidermis to the dermis. In dermatitis herpetiformis, the antigen is a transglutaminase.

The Pemphigus family

Pemphigus is often severe and potentially life-threatening. There are two main types. The most common is pemphigus vulgaris, which accounts for at least three-quarters of all cases, and for most of the deaths. Pemphigus vegetans is a rare variant of pemphigus vulgaris. The other important type of pemphigus, superficial pemphigus, also has two variants: the generalized foliaceus type and localized erythematosus type. A few drugs, led by penicillamine and angiotensin-converting enzyme inhibitors (ACE inhibitors), can trigger a pemphigus-like reaction, but autoantibodies are then seldom found. Finally, a rare type of pemphigus with severe mucosal erosions, paraneoplastic pemphigus, is associated with neoplasms such as thymoma, Castleman's tumour and lymphoma.

Cause

All types of pemphigus are autoimmune diseases in which pathogenic immunoglobulin G (IgG, predominantly IgG4) antibodies bind to antigens within the epidermis. The main target antigens are desmoglein 3 (in pemphigus vulgaris) and desmoglein 1 (in superficial pemphigus). Both are cell-adhesion molecules of the cadherin family (see Table 2.5), found in desmosomes. The antigen–antibody reaction interferes with adhesion, causing the keratinocytes to fall apart (acantholysis). Pemphigus vulgaris is particularly common in Ashkenazi Jews and people of Mediterranean or Indian origin. There is linkage between the disease and certain human leucocyte antigen (HLA) class II alleles. An endemic, superficial form of pemphigus foliaceus (fogo selvagem) is prevalent in certain areas of South America and Tunisia. It is postulated that a combination of genetic susceptibility (also

Clinical Dermatology, Fifth Edition. Richard B. Weller, Hamish J.A. Hunter and Margaret W. Mann.
© 2015 John Wiley & Sons, Ltd. Published 2015 by John Wiley & Sons, Ltd.

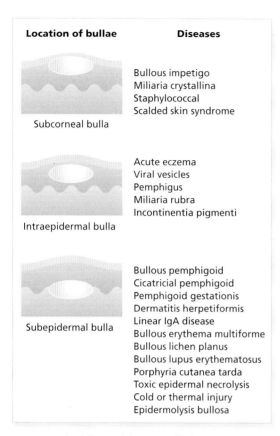

Location of bullae	Diseases
Subcorneal bulla	Bullous impetigo Miliaria crystallina Staphylococcal Scalded skin syndrome
Intraepidermal bulla	Acute eczema Viral vesicles Pemphigus Miliaria rubra Incontinentia pigmenti
Subepidermal bulla	Bullous pemphigoid Cicatricial pemphigoid Pemphigoid gestationis Dermatitis herpetiformis Linear IgA disease Bullous erythema multiforme Bullous lichen planus Bullous lupus erythematosus Porphyria cutanea tarda Toxic epidermal necrolysis Cold or thermal injury Epidermolysis bullosa

Figure 9.1 The differential diagnosis of bullous diseases based on the histological location of the blister.

linked to HLA class II alleles) and environmental exposure to a putative insect vector results in the disease.

Presentation

Pemphigus vulgaris is characterized by flaccid blisters of the skin (Figure 9.2) and mouth (Figure 9.3). The blisters rupture easily to leave widespread painful erosions. Most patients develop the mouth lesions first. Shearing stresses on normal skin can cause new erosions to form (a positive Nikolsky sign). In the vegetans variant (Figure 9.4), heaped up cauliflower-like weeping areas are present in the groin and body folds. The blisters in pemphigus foliaceus are so superficial, and rupture so easily, that the clinical picture is dominated more by weeping and crusted erosions than by blisters. In the rarer pemphigus erythematosus the rash may have a predilection for photo-exposed areas; on the face, lesions are often pink, rough and scaly.

Course

The course of all forms of pemphigus is prolonged, even with treatment, and the mortality rate of pemphigus vulgaris is still at least 15%. Most patients have a terrible time with weight gain and other side effects from systemic corticosteroids and from the lesions, which resist healing. However, about one-third of patients with pemphigus vulgaris will go into complete remission within 3 years. Superficial pemphigus is less severe. With modern treatments, most patients with pemphigus can live relatively normal lives, with occasional exacerbations.

Table 9.1 Distinguishing features of the three main immunobullous diseases.

	Age	Site of blisters	General health	Blisters in mouth	Nature of blisters	Circulating antibodies	Fixed antibodies	Treatment
Pemphigus	Middle age	Trunk flexures and scalp	Poor	Common	Superficial and flaccid	IgG to intercellular adhesion proteins	IgG in intercellular space	Steroids Immunosuppressives
Pemphigoid	Old	Often flexural	Good	Rare	Tense and blood-filled	IgG to basement membrane region	IgG at basement membrane	Steroids Immunosuppressives
Dermatitis herpetiformis	Primarily adults	Elbows, knees, upper back, buttocks	Itchy	Rare	Small, excoriated and grouped	IgG to the endomysium of muscle	IgA granular deposits in papillary dermis	Gluten-free diet Dapsone Sulphapyridine

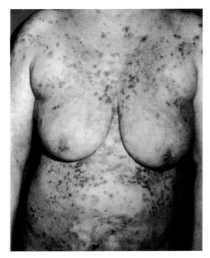

Figure 9.2 Pemphigus vulgaris: widespread erosions that have followed blisters.

Complications

Complications are inevitable with the high doses of steroids and immunosuppressive drugs that are needed to control the condition. Indeed, side effects of treatment are now the leading cause of death. Infections of all types are common. The large areas of denudation may become infected and smelly, and severe oral ulcers make eating painful.

Differential diagnosis

Widespread erosions may suggest a pyoderma, impetigo, epidermolysis bullosa or ecthyma. Mouth ulcers can be mistaken for aphthae, Behçet's disease or herpes simplex infection. Scalp erosions suggest bacterial or fungal infections. Pemphigus erythematosus is now considered as an overlap syndrome with lupus erythematosus.

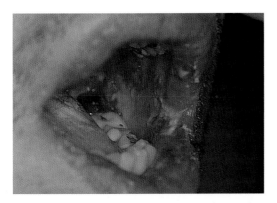

Figure 9.3 Painful sloughy mouth ulcers in pemphigus vulgaris.

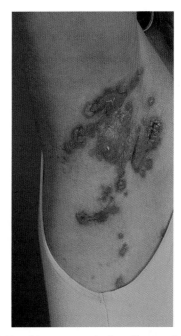

Figure 9.4 Pemphigus vegetans in the axilla, some intact blisters can be seen.

Investigations

Biopsy shows that the vesicles are intraepidermal, with rounded keratinocytes floating freely within the blister cavity (acantholysis). Direct immunofluorescence (p. 42) of adjacent normal skin shows intercellular epidermal deposits of IgG and C3 (Figure 9.5). The serum from a patient with pemphigus contains antibodies that bind to the desmogleins in the desmosomes of normal epidermis, so that indirect immunofluorescence (p. 42) or enzyme-linked immunosorbent assay (ELISA) assays can also be used to confirm the diagnosis. The titre of these antibodies correlates loosely with clinical activity and may guide changes in the dosage of systemic steroids.

Treatment

Because of the dangers of pemphigus vulgaris, and the difficulty in controlling it, patients should be treated by dermatologists. Resistant and severe cases need very high doses of systemic steroids, such as prednisolone (Formulary 2, p. 420) 60–180 mg/day. These 'industrial doses' work because prednisolone upregulates the expression of desmoglein molecules on the surfaces of keratinocytes, in addition to other effects above and beyond their anti-inflammatory ones. The dose is reduced only when new blisters stop appearing. Immunosuppressive agents, such as azathioprine, cyclophosphamide and mycophenylate

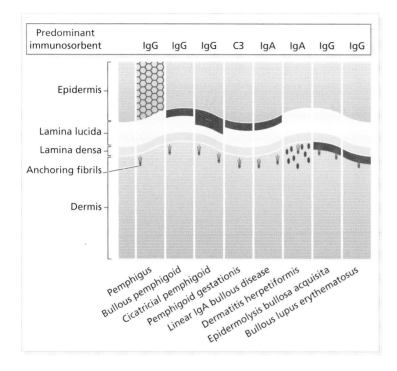

Figure 9.5 Immunofluorescence (red) in bullous diseases.

mofetil, are often used as steroid-sparing agents. As ever, the benefit of increasing immunosuppression has to be weighed up against the risk of treatment-associated adverse reactions. With long-term corticosteroid therapy being the norm it is worth commencing bone and gastric protection at the earliest opportunity. New and promising approaches include plasmapheresis, immunoadsorption and administration of intravenous immunoglobulin. Rituximab is a humanized murine monoclonal antibody to CD20 that may knock out B cells, pre-B cells and antibody production. Dapsone may sometimes be helpful, especially to allow healing. After control has been achieved, prolonged maintenance therapy and regular follow-up will be needed. In superficial pemphigus, smaller doses of systemic corticosteroids are usually needed, and the use of topical corticosteroids may help too.

Learning point

Pemphigus is more attacking than pemphigoid and needs higher doses of steroids to control it.

Hailey–Hailey disease

Hailey–Hailey disease (familial benign chronic pemphigus) is an autosomal dominant blistering condition result-

ing from mutations in the *ATP2C1* gene located on chromosome 3. The gene encodes a calcium–manganese pump essential for desmosomal adhesion. Mutations result in suprabasal keratinocyte acantholysis. Clinically, this manifests as flaccid vesicopustules and superficial erosions coalescing to form larger scaly circinate plaques. These have a predilection for sites of skin friction, typically the neck, submammary and intertriginous areas. Secondary infection, both fungal and bacterial, is common. There is no universally effective treatment. Mild cases can usually be managed with topical corticosteroids, antibiotics, antifungals or vitamin D analogues. More severe cases may require systemic therapy with ciclosporin, methotrexate, dapsone or retinoids. There are case reports of successful outcomes with various surgical and ablative laser procedures.

Other causes of subcorneal and intraepidermal blistering

Bullous impetigo (p. 215)

This is a common cause of blistering in children. The bullae erupt suddenly, are flaccid, often contain pus and are frequently grouped or located in body folds. Bullous impetigo is caused by *Staphylococcus aureus*.

Scalded skin syndrome (p. 217)

A toxin (exfoliatin) elaborated by some strains of *S. aureus* makes the skin painful and red; later it peels like a scald. The staphylococcus is usually hidden (e.g. conjunctiva, throat, wound, furuncle). The toxin causes dyshesion of desmoglein I, the same cadherin injured in pemphigus foliaceus.

Miliaria crystallina (p. 169)

Here sweat accumulates under the stratum corneum leading to the development of multitudes of uniformly spaced vesicles without underlying redness. Often this occurs after a fever or heavy exertion. The vesicles look like droplets of water lying on the surface, but the skin is dry to the touch. The disorder is self-limiting and needs no treatment.

Subcorneal pustular dermatosis

As its name implies, the lesions are small groups of pustules rather than vesicles. However, the pustules pout out of the skin in a way that suggests they were once vesicles (like the vesico-pustules of chickenpox). Oral dapsone (Formulary 2, p. 413) usually suppresses it. Many patients have IgA antibodies to intercellular epithelial antigens.

Acute dermatitis (see Chapter 7)

Severe acute eczema, especially of the contact allergic type, can be bullous. Plants such as poison ivy, poison oak or primula are common causes. The varied size of the vesicles, their close grouping, their asymmetry, their odd configurations (e.g. linear, square, rectilinear), their intense itch and a history of contact with plants are helpful guides to the diagnosis.

Pompholyx (p. 94)

In pompholyx, highly itchy small eczematous vesicles occur along the sides of the fingers, and sometimes also on the palms and soles. Some call it *dyshidrotic eczema*, but the vesicles are not related to sweating or sweat ducts. The disorder is very common, but its cause is not known.

Viral infections (see Chapter 16)

Some viruses create blisters in the skin by destroying epithelial cells. The vesicles of herpes simplex and zoster are the most common examples.

Subepidermal immunobullous disorders

These can be hard to separate on clinical grounds and only the two most important, pemphigoid and dermatitis herpetiformis, are described in detail here. Several others are mentioned briefly.

The Pemphigoid family

Bullous pemphigoid is an autoimmune disease. Serum from about 70% of patients contains antibodies that bind *in vitro* to normal skin at the basement membrane zone. However, their titre does not correlate with clinical disease activity. The IgG antibodies bind to two main antigens: most commonly to BP230 (which anchors keratin intermediate filaments to the hemidesmosome, p. 14), and less often to BP180 (a transmembrane molecule with one end within the hemidesmosome and the other bound to the lamina lucida). Complement is then activated (p. 24), starting an inflammatory cascade. Eosinophils often participate in the process causing the epidermis to separate from the dermis.

Presentation

Bullous pemphigoid is a chronic, usually itchy, blistering disease, mainly affecting the elderly (mean age of onset around 80 years). Usually, no precipitating factors can be found, but rarely drugs, ultraviolet radiation exposure or radiotherapy seem to play a part. Several neurological diseases may pre-date the onset of the disease; including cerebrovascular disease, Parkinson's disease, epilepsy and multiple sclerosis, and these are now considered risk factors for bullous pemphigoid. The skin often erupts with smooth itching red plaques in which tense vesicles and bullae form (Figure 9.6). Occasionally they arise from normal skin. The flexures are often affected; the mucous membranes usually are not. The Nikolsky test is negative. Denudation occurs only over small areas as blisters rupture, so the disorder would not be fatal were it not for its propensity to affect elderly people who may be already in poor health; factors carrying a high risk include old age, the need for high steroid dosage, and low serum albumin levels.

Course

Bullous pemphigoid is usually self-limiting and treatment can often be stopped after 1–2 years.

Complications

Untreated, the disease causes much discomfort and loss of fluid from ruptured bullae. Systemic steroids and immunosuppressive agents carry their usual complications if used long term (Formulary 2, p. 420 and p. 418, respectively).

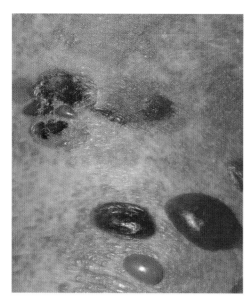

Figure 9.6 Numerous large tense blisters in an elderly person suggest pemphigoid.

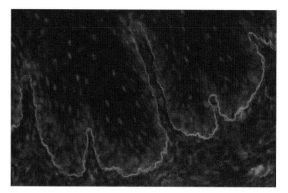

Figure 9.7 Indirect immunofluorescence using serum from a patient with pemphigoid, showing basement zone immunofluorescence.

Differential diagnosis

Most of the time, a clinical diagnosis proves correct. Bullous pemphigoid may look like other bullous diseases, especially epidermolysis bullosa acquisita, bullous lupus erythematosus, dermatitis herpetiformis, pemphigoid gestationis, bullous erythema multiforme and linear IgA bullous disease. Immunofluorescence helps to separate it from these (Figure 9.5).

Investigations

A subepidermal blister is often filled with eosinophils. Direct immunofluorescence shows a linear band of IgG and C3 along the basement membrane zone. Indirect immunofluorescence, using serum from the patient, identifies IgG antibodies that react with the basement membrane zone in some 70% of patients (Figure 9.7). Recently, an ELISA has been developed to measure serum antibodies to BP230 and BP180. Most patients have peripheral blood eosinophilia.

Treatment

Mild bullous pemphigoid can sometimes be controlled by the use of very potent topical steroids alone. However, in the acute phase, prednisolone or prednisone (Formulary 2, p. 420) at a dosage of 40–60mg/day is usually needed to control the eruption – although starting doses of over 0.75 mg/kg/day give no additional benefit. The dosage is reduced as soon as possible, and patients end up on a low maintenance regimen of systemic steroids, taken on alternate days until treatment is stopped. The addition of anti-inflammatory antibiotics and/or nicotinamide may confer further benefit. For non-responsive disease, immunosuppressive agents such as azathioprine, methotrexate or dapsone may be required. Again, if long-term corticosteroid therapy is required bone and gastric protection should be considered.

Learning points

1 Death is uncommon and the disease is self-limiting.
2 Some elderly people get fatal adverse effects from their systemic steroids. Reduce the dosage as soon as possible.

Pemphigoid gestationis (herpes gestationis)

This is pemphigoid occurring in pregnancy, or in the presence of a hydatidiform mole or a choriocarcinoma. Certain paternally derived histocompatability antigens carried by the fetus might provoke an autoimmune response directed towards BP180 in the skin of some mothers. As in bullous pemphigoid, most patients have linear deposits of C3 along the basement membrane zone (Figure 9.5), although IgG is detected less often. Clinically, pruritic papules and plaques are found in a peri-umbilical distribution; less common are the typical tense bullae found in bullous pemphigoid. The condition usually remits after the birth but may return in future pregnancies. It is not caused by a herpes virus. The name herpes gestationis should be discarded now so that the disease is not confused with herpes genitalis. Treatment is with topical or systemic steroids. Oral contraceptives should be avoided, because their hormones may precipitate the disease.

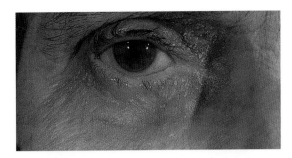

Figure 9.8 Long-standing mucous membrane pemphigoid. Adhesions are now forming between the upper and lower eyelids.

Mucous membrane pemphigoid (cicatricial pemphigoid) (Figure 9.8)

Like bullous pemphigoid itself, mucous membrane pemphigoid is an autoimmune skin disease showing IgG and C3 deposition at the basement membrane zone (Figure 9.5). The target antigens are often as in bullous pemphigoid (BP230 and BP180), but other antigens at the dermo-epidermal junction are sometimes targeted such as α6β4 integrin, laminin 332 and type VII collagen (in anchoring filaments). The finding of anti-laminin 332 antibodies should prompt a thorough search for occult malignancy; their presence may be associated with solid tumours. The condition differs from bullous pemphigoid in that its blisters and ulcers occur mainly on mucous membranes such as the conjunctivae, the mouth and genital tract. Bullae on the skin itself are less common (25–30% of cases). The condition also differs from bullous pemphigoid in that the lesions heal with scarring; around the eyes this may cause blindness, especially when the palpebral conjunctivae are affected (Figure 9.8). The condition tends to persist and treatment is relatively ineffective, although very potent local steroids, dapsone, systemic steroids and immunosuppressive agents are usually tried. Good eye hygiene and the removal of ingrowing eyelashes are important.

Linear IgA bullous disease

This is clinically similar to bullous pemphigoid, but affects children as well as adults. Blisters arise on urticarial plaques, and are more often grouped, and on extensor surfaces, than is the case with pemphigoid. The 'string of pearls sign', seen in some affected children, is the presence of blistering around the rim of polycyclic urticarial plaques. The conjunctivae may be involved. Again, the autoantibodies are directed against BP180 (BP 2 antigen).

Linear IgA bullous disease is, as its name implies, associated with linear deposits of IgA and C3 at the basement membrane zone (Figure 9.5). IgG is sometimes also found. The disorder responds well to oral dapsone (Formulary 2, p. 413).

Acquired epidermolysis bullosa (epidermolysis bullosa acquisita)

This can also resemble bullous pemphigoid, but has two important extra features: many of the blisters arise in response to trauma on otherwise normal skin; and milia are a feature of healing lesions. The target of the autoantibodies is type VII collagen in anchoring fibrils (Figure 9.5). The antigen lies on the dermal side of the lamina densa, in contrast to the bullous pemphigoid antigens, which lie on the epidermal side – a difference that can be demonstrated by immunofluorescence after the basement membrane is split at the lamina densa by incubating skin in a saline solution (the 'salt-split' technique). The condition responds poorly to systemic corticosteroids or immunosuppressive agents.

Dermatitis herpetiformis

Dermatitis herpetiformis is a very itchy chronic subepidermal vesicular disease, in which the vesicles erupt in groups as in herpes simplex – hence the name herpetiformis. It is most prevalent in northern European populations and has a male preponderance. Asians or African Americans are very rarely affected.

Cause

Gluten-sensitive enteropathy (sprue, adult coeliac disease), demonstrable by small bowel biopsy, is always present, but most patients do not have diarrhoea, constipation or malnutrition as the enteropathy is mild, patchy and involves only the proximal small intestine. A range of antibodies can be detected in serum, notably directed against tissue transglutaminase, reticulin, gliadin and endomysium – a component of smooth muscle. In a minority of patients with gluten-sensitive enteropathy, IgA antibodies against tissue transglutaminase cross-react with antigens of epidermal transglutaminase leading to granular deposits of IgA and then C3 in the tips of the dermal papillae and along the basement membrane (Figure 9.5). These induce a neutrophil-rich inflammation, which separates the epidermis from the dermis (a subepidermal cleft within the lamina lucida). The IgA deposits in skin clear slowly after the introduction of a gluten-free

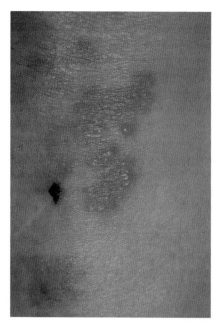

Figure 9.9 The typical small tense grouped itchy blisters of dermatitis herpetiformis.

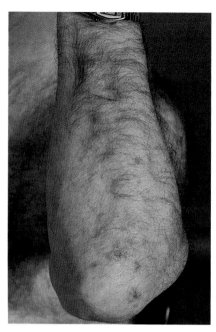

Figure 9.10 The itchy blisters of dermatitis herpetiformis favour the points of the elbows and knees, where they are quickly destroyed by scratching.

diet. There is a strong association with certain HLA types, particularly HLA-DQ2 and HLA-DQ8.

Presentation

The extremely itchy, grouped vesicles (Figure 9.9) and urticated papules develop in a symmetrical distribution over the elbows (Figure 9.10) knees, buttocks and shoulders. They are often broken by scratching before they reach any size. A typical patient therefore shows only grouped excoriations and erosions. Sometimes, a secondary eczematous dermatitis develops from fierce scratching. Thus, the name *dermatitis* comes from scratching, and *herpetiformis* comes from grouping of vesicles and crusts. Palmoplantar purpura and enamel defects of the secondary teeth are less commonly noted signs.

Course

The condition typically lasts for decades unless patients avoid gluten entirely.

Complications

The complications of gluten-sensitive enteropathy include diarrhoea, abdominal pain, anaemia and, rarely, malabsorption. Small bowel lymphomas have been reported,

and the use of a gluten-free diet may reduce this risk. There is a proven association with other autoimmune diseases, most commonly of the thyroid.

Differential diagnosis

The disorder masquerades as linear IgA bullous disease, scabies, an excoriated eczema, insect bites or neurodermatitis.

Investigations

If a vesicle can be biopsied before it is scratched away, the histology will be that of a subepidermal blister, with neutrophils packing the adjacent dermal papillae. Direct immunofluorescence of uninvolved skin shows granular deposits of IgA, and usually C3, in the dermal papillae and superficial dermis (Figure 9.5). Serum antibody tests for antiendomysial antibodies or tissue transglutaminase can help diagnose the enteropathy. Recent reports suggest that detection of IgA antiepidermal transglutaminase (anti-eTG) antibodies is the most sensitive and specific serum test for dermatitis herpetiformis. However, commercially available ELISA may not be routinely performed in all centres. Small bowel biopsy is no longer recommended as routine because the changes are often patchy and serum tests are more sensitive. Tests for malabsorption are seldom needed.

Treatment

The disorder responds to a gluten-free diet, which should be supervised by a dietitian. Adherence to this can be monitored using the titre of antibodies to antiendomysial antigens or to tissue transglutaminase, which fall if gluten is strictly avoided. The bowel changes revert quickly to normal but IgA deposits remain longer in the skin, so the skin disease can drag on for many months. Because of this, and because a gluten-free diet is hard to follow and enjoy, some patients prefer to combine the diet with dapsone (Formulary 2, p. 413) or sulfapyridine at the start, although both can cause severe rashes, haemolytic anaemia (especially in those with glucose-6-phosphate dehydrogenase deficiency), leucopenia, thrombocytopenia, methaemoglobinaemia and peripheral neuropathy. Regular blood checks are therefore necessary.

Learning points

1 Biopsy non-involved skin to demonstrate the diagnostic granular deposits of IgA in the dermal papillae.
2 The gluten enteropathy of dermatitis herpetiformis seldom causes frank malabsorption.
3 Dapsone works quickly and a gluten-free diet only very slowly. Combine the two at the start and slowly reduce the dapsone.

Other causes of subepidermal blisters

Porphyria cutanea tarda (p. 316)
Flacid bullae and erosions occur on the backs of the hands and on other areas exposed to sunlight.

Blisters in diabetes and renal disease
A few diabetics develop unexplained blisters on their legs or feet. The backs of the hands of patients with chronic renal failure may show changes rather like those of porphyria cutanea tarda (pseudoporphyria). Furosemide can contribute to blister formation.

Bullous lupus erythematosus
Vesicles and bullae may be seen in severe active systemic lupus erythematosus (p. 126). This disorder is uncommon and carries a high risk of kidney disease. Non-cutaneous manifestations of systemic lupus erythematosus do not respond to dapsone; however, the bullae do.

Bullous erythema multiforme

Bullous erythema multiforme is discussed in Chapter 8.

Stevens–Johnson syndrome/toxic epidermal necrolysis (Lyell's disease)

Cause
Stevens–Johnson syndrome (SJS) and toxic epidermal necrolysis (TEN) are now widely regarded as the same condition at either end of a spectrum of severity. TEN, the severest form of the disease has an incidence of about two cases per million population per year; with an overall mortality of 20–30%. Differentiation between the two conditions is based predominantly on the extent of skin detachment (1–10% SJS, 10–30% SJS/TEN overlap syndrome, >30% TEN).

It is now considered that the SJS/TEN spectrum of diseases usually represent a severe cutaneous adverse drug reaction; unlike erythema multiforme or erythema multiforme major which is a distinct condition often precipitated by infection (see Chapter 8). Infection, especially *Mycoplasma pneumoniae*, may precipitate SJS/TEN but this is far less common than the drug-associated aetiology. The most commonly implicated prescribed drugs are sulfonamides, antiepileptics, nevirapine, allopurinol, sulfasalazine and oxicam-nonsteroidal anti-inflammatory drugs (see Chapter 25). The usual interval between ingestion of the drug and development of TEN/SJS is between 4 and 28 days. Several genetic associations have now been established; the most well recognized being that of SJS/TEN in response to carbamazepine therapy in Han Chinese individuals carrying the HLA-B*1502 allele. Several other genetic associations between specific drugs and HLA antigens have been discovered; it is likely that many more will come to light with increasing use of pharmacogenomics.

The cellular mechanism by which drug exposure causes apoptosis (programmed cell death) and necrosis in TEN/SJS has yet to be fully elucidated. However, it is likely that cytotoxic T lymphocytes, natural killer cells and possibly keratinocytes produce excessive pro-apoptotic proteins such as Fas and granulysin. These combined with oxidative stress and defective regulation by the innate immune system culminate in keratinocyte apoptosis, inflammation and necrosis.

Presentation
There may be a prodromal period involving fever, cough and general malaise, which is followed by a painful

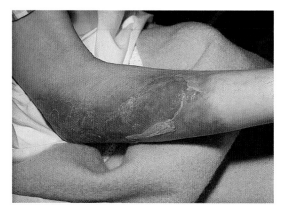

Figure 9.11 The burn-like appearance of toxic epidermal necrolysis.

macular exanthem. If this progresses, the skin becomes red, intensely painful, and detaches in sheets like a scald, leaving an eroded painful glistening surface (Figure 9.11). Nikolsky's sign is positive (p. 114). Usually, the skin signs start centrally (trunk and face) and spread to the extremities, in contrast to those of erythema multiforme, which initially favour acral sites. The mucous membranes are usually affected, including the mouth, eyes, gastrointestinal and genitourinary tracts and even the bronchial tree.

Course
The condition usually clears if the offending drug is stopped and if the patient lives. New epidermis grows out from hair follicles so that skin grafts are not usually needed. The disorder may come back if the drug is taken again. A toxic epidermal necrolysis-specific severity-of-illness score (SCORTEN) has been developed to grade the severity of SJS/TEN and predict its mortality (see *Further reading*).

Complications
Toxic epidermal necrolysis is a skin emergency and can be fatal. Infection, and the loss of fluids and electrolytes, are life-threatening, and the painful denuded skin surfaces make life a misery. Corneal scarring may remain when the acute episode has settled, resulting in permanent loss of vision.

Differential diagnosis
The epidermolysis of the staphylococcal scalded skin syndrome (p. 217) looks like TEN clinically, but only the stratum corneum is lost. Whereas TEN affects adults, the staphylococcal scalded skin syndrome is usually seen in infancy or early childhood. Histology differentiates the two. Pemphigus may also look similar, but starts more slowly and is more localized. Severe graft versus host reactions can also mimic this syndrome.

Investigations
Biopsy helps to confirm the diagnosis. The split is subepidermal in TEN, with extensive keratinocyte apoptosis and a sparse mononuclear infiltrate; the entire epidermis may be necrotic. A frozen section provides a quick answer if there is genuine difficulty in separating TEN from the scalded skin syndrome where the slit is subcorneal (p. 117). There are no tests to tell which drug caused the disease.

Treatment
The most important step in treating TEN/SJS is to identify and stop the culprit drug (see Chapter 25); otherwise treatment relies mainly on symptomatic management. The best practice involves a multidisciplinary team approach, with intensive nursing and medical support from multiple specialties, not least the dermatologist. Many patients are treated in units designed to deal with extensive thermal burns. Invasive monitoring with central and arterial lines may be required. Meticulous attention should be paid to fluid and electrolyte balance, wound care and infection control, pain management and nutritional support. Air suspension beds increase comfort. The weight of opinion has turned against the use of systemic corticosteroids. High-dose intravenous IgG seems more promising and ciclosporin treatment has been associated with decreased mortality rates. Plasmapheresis may remove triggering drugs, or inflammatory mediators.

> **Learning points**
> 1 The skin is programmed to die; treatments may not stop it.
> 2 Identify and stop the 'culprit' drug immediately.
> 3 This is an emergency. Death is common.
> 4 Refer the patient to a unit that treats thermal burns.

Epidermolysis bullosa (also known as the mechanobullous disorders)

There are many types of epidermolysis bullosa for which the underlying genetic defects and corresponding clinical phenotypes have now been established. Over 1000 gene mutations have been reported, affecting 15 structural proteins. Given the increased knowledge of these conditions,

Table 9.2 Simplified classification of epidermolysis bullosa.

Type	Mode of inheritance	Level of split	Mutations in
Epidermolysis bullosa simplex	Usually autosomal dominant	Intraepidermal	Keratins 5 and 14
Junctional epidermolysis bullosa	Autosomal recessive	Lamina lucida	Components of the hemidesmosome-anchoring filaments (e.g. laminins, integrins and bullous pemphigoid 180 molecule)
Dystrophic epidermolysis bullosa	Autosomal dominant	Beneath lamina densa	Type VII collagen
Dystrophic epidermolysis bullosa	Autosomal recessive	Beneath lamina densa	Type VII collagen
Kindler syndrome	Kindlin-1	Autosomal dominant	Mixed
Acquired epidermolysis bullosa	Not inherited	Dermal side of lamina densa	Nil

experts in the field published a consensus classification in 2008; they felt that this was comprehensive at the time of print and could be easily amended as further discoveries dictate. The full classification is outwith the remit of this book; rather we present an overview of the most common conditions. For more comprehensive reviews see *Further reading*.

The main types of epidermolysis bullosa are listed in Table 9.2. All are characterized by an inherited tendency to develop blisters after minimal trauma, although at different levels in the skin (Figure 9.12). The most severe types are usually caused by mutations resulting in very low levels or a complete absence of the corresponding structural protein. These have a catastrophic impact on the lives of patients. In contrast to this, the milder forms often have minimal impact on quality of life. The gold standard method for the diagnosis of epidermolysis bullosa was transmission electron microscopy; however, limited expertise and availability of this technique has seen it surpassed by immunofluorescence microscopy (IFM) with standardized antibodies against the various structural proteins. Mutation analysis is often very helpful but only available in specialist centres. Acquired epidermolysis bullosa is not inherited and is discussed earlier in this chapter.

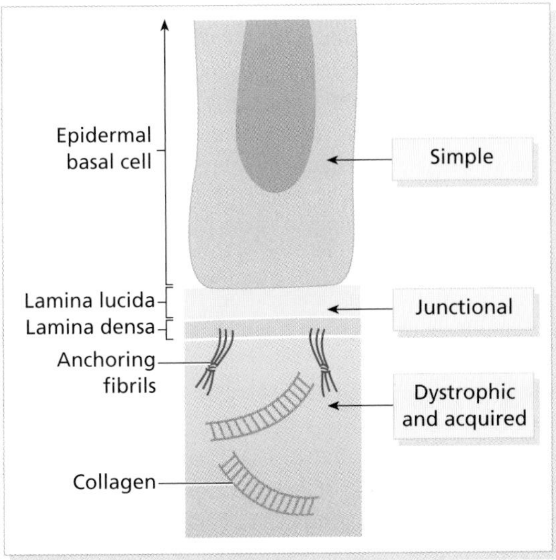

Epidermolysis bullosa simplex

Several subtypes are recognized of which the most common are epidermolysis bullosa simplex-localized (formerly Weber–Cockayne type), presenting in childhood with blistering at sites of trauma (hands, elbows and feet) and the Dowling–Meara type, featuring herpetiform blisters on the trunk. Most of these subtypes are inherited as autosomal dominant conditions and are caused by abnormalities in genes responsible for production of the paired keratins (K5 and K14) expressed in basal keratinocytes (see Figure 2.4). Linkage studies show that the genetic defects responsible for the most common types of simple epidermolysis bullosa lie on chromosomes 17 and 12. Rarer, more severe, types result from defects in the genes encoding desmosomal and hemidesmosomal proteins (see Figure 2.9) including plectin, α6β4 integrin, desmoplakin and plakophylin-1, respectively.

Blisters form within or just above the basal cell layers of the epidermis and so tend to heal without scarring.

Figure 9.12 Levels of blister formation in epidermolysis bullosa at the dermo-epidermal junction.

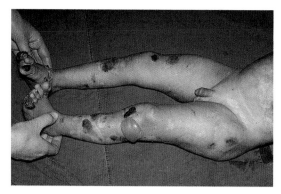

Figure 9.13 Junctional epidermolysis bullosa: minor trauma has caused large blisters and erosions which will heal slowly or not at all.

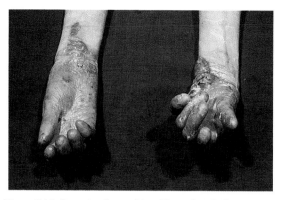

Figure 9.14 Recessive dystrophic epidermolysis bullosa: note large blood-filled blister. Scarring has led to fixed deformity of the fingers and loss of nails.

Nails and mucosae are not involved. The problems are made worse by sweating and ill-fitting shoes. Blistering can be minimized by avoiding trauma, wearing soft well-fitting shoes and using foot powder. Large blisters should be pricked with a sterile needle and dressed. Their roofs should not be removed. Local antibiotics may be needed.

Junctional epidermolysis bullosa

In these autosomal recessive conditions the separation occurs in the lamina lucida of the basement membrane, usually following mutations in the genes responsible for laminin-332 formation (p. 14; see Figure 2.9). The Herlitz type of junctional epidermolysis bullosa is rare, often lethal and evident at birth. The newborn child has large raw areas and flaccid blisters, which are slow to heal (Figure 9.13). The peri-oral and peri-anal skin is usually involved, as are the nails and oral mucous membrane. Other less severe types of junctional epidermolysis bullosa preserve a degree of laminin-332 function or result from mutations in the genes encoding type XVII collagen or α6β4 integrin.

Dystrophic epidermolysis bullosa

There are many subtypes, all of which probably result from abnormalities of type VII collagen, the major structural component of anchoring fibrils.

Dominant dystrophic epidermolysis bullosa

In the autosomal dominant type blisters appear in late infancy. They are most common on friction sites (e.g. the knees, elbows and fingers), healing with scarring and milia formation. The nails may be deformed or even lost.

The mouth is not affected. The only treatment is to avoid trauma and to dress the blistered areas.

Recessive dystrophic epidermolysis bullosa

Recessive dystrophic epidermolysis bullosa (generalized severe subtype) is a tragic form of epidermolysis bullosa. Extensive, sometimes haemorrhagic, subepidermal blisters start in infancy, and heal with scarring; this can be so severe that the nails are lost and webs form between the digits (Figure 9.14). The hands and feet may become useless balls, having lost all fingers and toes. The teeth, mouth and upper part of the oesophagus are all affected; oesophageal strictures may form. Squamous cell carcinomas of the skin and renal failure are late complications. It is especially important to minimize trauma, to maintain nutrition, to prevent contractures and web formation between the digits, and to combat anaemia and secondary infection. Referral to centres with expertise in management of these patients is strongly recommended.

Kindler syndrome

Recently added to the classification, this autosomal recessive condition results from mutations in the *KIND1* gene, encoding the protein kindlin-1. The split in the skin in kindler syndrome can be at any level (intraepidermal, junctional or sub-lamina densa) hence, it is classified separately from the above conditions. It presents with generalized blistering at birth, atrophic scarring, poikiloderma and photosensitivity. Other rare non-cutaneous features include mental retardation, bone abnormalities and involvement of the genitourinary and gastrointestinal tracts.

Treatment

Despite tremendous advances in the characterization of the molecular defects and clinical correlates in epidermolysis bullosa, effective therapies for any of the subtypes have yet to be established. The mainstays of treatment are avoidance of skin trauma, meticulous wound care, adequate pain relief and monitoring for secondary complications. Treatment of recessive dystrophic epidermolysis bullosa with phenytoin, which reduces the raised dermal collagenase levels found in this variant, and systemic steroids are disappointing. However, there is hope on the horizon. Gene therapy to replace the mutated DNA may be possible if a safe vector can be found to insert the 'corrected' sequence. Silencing autosomal dominant inherited mutations with small interfering RNA (siRNA) also shows promise. Cell therapies with keratinocyte, dermal fibroblast, bone marrow-derived stem cell or patient-specific induced pluripotent stem cell injections may be useful. Bone marrow transplantation has proved effective in small clinical trials but has a significant risk of transplant-related morbidity and mortality. Finally, novel methods of topical and/or systemic protein replacement therapies may be realistic options in the future.

Accurate diagnosis of the exact type of epidermolysis bullosa may be very difficult in the neonatal period but is essential to guide parents and families regarding prognosis and heritability of the condition. Prenatal testing and preimplantation diagnosis (in assisted pregnancies) is now possible for many of these conditions. National registers provide an exceptional resource of data and tissue for research. Patient support groups are a vital source of research funding and produce a wealth of easily accessible information for patients, families and healthcare professionals alike; the most well known of which is the Dystrophic Epidermolysis Bullosa Research Association (DebRA) (www.debra-international.org, www.debra.org.uk, www.debra.org).

Further reading

Bastuji-Garin S, Fouchard N, Bertocchi M, *et al.* (2000) SCORTEN: A severity-of-illness score for toxic epidermal necrolysis. *Journal of Investigative Dermatology* **115**, 149–153.

Bolotin D, Petronic-Rosic V. (2011) Dermatitis herpetiformis, Part I. Epidemiology, pathogenesis and clinical presentation. *Journal of the American Academy of Dermatology* **64**, 1017–1024.

Bolotin D, Petronic-Rosic V. (2011) Dermatitis herpetiformis, Part II. Diagnosis, management and prognosis. *Journal of the American Academy of Dermatology* **64**, 1027–1033.

Burge SM. (1992) Hailey–Hailey disease: the clinical features response to treatment and prognosis. *British Journal of Dermatology* **126**, 275–282.

Bystryn JC, Rudolph JL. (2005) Pemphigus. *Lancet* **366**, 61–73.

Downey A, Jackson C, Harun N, Cooper A. (2012) Toxic epidermal necrolysis: review of pathogenesis and management. *Journal of the American Academy of Dermatology* **66**, 995–1003.

Fassihi H, Wong T, Wessagowit V, McGrath JA, Mellerio JE. (2006) Target proteins in inherited and acquired blistering skin disorders. *Clinical and Experimental Dermatology* **31**, 252–259.

Fine JD, Eady, RAJ, Bauer EA, *et al.* (2008) The classification of inherited epidermolysis bullosa (EB): report of the third international consensus meeting on diagnosis and classification of EB. *Journal of the American Academy of Dermatology* **58**, 931–950.

Harman KE, Albert S, Black MM. (2003) Guidelines for the management of pemphigus vulgaris. *British Journal of Dermatology* **149**, 926–937.

Intong LRA, Murrell DF. (2012) Inherited epidermolysis bullosa: new diagnostic criteria and classification. *Clinics in Dermatology* **30**, 70–77.

Knudson RM, Kalaaji AN, Bruce AJ. (2010) The management of mucous membrane pemphigoid and pemphigus. *Dermatologic Therapy* **23**, 268–280.

Martin LK, Werth VP, Villanueva EV, Murrell DF. (2011) A systematic review of randomized controlled trials for pemphigus vulgaris and pemphigus foliaceous. *Journal of the American Academy of Dermatology* **64**, 903–908.

Mockenhaupt M, Viboud C, Dunant A, *et al.* (2008) Stevens–Johnson syndrome and toxic epidermal necrolysis: assessment of medication risks with emphasis on recently marketed drugs. The EuroScar study. *Journal of Investigative Dermatology* **128**, 35–44.

Pirmohamed M, Friedmann PS, Molokhia M, *et al.* (2011) Phenotype standardization for immune-mediated drug-induced skin injury. *Clinical Pharmacology and Therapeutics* **89**, 896–901.

Schmidt E, Zillikens D. (2013) Pemphigoid diseases. *Lancet* **381**, 320–332.

Uitto J, Christiano AM, McLean WHI, McGrath JA. (2012) Novel molecular therapies for heritable skin disorders. *Journal of Investigative Dermatology* **132**, 820–828.

Uitto J, McGrath JA, Rodeck U, Bruckner-Tuderman L, Robinson C. (2010) Progress in epidermolysis bullosa research: toward treatment and cure. *Journal of Investigative Dermatology* **130**, 1778–1784.

Venning VA, Taghipour K, Mohd Mustapa MF, Highet AS, Kirtschig G. (2012) British Association of Dermatologists' guidelines for the management of bullous pemphigoid 2012. *British Journal of Dermatology* **167**, 1200–1214.

10 Connective Tissue Disorders

The cardinal feature of these conditions is inflammation in the connective tissues which leads to dermal atrophy or sclerosis, to arthritis, and sometimes to abnormalities in other organs. In addition, antibodies form against normal tissues and cellular components; these disorders are therefore classed as autoimmune. Many have difficulty in remembering which antibody features in which condition; Table 10.1 should help here.

The main connective tissue disorders present as a spectrum ranging from the benign cutaneous variants to severe multisystem diseases (Table 10.2).

Lupus erythematosus

Lupus erythematosus (LE) is a good example of such a spectrum, ranging from the purely cutaneous type (discoid LE), through patterns associated with some internal problems (and subacute cutaneous LE), to a severe multisystem disease (systemic lupus erythematosus, SLE; Table 10.2). It is characterized by loss of tolerance to nuclear self antigens, with the subsequent development of pathogenic autoantibodies which damage the skin an other organs.

Systemic lupus erythematosus

Cause
Variations in the major histocompatibility complex (MHC) are the most important genetic risk factor for the development of SLE, and a number of non-MHC genetic variants also play a part. Exposure to sunlight and artificial ultraviolet radiation (UVR) may precipitate the disease or lead to flare ups, probably by exposing previously hidden nuclear or cytoplasmic antigens to which autoantibodies are formed. Such autoantibodies to DNA, nuclear proteins and other normal antigens are typical of LE, and immune complexes formed from these are deposited in the tissues or found in the serum.

Hydralazine and procainamide are the most likely drugs to trigger SLE, while isoniazid, methyldopa, quinidine, minocycline, chlorpromazine and anti-tumour necrosis factor (anti-TNF) agents precipitate the disease just occasionally.

Presentation
Typically, but not always, the onset is acute. SLE is an uncommon disorder, affecting women more often than men (in a ratio of about 8 : 1). The classic rash of acute SLE is an erythema of the cheeks and nose in the rough shape of a butterfly (Figures 10.1 and 10.2), with facial swelling. Blisters occur rarely, and when they do they signify very active systemic disease. Some patients develop widespread discoid or annular papulosquamous plaques very like those of discoid LE; others, about 20% of patients, have no skin disease at any stage.

Other dermatological features include peri-ungual telangiectasia (see Figure 10.7), erythema over the digits, hair fall (especially at the frontal margin of the scalp) and photosensitivity. Ulcers may occur on the palate, tongue or buccal mucosa.

Course
The skin changes may be transient, continuous or recurrent; they correlate well with the activity of the systemic disease. Acute SLE may be associated with fever, arthritis, nephritis, polyarteritis, pleurisy, pneumonitis, pericarditis, myocarditis and involvement of the central nervous system. Internal involvement can be fatal, but about three-quarters of patients survive for 15 years. Renal involvement suggests a poorer prognosis.

Complications
The skin disease may cause scarring or hyperpigmentation, but the main dangers lie with damage to other organs and the side effects of treatment, especially systemic steroids.

Clinical Dermatology, Fifth Edition. Richard B. Weller, Hamish J.A. Hunter and Margaret W. Mann.
© 2015 John Wiley & Sons, Ltd. Published 2015 by John Wiley & Sons, Ltd.

Table 10.1 Some important associations with non-organ-specific antibodies.

Disease	Autoantibody	Frequency
Systemic lupus erythematosus	Double-stranded DNA	50–70%
	Sm antigens (U1, U2, etc.)	15–30%
	Phospholipid	10–20%
Drug-induced lupus	Nuclear histones	Common
Subacute cutaneous Lupus	SS-A(Ro)	50–70%
	SS-B(La)	20–30%
Dermatomyositis	Jo-1	20–30%
	Mi-2	(5–10%)
Systemic sclerosis	SCL–70 (topoisomerase 1)	20–30%
CREST syndrome	Centromere	20–30%
Mixed connective tissue disease	U1-RNP	100%
Lichen sclerosis	Extracellular matrix protein 1	Uncertain

Differential diagnosis

SLE is a great imitator. Its malar rash can be confused with sunburn, polymorphic light eruption (p. 263) and rosacea (p. 164), but is more livid in colour and swollen in texture.

The discoid lesions are distinctive, but are also seen in discoid LE and in subacute cutaneous LE. Occasionally, they look like psoriasis or lichen planus (p. 69). The hair fall suggests telogen effluvium (p. 178). Plaques on the scalp

Table 10.2 Classification of connective tissue disease.

Localized disease	Intermediate type	Aggressive multisystem disease
Discoid lupus erythematosus	Subacute lupus erythematosus	Systemic lupus erythematosus
	Juvenile dermatomyositis	Adult dermatomyositis
Localized scleroderma	Diffuse scleroderma	
Morphoea	CREST syndrome	Systemic sclerosis

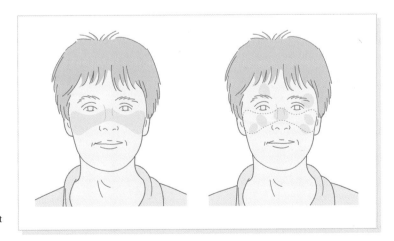

Figure 10.1 In systemic lupus erythematosus (SLE) (left) the eruption is often just an erythema, sometimes transient, but occupying most of the 'butterfly' area with sparing of the nasolabial fold. In discoid LE (right) the fixed scaling and scarring plaques may occur in the butterfly area (dotted line), but can occur outside it too.

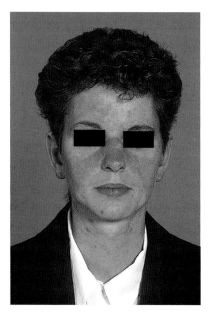

Figure 10.2 Erythema in the butterfly area, suggestive of SLE.

may cause a scarring alopecia. SLE should be suspected when a characteristic rash is combined with fever, malaise and internal disease (Table 10.3).

Investigations

Conduct a full physical examination, looking for internal disease. Biopsy of skin lesions is worthwhile because the pathology and immunopathology are distinctive. There is usually some thinning of the epidermis, liquefaction degeneration of epidermal basal cells and a mild perivascular mononuclear cell infiltrate. Direct immunofluorescence is helpful: immunoglobulin G (IgG), IgM, IgA

Table 10.3 Criteria for the diagnosis of systemic lupus erythematosus (SLE) (must have at least four).

Malar rash
Discoid plaques
Photosensitivity
Mouth ulcers
Arthritis
Serositis
Renal disorder
Neurological disorder
Haematological disorder
Immunological disorder
Antinuclear antibodies (ANA)

Table 10.4 Investigations in systemic lupus erythematosus (SLE).

Test	Usual findings
Skin biopsy	Degeneration of basal cells, epidermal thinning, inflammation around appendages
Skin immunofluorescence	Fibrillar or granular deposits of IgG, IgM, IgA and/or C3 alone in basement membrane zone
Haematology	Anaemia, raised ESR, thrombocytopenia, decreased white cell count
Immunology	Antinuclear antibody (higher titres typical of SLE rather than cutaneous LE), antibodies to double-stranded DNA, false positive tests for syphilis, low total complement level, lupus anticoagulant factor, ENA screen, sm antibody
Urine analysis	Proteinuria or haematuria, often with casts if kidneys involved
Tests for function of other organs	As indicated by history, but always test kidney and liver function

ENA, extractable nuclear antigens; ESR, erythrocyte sedimentation rate; Ig, immunoglobulin; LE, lupus erythematosus.

and C3 are found individually or together in a band-like or granular pattern at the dermo-epidermal junction of involved skin and often uninvolved skin as well. Relevant laboratory tests are listed in Table 10.4.

Treatment

Systemic steroids are helpful in gaining control of acute exacerbations, but should not be used for routine use because of the risk of adverse effects. Large doses of prednisolone (Formulary 2, p. 419) are often needed to achieve control, as assessed by symptoms, signs, erythrocyte sedimentation rate (ESR), total complement level and tests of organ function. Having gained control with systemic steroids, slower acting immunosuppressive agents, such as methotrexate, azathioprine (Formulary 2, p. 418), cyclophosphamide and other support drugs (e.g.

antihypertensive therapy or anticonvulsants) can be introduced. Antimalarial drugs may help some patients with marked photosensitivity, but the effectiveness of these is reduced in smokers. Sunscreen and appropriate clothing should reduce UV-induced flares. Long-term and regular follow up is necessary and the disease should be managed in conjunction with a rheumatologist.

Learning points

1 Do not wait for the laboratory to confirm that your patient has severe systemic lupus erythematosus (SLE). Use systemic steroids quickly if indicated by clinical findings.
2 A person with aching joints and small amounts of antinuclear antibodies probably does not have SLE.
3 Once committed to systemic steroids, adjust the dosage on clinical rather than laboratory grounds.
4 There are other causes of scleroderma besides diffuse sclerosis.

Subacute cutaneous lupus erythematosus

This is less severe than acute SLE. Sometimes only the skin is affected but about half of patients also have marked systemic disease. While the aetiology is not fully understood, clues have been given by experiments *in vivo*. Autoantibodies to SSA(Ro) are particularly common in subacute cutaneous LE, and blebs containing SSA(Ro) and other intracellular antigens form on the nuclear surface of irradiated keratinocytes. SSA(Ro) autoantibodies can activate complement. Antibody-dependent cellular cytotoxicity and autoantibody binding to SSA(Ro) are enhanced by oestradiol, perhaps accounting for the increased prevalence of subacute cutaneous LE in women. Unusually, drugs may cause subacute cutaneous LE, producing a more widespread rash than in the idiopathic disease.

Presentation

Patients with subacute cutaneous LE are often photosensitive. The skin lesions are sharply marginated psoriasiform plaques, sometimes annular, lying on the forehead, nose, cheeks, chest, hands and sun-exposed surfaces of the arms and forearms. They tend to be symmetrical and are hard to tell from discoid LE, or SLE with widespread discoid lesions.

Course

As in SLE, the course is prolonged. The skin lesions are slow to clear but, in contrast to discoid LE, do so with little or no scarring.

Complications

Systemic disease is frequent, but not usually serious. SSA(Ro) can cross the placenta and children born to mothers who have, or have had, this condition are liable to neonatal LE with transient annular skin lesions and permanent heart block.

Differential diagnosis

The morphology is characteristic, but lesions can be mistaken for psoriasis or widespread discoid LE. Annular lesions may resemble tinea corporis (p. 240) or figurate erythemas (p. 141).

Investigations

Patients with subacute cutaneous LE should be evaluated in the same way as those with acute SLE, although deposits of immunoglobulins in the skin and antinuclear antibodies in serum are present less often. Many have antibodies to the cytoplasmic antigen SS-A(Ro) and SS-B(La).

Treatment

Subacute cutaneous LE does better with antimalarials, such as hydroxychloroquine (Formulary 2, p. 424), than acute SLE. Moderate potency topical corticosteroid creams help, and oral retinoids (Formulary 2, p. 420) are also effective in some cases. Systemic steroids may be needed too, especially if there are signs of internal disease.

Discoid lupus erythematosus

This is the most common form of LE. Patients with discoid LE may have one or two plaques only, or many in several areas. The cause is also unknown but UVR is one factor.

Presentation

Plaques show erythema, scaling, follicular plugging (like a nutmeg grater), scarring and atrophy, telangiectasia, hypopigmentation and a peripheral zone of hyperpigmentation. They are well demarcated and lie mostly on sun-exposed skin of the scalp, face and ears (Figures 10.1 and 10.3). In one variant (chilblain LE) dusky lesions appear on the fingers and toes.

Course

The disease may spread relentlessly, but in about half of the cases the disease goes into remission over the course of several years. Scarring is common and hair may be lost permanently if there is scarring in the scalp (Figure 10.4).

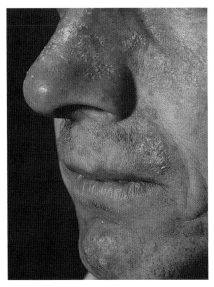

Figure 10.3 Red scaly fixed plaques of discoid lupus erythematosus (LE). This degree of scaling is not uncommon in the active stage. Follicular plugging is seen on the nose.

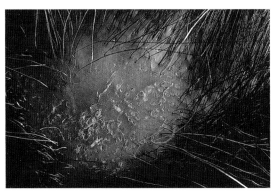

Figure 10.4 Discoid LE of the scalp leading to permanent hair loss. Note the marked follicular plugging.

Whiteness remains after the inflammation has cleared, and hypopigmentation is common in dark-skinned people. Discoid LE rarely progresses to SLE.

Differential diagnosis

Psoriasis is hard to tell from discoid LE when its plaques first arise but psoriasis has larger thicker scales, and later it is usually symmetrical and affects different sites from those of discoid LE. Discoid LE is common on the face and ears, and on sun-exposed areas, whereas psoriasis favours the elbows, knees, scalp and sacrum. Discoid LE is far more prone than psoriasis to scar and cause hair loss.

Investigations

Most patients with discoid LE remain well. However, screening for SLE and internal disease is still worthwhile. A skin biopsy is most helpful if taken from an untreated plaque where appendages are still present (Figure 10.5). Direct immunofluorescence shows deposits of IgG, IgM, IgA and C3 at the basement membrane zone.

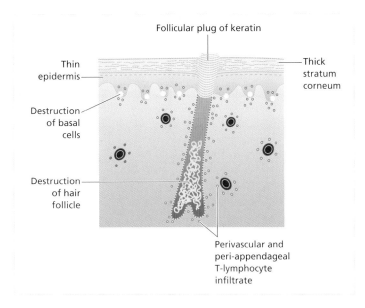

Follicular plug of keratin

Thin epidermis

Thick stratum corneum

Destruction of basal cells

Destruction of hair follicle

Perivascular and peri-appendageal T-lymphocyte infiltrate

Figure 10.5 The histology of discoid LE.

Table 10.5 Factors distinguishing the different types of lupus erythematosus (LE).

	Antinuclear antibodies	Sun sensitivity	Internal organ involvement
Systemic LE	Often against DNA++++	+++	++
Subacute LE	Often against SSA+	++++	+
Discoid LE	Often other+/−	+	−

Biopsies for direct immunofluorescence are best taken from older untreated plaques. Blood tests are usually normal but occasionally serum contains antinuclear antibodies (Table 10.5).

Treatment

Discoid LE needs potent or very potent topical corticosteroids (Formulary 1, p. 401). In this condition, it is justifiable to use them on the face, as the risk of scarring is worse than that of atrophy. Topical steroids should be applied twice daily until the lesions disappear or side effects, such as atrophy, develop. Weaker preparations can then be used for maintenance. An alternative to potent topical corticosteroids is the topical calcineurin inhibitor tacrolimus. This does not induce atrophy and is thus particularly useful for treating facial lesions. It is less effective on thick hyperkeratotic lesions. Topical retinoids such as tretinoin or tazarotene may be useful for these. Sun avoidance and screens are also important. Stubborn and widespread lesions improve in about half of patients treated with oral antimalarials such as hydroxychloroquine (Formulary 2, p. 424) although rarely these cause irreversible eye damage. The eyes should therefore be tested before and at intervals during treatment. Acitretin (Formulary 2, p. 420) has a similar efficacy to hydroxychloroquine, although with more adverse effects.

Tumid lupus erythematosus

This is a dermal form of discoid lupus erythematosus. The epidermis remains smooth although the blood vessels and adnexae are surrounded by a lymphocytic infiltrate very similar to that seen in discoid LE. The lesions are smooth tumid round violaceous plaques, usually on the face. Treatment is with oral antimalarials. Jessner's lymphocytic infiltration is viewed by some as a photosensitive form of tumid LE.

Dermatomyositis

Dermatomyositis is a subset of polymyositis with distinctive skin changes. There are adult and juvenile types (Table 10.2). The cause is unknown but an autoimmune mechanism seems likely. When starting after the age of 40, dermatomyositis may signal an internal malignancy. Presumably, the epitopes of some tumour antigens are so similar to those of muscle antigens that immune reactions directed against the tumour cross-react with muscle cells and initiate the disease in a few adults with internal malignancy.

Presentation

The skin signs are characteristic. Typical patients have a faint lilac discoloration around their eyes (sometimes called heliotrope because of the colour of the flower). This is associated with malar erythema and oedema (Figure 10.6) and, sometimes, less striking poikiloderma (pigmentary variation, epidermal atrophy and telangiectasia) of the neck and presternal area (shawl sign). Most patients also develop lilac slightly atrophic scaly papules over the knuckles of their fingers (Gottron's papules), streaks of erythema over the extensor tendons of the hand, periungual telangiectasia and ragged cuticles (Figure 10.7). The skin signs usually appear at the same time as the muscle symptoms but, occasionally, appear months or even years earlier. Many, but not all, patients have weakness of proximal muscles. Climbing stairs, getting up from chairs and combing the hair become difficult. In amyopathic dermatomyositis, a less common variation, the skin signs appear in isolation.

In juvenile dermatomyositis subcutaneous calcification is common.

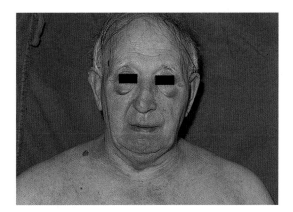

Figure 10.6 Acute dermatomyositis: oedematous purple face with erythema on presternal area. Severe progressive muscle weakness, but no underlying tumour was found.

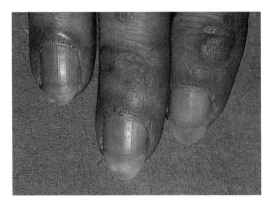

Figure 10.7 Erythema and telangiectasia of the nail folds are important clues to systemic connective tissue disorders. This patient has dermatomyositis. Note Gottron's papules over the knuckles.

Course

In children the disorder is often self-limiting, but in adults it may be prolonged and progressive. Raynaud's phenomenon, arthralgia, dysphagia and calcinosis may follow. The rash may become scaly and, rarely, itchy; eventually that on the light-exposed areas and overlying involved muscles develops poikiloderma (p. 277). Features of mixed connective disease (see *Mixed connective tissue disease*) may develop. The presence of calcinosis suggests a good prognosis.

Complications

Myositis may lead to permanent weakness and immobility, and inflammation to contractures or cutaneous calcinosis. Some die from progessive and severe myopathy.

Differential diagnosis

Other connective tissue disorders may look similar, particularly mixed connective tissue disease (p. 136) and SLE. In LE, the finger lesions favour the skin between the knuckles whereas in dermatomyositis the knuckles are preferred. Toxoplasmosis may cause a dermatomyositis-like syndrome. Myopathy can be a side effect of systemic steroids, so weakness is not always caused by the disease itself.

Investigations

Up to 25% of adults over the age of 40 with dermatomyositis also have an underlying malignancy. Their dermatomyositis coincides with the onset of the tumour and may improve if it is removed. Adult dermatomyositis or polymyositis therefore requires a search for such an underlying malignancy. In women, the ovaries are a favourite hiding place, but breast, gastrointestinal tract and lung cancers are also common. The levels of muscle enzymes such as aldolase and creatinine kinase are often elevated. Electromyography (EMG) detects muscle abnormalities, and biopsy of an affected muscle shows inflammation and destruction. Magnetic resonance imaging is increasingly used to non-invasively detect inflammation in clinically involved muscles. The ESR is sometimes normal and antinuclear antibodies may not be detected. The presence of Jo-1 antibodies in plasma suggests high risk for myositis, arthritis and interstitial lung disease. Mi-2 antinuclear antibody, if found, indicates a good prognosis. An isolated skin biopsy is not particularly helpful diagnostically, and shows the same histological features as cutaneous LE.

Treatment

Systemic steroids, often in high doses (e.g. prednisolone 60 mg/day for an average adult; Formulary 2, p. 419), are the cornerstone of treatment and protect the muscles from destruction. A maintenance regimen may be needed for several years and thus concomitant osteoporosis prevention with calcium, vitamin D and possibly bisphosphonates will almost certainly be required. Immunosuppressive agents, such as azathioprine (Formulary 2, p. 418) or methotrexate (Formulary 2, p. 419), also help to control the condition and to reduce the high steroid dose. Maintenance treatment is adjusted according to clinical response and creatinine kinase level. Some case reports show benefit from intravenous gammaglobulin infusions or cyclophosphamide, but good clinical trial data are generally lacking in dermatomyositis treatment. Muscle disease usually responds much better than skin disease, but avoidance of sunlight will prevent UV-induced flares of skin disease. Long-term follow up is necessary, although the increased risk of underlying malignancy reverts to that of the age-matched population 2 years after diagnosis.

> **Learning point**
>
> Hunt for internal malignancy in the middle aged and elderly, but not in juvenile cases.

Systemic sclerosis

Systemic sclerosis (scleroderma) can affect a number of different organs, but almost always affects the skin

Table 10.6 Differential diagnosis of sclerosis.

Diffuse
Diffuse scleroderma (systemic sclerosis)
Limited scleroderma (CREST).
Diabetic sclerodactyly
Chronic graft versus host reaction
Chronic vibration exposure
Phenylketonuria
Porphyria cutanea tarda
Chemicals – polyvinylchloride monomers
Drugs – bleomycin, pentazocine, taxanes
Amyloidosis
Nephrogenic sclerosing dermopathy
Progeria
Werner's syndrome

Localized
Lichen sclerosus
Morphoea
Morphoea profunda
Fasciitis with eosinophilia
Pansclerotic morphoea
Linear morphoea
En coup de sabre
Injections (silicone, paraffin, vitamin K)
Trauma
Radiation therapy

Table 10.7 Skin signs of diffuse scleroderma.

Raynaud's phenomenon (95%)
Sclerosis (especially hands and fingers)
Diffuse darkening (hyperpigmentation)
Pinched nose
Mask-like face
Decreased oral aperture
Square mat telangiectasias
Thin lips
Prominent periungual capillaries
Nail abnormalities (pterygium)
Calcinosis cutis
Painful digital ulcers

which develops reduced elasticity, thickening and hardening (sclerosis). Vascular damage and altered immune reponses are other features of the disease. The pattern of organ involvement, speed of progress and prognosis separate the disease into two subtypes: diffuse cutaneous (dcSSc) and localized cutaneous systemic sclerosis (lcSSc). Table 10.6 lists the differential diagnosis.

Cause
Systemic sclerosis is an autoimmune condition, but beyond this, the aetiology is complex. Genetic studies show that the variants in the MHC region, the CD 247 gene (which codes for part of a T-cell receptor) the interferon regulatory factor 5 gene and the STAT4 gene are all linked to the disease. Variants in these genes, all of which alter immune response are not individually strong risk factors for systemic sclerosis, so presumably unknown environmental factors acting on a background of this genetic predisposition are needed to initiate the disease. A vascular phase often preceeds the sclerosis. Adhesion molecules are upregulated on endothelial cells and chemotactic cytokines synthesized and both innate and adaptive arms of the immune system are activated. An oligoclonal CD4$^+$ T lymphocyte and macrophage tissue infiltration follows with high levels of interlukin 4 (IL-4) and transforming growth factor β (TGF-β) being produced. Increased levels of growth factors induce fibroblasts to make collagen. TGF-α promotes synthesis of collagen and matrix proteins, decreases metalloproteinases that degrade collagen and keeps fibroblasts in an active state.

A diffuse sclerosis-like syndrome is a feature of the chronic graft versus host disease after allogeneic bone marrow transplantation (Table 10.7). This has lead to speculation that diffuse sclerosis may occur by similar mechanisms, perhaps from fetus-derived lymphocytes that cross the placenta during pregnancy, reactivating in a mother later in her life.

Localized cutaneous systemic sclerosis (CREST syndrome)
In lcSSc, the skin disease is usually confined to the extremities and face, and onset is slow. Raynaud's phenomenon often precedes the skin changes in contrast with dcSSc. The fingers become immobile, hard and shiny (sclerodactyly) and abnormal calcium deposition occurs over pressure points (calcinosis). Other vascular features of this form of systemic sclerosis include pulmonary artery hypertension, digital ulceration and renal crises, but despite this the prognosis is relatively good. LcSSc used to be known as CREST (standing for calcinosis, Raynaud's phenomenon, oesophageal dysmotility, sclerodactyly and telangiectasia). Telangiectasia is periungual on the fingers and flat, mat-like or rectangular on the face. Some patients produce anticentromere antibodies.

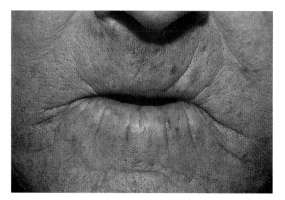

Figure 10.8 Systemic sclerosis: radial furrowing around the mouth.

Diffuse cutaneous systemic sclerosis

This form of systemic sclerosis shares some features with lcSSc such as Raynaud phenomenon and sclerodactyly, but the onset of disease is more rapid, and Raynaud's phenomenon occurs concurrently with sclerodactyly. Anti-DNA topo I (anti-Scl-70) antibodies are found.

Skin involvement is more widespread than in lcSSc and as the disease progresses, sclerosis spreads to the face, scalp and trunk. Sclerotic skin can become hypo or hyperpigmented and itchy early in the disease. Periungual telangiectasia is common. The nose becomes beak-like, and wrinkles radiate around the mouth (Figures 10.8–10.10). Loss of hair follicles and sebaceous glands in affected areas of skin leads to alopecia and dryness. Most have abnormalities of the gut including dysphagia, oesophagitis, constipation, diarrhoea and malabsorption. Interstitial lung disease leads to dyspnoea; fibrosis of the heart and pulmonary hypertension to congestive failure. The kidneys are involved late, but this has a grave prognosis from malignant hypertension.

Complications

Most complications are caused by the involvement of organs other than the skin, but ulcers of the fingertips and calcinosis are distressing (Figure 10.11). Hard skin immobilizes the joints and leads to contractures.

Differential diagnosis

Other causes of Raynaud's phenomenon are given in Table 11.4. The differential diagnosis includes chilblains (p. 140) and erythromelalgia (p. 140). The sclerosis should be distinguished from that of widespread morphoea, porphyria cutanea tarda, mixed connective tissue disease,

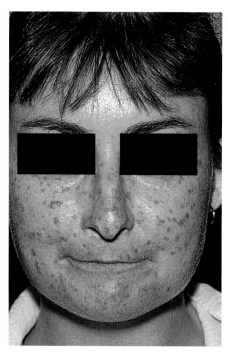

Figure 10.9 Mat-like telangiectasia seen in a patient with systemic sclerosis.

eosinophilic fasciitis, diabetic sclerodactyly and an acute arthritis with swollen fingers. Rarely, the disease is mimicked by progeria, scleromyxoedema, amyloidosis or carcinoid syndrome. A more complete differential diagnosis is given in Table 10.6. Nephrogenic sclerosing dermopathy, as the name suggests, occurs in some patients with renal disease undergoing dialysis. Its cause may be erythropoietin used to treat coexisting anaemias or gadolinium used in radiological scans. Similar syndromes have been reported following ingestion of adulterated rape seed oil, dimerised L-tryptophan, and treatment with the antitumour agent, bleomycin.

Investigations

The diagnosis is made clinically because histological abnormalities are seldom present until the physical signs are well established. Laboratory tests should include a fluorescent antinuclear antibody test and the evaluation of the heart, kidney, lungs, joints and muscles. Barium studies are best avoided as obstruction may follow poor evacuation. Other contrast media are available. X-rays of the hands, measurement of muscle enzymes and immunoglobulin levels, and a blood count, ESR and test

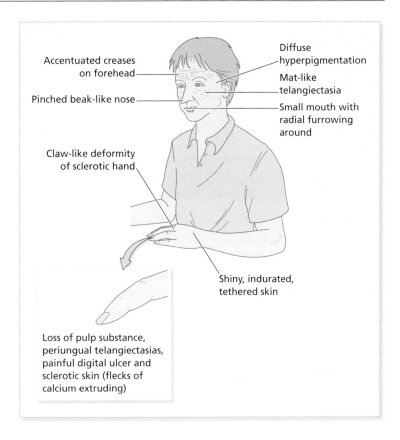

Diffuse hyperpigmentation

Mat-like telangiectasia

Small mouth with radial furrowing around

Accentuated creases on forehead

Pinched beak-like nose

Claw-like deformity of sclerotic hand

Shiny, indurated, tethered skin

Loss of pulp substance, periungual telangiectasias, painful digital ulcer and sclerotic skin (flecks of calcium extruding)

Figure 10.10 Signs of systemic sclerosis.

for the scleroderma-associated antibody Scl-70 are also worthwhile.

Treatment

This is unsatisfactory. The calcium channel blocker nifedipine or the guanylate cyclase inhibitor sildenafil

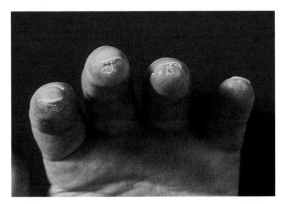

Figure 10.11 Loss of fingertip pulp, and extrusion of chalky material.

may help Raynaud's phenomenon (p. 143). Systemic steroids, methotrexate, mycophenolate mofetil, salicylates and antimalarials are used, but are not of proven value. D-penicillamine has many adverse effects, especially on renal function. Physiotherapy is helpful; photopheresis is experimental. Recently, there have been promising reports of the efficacy of UVA-1 (340–400 nm) phototherapy for affected skin in systemic sclerosis. Antagonists to endothelin receptors such as bosentan reduce risks from pulmonary hypertension.

Localized scleroderma

Sometimes only areas of skin become sclerotic. The differential diagnosis is listed in Table 10.6. Some people view lichen sclerosis, morphoea, morphoea profunda, eosinophic fasciitis and pansclerotic morphoea as a spectrum of localized sclerosis based on the level of sclerosis in the skin. Overlaps occur.

Morphoea

Morphoea is a localized form of diffuse sclerosis with pale indurated plaques on the skin but no internal sclerosis

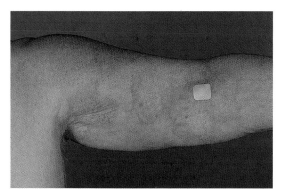

Figure 10.12 Morphoea. Pale indurated plaques on the arm, showing a purplish rim.

(Figures 10.12 and 10.13). Many plaques are surrounded by a violaceous halo. Its prognosis is usually good, and the fibrosis slowly clears leaving slight depression and hyperpigmentation. In pansclerotic morphoea, contractures can cause marked disability. A rare type may lead to arrest of growth of the underlying bones causing, for example, facial hemiatrophy or shortening of a limb. Little is known about the cause, except that Lyme borreliosis may be associated with the disease in Europe but not in the Americas. Treatments work slowly, if at all. Phototherapy with UVA or long wavelength UVA (UVA-1), topical calcipotriol (calcipotriene), topical tacrolimus and systemic methotrexate, with or without corticosteroids, have all shown some efficacy in clinical studies.

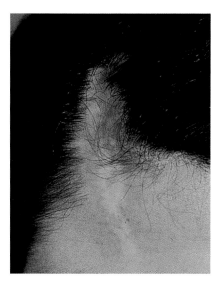

Figure 10.13 Morphoea (en coup de sabre type) on the forehead. In a young child this can lead to facial hemiatrophy.

Diffuse fasciitis with eosinophilia (eosinophilic fasciitis)

Localized areas of skin become indurated, sometimes after an upper respiratory tract infection or prolonged severe exercise. Hypergammaglobulinaemia and eosinophilia are present and a deep skin biopsy, which includes muscle, shows that the fascia overlying the muscle is thickened. Despite its common name *eosinophilic fasciitis* and despite a profound eosinophilia in the peripheral blood, the fascia is neither eosinophilic nor permeated by eosinophils. The disease responds promptly to systemic steroids; the long-term prognosis is good but disability in the short term can be severe.

Lichen sclerosus

Many think that this condition is related to morphoea, with which it may coexist. However, its patches are non-indurated white shiny macules (Figure 10.14), sometimes with obvious plugging in the follicular openings. Women are affected far more often than men and, although any area of skin can be involved, the classic ivory-coloured lesions often surround the vulva and anus. Intractable itching is common in these areas and the development of vulval carcinoma is a risk. In men, the condition may cause stenosis of the urethral meatus, and adhesions between the foreskin and glans of the penis (see Chapter 13). Patients with lichen sclerosus may have antibodies to extracellular matrix protein 1.

Mixed connective tissue disease

This is an overlap between SLE and either scleroderma or dermatomyositis.

Presentation

As in LE, women are affected more often than men. A wide range of clinical features are seen, but the most

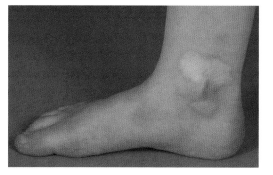

Figure 10.14 Lichen sclerosus. Follicular hyperkeratosis differentiates this from morphoea.

common presentations include swollen hands and sclero-dactyly, Raynaud's phenomenon, oesophageal dysmotility and muscle disorders. Alopecia is mild and the hair fall mimics telogen effluvium. Peri-ungual telangiectasia and pigmentary disturbances are common. About 25% of patients have a small vessel vasculitis with palpable purpura, leg ulcers and painful dermal nodules on the hands or elbows. Headaches, weakness, fatigue, lymph node enlargement or hoarseness occur in about one in three patients; renal and central nervous system disease are less common. Pulmonary involvement occurs in 85% of patients, and the development of pulmonary artery hypertension has the most grave prognosis.

Course

The disorder is chronic, and usually turns into either SLE or systemic sclerosis.

Differential diagnosis

The disorder can be confused with SLE, dermatomyositis, polymyositis, systemic sclerosis and other sclerosing processes such as porphyria cutanea tarda (p. 316). The diagnosis of mixed connective tissue disease is usually based on the combination of positive serology combined with three or four clinical criteria.

Investigations

Patients with mixed connective tissue disease have antibodies in high titre directed against anti-U1 small nuclear (sn) anti-ribonucleoprotein (anti-RNP) antibodies. These give a speckled pattern when serum is reacted against nuclei and detected by indirect immunofluorescence.

Treatment

No good clinical trial data exist, so treatment is chosen dependent upon which organs are involved. Inflammatory disease usually requires systemic steroids. Sclerodermatous changes such as oesophageal motility problems, sclerodactyly and Raynaud's phenomenon are best treated with cytotoxic immunosuppressive agents such as cyclophosphamide. Non-steroidal anti-inflammatory drugs (NSAIDs) help with arthralgia, myalgia and swelling of the hands.

Other connective tissue diseases

Rheumatoid arthritis

Most patients with rheumatoid arthritis have no skin disease, but some have tiny fingertip infarcts, purpura, ulcers, palmar or peri-ungual erythema, or pyoderma gangrenosum. The most common skin manifestations are marble-like nodules near joints. These are always associated with the presence of rheumatoid factor. Some patients with rheumatoid arthritis have a vasculitis of larger blood vessels with deep 'punched out' ulcers on the legs.

Reactive arthritis (Reiter's syndrome)

Reiter's syndrome, precipitated by non-specific urethritis or dysentery, combines skin lesions, arthropathy, conjunctivitis, balanitis, mucositis and spondylitis. Arthritis is the most severe element. It is particularly common in men bearing the HLA B27 genotype. The skin lesions (keratoderma blenorrhagicum) are psoriasis-like red scaling plaques, often studded with vesicles and pustules, seen most often on the feet. The toes are red and swollen, and the nails thicken. Psoriasiform plaques may also occur on the penis and scrotum, with redness near the penile meatus. Sometimes, nearly the whole skin may be afflicted, and Reiter's syndrome should be considered in the differential diagnosis of erythroderma. Topical steroids, systemic retinoids and systemic NSAIDs help, but many patients need methotrexate(Formulary 2, p. 419), and/or systemic steroids.

Relapsing polychondritis

This process can affect any cartilage as the disorder is apparently caused by autoimmunity to type II collagen. The ears are the usual target, and often just one ear is involved at the start. The overlying skin becomes red, swollen and tender. Exacerbations and remissions may occur spontaneously. The cartilage of the nose and the tracheo-bronchial tree may be involved, so that patients develop floppy ears, a saddle nose, hoarseness, stridor and respiratory insufficiency. Aortic aneurysms are also seen. Treatment is with systemic steroids and NSAIDs and there are a number of reports of benefit from TNF-α blockers. Tracheostomy may be necessary.

Behçet's syndrome

Behçet's syndrome is discussed in Chapter 13.

Polyarteritis nodosa

This is discussed in Chapter 8 but is considered by some to be a connective tissue disorder.

Table 10.8 Causes of panniculitis.

Infections, including cellulitis
Traumatic
Foreign bodies
Erythema nodosum (p. 107)
Erythema nodosum leprosum (leprosy)
Nodular vasculitis (p. 108)
Erythema induratum
Weber–Christian type
Polyarteritis nodosa (p. 110)
Associated with pancreatitis
Associated with SLE (lupus profundus)
Panniculitis-like subcutaneous T-cell lymphoma
Morphoea profunda (deep morphoea)
Cold-induced
Withdrawal of systemic steroids
Calciphylaxis
Superficial and migratory thrombophlebitis
Dermatoliposclerosis
Deficiency of α_1-antitrypsin
Dermatoliposclerosis
Gout
Traumatic fat necrosis
Factitial (e.g. from injection of milk)

Panniculitis

Panniculitis is an inflammation of the subcutaneous fat. It includes a number of diseases with different causes but a similar appearance: some are listed in Table 10.8.

Presentation

Most patients have tender ill-defined red nodules and indurated plaques on the lower legs, thighs and buttocks.

Differential diagnosis

Diagnosis can be tricky. Usually, the diagnosis is made from clinical suspicion linked to findings from the laboratories. If the panniculitis is unilateral, consider infection (including cellulitis), foreign bodies and phlebitis. If there is ulceration, consider lupus profundus, panniculitis-like subcutaneous T-cell lymphoma, polyarteritis and nodular vasculitis. The discharge from the ulcers associated with pancreatitis and α_1-antitrypsin deficiency often drain as an oily saponified fat. The most common bilateral panniculitis is erythema nodosum (p. 107). Calcifying panniculitis (calciphylaxis) usually occurs in the setting of haemodialysis, end stage renal failure and secondary hyperparathyroidism. It presents acutely as livedo, stellate necrosis and eventual deep ulcerations.

Course

This depends upon the cause. Migratory thrombophlebitis may be associated with underlying malignancy. In lupus profundus, a panniculitis is associated with discoid or systemic lupus erythematosus. Watch out if you suspect this, because subcutaneous T-cell lymphomas look like lupus profundus clinically and even histologically, but can cause rapid death. Causes of erythema nodosum are discussed in Chapter 8. Erythema induratum may be caused by tuberculosis. Erythema nodosum leprosum is a reactional state in leprosy (p. 225). Patients with pancreatitis may liberate enough lipase into the systemic circulation to cause cutaneous fat to liquefy and discharge through the overlying skin. The Weber–Christian variant is associated with fever, but its cause is unknown.

Investigations

The type of panniculitis can sometimes be identified by skin biopsy, which must include subcutaneous fat. Inflamed fat usually pulls easily off the dermis and punch biopsies are usually inadaquate. An incisional biopsy with scalpel can better provide adequate fatty tissue. When performing an incisional biopsy, ensure that there is enough extra tissue for culture for bacteria (including acid-fast organisms) and fungi. The pathologists often start by classifying panicultis as septal (if the inflammation is mostly around the fibrous septae that separate fat lobules) or lobular (if the inflammation is primarily in the fat). They also note whether or not vascultitis is present. A complete blood count, ESR, chest X-ray, serum α_1-antitrypsin and tests for antinuclear antibodies are often needed. Patients with pancreatitis have elevated levels of amylase and lipase and abnormal tomography scans.

Treatment

This depends upon the cause. Rest, elevation of affected extremities and local heat often help symptoms. NSAIDs may also help in the absence of specific therapy.

Further reading

Jessop S, Whitelaw DA, Delamere FM. (2009) Drugs for discoid lupus erythematosus. *Cochrane Database Systematic Reviews* **4**, CD002954.
Krieg T, Takehara K. (2009) Skin disease: a cardinal feature of systemic sclerosis. *Rheumatology* **48**, iii14–iii18.
Liu Z, Davidson A. (2012) Taming lupus: a new understanding of pathogenesis is leading to clinical advances. *Nature Medicine* **18**, 871–882.

Ortega-Hernandez OD, Shoenfeld Y. (2012) Mixed connective tissue disease: an overview of clinical manifestations, diagnosis and treatment. *Best Practice and Research: Clinical Rheumatology* **26**, 61–72.

Patterson JW. (1991) Differential diagnosis of panniculitis. *Advances in Dermatology* **6**, 309–329.

Strowd LC, Jorizzo JL. (2013) Review of dermatomyositis: establishing the diagnosis and treatment algorithm. *Journal of Dermatological Treatment* **24**, 418–421.

Varga J. (2008) Systemic sclerosis: an update. *Bulletin of the NYU Hospital for Joint Diseases* **66**, 198–202.

Vedove C, Del Giglio M, Schena D, Girolomoni G. (2009) Drug-induced lupus erythematosus. *Archives of Dermatological Research* **301**, 99–105.

Walling HW, Sontheimer RD. (2009) Cutaneous lupus erythematosus issues in diagnosis and treatment. *American Journal of Clinical Dermatology* **10**, 365–381.

Wu IB, Schwartz RA. (2008) Reiter's syndrome: the classic triad and more. *Journal of the American Academy of Dermatology* **59**, 113–121.

Zwischenberger BA, Jacobe HT. (2011) A systematic review of morphea treatments and therapeutic algorithm. *Journal of the American Academy of Dermatology* **65**, 925–941.

11 Disorders of Blood Vessels and Lymphatics

Disorders of blood vessels and lymphatics can be grouped into functional and structural diseases. In functional diseases, abnormalities of flow are reversible, and there is no vessel wall damage (e.g. in urticaria; discussed in Chapter 8). The diseases of structure include the many types of vasculitis, some of which, with an immunological basis, are also covered in Chapter 8. For convenience, disorders of the blood vessels are grouped according to the size and type of the vessels affected.

Disorders involving small blood vessels

Acrocyanosis

This type of 'poor circulation', often familial, is more common in females than males. The hands, feet, nose, ears and cheeks become blue–red and cold. The palms are often cold and clammy. The condition is caused by arteriolar constriction and dilatation of the subpapillary venous plexus, and to cold-induced increases in blood viscosity. Patients have normal peripheral pulses, in contrast to those with peripheral arterial occlusive disease. The best answers are warm clothes and avoidance of cold.

Erythrocyanosis

This occurs in fat, often young, women. Purple–red mottled discoloration is seen over the fatty areas such as the buttocks, thighs and lower legs. Cold provokes it and causes an unpleasant burning sensation. Most young people outgrow the condition, but an area of acrocyanosis or erythrocyanosis may be the site where other disorders will settle in the future (e.g. perniosis, erythema induratum, lupus erythematosus, sarcoidosis, cutaneous tuberculosis and leprosy). Weight reduction is often recommended.

Perniosis (chilblains)

In this common, sometimes familial, condition, inflamed purple–pink swellings appear on the fingers, toes and, rarely, ears (Figure 11.1). They are painful, and itchy or burning on rewarming. Occasionally, they ulcerate. It tends to affect young to middle aged white women during winter, particularly on exposure to cold damp nonfreezing temperatures. Chilblains are caused by a combination of arteriolar and venular constriction, the latter predominating on rewarming with exudation of fluid into the tissues. Lesions usually resolve in 1–3 weeks. Warm clothing and avoidance of precipitating conditions help. Topical remedies rarely work, but the oral calcium channel blocker nifedipine may be useful. The blood pressure should be monitored at the start of treatment and at return visits. The vasodilator nicotinamide (500 mg three times daily) may be helpful alone or in addition to calcium channel blockers. Sympathectomy may be advised in severe cases.

Erythromelalgia

This is a rare paroxysmal condition in which the extremities (most commonly the feet) become red, hot, swollen and painful when exposed to heat, and relieved by cooling. The condition may be sporadic or familial. Secondary erythromelalgia is associated with a myeloproliferative disease (e.g. polycythaemia rubra vera or thrombocythaemia), lupus erythematosus, rheumatoid arthritis, diabetes, degenerative peripheral vascular disease or hypertension. Elevation and cooling of the extremities can be helpful. Small doses of aspirin give symptomatic relief. Topical therapies include capsaicin cream and lidocaine patch. Alternatives include nonsteroidal anti-inflammatory drugs (NSAIDs), gabapentin,

Clinical Dermatology, Fifth Edition. Richard B. Weller, Hamish J.A. Hunter and Margaret W. Mann.
© 2015 John Wiley & Sons, Ltd. Published 2015 by John Wiley & Sons, Ltd.

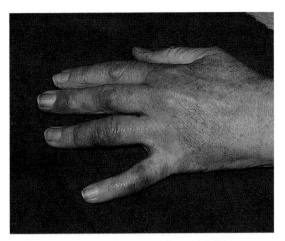

Figure 11.1 The typical purplish swellings of chilblains.

beta-blockers, pentoxifylline and the serotonin re-uptake inhibitor venlafaxine.

Erythemas

Erythema accompanies all inflammatory skin conditions, but the term 'the erythemas' is usually applied to a group of conditions with redness but without primary scaling. Such areas are seen in some bacterial and viral infections such as toxic shock syndrome and measles. Drugs are another common cause (see Chapter 25). If no cause is obvious, the rash is often called a 'toxic' or 'reactive' erythema.

When erythema is associated with oedema (*urticated erythema*) it becomes palpable.

Figurate erythemas

These are chronic eruptions, made up of bizarre serpiginous and erythematous rings. In the past most carried Latin labels; happily, these eruptions are now grouped under the general term of *figurate erythemas*. Underlying malignancy, a connective tissue disorder, a bacterial, viral, fungal or yeast infection, parasitic and worm infestation, drug sensitivity and rheumatic heart disease should be excluded, but often the cause remains obscure.

Palmar erythema

This may be an isolated finding in a normal person or be familial. It occurs in at least 30% of pregnant women. It can be associated with liver disease and rheumatoid arthritis. Often associated with spider telangiectases (see

Telangiectases), it may be caused by increased circulating oestrogens.

Telangiectases

This term refers to permanently dilated and visible small vessels in the skin. They appear as linear, punctate or stellate crimson–purple markings. They can occur as a primary process or secondary to an underlying systemic disease or physical damage to the skin. The common causes are given in Table 11.1.

Spider naevi

These stellate telangiectases do look rather like spiders, with legs radiating from a central, often palpable, feeding vessel. If the diagnosis is in doubt, press on the central feeding vessel with the corner of a glass slide and the entire lesion will disappear. Spider naevi are seen frequently on the faces of normal children, and may erupt in pregnancy or be the presenting sign of liver disease, with many lesions on the upper trunk. Liver function should be checked in those with many spider naevi. The central vessel can be destroyed by electrodessication without local anaesthesia or with a vascular laser (p. 380).

Livedo reticularis

This cyanosis of the skin is net-like (reticulated) or marbled and caused by stasis in the capillaries furthest from their arterial supply: at the periphery of the inverted cone supplied by a dermal arteriole (see Figure 2.1). It may be widespread or localized. *Cutis marmorata* is the name given to the mottling of the skin seen in many normal children. It is a physiologic vasospastic response to cold exposure and disappears on warming, whereas true livedo reticularis remains.

The causes of livedo reticularis are listed in Table 11.2. Livedo vasculitis and cutaneous polyarteritis are forms of vasculitis associated with livedo reticularis (see Chapter 8). Localized forms suggest localized blood vessel injury, for example from cholesterol emboli.

Antiphospholipid syndrome

Some patients with an apparently idiopathic livedo reticularis develop progressive disease in their peripheral, cerebral, coronary and renal arteries. Others, usually women, have multiple arterial or venous thromboembolic episodes accompanying livedo reticularis. Recurrent spontaneous abortions and intrauterine fetal growth retardation are also features. Prolongation of the activated partial thromboplastin time (APTT) and the presence of

Table 11.1 Causes of telangiectasia.

Primary telangiectasia	
Hereditary haemorrhagic telangiectasia	Autosomal dominant
	Nose and gastointestinal bleeds
	Lesions on face, lips, and hands
	Variable involvement of the lungs, liver and CNS
Ataxia telangiectasia	Autosomal recessive
	Telangiectases develop between the ages of 3 and 5 years
	Cerebellar ataxia
	Recurrent respiratory infections
	Immunological abnormalities
Generalized essential telangiectasia	Typically affects adult women, may commence in childhood
	Multiple lesions on legs
	Runs benign course
	No other associations
Unilateral naevoid telangiectasia	Unilateral distribution of telangiectases
	May occur in pregnancy or in females on oral contraceptive
Secondary telangiectasia	
Rosacea	Associated with centrofacial erythema (erythematotelangiectatic subtype)
Sun-damaged skin	
Atrophy	Seen on exposed skin of elderly, after topical steroid applications, after radiation therapy, and with poikiloderma
Connective tissue disorders	Always worth inspecting nail folds
	Mat-like on the face in systemic sclerosis
Prolonged vasodilatation	For example, with venous hypertension
Mastocytosis	Accompanying a rare and diffuse variant
Liver disease	Multiple spider telangiectases are common
Drugs	Nifedipine
Tumours	A tell-tale sign in nodular basal cell carcinomas

Table 11.2 Common causes of livedo reticularis.

Physiological	Cutis marmorata/ physiologic livedo reticularis
Vessel wall disease	Atherosclerosis
	Connective tissue disorders (especially polyarteritis, livedo vasculitis and systemic lupus erythematosus)
Vessel obstruction	Embolic (cholesterol, septic emboli)
	Calciphylaxis
Hyperviscosity states	Polycythaemia/thrombocythaemia
	Macroglobulinaemia
Cryopathies	Cryoglobulinaemia
	Cold agglutininaemia
	Cryofibrinogenaemia
Hypercoagulability	Antiphospholipid syndrome
	Sneddon's syndrome
Medications	Amantadine, minocycline, quinidine, catecholamines
Congenital	
Idiopathic	

antiphospholipid antibodies (either anticardiolipin antibody or lupus anticoagulant, or both) help to identify this syndrome. Systemic lupus erythematosus should be excluded (p. 126).

Erythema ab igne

This appearance is also determined by the underlying vascular network. Its brownish pigmented, reticulated erythema, with variable scaling, is caused by damage from long-term exposure to local heat or infrared source – usually from an open fire, hot water bottle, heating pad or, in recent years, laptop computer. If on one side of the leg, it gives a clue to the side of the fire on which granny likes to sit (Figure 11.2). The condition has become less common with the advent of central heating.

Flushing

This transient vasodilatation of the face may spread to the neck, upper chest and, more rarely, other parts of the body. There is no sharp distinction between flushing and blushing apart from the emotional provocation of the latter. The mechanism varies with the many causes that are listed in Table 11.3. Paroxysmal flushing ('hot flushes'), common at the menopause, is associated with the pulsatile release of luteinizing hormone from the pituitary, as a consequence of low circulating oestrogens and failure of normal

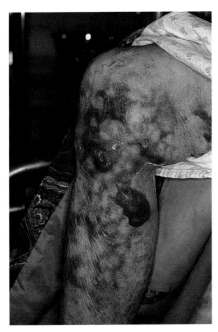

Figure 11.2 Erythema ab igne: this patient persisted in sitting too close to an open fire and burned herself.

Table 11.3 Causes of flushing.

Physiological	Emotional (blushing)
	Menopausal ('hot flushes')
	Exercise
Foods	Hot drinks
	Spicy foods
	Additives (monosodium glutamate)
	Alcohol (especially in Oriental people)
Drugs	Vasodilatators including nicotinic acid, hydralazine
	Nitrates and sildenafil
	Calcium channel blockers including nifedipine
	Disulfiram or chlorpropamide + alcohol
	Cholinergic agents
Pathological	Mastocytosis
	Carcinoid tumours – with asthma and diarrhoea
	Phaeochromocytoma (type producing adrenaline) – with episodic headaches (caused by transient hypertension) and palpitations
	Dumping syndrome
	Migraine headaches

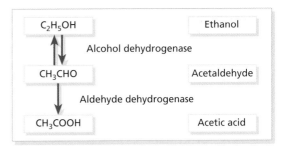

Figure 11.3 The metabolism of ethanol.

negative feedback. However, luteinizing hormone itself cannot be responsible for flushing as this can occur after hypophysectomy. It is possible that menopausal flushing is mediated by central mechanisms involving encephalins. Hot flushes can usually be helped by oestrogen replacement, clonidine or serotonin reuptake inhibitors.

Alcohol-induced flushing is caused by the vasodilatory effects of alcohol and accumulation of acetaldehyde. Ethanol is broken down to acetaldehyde by alcohol dehydrogenase and acetaldehyde is metabolized to acetic acid by aldehyde dehydrogenase (Figure 11.3). This condition is most prevalent in Japanese, Chinese and Koreans, as they have a high-activity variant of alcohol dehydrogenase and defective aldehyde dehydrogenase. Disulfiram (Antabuse) and, to a lesser extent, chlorpropamide inhibit aldehyde dehydrogenase so that some individuals taking these drugs may flush.

Arterial disease

Raynaud's phenomenon

This is a common paroxysmal vasospasm of the digital arteries provoked by cold or, rarely, emotional stress. The result is a characteristic progression of white, blue and red discoloration of the fingers. At first, the top of one or more fingers becomes white due to vasoconstriction. A painful cyanosis then appears as the residual blood in the finger desaturates. On rewarming, the rapid reperfusion of the digit turns the area red before the hands return to their normal colour.

Raynaud's disease, often familial and typically affecting adolescent women, is the name given when no cause can be found. In contrast, secondary Raynaud's phenomenon affects women over age 25 and is associated with an underlying systemic disease, usually scleroderma. The presence of other signs of connective tissue disease, including prominent dilated nailfold capillaries (see

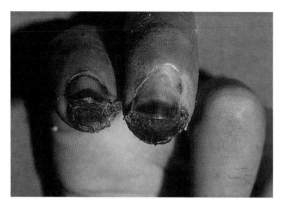

Figure 11.4 Digital gangrene. In this case caused by frostbite.

Figure 10.7), sclerodactyly and positive autoantibodies, can distinguish secondary from primary Raynaud's phenomenon. In severe cases of secondary Raynaud's, the fingers lose pulp substance, ulcerate or become gangrenous (Figure 11.4). Some causes are listed in Table 11.4.

The main treatment is to protect the vulnerable digits from cold. Warm clothing reduces the need for peripheral vasoconstriction to conserve heat. Smoking should be abandoned. Second-line therapy is with vasodilators,

Table 11.4 Causes of Raynaud's phenomenon.

Familial	Raynaud's disease (idiopathic)
Connective tissue diseases	Systemic sclerosis
	Lupus erythematosus
	Dermatomyositis
	Mixed connective tissue disease
Arterial occlusion	Thoracic outlet syndrome
	Atherosclerosis
	Endarteritis obliterans (Buerger disease)
Repeated trauma	Pneumatic hammer/drill operators ('vibration white finger')
Hyperviscosity	Polycythaemia
	Macroglobulinaemia
Cryopathies	Cryoglobulinaemia
	Cryofibrinogenaemia
	Cold agglutinaemia
Neurological disease	Peripheral neuropathy
	Syringomyelia
Toxins	Ergot
	Vinyl-chloride

the most effective being calcium channel blockers (e.g. nifedipine 10–30 mg three times daily) for patients with primary Raynaud's disease. Patients should be warned about dizziness caused by postural hypotension. Initially, it is worth giving nifedipine as a 5-mg test dose with monitoring of the blood pressure in the clinic. If this is tolerated satisfactorily the starting dosage should be 5 mg/day, increasing by 5 mg every 5 days until a therapeutic dose is achieved (e.g. 5–20 mg three times daily) or until intolerable side effects occur. The blood pressure should be monitored before each incremental increase in the dosage. Diltiazem (30–60 mg three times daily) is less effective than nifedipine but has fewer side effects. The systemic vasodilator inositol nicotinate may help, and a combination of low dose acetylsalicylic acid and the antiplatelet drug dipyridamole is also worth trying. Sustained release glycerol trinitrate patches, applied once daily, may reduce the severity and frequency of attacks and allow reduction in the dosage of calcium channel blockers and vasodilators. Slow intravenous infusions with prostaglandin analogues, which are potent vasodilators and inhibitors of platelet aggregation, help some severe cases. Endothelin receptor antagonists (bosentan) and phosphodiesterase inhibitors (sildenafil) have also been used with varying success.

Polyarteritis nodosa
This is discussed in Chapter 8, p. 110.

Temporal arteritis
This condition, also termed giant cell arteritis, is a vasculitis of the large and middle-sized blood vessels of the head and neck. It affects elderly people and may be associated with polymyalgia rheumatica. The classic site is the temporal arteries, which become tender and pulseless, in association with severe headaches, jaw claudication and constitutional symptoms (malaise, fever, weight loss). Rarely, necrotic ulcers appear on the scalp. Blindness may follow if the ophthalmic arteries are involved and, to reduce this risk, systemic steroids should be given as soon as the diagnosis has been made. A temporal artery biopsy is the gold standard test for diagnosis. In active phases the erythrocyte sedimentation rate (ESR) is high and its level can be used to guide treatment, which is often prolonged.

Atherosclerosis
This occlusive disease, most common in developed countries, is not discussed in detail here, but involvement of the

large arteries of the legs is of concern to dermatologists. It may cause intermittent claudication, nocturnal cramps, ulcers or gangrene. These may develop slowly over the years or within minutes if a thrombus forms on an atheromatous plaque. The feet are cold and pale, the skin is often atrophic, with little hair, and peripheral pulses are diminished or absent.

Investigations should include urine testing to exclude diabetes mellitus. Fasting plasma lipids (cholesterol, triglycerides and lipoproteins) should be checked in the young, especially if there is a family history of vascular disease. Doppler ultrasound measurements help to distinguish atherosclerotic from venous leg ulcers in the elderly (see *Venous hypertension: investigations*). Complete assessment is best carried out by a specialist in peripheral vascular disease or a vascular surgeon.

Arterial emboli

Emboli may lodge in arteries supplying the skin and cause gangrene, ulcers or necrotic papules, depending on the size of the vessel obstructed. Causes include dislodged thrombi (usually from areas of atherosclerosis), fat emboli (after major trauma), infected emboli (e.g. gonococcal septicaemia or subacute bacterial endocarditis) and tumour emboli.

Pressure sores (Figure 11.5)

Sustained or repeated pressure on skin over bony prominences can cause ischaemia and pressure sores. These are common in patients over 70 years old who are confined to hospital, especially those with a fractured neck of femur. The morbidity and mortality of those with deep ulcers is high.

Cause

The skin and underlying tissues need to be continually nourished with oxygen and nutrients. Pressure prevents adequate blood flow, and if prolonged can lead to tissue death. Healthy people get neurological signals that cause them to shift position. The main factors responsible for pressure sores are:
1 Prolonged immobility and recumbency (e.g. caused by paraplegia, arthritis or senility).
2 Vascular disease (e.g. atherosclerosis).
3 Neurological disease causing diminished sensation (e.g. in paraplegia).
4 Malnutrition, severe systemic disease and general debility.

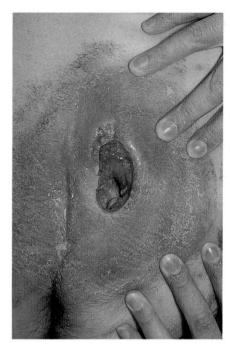

Figure 11.5 A deep pressure sore on the buttock.

Clinical features

The sore begins as an area of erythema which progresses to a superficial blister or erosion. If pressure continues, deeper damage occurs with the development of a black eschar which, when removed or shed, reveals a deep ulcer, often colonized by *Pseudomonas aeruginosa*. The skin overlying bony prominences, such as the sacrum, greater trochanter, ischial tuberosity, the heel and the lateral malleolus, is especially at risk.

Management

The following are important.
1 Prevention: by turning recumbent patients regularly and using antipressure mattresses and positioning devices such as foam wedges for susceptible patients.
2 Treatment of malnutrition and the general condition.
3 Debridement: regular cleansing with normal saline or 0.5% aqueous silver nitrate. Antibacterial preparations locally (Formulary 1, p. 404). Absorbent dressings (Formulary 1, p. 408). Hydrocolloid wafer dressings if there is no infection. Appropriate systemic antibiotic if an infection is spreading.
4 Plastic surgical reconstruction may be indicated in the young when the ulcer is clean.

Venous disease

Deep vein thrombosis

The common causes are listed in Table 11.5.

The onset may be 'silent' or heralded by pain in the calf, often about 10 days after immobilization following surgery or a long haul aeroplane flight, parturition or an infection. The leg becomes swollen and cyanotic distal to the thrombus. The calf may hurt when handled or if the foot is dorsiflexed (Homan's sign). Sometimes a pulmonary embolus is the first sign of a silent deep vein thrombosis (DVT).

A patient suspected of a DVT should be assessed for their pretest probability of an acute DVT using a validated scoring system. If the clinical suspicion is low, a negative D-dimer assay is useful to exclude DVT with-out the need for imaging studies. Suitable investigations include compression ultrasonography, which can only detect thrombi in large veins at, or above, the popliteal fossa, ^{125}I-fibrinogen isotope leg scanning, computerized tomography and magnetic resonance imaging. These have largely replaced venography to diagnose DVT.

Treatment is anticoagulation with unfractionated heparin or low molecular weight heparin and later with a coumarin. The value of thrombolytic regimens has yet to be assessed properly. Prevention is important. DVT after a surgical operation is less frequent now, with early postoperative mobilization, regular leg exercises, the use of elastic stockings over the operative period and prophylaxis with low dose heparin. There is no evidence that aspirin taken before a long flight reduces the incidence of DVTs, but elastic stockings and leg exercises during the flight are sensible precautions.

Table 11.5 Some causes of deep vein thrombosis.

Abnormalities of the vein wall	Trauma (surgery and injuries)
	Chemicals (intravenous infusions)
	Neighbouring infection (e.g. in leg ulcer)
	Tumour (local invasion)
Abnormalities of blood flow	Stasis (immobility, operations, long aircraft flights, pressure, pregnancy, myocardial infarction, heart failure, incompetent valves)
	Impaired venous return
Abnormalities of clotting	Platelets increased or sticky (thrombocythaemia, polycythaemia vera, leukaemia, trauma, splenectomy)
	Decreased fibrinolysis (postoperative)
	Deficiency of clotting factors (e.g. antithrombin, proteins C and S, factor V Leiden)
	Alteration in clotting factors (oral contraceptive, infection, leukaemia, pregnancy, shock and haemorrhage)
	Antiphospholipid antibody
	Prothrombin gene mutation
Unknown mechanisms	Malignancy (thrombophlebitis migrans)
	Smoking
	Behçet's syndrome
	Inflammatory bowel disease

Thrombophlebitis

This is inflammation in a thrombosed vein characterized by pain, erythema and tenderness at the sites of inflammation. If the affected vein is varicose or superficial it will be red and feel like a tender cord. The leg may be diffusely inflamed, making a distinction from cellulitis (p. 218) difficult. There may be fever, leucocytosis and a high ESR. Thrombophlebitis typically occurs in the setting of varicose veins, hypercoagulable states, pregnancy and infections. Patients with intravenous catheters and recent trauma or immobilization are also at higher risks for thrombophlebitis. Most cases are self-limiting and resolve spontaneously within 2 weeks. Migratory superficial thrombophlebitis (Trousseau's sign), in which recurrent episodes affect multiple segments of the veins, should arouse suspicion of an underlying malignancy (most commonly pancreas, lung, gastrointestinal, ovary, and prostate) or systemic disorders (Buerger, Beçhet, systemic lupus and collagen vascular disease).

Treatment is based on NSAIDs for analgesic and anti-inflammatory effects, elastic compression and mobilization. Mild exercise such as walking reduces pain and the potential for propagation of the thrombus. Only in cases of severe pain is bed rest recommended. Patients with recurrent superficial thrombophlebitis from varicose veins may benefit from daily use of compression stockings and surgical treatment of the varicosities (p. 330). Antibiotics rarely help. Anticoagulation is not necessary unless thrombophlebitis is associated with DVT or in association with neoplastic and systemic disorders.

Venous hypertension, the gravitational syndrome and venous leg ulceration

Venous leg ulcers represent the end stage of chronic venous hypertension. Other signs of chronic venous hypertension include palpable varicosities, oedema, stasis dermatitis, hyperpigmentation and lipodermatosclerosis. Venous ulcers have an estimated prevalence of around 1%, are more common in women than in men and account for some 85% of all leg ulcers seen in the United Kingdom and United States.

Cause

Satisfactory venous drainage of the leg requires three sets of veins: deep veins surrounded by muscles; superficial veins; and the veins connecting these together – the perforating or communicating veins (Figure 11.6). When the leg muscles contract, blood in the deep veins is squeezed back, against gravity, to the heart (the calf muscle pump); reflux is prevented by valves. When the muscles relax, with the help of gravity, blood from the superficial veins passes into the deep veins via the communicating vessels. If the valves in the deep and communicating veins are incompetent, the calf muscle pump now pushes blood

into the superficial veins, where the pressure remains high (venous hypertension) instead of dropping during exercise. This persisting venous hypertension enlarges the capillary bed, leading to extravasation of erythrocytes and accumulation of leucocytes and inflammatory cytokines including transforming growth factor-β_1 (TGF-β_1). This prompts a cascade of events, including the release of oxygen free radicals and matrix metalloproteinases, which causes local tissue destruction, fibrosis and ulceration.

Patients with these changes develop lipodermatosclerosis (see *Clinical features*) and have a high serum fibrinogen and reduced blood fibrinolytic activity. The combination of pressure, shearing force (as generated by sliding down a bed), friction and moisture on this background all greatly increase the risks of developing an ulcer. Figure 11.7 shows the factors causing venous ulceration.

Clinical features

Patients with venous hypertension often complain of pain, burning, aching, heaviness, itching, cramping, swelling and restless legs. These symptoms generally worsen after prolonged standing and at the end of the day.

On clinical examination, signs of venous hypertension include:

1 Red or bluish discoloration especially over the medial malleolus (*corona phlebectasia*);
2 Oedema;
3 Loss of hair;
4 Brown pigmentation (mainly haemosiderin from the breakdown of extravasated red blood cells) and scattered petechiae;
5 Prominent varicose veins and incompetent perforating branches (blowouts) between the superficial and deep veins, which are best felt with the patient standing;
6 Atrophie blanche (ivory white scarring with dilated capillary loops; Figure 11.8); and
7 Induration, caused by fibrosis and oedema of the dermis and subcutis – sometimes called lipodermatosclerosis. Prolonged lipodermatosclerosis is classically described as a plaque of indurated hyperpigmented bound-down skin around the midcalf resembling an inverted champagne bottle.

Ulceration is most common found in the gaiter area, from the mid-calf to the medial malleolus (Figure 11.9). In contrast to arterial ulcers, which are usually deep and round, with a punched out appearance, venous ulcers are often large but shallow, with prominent granulation tissue in their bases. Under favourable conditions the exudative

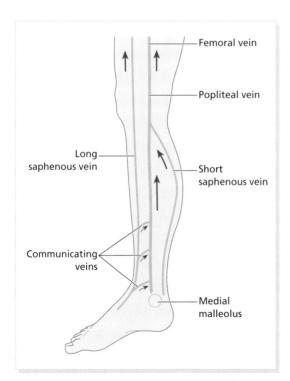

Figure 11.6 The direction of blood flow in normal leg veins.

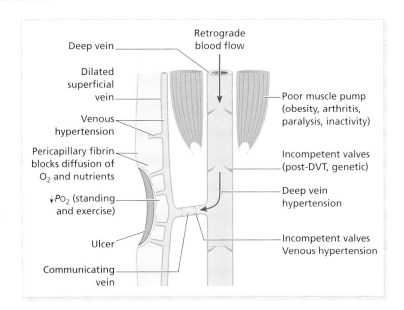

Figure 11.7 Factors causing venous leg ulceration.

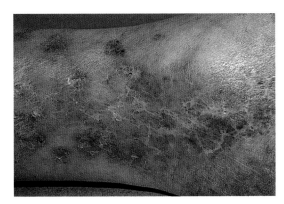

Figure 11.8 Irregular areas of whitish scarring and dilated capillary loops – the changes of atrophic blanche.

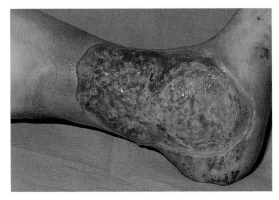

Figure 11.9 Large venous ulcer overlying the medial malleolus.

phase gives way to a granulating and healing phase, signalled by a blurring of the ulcer margin, ingrowth of skin from it and the appearance of scattered small grey epithelial islands over the base.

Complications

Bacterial superinfection is inevitable in a long-standing ulcer, but needs systemic antibiotics only if there is pyrexia, a purulent discharge, rapid extension or an increase in pain, cellulitis, lymphangitis or septicaemia.

Eczema (p. 95) is common around venous ulcers. Allergic contact dermatitis (p. 84) is a common complication and should be suspected if the rash worsens, itches or fails to improve with local treatment. Lanolin, parabens (a preservative) and neomycin are the most common culprits.

Malignant change can occur. If an ulcer has a hyperplastic base or a rolled edge, biopsy may be needed to rule out a squamous cell carcinoma (Figure 11.10).

Differential diagnosis

The main causes of leg ulceration are given in Table 11.6. The most important differences between venous and other leg ulcers are the following.

Atherosclerotic. These ulcers are more common on the toes, dorsum of foot, heel, calf and shin, and are unrelated to perforating veins. Their edges are often sharply defined, their outline may be polycyclic and the ulcers may be deep

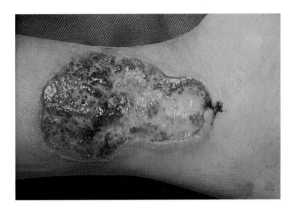

Figure 11.10 Chronic ulcer failing to respond to treatment. Biopsy, taken from rolled edge, excluded malignant change.

and gangrenous. Islands of intact skin are characteristically seen within the ulcer. Claudication may be present and peripheral pulses absent.

Vasculitic. These ulcers start as painful palpable purpuric lesions, turning into small punched-out ulcers. The involvement of larger vessels is heralded by livedo and painful nodules that may ulcerate. Some times a digit may become gangrenous. The intractable deep sharply demarcated ulcers of rheumatoid arthritis are caused by an underlying vasculitis (Figure 11.11).

Thrombotic ulcers. Skin infarction (Figure 11.12), leading to ulceration, may be caused by embolism or by the increased coagulability of polycythaemia or cryoglobulinaemia.

Infective ulcers. Infection is now a rare cause of leg ulcers in the United Kingdom but ulcers caused by tuberculosis, leprosy, atypical mycobacteria, diphtheria and deep fungal infections, such as sporotrichosis or chromoblastomycosis, are still seen in the tropics.

Panniculitic ulcers. These may appear at odd sites, such as the thighs, buttocks or backs of the calves. The most common types of panniculitis that ulcerate are lupus panniculitis, panniculitic T-cell lymphoma, pancreatic panniculitis and erythema induratum (p. 138).

Malignant ulcers. Those caused by a squamous cell carcinoma (p. 292) are the most common, but both malignant melanomas (p. 294) and basal cell carcinomas (p. 291) can present as flat lesions, which expand, crust and ulcerate.

Table 11.6 Causes of leg ulceration.

Vascular	Venous hypertension (Table 11.5)
Arterial disease	Atherosclerosis
	Buerger's disease
	Giant cell arteritis
	Polyarteritis nodosa
	Systemic sclerosis
Small vessel disease	Diabetes mellitus
	Systemic lupus erythematosus
	Rheumatoid arthritis
	Systemic sclerosis
	Allergic vasculitis
	Wegener's granulomatosis
Neuropathic	Diabetes mellitus
	Peripheral neuropathy
	Leprosy
	Syphilis
	Syringomyelia
Haematologic	Immune complex disease
	Polycythaemia vera
	Sickle cell anaemia
	Cryoglobulinaemia
	Peripheral neuropathy
Infection	Osteomyelitis
	'Tropical ulcer'
	Tuberculosis
	Deep fungal infections
Tumour	Squamous cell carcinoma
	Malignant melanoma
	Kaposi's sarcoma
	Basal cell carcinoma
Trauma	Pressure (decubitus)
	Injury
	Artefact
	Iatrogenic

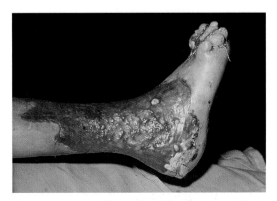

Figure 11.11 Large, shallow and recalcitrant ulcer complicating rheumatoid arthritis.

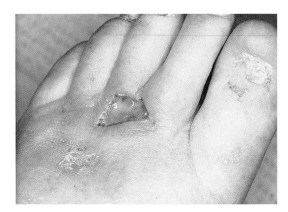

Figure 11.12 This ulcer on the foot was not caused by venous insufficiency but cryoglobulins were detected.

Furthermore, squamous cell carcinoma can arise in any long-standing ulcer, whatever its cause. Ulcers form over CD30 anaplastic large cell lymphomas, panniculitic T-cell lymphomas and tumour stage mycosis fungoides (p. 307).

Pyoderma gangrenosum (p. 321). These large and rapidly spreading ulcers may be circular or polycyclic, and have a blue, indurated, undermined or pustular margin. Pyoderma gangrenosum may complicate rheumatoid arthritis, Crohn's disease, ulcerative colitis or blood dyscrasias.

Investigations

Most chronic leg ulcers are venous in origin, but other causes should be considered if the signs are atypical. The two most common causes of leg ulceration after venous disease are arterial insufficiency and neuropathic diseases. In patients with venous ulcers, a search for contributory factors to leg oedema and poor wound healing is always worthwhile. Factors such as obesity, peripheral artery disease, immunosuppression, malnutrition, diabetes, cardiac failure or arthritis should not be overlooked. Investigations should include the following:
- Blood glucose.
- Full blood count to detect anaemia, which will delay healing.
- Swabbing for pathogens (see *Bacterial superinfection* above).
- Colour flow duplex ultrasound is the gold standard in the diagnosis of venous incompetence and has replaced the use of venography and measuring ambulatory venous pressure. Duplex ultrasound can assess both reflux and obstruction in the deep, superficial and perforator vein systems.
- Doppler ultrasound may help to assess arterial circulation when atherosclerosis is likely. It seldom helps if the dorsalis pedis or posterior tibial pulses can easily be felt. If the maximal systolic ankle pressure divided by the systolic brachial pressure (*ankle brachial pressure index*) is greater than 0.8, the ulcer is unlikely to be caused by arterial disease.
- Cardiac evaluation for congestive failure.

Treatment

Venous ulcers will not heal if the leg remains swollen and the patient chair-bound. Pressure bandages, leg elevation, weight reduction and walking exercise take priority over other measures but not for atherosclerotic ulcers with an already precarious arterial supply. A common error is to use local treatment that is too elaborate. As a last resort, admission to hospital for elevation and intensive treatment may be needed, but the results are not encouraging; patients may stay in the ward for many months only to have their apparently well-healed ulcers break down rapidly when they go home as a result of non-compliance with therapy.

The list of therapies is extensive. They can be divided into the following categories: physical, local, oral and surgical.

Physical measures

Compression bandages and stockings
Compression therapy is the mainstay of treatment in venous leg ulcers and has been well validated in randomized trials. Prior to starting compression therapy, care must be taken to ensure that the arterial supply is satisfactory and not compromised. Compression bandaging, with the compression graduated so that it is greatest at the ankle and least at the top of the bandage, reduces oedema and aids venous return. The bandages are applied over the ulcer dressing, from the forefoot to just below the knee. Self-adhesive bandages are convenient and have largely replaced elasticated bandages. Bandages can stay on for 2–7 days at a time and are left on at night. Various compression bandaging systems are available, comprising two or three extensible bandages applied over a layer of orthopaedic wool. These require changing only once a week and are very effective. The combined layers give a 40–50 mmHg compression at the ankle.

Once an ulcer has healed, a graduated compression stocking from toes to knee (or preferably thigh), should be prescribed, preferably of class 3, providing pressures of 25–35 mmHg at the ankle. A foam or felt pad may be worn under the stockings to protect vulnerable areas against minor trauma. The stocking should be put on before rising from bed. Compression stockings are effective but compliance on a daily basis is essential.

For patients unwilling or unable to use compression stockings because of arthritis or other medical conditions, inelastic stockings are an alternative compression device. These consist of multiple adjustable compression bands held in place with Velcro. Alternatively, intermittent pneumatic compression device can be used in patients who are unable to walk. These devices sequentially inflate and deflate to encourage venous return, thereby reducing oedema.

Elevation of the affected limb
Preferably above the hips, this aids venous drainage, decreases oedema and raises oxygen tension in the limb. Patients should rest with their bodies horizontal and their legs up for at least 2 hours every afternoon. The foot of the bed should be raised by at least 15 cm; it is not enough just to put a pillow under the feet.

Walking
Walking, in moderation, is beneficial, but prolonged standing or sitting with dependent legs is not.

Physiotherapy
Some physiotherapists are good at persuading venous ulcers to heal. Their secret lies in better compliance with therapies such as leg exercises, elevation, gentle massage, intermittent pneumatic compression and graduated compression bandaging. They also teach patients tricks to help them pull on tighter stockings.

Diet
Many patients are obese and should lose weight. At the same time, adequate nutrition is essential for wound healing. Studies have shown that inadequate intake of protein, vitamin C and zinc may prevent wound healing.

Local wound therapy
Remember that many ulcers will heal with no treatment at all but, if their blood flow is compromised, they will not heal despite meticulous care. In venous ulceration, the blood flow is always compromised. Therefore any local wound care therapy must include compression.

Local wound care should be chosen to:
- Maintain a moist environment;
- Absorb excess exudates;
- Reduce the pain;
- Control the odour;
- Protect the surrounding skin;
- Remove surface debris;
- Promote re-epithelialization; and
- Make optimal use of nursing time.

There are many preparations to choose from; those we have found most useful are listed in Formulary 1 (p. 407). Keep in mind that there is insufficient evidence that any particular type of wound dressing is superior in wound healing when used beneath compression. The choice of wound dressing largely depends on patient's comfort and the amount of exudate in the wound.

Clean ulcers (Figure 11.13)
Low-adherent dressings are useful in patients with fragile skin. They reduce adherence at the wound bed and allow passage of exudate to an overlying dressing. They are usually made of paraffin tulle, either plain or impregnated with various agents (e.g. chlorhexidine, xeroform, povidone iodine) and need be changed only once or twice a week. The area should be cleaned gently with saline before the next dressing is applied. Sometimes immersing the whole ulcer in a tub of warm water helps to loosen or dissolve adherent crusts.

Semipermeable films (e.g. OpSite, Tegaderm, Mefilm) are porous to air and water vapour, but not fluids or bacteria, and are suitable for shallow ulcers with low to medium exudate, in which they encourage a moist wound

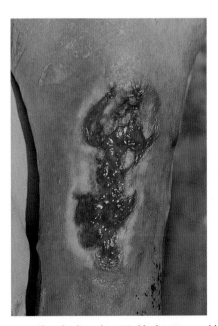

Figure 11.13 Clean healing ulcer. Weekly dressing would be suitable.

environment and allow healing cytokines in the exudates to do their work. More heavily exudative wounds can be dressed with either alginate or foam dressings. Alginates (e.g. Kaltostat, Tegagen, Sorbsan), produced from the naturally occurring alginic acid found in brown seaweed are biodegradable and highly absorbent. They are useful in cavities or undermined wounds but need to be changed daily or they may cause maceration of the surrounding tissues. Foam dressings are made from polyurethane or silicon. They produce a moist environment by absorbing exudates into the cells of the foam and keeping excess fluid from the surrounding skin.

Necrotic or sloughy wounds should be treated with hydrogel dressings, which promote a moist wound environment, and subsequent debridement of non-viable tissue. Hydrocolloid sheets (e.g. DuoDERM, Granuflex) are almost impermeable to water vapour, and can rehydrate dry eschar while hydrocolloid fibres (e.g. Aquacel) are highly absorbent for exudative wounds.

Medicated bandages (Formulary 1, p. 408) based on zinc oxide paste, with ichthammol, or with calamine and clioquinol, are useful when there is much surrounding eczema, and can be used for all types of ulcers, even infected exuding ones. The bandage is applied in strips from the foot to below the knee. Worsening of eczema under a medicated bandage may signal the development of allergic contact dermatitis to a component of the paste, most often parabens (a preservative) or cetostearyl alcohols.

Infected ulcers (Figure 11.14)
Most patients will be helped with local treatment alone.

Infected ulcers have to be cleaned and dressed more often than clean ones, sometimes even twice daily. Useful preparations include 0.5% silver nitrate, 0.25% sodium hypochlorite, 0.25% acetic acid, potassium permanganate (1 in 10 000 dilution) and 5% hydrogen peroxide, all made up in aqueous solution, and applied as compresses with or without occlusion. Helpful creams and lotions include 1.5% hydrogen peroxide, 20% benzoyl peroxide, 1% silver sulfadiazine, 10% povidone-iodine (Formulary 1, p. 407). The main function of starch polymer beads within cadexomer iodine is to absorb exudate. Although antibiotic tulles are easy to apply and are well tolerated, they should not be used for long periods as they can induce bacterial resistance and sensitize. Resistance is not such a problem with povidone-iodine, and a readily applied non-adherent dressing impregnated with this antiseptic may be useful. Surrounding eczema is helped by weak or moderate strength local steroids, which must never be put on the

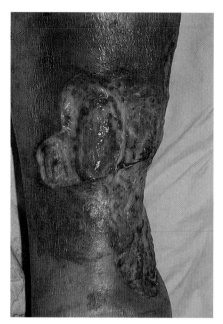

Figure 11.14 Infected ulcer with sloughing. Tendon visible at bottom of figure. Hospital admission and frequent dressings needed to save leg.

ulcer itself. Lassar's paste, zinc cream or paste bandages (see *Clean ulcers*) are suitable alternatives.

Oral and/or intravenous treatment
The following may be helpful.

Diuretics. Pressure bandaging is more important as the oedema associated with venous ulceration is largely mechanical. Diuretics will combat the oedema of cardiac failure.

Analgesics. Adequate analgesia is important. Aspirin may not be well tolerated by the elderly. Paracetamol (acetaminophen in the United States) or ibuprofen are often adequate but dihydrocodeine may be required. Analgesia may be needed only when the dressing is changed.

Antibiotics. Just because bacteria can be isolated from an ulcer does not mean that antibiotics should be prescribed. Ulcers need not be 'sterilized' by local or systemic antibiotics. Short courses of systemic antibiotics should be reserved for spreading infections characterized by an enlarging ulcer, increased redness around the ulcer and lymphangitis. Sometimes they are tried for pain or even odour. Bacteriological guidance is needed and the drugs used include erythromycin and flucloxacillin (streptococcal or staphylococcal cellulitis), metronidazole (*Bacteroides* infection) and ciprofloxacin (*Pseudomonas aeruginosa* infection). Bacterial infection may prejudice the outcome of skin grafting.

Ferrous sulfate and folic acid. For anaemia.

Zinc sulfate. May help to promote healing, especially if the plasma zinc level is low.

Pentoxifylline is fibrinolytic, increases the deformability of red and white blood cells, decreases blood viscosity and diminishes platelet adhesiveness. It may speed the healing of venous ulcers if used with compression bandages.

Prostagladin E_1 (PGE$_1$) administered intravenously over 3–6 weeks has been shown in several trials to improve symptoms of venous insufficiency, reduce oedema and heal venous ulcers.

Surgery (see also p. 330)

If superficial venous reflux is demonstrated on duplex ultrasound, patients with chronic venous insufficiency will generally benefit from surgical treatment. Several randomized trials have shown quicker healing time and lower rates of recurrence of venous ulcers in patients who had surgical treatment in comparison with compression stockings.

Newer minimally invasive surgical techniques for the treatment of superficial venous reflux have changed our approach to the treatment of venous ulcers. In the past, surgical management consisted of ligation and stripping, which was associated with higher morbidity and usually a treatment of last resort. In the last decade, saphenous vein incompetence has been managed with endovenous laser or radiofrequency ablation. Combined with local tumescent anaesthesia, these minimally invasive techniques have outperformed traditional ligation and stripping. Patients can walk immediately after the endovenous ablation and most patients can resume normal activities within 24–48 hours. A radiofrequency catheter or laser fiber is introduced into the saphenous vein under ultrasound guidance and placed at the sapheno-femoral junction. The device is turned on and gradually withdrawn along the length of the vessel resulting in a controlled fibrosis of the treated vein. Varicose veins, especially elevated vessels larger than 4 mm in diameter, can be treated using ambulatory microphlebectomy. Veins are permanently removed using a vein hook through small incisions (1–2 mm in length).

Chemical ablation of the saphenous vein with foam sclerotherapy has also been shown to be an effective treatment for venous reflux. The aim of sclerotherapy is the fibrous occlusion of the vessel lumen. Rather than merely thrombosing a vessel which may be amenable to recanalization, sclerosing a vessel transforms it into a fibrous cord, which cannot be recanalized. Foam sclerotherapy is more efficacious for larger diameter vessels because the bubbles mechanically displace blood, thereby maximizing the contact time and surface area between the sclerosant and the vein endothelium. Foam sclerosants are mixtures of gas with a liquid solution with surfactant properties such as polidocanol or sodium tetradecyl sulfate. The sclerosant is injected under ultrasound guidance into the diseased vein. Compression is then applied to ensure more direct apposition of the treated vein walls to encourage sclerosis of the vessel.

Patients with non-healing venous ulcer may benefit from autologous pinch, split-thickness or mesh grafts. Human skin equivalents comprising a cultured bilayer of epidermal keratinocytes and dermal fibroblasts have been used as grafts with promising results, but this treatment is not widely available. Remember, the cause of the ulcer and slow healing is venous hypertension. Skin grafting, like local topical therapy, will not be successful if the skin continues to be deprived of essential nutrients. Surgical intervention to treat the underlying venous insufficiency is important to prevent recurrence of the ulcer.

Patients with atherosclerotic ulcers should see a vascular surgeon for assessment. Some blockages are surgically remediable.

Purpura

Purpura (Figure 11.15), petechiae and ecchymoses may be caused by a coagulation or platelet disorder, or by an

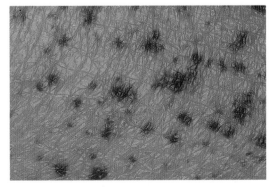

Figure 11.15 Typical purpura, which is not abolished by pressure.

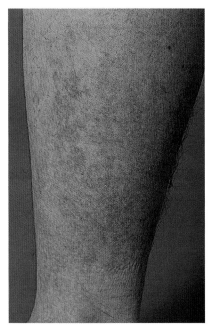

Figure 11.16 This gingery colour is typical of haemosiderin rather than melanin. It is caused by capillary fragility.

abnormality of the vessel wall or the surrounding dermis (Figure 11.16). Some common causes are listed in Table 11.7. In general, coagulation defects give rise to ecchymoses and external bleeding. Platelet defects present more often as purpura, although bleeding and ecchymoses can still occur. Vasculitis of small vessels causes purpura, often palpable and painful, but not bleeding; this is discussed in Chapter 8. Purpura from vasodilatation and gravity is seen in many diseases of the legs, especially in the elderly (defective dermis around the blood vessels), and seldom requires extensive investigation.

Cryoglobulinaemia is a rare cause of purpura, which is most prominent on exposed parts. It may also cause cold urticaria (p. 149) and livedo reticularis (p. 141). The condition may be idiopathic, or secondary to myeloma, leukaemia, hepatitis C infection or an autoimmune disease.

Investigations

The most common cause of purpura is trauma, especially to the thin sun-damaged skin of elderly forearms (senile purpura). When purpura has no obvious cause, investigations should include a platelet count, prothrombin time, APTT, a full blood count and biochemical screen. Electrophoresis is needed to exclude

Table 11.7 Causes of intracutaneous bleeding.

Coagulation defects	Inherited defects (e.g. haemophilia, Christmas disease)
	Connective tissue disorders
	Disseminated intravascular coagulation
	Paraproteinaemias (e.g. macroglobulinaemia)
	Acquired defects (e.g. liver disease, anticoagulant therapy, vitamin K deficiency, drugs)
Platelet defects	Thrombocytopenia
	Idiopathic
	Connective tissue disorders, especially lupus erythematosus
	Disseminated intravascular coagulation
	Haemolytic anaemia
	Hypersplenism
	Giant haemangiomas (Kasabach–Merritt syndrome)
	Bone marrow damage (cytostatic drugs, leukaemia, carcinoma)
	Drugs (quinine, aspirin, thiazides and sulfonamides)
Abnormal function	von Willebrand disease
	Drugs (e.g. aspirin)
Vascular defect	Raised intravascular pressure (coughing, vomiting, venous hypertension, gravitational)
	Vasculitis (including Henoch–Schönlein purpura)
	Infections (e.g. meningococcal septicaemia, Rocky Mountain spotted fever)
	Drugs (carbromal, aspirin, sulfonamides, quinine, phenylbutazone and gold salts)
	Painful bruising syndrome
Idiopathic	Progressive pigmented dermatoses (Figure 11.16)
Lack of support from surrounding dermis	Senile purpura
	Topical or systemic corticosteroid therapy
	Scurvy (perifollicular purpura)
	Lichen sclerosus et atrophicus
	Systemic amyloidosis

hypergammaglobulinaemia and paraproteinaemia. Cryo-globulinaemia should also be excluded. To help detect a consumptive coagulopathy, a coagulation screen, including measurement of fibrinogen and fibrin degradation products, may be necessary. The bleeding time, and a Hess tourniquet test for capillary fragility, are rarely helpful. Skin biopsy will confirm a small vessel vasculitis, if the purpura is palpable.

Treatment

Treat the underlying condition. Replacement of relevant blood constituents may be needed initially. Systemic steroids are usually effective in vasculitis (see Chapter 8).

Disorders of the lymphatics

Lymphoedema

The skin overlying chronic lymphoedema is firm and pits poorly. Long-standing lymphoedema may lead to gross, almost furry, hyperkeratosis, as in the so-called 'mossy foot'.

Cause

Lymphoedema may be primary or secondary. The primary forms are developmental defects, although signs may only appear in early puberty or even in adulthood. Sometimes lymphoedema involves only one leg. Secondary causes are listed in Table 11.8.

Table 11.8 Causes of secondary lymphoedema.

Recurrent lymphangitis	Erysipelas
	Infected pompholyx
Lymphatic obstruction	Filariasis
	Granuloma inguinale
	Tuberculosis
	Tumour
Lymphatic destruction	Surgery
	Radiation therapy
	Tumour
Uncertain aetiology	Rosacea
	Melkersson–Rosenthal syndrome (facial nerve palsy, fissuring of tongue and lymphoedema of lip)
	Yellow nail syndrome

Treatment

Complete decongestive therapy is the best treatment. This consists of multilayer compression bandaging, manual lymphatic drainage by an experienced physiotherapist, exercise and skin care. Prevention of infection is essential to prevent continued lymphatic damage and antibiotics should be given at the first sign of lymphangitis or erysipelas. If erysipelas recurs, long-term penicillin should be given. Surgery occasionally helps to remove an obstruction or restore drainage.

Lymphangitis

This streptococcal infection of the lymphatics may occur without any lymphoedema. A tender red line extends proximally. Penicillin flucloxacillin, cephalexin and erythromycin are usually effective.

Learning points

1 An ulcer will never heal, whatever you put on it, if the ankle is oedematous or the blood flow is inadequate.
2 Support stockings are better than fancy creams.
3 Watch out for contact allergy to local applications.
4 Never put topical steroids on ulcers.
5 Most ulcers, despite positive bacteriology, are not much helped by systemic antibiotics.
6 Avoid compression bandaging if the arterial supply is compromised.

Further reading

Douglas WS, Simpson NB. (1995) Guidelines for the management of chronic venous ulceration: report of a multidisciplinary workshop. *British Journal of Dermatology* **132**, 446–452.

Lymphoedema Framework. (2006) *Best Practice for the Management of Lymphoedema. International consensus.* London: MEP Ltd.

Palfreyman SSJ, Nelson EA, Lochiel R, Michaels JA. (2006). Dressings for healing venous leg ulcers. *Cochrane Database of Systematic Reviews* **3**, CD001103.

Takahashi PY, Kiemele LJ, Jones JP Jr. (2004) Wound care for elderly patients: advances and clinical applications for practicing physicians. *Mayo Clinic Proceedings* **79**, 260–267.

Valencia IC, Falabella A, Kirsner RS, Eaglstein WH. (2001) Chronic venous insufficiency and venous leg ulceration. *Journal of the American Academy of Dermatology* **44**, 401–421.

Word R. (2010) Medical and surgical therapy for advanced chronic venous insufficiency. *Surgical Clinics of North America* **90**, 1195–1214.

12 Sebaceous and Sweat Gland Disorders

Sebaceous glands

Most sebaceous glands develop embryologically from hair germs, but a few free glands arise from the epidermis. Those associated with hairs lie in the obtuse angle between the follicle and the epidermis (see Figure 13.1). The glands themselves are multilobed and contain cells full of lipid, which are shed whole (holocrine secretion) during secretion so that sebum contains their remnants in a complex mixture of triglycerides, free fatty acids, wax esters, squalene and cholesterol. Sebum is discharged into the upper part of the hair follicle. It lubricates and waterproofs the skin, and protects it from drying; it is also mildly bacteriocidal and fungistatic. Sebaceous follicles are most commonly found on the face, behind the ears, and on the upper chest and back. Free sebaceous glands not associated with hair follicles may be found in the eyelid (meibomian glands), mucous membranes (Fordyce spots), nipple, peri-anal region and genitalia.

Androgenic hormones, especially dihydrotestosterone, stimulate sebaceous gland activity. Human sebaceous glands contain 5α-reductase, 3α- and 17α-hydroxysteroid dehydrogenase, which convert weaker androgens to dihydrotestosterone, which in turn binds to specific receptors in sebaceous glands, increasing sebum secretion. The sebaceous glands react to maternal androgens for a short time after birth, and then lie dormant until puberty when a surge of androgens produces a sudden increase in sebum excretion and sets the stage for acne.

Acne

Acne is a disorder of the pilosebaceous apparatus characterized by comedones, papules, pustules, cysts and scars.

Prevalence
Nearly all teenagers have some acne (acne vulgaris). It affects the sexes equally, starting usually between the ages of 12 and 14 years, tending to be earlier in females. The peak age for severity in females is 16–17 and in males 17–19 years. Variants of acne are much less common.

Cause

Acne vulgaris
Many factors combine to cause acne (Figure 12.1), characterized by chronic inflammation around pilosebaceous follicles.
- *Sebum over-production.* Sebum excretion is increased. However, this alone need not cause acne; patients with acromegaly, or with Parkinson's disease, have high sebum excretion rates but no acne. Furthermore, sebum excretion often remains high long after the acne has gone away.
- *Hormonal.* Androgens (from the testes, ovaries, adrenals and sebaceous glands themselves) are the main stimulants of sebum excretion, although other hormones (e.g. thyroid hormones and growth hormone) have minor effects too. Those castrated before puberty, or with androgen insensitivity, never develop acne. In acne, the sebaceous glands respond excessively to what are usually normal levels of these hormones (increased target organ sensitivity). This may be caused by 5α-reductase activity being higher in the target sebaceous glands than in other parts of the body. Fifty per cent of females with acne have slightly raised free testosterone levels – usually because of a low level of sex hormone binding globulin rather than a high total testosterone – but this is still only a fraction of the concentration in males, and its relevance is debatable.

Clinical Dermatology, Fifth Edition. Richard B. Weller, Hamish J.A. Hunter and Margaret W. Mann.
© 2015 John Wiley & Sons, Ltd. Published 2015 by John Wiley & Sons, Ltd.

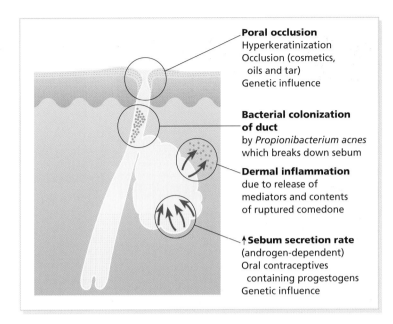

Poral occlusion
Hyperkeratinization
Occlusion (cosmetics,
   oils and tar)
Genetic influence

**Bacterial colonization
of duct**
by *Propionibacterium acnes*
which breaks down sebum

Dermal inflammation
due to release of
mediators and contents
of ruptured comedone

↑**Sebum secretion rate**
(androgen-dependent)
Oral contraceptives
   containing progestogens
Genetic influence

Figure 12.1 Factors causing acne.

• *Poral occlusion.* Both genetic and environmental factors (e.g. some cosmetics) cause the epithelium to overgrow the follicular surface. Follicles then retain sebum that has an increased concentration of bacteria and free fatty acids. Rupture of these follicles is associated with intense inflammation and tissue damage, mediated by oxygen free radicals and enzymes such as elastase, released by white cells.

• *Increased bacterial colonization.* *Propionibacterium acnes*, a normal skin commensal, plays a pathogenic part. It colonizes the pilosebaceous ducts, breaks down triglycerides releasing free fatty acids, and induces the ductal epithelium to secrete pro-inflammatory cytokines via activation of Toll-like receptor 2 (TLR2) pathway. Activated neutrophils release lysosomal enzymes which lead to follicular rupture. The release of follicular content results in a foreign body reaction which furthers the inflammatory reaction.

• *Genetic.* The condition is familial in about half of those with acne. There is a high concordance of the sebum excretion rate and acne in monozygotic, but not dizygotic, twins. Further studies are required to determine the precise mode of inheritance.

• *Diet.* Recent systematic reviews of diet on acne suggest that dairy products (particularly milk) and high glycaemic load may be associated with increased risk and severity of acne. Prospective studies are needed to determine if a low glycaemic diet and reduced dairy intake may help acne.

Presentation

Common type

Lesions are confined to the face, shoulders, upper chest and back. Seborrhoea (a greasy skin; Figure 12.2) is often present. Open comedones (blackheads), because of the plugging by keratin and sebum of the pilosebaceous orifice, or closed comedones (whiteheads), caused by overgrowth of the follicle openings by surrounding epithelium, are always seen. Inflammatory papules, nodules and cysts occur (Figures 12.3 and 12.4), with one or two types of lesion predominating. Depressed or hypertrophic scarring and post-inflammatory hyperpigmentation can follow.

Conglobate (gathered into balls; from the Latin *globus* meaning 'ball') is the name given to a severe form of acne with all of the above features as well as abscesses

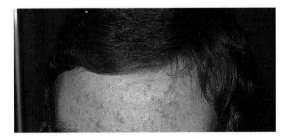

Figure 12.2 The seborrhoea, comedones and scattered inflammatory papules of teenage acne.

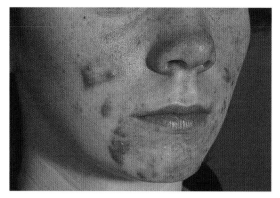

Figure 12.3 Prominent and inflamed cysts are the main features here.

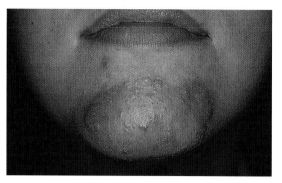

Figure 12.5 Late-onset acne in a woman. Often localized to the chin.

or cysts with intercommunicating sinuses that contain thick serosanguinous fluid or pus. On resolution, it leaves deeply pitted or hypertrophic scars, sometimes joined by keloidal bridges. Although hyperpigmentation is usually transient, it can persist, particularly in those with an already dark skin. Psychological depression is common in persistent acne, which need not necessarily be severe.

Variants of acne

• *Neonatal acne.* This occurs in more than 20% of healthy newborn babies between 2 weeks to 3 months of age. It may follow transplacental stimulation of a child's sebaceous glands by maternal androgens.

• *Infantile acne.* This rare type of acne is present at 3–6 months of age and typically resolves in 12 months. It is more common in males and may last up to 3 years. Its morphology is like that of common acne and it may

be the forerunner of severe acne in adolescence. Maternal hormones have a minor role at this age. Rather, the immature infantile adrenal gland produces elevated dehydroepiandrosterone (DHEA) and delayed maturation of the gonadal feedback system results in increased levels of luteinizing hormone (LH), follicle-stimulating hormone (FSH) and testosterone.

• *Late onset.* This occurs mainly in women and is often limited to the chin and jawline (Figure 12.5). Nodular and cystic lesions predominate. It is stubborn and persistent.

• *Acne fulminans.* Acne fulminans is a rare variant in which conglobate acne is accompanied by fever, joint pains and a high erythrocyte sedimentation rate (ESR).

• *Mechanical.* Excessive scrubbing, picking or the rubbing of chin straps or a fiddle (Figure 12.6) can rupture occluded follicles.

• *Tropical.* Heat and humidity are responsible for this variant, which affects Caucasoids with a tendency to acne. This occurs mainly on the trunk and may be conglobate. Sweat causes follicular occlusion by causing the perifollicular epidermis to swell.

• *Excoriated.* This is most common in young girls. Obsessional picking or rubbing leaves discrete denuded areas.

• *Exogenous.* Tars, chlorinated hydrocarbons, oils and oily cosmetics may induce comedone formation or precipitate inflammation around vellous hair follicles. Suspicion should be raised if the distribution is odd or if comedones predominate (Figure 12.7).

• *Drug-induced* (Figure 12.8). Corticosteroids, androgenic and anabolic steroids, gonadotrophins, oral contraceptives, lithium, iodides, bromides, antituberculosis and anticonvulsant therapy can all cause an acneiform rash. Follicular acneiform eruption has commonly been reported in patients receiving inhibitors of the epidermal

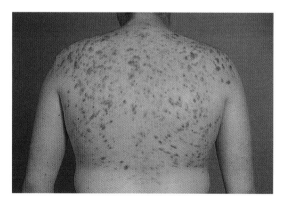

Figure 12.4 Conglobate acne with inflammatory nodules, pustulocystic lesions and depressed scars.

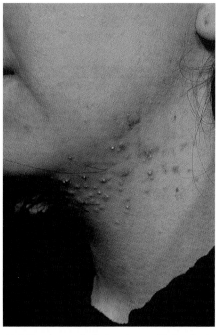

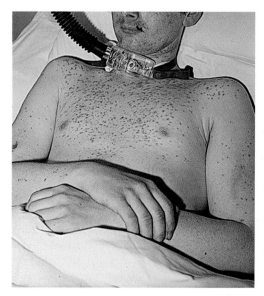

Figure 12.8 Steroid-induced acne in a seriously ill patient.

Figure 12.6 Papulopustular lesions in an odd distribution. The patient played the violin ('fiddler's neck').

growth factor receptor (EGF-R). Suspicion should be raised when acne, dominated by monomorphous papulo-pustules rather than comedones, appears suddenly in a non-teenager and coincides with the prescription of a drug known to cause acneiform lesions.

• *Follicular occlusion tetrad.* Severe nodulocystic acne can be associated with dissecting cellulitis of the scalp, suppu-rative hidradenitis and pilonidal cysts.

• *Polycystic ovarian syndrome.* Consider this in obese females with oligomenorrhoea or secondary amenor-rhoea or infertility. Glucose intolerance, dyslipidaemia, hirsutism and hypertension may be other features. Acne accompanying the polycystic ovarian syndrome is caused by modestly raised circulating androgen levels.

• *Congenital adrenal hyperplasia.* Hyperpigmentation, ambiguous genitalia, history of salt-wasting in childhood and a Jewish background are all clues to this rare diagnosis caused by 21-hydroxylase deficiency.

• *Androgen-secreting tumours.* These cause the rapid onset of virilization (clitoromegaly, deepening of voice, breast atrophy, male pattern balding and hirsutism) as well as acne.

Course

Acne vulgaris clears by the age of 23–25 years in 90% of patients, but some 5% of women and 1% of men still need treatment in their thirties or even forties.

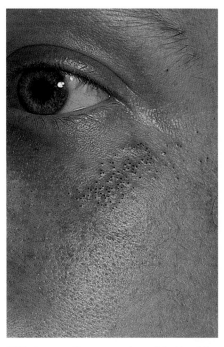

Figure 12.7 A group of open comedones (blackheads) following the use of a greasy cosmetic.

Investigations

None are usually necessary. Cultures are occasionally needed to exclude a pyogenic infection, an anaerobic infection or Gram-negative folliculitis. Only a few laboratories routinely culture *P. acnes* and test its sensitivity to antibiotics.

Any acne, including infantile acne, which is associated with virilization, needs investigation to exclude an androgen-secreting tumour of the adrenals, ovaries or testes, and to rule out congenital adrenal hyperplasia caused by 21-hydroxylase deficiency. Tests should then include the measurement of plasma levels of total and free testosterone, sex hormone binding globulin, LH, FSH, DHEA sulfate, androstenedione, 17-hydroxyprogesterone, urinary free cortisol and, depending on the results, ultrasound examination or computed tomography scan of the ovaries and adrenals. Female patients should not be taking the oral contraceptive pill when these hormone levels are measured. Congenital adrenal hyperplasia is associated with high levels of 17-hydroxyprogesterone, and androgen secreting tumours with high androgen levels.

Polycystic ovarian syndrome is characterized by modestly elevated testosterone, androstenedione and DHEA sulfate levels, a reduced sex hormone binding level and an LH : FSH ratio of greater than 2.5 : 1. Pelvic ultrasound may reveal multiple small ovarian cysts, although some patients with acne have ovarian cysts without biochemical evidence of the polycystic ovarian syndrome.

Differential diagnosis

Rosacea (see *Rosacea*) affects older individuals. Comedones are absent, the papules and pustules occur only on the face and the rash has a centrofacial erythematous background. Pyogenic folliculitis can be excluded by culture. Hidradenitis suppurativa (see *Hidradenitis suppurativa*) is associated with acne conglobata, but attacks the axillae and groin. Pseudofolliculitis barbae and acne keloidalis nuchae, caused by ingrowing hairs, occur on the necks and scalps of men with curly facial hair and clears up if shaving is stopped. Always suspect cosmetic acne, especially in post-adolescent women with acne limited to the face.

Treatment

Acne frequently has marked psychological effects. Even mild acne can have significant impact on self-esteem and quality of life. An optimistic approach is essential, and regular encouragement worthwhile.

Occasionally, an underlying cause (see *Variants of acne*) is found; this should be removed or treated.

At some time most teenagers try antiacne preparations bought from their pharmacist. Local treatment is the standard of care for most patients with comedo-papular acne, although both local and systemic treatments are needed for pustulocystic scarring acne (Figure 12.9).

Local treatment (Formulary 1, p. 405)

1 Regular gentle cleansing with soap and water should be encouraged, to remove surface sebum.

2 Salicylic acid is widely available as an over-the-counter acne treatment; it is a mild comedolytic agent.

3 The antibacterial agent benzoyl peroxide is applied only at night initially, but can be used twice daily if this does not cause too much dryness and irritation. It is most effective for inflammatory lesions and is not affected by

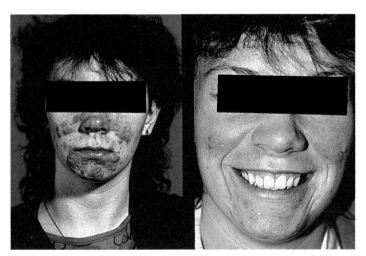

Figure 12.9 A successful systemic treatment of acne – the picture tells its own story.

propionibacterial antibiotic resistance. It is wise to start with a 2.5 or 5% preparation, moving up to 10% if necessary. Benzoyl peroxide bleaches coloured materials, particularly towels and flannels.

4 The vitamin A (retinol) analogues (tretinoin, isotretinoin, adapalene, tazarotene) normalize follicular keratinization, down-regulate TLR 2 expression and reduce sebum production. Retinoids are especially effective against comedones. Patients should be warned about skin irritation (start with small amounts) and photosensitivity. Concomitant eczema is usually a contraindication to their use. Tretinoin can be prescribed as a lotion, cream or gel. Patients with oily skin may prefer gels which are drying, while those with sensitive skin tend to prefer the more emollient creams. Newer preparations (in the United States) use microspheres (Retin-A micro) or specially formulated bases (Avita, Avage) that minimize irritation. The weakest preparation should be used first, and applied every 2–3 nights, increasing frequency after several weeks as tolerated. Sometimes, after a week or two, it will have to be stopped temporarily because of irritation. The combination of benzoyl peroxide in the morning and tretinoin at night has many advocates.

• Isotretinoin 0.05% is made up in a gel base (not available in United States) and applied once or twice daily. It irritates less than the same concentration of tretinoin.

• Adapalene (0.1% gel) is a retinoid-like drug indicated for mild to moderate acne. Compared with tretinoin, it is a milder comedolytic but also better tolerated.

• Tazarotene (0.1% gel), applied once daily, was found in one study to be more effective than tretinoin (0.1% microsponge).

Topical retinoids should not be prescribed for pregnant woman with acne.

5 Azelaic acid is bacteriocidal for *P. acnes*: it is also anti-inflammatory and inhibits the formation of comedones by reducing the proliferation of keratinocytes. It should be applied twice daily. It is often used in darker skin patients as it may help to lighten post-inflammatory hyperpigmentation.

6 Topical antibiotics include topical clindamycin, erythromycin and sulfacetamide (Formulary 1, p. 405) but antibacterial resistance of *P. acnes* is a growing problem, with most erythromycin-resistant strains being cross-resistant to clindamycin. Combining antibiotics with benzoyl peroxide reduces *P. acnes* numbers and the likelihood of resistant strains emerging (Formulary 1, p. 405). The addition of zinc acetate complex to erythromycin enhances the anti-inflammatory effect of the antibiotic.

7 Topical dapsone 5% gel is a newer option for treating acne. It is safe in patients with a deficiency in glucose-6-phosphate dehydrogenase.

8 Cosmetic camouflage help some patients, especially females, whose scarring is unsightly. Cover-ups also obscure post-inflammatory pigmentation. A range of makeup is available in the United Kingdom and the United States (Formulary 1, p. 399).

Systemic treatment (Formulary 2, p. 411)

Antibiotics
The prevalence of antibiotic-resistant *P. acnes*, particularly to erythromycin, is rising even in patients never previously exposed to it. As well as reducing *P. acnes* numbers, antibiotics also have a direct anti-inflammatory effect so will continue to be beneficial, but wherever possible they should be used in combination with topical benzoyl peroxide or retinoids to limit colonization by antibiotic-resistant bacteria.

Tetracyclines
• An average starting dosage for an adult of oxytetracycline or tetracycline is 500 mg twice daily, but up to 1.5 g/day may be needed in resistant cases. The antibiotic should not be used for less than 3 months and may be needed for a year or two, or even longer. It should be taken on an empty stomach, 1 hour before meals or 4 hours after food, as the absorption of these tetracyclines is decreased by milk, antacids and calcium, iron and magnesium salts. The dosage should be tapered in line with clinical improvement, an average maintenance dosage being 250–500 mg/day. Even with long courses, serious side-effects are rare, although candidal vulvovaginitis may force a change to a narrower spectrum antibiotic such as erythromycin.

• Doxycycline, 100 mg once or twice daily, is a cheaper alternative to minocycline, but more frequently associated with phototoxic skin reactions. A new low dose preparation (40 mg; Oracea, United States) is given once daily and inhibits acne by stopping inflammation in and around the pilosebaceous follicles without apparently affecting the bacterial flora of the vagina or elsewhere.

• Minocycline, 50 mg twice or 100 mg once daily (in a modified release preparation), has the same efficacy as other tetracyclines. Absorption is not significantly affected by food or drink. It carries the risk of causing a lupus-like syndrome and also pigmentation, and is thus not recommended as a first-line treatment.

Tetracyclines should not be taken in pregnancy or by children under 9 years as they are deposited in growing bone and developing teeth, causing stained teeth and dental hypoplasia. Rarely, the long-term administration of minocycline causes a greyish pigmentation, like a bruise, especially on the faces of those with actinic damage and over the shins.

Erythromycin (dosage as for oxytetracycline) is the next antibiotic of choice but is preferable to tetracyclines in women who might become pregnant. Its major drawbacks are nausea and the widespread development of resistant Propionibacteria, which leads to therapeutic failure.

Trimethoprim is used with or without sulfamethoxazole by some as a third-line antibiotic for acne, when a tetracycline and erythromycin have not helped. White blood cell counts should be monitored. Ampicillin is another alternative.

Learning points

1 Never prescribe short courses of many different antibiotics.
2 Patients should use a topical retinoid or benzoyl peroxide when they are on antibiotics.
3 Avoid tetracyclines in children and pregnant women.
4 Make sure that females with acne are not pregnant before you prescribe isotretinoin. Only prescribe 1 month of isotretinoin at a time, after confirming a negative pregnancy test. Avoid pregnancy for 3 months after stopping treatment.
5 Look out for depression in patients taking isotretinoin. If it occurs, stop the drug immediately, seek specialist advice and review your therapeutic options.

Hormonal treatment

Hormonal therapy can be very effective for female patients with acne, even if their serum androgen levels are normal. They tend to work best in adult women with persistent inflammatory papules involving the chin and jawline who report flares around their menstrual cycle.

Co-cyprindiol, a combined antiandrogen–oestrogen treatment (Dianette: 2 mg cyproterone acetate and 0.035 mg ethinylestradiol), is available in many countries and may help persistent acne in women. Monitoring is as for any patient on an oral contraceptive pill (OCP), and further contraceptive measures are unnecessary. The incidence of venous thrombo-embolism is higher than for the low dose OCP, and the course should not go on for more than 3 months after the acne has cleared, at which point the drug should be replaced by a low oestrogen/low progestogen oral contraceptive. These drugs are not for males.

A number of combined oral contraceptives have been shown to improve acne. They reduce ovarian androgen synthesis and, by increasing sex hormone binding globulin, reduce free testosterone levels and sebum production. Ethinyl estradiol 35 μg/norgestimate (Ortho Tri-Cyclen) and ethinyl estradiol 20–35 μg/norethindrone acetate (Estrostep) have been approved for use in acne in the United States.

Spironolactone blocks the androgen receptor and inhibits 5α-reductase, thus reducing sebum production. It may be added to the OCP after 3 months if there has been an inadequate response. The usual dose is 25–100 mg/day with food. In older patients, or those with concomitant medical problems, serum electrolytes should be checked as it may cause hyperkalaemia. Pregnancy should be avoided as there is a risk of causing abnormalities of the fetal male genitalia.

Isotretinoin (13-*cis*-retinoic acid; Formulary 2, p. 422) is an oral retinoid that inhibits sebum excretion, the growth of *P. acnes* and acute inflammatory processes. The drug is usually reserved for severe nodulocystic acne, unresponsive to the measures outlined above. It is routinely given for 4–6 months, in a dosage of 0.5–2 mg/kg body weight/day. Young men with truncal acne may require higher dosage while patients with side effects may benefit from a lower daily dose given over a longer period of time. Patients with severe acne may notice a flare on initiation of isotretinoin, but this effect is usually short lived and the drug can be continued. A lower starting dose and concomitant administration of prednisone may prevent severe flares during the first few months. It is because of its early side effects that some dermatologists start isotretinoin in a low dose (e.g. 20 mg/day) and then work up to the target dose if no significant side effects are reported at review during the first month of treatment. The goal is to achieve a total cumulative dose of 120–150 mg/kg to reduce the risk of relapse. A full blood count, liver function tests and fasting lipid levels should be checked before the start of the course, and then 1 and 4 months after starting the drug. The drug seldom has to be stopped, although abnormalities of liver function rarely limit treatment.

Isotretinoin is highly teratogenic: various national programmes (iPledge in the USA, Pregnancy Prevention Programme in UK) have been instituted to reduce the risk of women becoming pregnant while taking isotretinoin. Tests for pregnancy are carried out monthly while the drug is being taken, and only a single month's supply of the drug should be prescribed at a time, on receipt of a negative pregnancy test. The recommendations in the United States are especially stringent. Patient, physician and dispensing pharmacy must all be registered with the iPLEDGE programme and, as in the United Kingdom, prescriptions are given 1 month at a time on receipt of a negative pregnancy test. Two separate effective forms of birth control must be used at the same time for at least 1 month before starting isotretinoin, throughout treatment and for 1 month after stopping it. Treatment should start on day 3 of the patient's next menstrual cycle following a negative pregnancy test.

Depression, sometimes leading to suicide, is a rare accompaniment of treatment although causality has yet to be confirmed in a large controlled study. Nevertheless, patients and their family doctors should be warned about the possible appearance or worsening of depression before starting a course of isotretinoin, and patients should be asked to sign a document that indicates that the issue of adverse psychiatric events has been discussed. A review of signs and symptoms of depression and suicidal ideation should be performed at every visit and the drug should be stopped immediately if there is any concern. This potentially severe accompaniment of isotretinoin treatment has to be balanced against its remarkable efficacy in severe acne. Isotretinoin has been available in Europe for the treatment acne since 1971 and the lives of most patients with conglobate acne have been transformed after successful treatment with isotretinoin.

Other side effects of isotretinoin include dry skin, dry and inflamed lips and eyes, nosebleeds, facial erythema, muscle aches, hyperlipidaemia and hair loss; these are reversible and often tolerable, especially if the acne is doing well. Rarer and potentially more serious side effects include changes in night-time vision, pseudotumor cerebri, pancreatitis, hepatotoxicity, blood dyscrasias, hyperostosis and hearing loss. Early review appointments (e.g. at 1 and 2 weeks into treatment) are comforting to both patient and doctor. A useful 'avoidance list' for patients taking isotretinoin is given in Table 12.1.

Physical treatment

Epidermabrasion with gritty soaps peel off more of the stratum corneum than they open comedones, may cause irritation and are not generally recommended.

Chemical peels are a useful adjunct to medical acne treatment. The comedolytic effects include decreasing corneocyte cohesion at the follicular opening and assisting in comedo plug extrusion. β-hydroxy acids (salicylic acid, β-lipohydroxy acid; LHA) are more efficacious

Table 12.1 Avoidance list for patients taking isotretinoin.

Avoid	Reason
Pregnancy	Teratogenicity
Breastfeeding	Unknown effect on baby
Giving blood	Teratogenicity in recipient
Uncontrolled hyperlipidaemia	Additive side effects
Taking vitamin A and hypervitaminosis A	Additive side effects
Cosmetic procedures	Increased scarring
Excessive natural or artificial UVR	Photosensitivity
Oral contraceptive with low dose of progesterone – 'minipills'	Ineffective contraception
Concomitant antibiotics, unless with permission of prescribing doctor	Intracranial hypertension

because of their lipophilicity, which preferentially target the lipid-filled sebaceous follicles.

For deep persistent comedones, extraction with an 18-gauge needle or No. 11 blade and a comedo extractor may aid in their rapid resolution. This can be used in conjunction with topical retinoids.

Cysts can be incised and drained with or without a local anaesthetic. Intralesional injections of 0.1 mL triamcinolone acetonide (2.5–10 mg/mL) hasten the resolution of stubborn cysts, but can leave atrophy.

Treatment with light and laser therapies

Light and laser treatments offer an alternative for patients who are refractory to traditional topical therapy, cannot tolerate side effects from systemic therapy, have concerns about antibiotic resistance or are adverse to prescription medication. Light and laser treatments reduce acne by photoactivation of porphyrins naturally produced by *P. acnes*, leading to reduction in the growth of *P. acnes*. These treatments have been shown to have short-term improvements over placebo in small trials, although more robust controlled trials comparing light with conventional treatments need to be carried out. The combination of red and blue light may provide some benefit in mild inflammatory acne. Current studies using intense pulsed light (IPL) have led to mixed results. Some studies suggest IPL may reduce

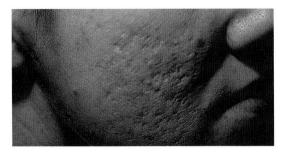

Figure 12.10 Acne scarring: worth treating a test area with a resurfacing laser.

both inflammatory and non-inflammatory lesions, while others have shown benefit in non-inflammatory lesions only. Pulsed dye 585 nm laser has been tried with some benefit, but there are no data on long-term outcomes. Photodynamic therapy may reduce acne lesion count, but results are no better than topical retinoids, and the side effects (redness, swelling, pain and exfoliation) may limit its use.

Acne scar treatment

Scarring caused by acne is often bothersome to patients but treatment can be challenging. Acne scarring can be classified based on colour and texture and treatment modalities including topical, surgical and laser therapy used to improve their appearance (Figure 12.10).

Colour

Erythema from dilated capillaries is not uncommon after inflammatory acne lesions. This generally resolves over time but pulsed dye laser (PDL, 585 or 595 nm) can safely reduce vascularity by targeting oxyhaemoglobin within red blood cells. IPL has also been shown to reduce erythema but must be used with caution in patients with darker skin types.

Post-inflammatory hyperpigmentation is particularly common after acne in darker skinned individuals. This often improves with time, but sun avoidance and the use of hydroquinone can help to speed resolution. Various lasers, including short pulse Q-switched lasers (ruby 694 nm, alexandrite 755 nm and Nd:YAG 1064 nm) are useful for treating skin pigmentation.

Texture

Elevated or hypertrophic scars can be treated with topical and intralesional corticosteroids. Recent studies have shown beneficial effects of fractionated ablative lasers

in softening elevated scars by ablating channels of condensed collagen that contribute to the scar's thickness.

Atrophic scars such as ice-pick and boxcar scars can be treated with surgical excision, dermabrasion, lasers and dermal fillers. Deeply bound rolled acne scars are best treated with surgical subcisions to loosen the tethering effect.

Dermabrasion helps to smooth out depressed scars by blending in the transition between the indentation and surrounding normal tissue. A high-speed rotating wire brush planes down to a bleeding dermis. Dermabrasion should not be carried out if there are any active lesions and does not help depressed 'ice-pick' scars, which may best be removed with a small punch. Unsightly hyperpigmentation may follow in darker skins. Microdermabrasion is well tolerated but its effects are usually transient.

Skin resurfacing with fractionated ablative lasers is rapidly replacing confluent ablative CO_2 and erbium resurfacing as the best treatment for post-acne scarring. The procedure, which should be delayed until the acne is quiescent, is usually performed under local anaesthesia. Unlike traditional confluent ablative laser, fractionated laser creates microscopic columns of thermal injury on the skin, causing skin tightening and collagen remodelling while reducing the amount of time for re-epithelization.

Collagen or hyaluronic acid dermal fillers can be injected into depressed scars to temporarily improve their appearance. Patients with a history of any autoimmune disorder are excluded from this treatment. Shallow atrophic lesions do better than discrete 'ice-pick' scars. The procedure is expensive and has to be repeated every 6 months as the filler is reabsorbed.

Rosacea

Rosacea affects the face of adults, usually women. Although its peak incidence is in the thirties and forties, it can also be seen in the young or old. Rosacea is more common in fair-skinned individuals. It may coexist with acne but is distinct from it.

Cause and histopathology

The cause is still unknown. Both genetic and environmental factors seem to have a role. Rosacea is often seen in those who flush easily in response to warmth, sunlight, spicy food, alcohol or embarrassment. Some authors have speculated that the persistent blood vessel dilatation compounded by chronic sun damage to the surrounding connective tissues may induce an inflammatory response,

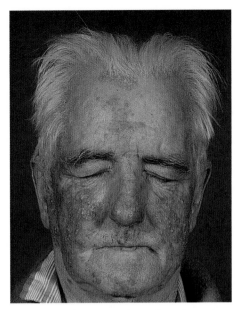

Figure 12.11 Typical rosacea with papules and pustules on a background of erythema. Note the patient also has a patch of scaly seborrhoeic eczema on his brow.

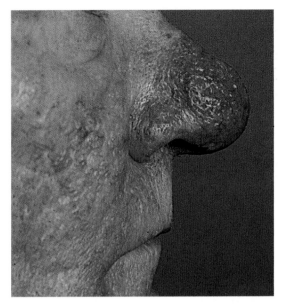

Figure 12.12 Marked rhinophyma.

setting off papules and pustules. Recent studies have shown rosacea patients express abnormally high levels of cathelicidin, an antimicrobial peptide, which promotes inflammation and vasodilatation. A pathogenic role for the hair follicle mite, *Demodex folliculorum*, or for *Helicobacter pylori* infection of the gastric mucosa has not been proved.

Clinical course and complications

The cheeks, nose, centre of forehead and chin are most commonly affected; the peri-orbital and peri-oral areas are spared (Figure 12.11). Intermittent flushing is followed by a fixed erythema and telangiectases. Discrete domed inflamed papules, papulo-pustules and, rarely, plaques or nodules develop. Rosacea, unlike acne, has no comedones or seborrhoea. It is usually symmetrical. Its course is prolonged, with exacerbations and remissions. Granulomatous rosacea is a variant of rosacea in which patients have persistent hard red–brown discrete papules and nodules. Some patients treated with potent topical steroids develop a rebound flare of pustules, worse than the original rosacea, when this treatment is stopped.

Rosacea is generally classified into four major subtypes. Many patients have only red skin or flushing and the disease does not necessarily progress.

1 Erythematotelangiectatic rosacea is characterized predominantly by its vascular features of flushing and fixed erythema, with or without telangiectasia.
2 Papulopustular rosacea consists of fixed erythema with inflammatory papules and/or pustules.
3 Phymatous rosacea, more common in males, is a result of overgrowth of sebaceous glands and connective tissue. It predominately affects the nose (rhinophyma) but can develop in extranasal sites such as the chin, forehead, cheeks or ears (Figure 12.12).
4 Ocular rosacea is frequently undiagnosed but quite common, with up to 50% of rosacea patients affected. Complications include blepharitis, conjunctivitis and, occasionally, keratitis.

Differential diagnosis

Acne has already been mentioned. Rosacea differs from it by its background of erythema and telangiectases, and by the absence of comedones. The distribution of the lesions is different too, as rosacea affects the central face but not the trunk. Also rosacea usually appears after adolescence. Sun-damaged skin with or without acne cosmetica causes most diagnostic difficulty. Remember, rosacea affects primarily the central, less mobile parts of the face, whereas sun damage and acne cosmetica are more generalized over the face. Seborrhoeic eczema, peri-oral dermatitis (Figure 12.13), systemic lupus erythematosus (p. 126) and

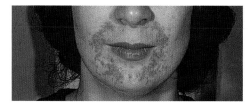

Figure 12.13 A peri-oral dermatitis following withdrawal of the potent topical steroid that had been wrongly used to treat seborrhoeic eczema.

photodermatitis should be considered, but do not show the papulo-pustules of rosacea. The flushing of rosacea can be confused with menopausal symptoms and, rarely, with the carcinoid syndrome. Superior vena caval obstruction has occasionally been mistaken for lymphoedematous rosacea.

Treatment

Treatment is best directed toward the subtype (Table 12.2). For papulo-pustular rosacea, tetracyclines, prescribed as for acne (p. 412), are the traditional treatment and are usually effective. Erythromycin is the antibiotic of second choice. Antiobiotics are used for their anti-inflammatory properties rather than antimicrobial effects. Courses should last for at least 10 weeks and,

Table 12.2 Overview of first-line treatments for rosacea based on subtype.

Erythromatotelangiectatic type	Topical metronidazole
	Topical azeleic acid
	Decrease flushing
	Cover-up makeup
	Colour-correcting gels (green)
	Pulsed dye laser and intense pulsed light
Papulospustular type	Combination of topical agent with oral antibiotic
	Topical metronidazole
	Topical azeleic acid
	Topical sulfacetamide/sulfur
	Oral tetracyclines
Phymatous type	Ablative lasers
	Electrosurgery
Ocular type	Oral doxycycline
	Artifical tears
	Lid cleansing

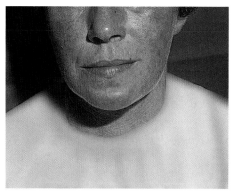

Figure 12.14 The result of the prolonged use of potent topical steroids for rosacea. Note the extreme telangiectasia.

after gaining control with 500–1000 mg/day, the dosage can be cut to 250 mg/day. The condition recurs in about half of the patients within 2 years, but repeated antibiotic courses, rather than prolonged maintenance ones, are generally recommended. To reduce the risk of bacterial resistance, some dermatologists have advocated the use of sub-antimicrobial dosage of doxycyclines (e.g. 40 mg extended release once daily). Topical 0.75% metronidazole gel (Formulary 1, p. 406), 15% azelaic acid, and sulfacetamide/sulfur lotions (United States only) applied sparingly once or twice daily, are nearly as effective as oral tetracycline and often prolong remission. They can be tried before systemic treatment and are especially useful in treating 'stuttering' recurrent lesions that do not then need repeated systemic courses of antibiotics. Rarely, systemic metronidazole or isotretinoin (p. 422) is needed for stubborn rosacea. Rosacea and topical steroids go badly together (Figure 12.14). Sunscreens help rosacea if sun exposure is an aggravating factor, but changes in diet or drinking habits are seldom of value. Erythematotelangiectatic rosacea responds well to treatment with vascular lasers or intense pulsed light sources. Measures to decrease flushing also help. Various techniques can be used to improve the appearance of disfiguring rhinophymas including surgical excision, electrocautery and either erbium or CO_2 laser ablation (Figure 27.19).

Learning point

Never put strong topical steroids on rosacea. If you do, red faces, skin addiction, rebound flares and a cross dermatologist will all figure in your nightmares.

Sweat glands

Eccrine sweat glands

There are 2–3 million sweat glands distributed all over the body surface but they are most numerous on the palms, soles and axillae. The tightly coiled glands lie deep in the dermis, and the emerging duct passes to the surface by penetrating the epidermis in a corkscrew fashion. Sweat is formed in the coiled gland by active secretion, involving the sodium pump. Some damage occurs to the membrane of the secretory cells during sweating. Initially, sweat is isotonic with plasma but, under normal conditions, it becomes hypotonic by the time it is discharged at the surface, after the tubular resorption of electrolytes and water under the influence of aldosterone and antidiuretic hormone.

In some ways the eccrine sweat duct is like a renal tubule. The pH of sweat is between 4.0 and 6.8; it contains sodium, potassium chloride, lactate, urea and ammonia. The concentration of sodium chloride in sweat is increased in cystic fibrosis, and sweat can be analysed when this is suspected.

Sweat glands have an important role in temperature control, the skin surface being cooled by evaporation. Up to 10 L/day of sweat can be excreted. Three stimuli induce sweating:

1 Thermal sweating is a reflex response to a raised environmental temperature and occurs all over the body, especially the chest, back, forehead, scalp and axillae.

2 Emotional sweating is provoked by fear or anxiety and is seen mainly on the palms, soles and axillae.

3 Gustatory sweating is provoked by hot spicy foods and affects the face.

The eccrine sweat glands are innervated by cholinergic fibres of the sympathetic nervous system. Sweating can therefore be induced by cholinergic, and blocked by anticholinergic drugs. Central control of sweating resides in the preoptic hypothalamic sweat centre.

Clinical disorders can follow increased or decreased sweating, or blockage of sweat gland ducts.

Generalized hyperhidrosis/thermal hyperhidrosis

The 'thermostat' for sweating lies in the preoptic area of the hypothalamus. Sweating follows any rise in body temperature, whether this is caused by exercise, environmental heat or an illness. The sweating in acute infections, and in some chronic illnesses (e.g. Hodgkin's disease), may be a result of a lowering of the 'set' of this thermostat.

Other causes of general hyperhidrosis

• Emotional stimuli, hypoglycaemia, opiate withdrawal and shock cause sweating by a direct or reflex stimulation of the sympathetic system at hypothalamic or higher centres. Sweating accompanied by a general sympathetic discharge occurs on a cold pale skin.

• Lesions of the central nervous system (e.g. a cerebral tumour or cerebrovascular accident) can cause generalized sweating, presumably by interfering directly with the hypothalamic centre.

• Phaeochromocytoma, the carcinoid syndrome, diabetes mellitus, thyrotoxicosis, Cushing's syndrome and the hot flushes of menopausal women have all been associated with general sweating. The mechanisms are not clear.

Local hyperhidrosis (Figure 12.15)

Local hyperhidrosis plagues many young adults. The most common areas to be affected are the palms, soles and axillae. Too much sweating there is embarrassing, if not socially crippling. A sodden shirt in contact with a dripping armpit, a wet handshake and stinking feet are hard crosses to bear. Seldom is any cause found, but organic disease, especially thyrotoxicosis, acromegaly, tuberculosis and Hodgkin's disease should be considered. A blatant anxiety state is occasionally present, but more often an otherwise normal person is understandably concerned about his or her antisocial condition. A vicious circle emerges, in which increased anxiety drives further sweating.

These problems may be no more than one end of the normal physiological range. How many students sitting examinations have to dry their hands before putting pen to paper? It is only when the sweating is gross, or

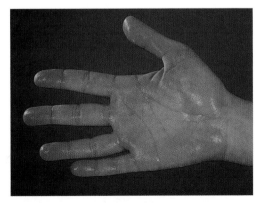

Figure 12.15 Severe palmar hyperhidrosis demanding treatment.

continuous, that medical advice is sought. Such sweating is often precipitated by emotional stimuli and stops during sleep.

Treatment

Topical applications. The first-line treatment for axillary hyperhidrosis is 20% aluminium chloride hexahydrate in an alcohol base (Formulary 1, p. 400). At first it is applied to the dry axillae every night and treated skin washed the following morning. Soon the interval can be increased, and many need the preparation only once or twice a week. The frequency may have to be cut down if the preparation irritates the skin, which is most likely if it is applied after shaving or when the skin is wet. Aluminium chloride also helps hyperhidrosis of the palms and soles, but it is less effective there.

Potassium permanganate soaks (1 : 10 000 aqueous solution) combat the bacterial superinfection of sweaty feet that is responsible for their foul smell. Patients should soak their feet for 15 minutes twice a day until the smell has improved and be warned that potassium permanganate stains the skin and everything else brown. Occasionally, glutaraldehyde solutions are used instead, but allergy and yellow-stained skin are potential complications. Topical clindamycin is also effective.

Iontophoresis. This is the passage of a low-voltage direct current across the skin. Iontophoresis with tap water or with the anticholinergic drug glycopyrronium bromide (glycopyrolate, United States) may help palmar or plantar hyperhidrosis (Formulary 1, p. 400). Patients attend two or three times a week for treatment until the condition improves. Repeated courses or maintenance therapy may be required.

Botulinum toxin. This binds to presynaptic nerve membranes and then inhibits the release of acetylcholine. It is now the treatment of choice for severe axillary or plantar hyperhidrosis, unresponsive to medical measures. Botulinum toxin is also effective for palmar hyperhidrosis but patients must be cautioned regarding the potential transient weakness to the intrinsic muscles of the hand. Subdermal aliquots of the toxin are injected into the hyperhidrotic area and sweating is abolished after a delay of 3–5 days. Repeat injections every 6–9 months are necessary as the sweating returns when the toxin has gone. Antibodies may form against the toxin and diminish its long-term effectiveness.

Systemic treatment. Oral anticholinergic agents such as propantheline bromide and glycopyrolate (United States) are sometimes tried. High doses are often required to control hyperhidrosis and their systemic side effects limit their value.

Surgery. This is used less nowadays as the above measures are usually effective. However, recalcitrant axillary hyperhidrosis can be treated by removing the vault of the axilla, which bears most of the sweat glands. These can be identified preoperatively by applying starch and iodine, which interact with sweat to colour the sweat gland openings blue. Thoracoscopic sympathetic trunkotomy (between the first and second thoracic ganglia) is effective for severe palmar hyperhidrosis alone but may cause compensatory hyperhidrosis and is considered a last resort.

Hypohidrosis and anhidrosis

Anhidrosis caused by abnormality of the sweat glands

Heat stroke. Caused by sweat gland exhaustion, this is a medical emergency seen most often in elderly people moving to a hot climate. It can also occur in the young, during or after prolonged exercise, especially in hot climates. Patients present with hyperthermia, dry skin, weakness, headache, cramps and confusion, leading to vomiting, hypotension, oliguria, metabolic acidosis, hyperkalaemia, delirium and death. They should be cooled down immediately with tepid water, and fluids and electrolytes must be replaced.

Hypohidrotic ectodermal dysplasia. This rare disorder is inherited as an X-linked recessive trait, in which the sweat glands are either absent or decreased. Affected boys have a characteristic facial appearance, with poor hair and teeth (Figure 13.13), and are intolerant of heat.

Prematurity. The sweat glands function poorly in premature babies nursed in incubators and hot nurseries.

Anhidrosis caused by abnormalities of the nervous system

Anhidrosis may follow abnormalities anywhere in the sympathetic system, from the hypothalamus to the peripheral nerves. It can therefore be a feature of multiple sclerosis, a cerebral tumour, trauma, Horner's syndrome or peripheral neuropathy (e.g. leprosy, alcoholic neuropathy and diabetes). Patients with widespread anhidrosis are heat-intolerant, developing nausea, dizziness, tachycardia and hyperthermia in hot surroundings.

Anhidrosis or hypohidrosis caused by skin disease

Local hypohidrosis has been reported in many skin diseases, especially those that scar (e.g. lupus erythematosus and morphoea). It may be a feature of Sjögren's syndrome, ichthyosis, psoriasis and miliaria profunda (see *Interference with sweat delivery*).

Interference with sweat delivery

Miliaria. This is the result of plugging or rupture of sweat ducts. It occurs in hot humid climates, at any age, and is common in over-clothed infants in hot nurseries. The physical signs depend on where the ducts are blocked.

Miliaria crystallina. This presents as tiny clear non-inflamed vesicles that look like dew. This is the most superficial type in which the location of obstruction is in the stratum corneum.

Miliaria rubra (prickly heat). Tiny erythematous and very itchy papules from obstruction of eccrine glands in the mid-epidermis.

Miliaria profunda. These consist of larger erythematous papules or pustules. This is the deepest type.

The best treatment is to move to a cooler climate or into air conditioning. Clothing that prevents the evaporation of sweat (e.g. nylon shirts) should be avoided; cotton is best. Claims have been made for ascorbic acid by mouth, but in our hands it rarely if ever helps. Salicylic acid 2% in isopropyl alcohol applied daily to prone areas has been advocated for prevention. Topical steroids reduce irritation but should only be used briefly. Calamine lotion cools and soothes.

Apocrine sweat glands

Apocrine glands are limited to the axillae, nipples, periumbilical area, perineum and genitalia. The coiled tubular glands (larger than eccrine glands) lie deep in the dermis, and during sweating the luminal part of their cells is lost (decapitation secretion). Apocrine sweat passes via the duct into the midportion of the hair follicle. The action of bacteria on apocrine sweat is responsible for body odour. The glands are innervated by adrenergic fibres of the sympathetic nervous system.

Hidradenitis suppurativa (apocrine acne)

This is a severe chronic suppurative disorder of the apocrine glands. Many papules, pustules, comedones, cysts, sinuses and scars occur in the axillae, groin and perianal areas. The condition may coexist with conglobate acne. Its cause is unknown, but an underlying follicular abnormality seems likely. In about one-third of cases there is a family history, and various mutations of the γ secretase gene complex have now been identified in some patients. Although probably not an immunodeficiency or a primary infection of the apocrine glands, *Staphylococcus aureus*, anaerobic streptococci and *Bacterioides* spp. are frequently present.

Treatment is unsatisfactory but should be as for acne vulgaris in the first instance. Obesity and cigarette smoking are associated with worse disease and weight loss and smoking cessation should be advised where relevant. Systemic antibiotics help early lesions to resolve but are ineffective for chronic draining abscesses and sinuses. Incision and drainage of abscesses, and injections of intralesional triamcinolone (5–10 mg/mL) may reduce the incidence of deforming scars and sinus formation. Topical clindamycin has been shown to prevent new lesions from forming. Infliximab has been used with success; just why it works is uncertain. Systemic antiandrogens help some women and oral retinoids may also help. Severe cases need plastic surgery to remove large areas of affected skin, but patients are often grateful for it, because the disease is painful, messy, unsightly, and smelly too.

Fox–Fordyce disease

This rare disease of the apocrine ducts is comparable to miliaria rubra of the eccrine duct. It occurs in women after puberty. Itchy skin-coloured or light brown papules appear in the axillae and other areas where apocrine glands are found, such as the breasts and vulva. Treatment is not usually necessary but removal of the affected skin, or electrodessication of the most irritable lesions, can be considered.

Learning point

Aluminium chloride hexahydrate 20% in an alcohol base has now taken over from anticholinergic drugs and surgery for most patients with sweaty armpits and hands. Be sure the skin is dry before it is applied – use a hairdryer if necessary. Botulium toxin is an effective treatment for patients who fail topical therapy.

Further reading

Collin J, Whatling P. (2000) Treating hyperhidrosis. *British Medical Journal* **320**, 1221–1222.

Dahl MV. (2001) Pathogenesis of rosacea. *Advances in Dermatology* **17**, 29–45.

James WD. (2005) Clinical practice. Acne. *New England Journal of Medicine* **352**, 1463–1472.

Kreyden OP, Böni R, Burg G. (2001) *Hyper-hidrosis and Botulinum Toxin in Dermatology.* Karger, Basel.

Mortimer PS, Lunniss PJ. (2000) Hidradenitis suppurativa. *Journal of the Royal Society of Medicine* **93**, 420–422.

Smith EV, Grindlay DJC, Williams HC. (2011) What's new in acne? An analysis of systematic reviews published in 2009–2010. *Clinical and Experimental Dermatology* **36**, 119–123.

Van Zuuren EJ, Kramer S, Carter B, Graber MA, Fedorowicz Z. (2011) Interventions for rosacea. *Cochrane Database Systematic Reviews* **3**, CD003262.

Wilkin J, Dahl MV, Detmar M, *et al.* (2002) Standard classification of rosacea: Report of the National Rosacea Society Expert Committee on the Classification and Staging of Rosacea. *Journal of the American Academy of Dermatology* **46**, 584–587.

13 Regional Dermatology

The hair

Hair is human plumage: we need just the right amount, in the right places. The twin torments of having too much or too little hair can be understood only when seen against the background of the formation and activity of normal hair follicles.

Hair follicles form before the ninth week of fetal life when the hair germ, a solid cylinder of cells, grows obliquely down into the dermis. Here it is met by a cluster of mesenchymal cells (the placode) bulging into the lower part of the hair germ to form the hair papilla. Eventually, the papilla contains blood vessels bringing nutrients to the hair matrix. The sebaceous gland is an outgrowth at the side of the hair germ, establishing early the two parts of the pilosebaceous unit. The hair matrix, the germinative part of the follicle, is equivalent to the basal cells of the epidermis. Adjacent to the sebaceous gland is the region of insertion of the arrector pili muscle called the bulge. This area contains hair follicle stem cells which presumably can regenerate the entire hair follicle and sebaceous gland. Damage to this area will cause permanent hair loss.

Melanocytes migrate into the matrix and are responsible for the different colours of hair (eumelanin, brown and black; phaeomelanin and trichochromes, red). Grey or white hair is caused by low pigment production, and the filling of the cells in the hair medulla with minute air bubbles that reflect light.

The structure of a typical hair follicle is shown in Figure 13.1.

Classification

Hairs are classified into three main types.

1 *Lanugo hairs*: fine long hairs covering the fetus, but shed about 1 month before birth.

2 *Vellus hairs*: fine short unmedullated hairs covering much of the body surface. They replace the lanugo hairs just before birth.

3 *Terminal hairs*: long coarse medullated hairs seen, for example, in the scalp or pubic regions. Their growth is often influenced by circulating androgen levels.

Terminal hairs convert to vellus hairs in male-pattern alopecia, and vellus to terminal hairs in hirsutism. The lips, glans penis, labia minora, palms and soles remain free of hair follicles.

The hair cycle

Each follicle passes, independently of its neighbours, through regular cycles of growth and shedding. There are three phases of follicular activity (Figure 13.2).

1 *Anagen*: the active phase of hair production.

2 *Catagen*: a short phase of conversion from active growth to the resting phase. Growth stops, and the end of the hair becomes club-shaped.

3 *Telogen*: a resting phase at the end of which the club hair is shed.

The duration of each of these stages varies from region to region. On the scalp (Figure 13.3), said to contain an average of 100 000 hairs, anagen lasts for up to 5 years, catagen for about 2 weeks and telogen for about 3 months. As many as 100 hairs may be shed from the normal scalp every day as a normal consequence of cycling. The proportion of hairs in the growing and resting stages can be estimated by looking at plucked hairs (a trichogram). On the scalp, about 85% are normally in anagen and 15% in the telogen phase. The length of hair is determined by the duration of anagen (e.g. the hairs of the eyebrows have shorter cycles than those of the scalp).

Each hair follicle goes through its growth cycles out of phase with its neighbours, so there is no moulting period. However, if many pass into the resting phase (telogen) at the same time, then a correspondingly large number will be shed 2–3 months later (see *Telogen effluvium*).

There are important racial differences in hair (see Chapter 14). Asians tend to have straight hair, Negroids woolly hair and Europeans wavy hair. These differences

Clinical Dermatology, Fifth Edition. Richard B. Weller, Hamish J.A. Hunter and Margaret W. Mann.
© 2015 John Wiley & Sons, Ltd. Published 2015 by John Wiley & Sons, Ltd.

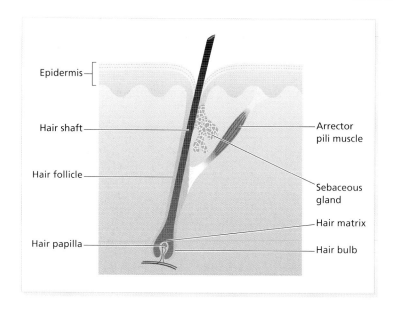

Figure 13.1 Anatomy of the hair follicle.

are associated with different cross-sectional shapes (round, flattened, etc.). Asians have less facial and body hair than Mediterranean people who also have more hair than northern Europeans.

Alopecia

The term means loss of hair and alopecia has many causes and patterns. One convenient division is into localized and diffuse types. It is also important to decide whether or not the hair follicles have been replaced by scar tissue; if they have, regrowth cannot occur. The presence of any disease of the skin itself should also be noted.

Localized alopecia

Some of the most common types are listed in Table 13.1; only a few are dealt with in detail.

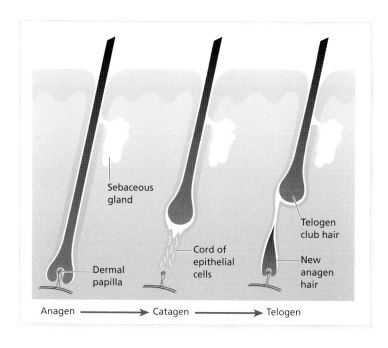

Figure 13.2 The hair cycle.

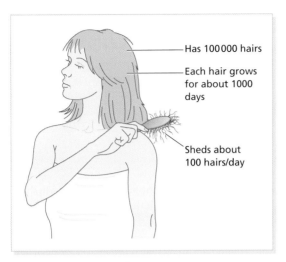

Figure 13.3 An average scalp.

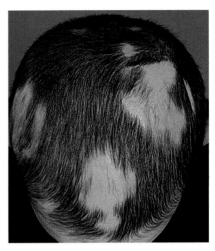

Figure 13.4 The characteristic uninflamed patches of alopecia areata.

Alopecia areata

The lifetime risk of getting alopecia areata is about 2% and, by a coincidence, it is the reason for about 2% of consultations in our skin clinics.

Cause

An immunological basis is suspected because of an association with autoimmune diseases such as Hashimoto's thyroiditis, atopy, vitiligo, inflammatory bowel disease and autoimmune polyendocrinopathy syndrome. Histologically, T lymphocytes cluster like a swarm of bees around affected hair bulbs, having been attracted and made to divide by cytokines from the dermal papilla.

Table 13.1 Causes of localized alopecia.

Non-scarring	Scarring
Alopecia areata	Burns, radiodermatitis
Androgenetic	Aplasia cutis
Scalp ringworm (human)	Kerion
Hair-pulling habit	Carbuncle
Traction alopecia	Cicatricial basal cell carcinoma
	Lichen planus
	Lupus erythematosus
	Necrobiosis
	Sarcoidosis
	Central centrifugal cicatricial alopecia

Alopecia areata is probably inherited as a complex genetic trait, sometimes HLA-DQ3, -DR11 or -DR4 act as susceptibility factors, with an increased occurrence in the first-degree relatives of affected subjects and twin concordance. It affects some 10% of patients with Down's syndrome – suggesting the involvement of genes on chromosome 21. Environmental factors may trigger alopecia areata in the genetically predisposed.

Presentation

A typical patch is uninflamed, with no scaling, but with empty hair follicles (Figure 13.4). Pathognomonic 'exclamation-mark' hairs may be seen around the edge of enlarging areas. They are broken off about 4 mm from the scalp, with the proximal end more narrowed and less pigmented (Figures 13.5 and 13.6). Patches are most common in the scalp and beard but other areas, especially the eyelashes and eyebrows, can be affected too. An uncommon diffuse pattern is recognized, with exclamation-mark hairs scattered widely over a diffusely thinned scalp. Up to 50% of patients show fine pitting or wrinkling of the nails.

Course

The outcome is unpredictable. In a first attack, regrowth is usual within a few months. New hairs appear in the centre of patches as fine pale down, and gradually regain their normal thickness and colour, although the new hair may remain white in older patients. Fifty percent of cases resolve spontaneously without treatment in

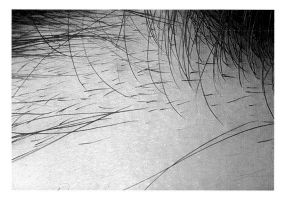

Figure 13.5 Exclamation-mark hairs: pathognomonic of alopecia areata.

1 year, and only 10% go on to develop severe chronic disease. Subsequent episodes tend to be more extensive and regrowth is slower. Hair loss in some areas may coexist with regrowth in others. A few of those patients who go on to have chronic disease lose all the hair from their heads (alopecia totalis) or from the whole skin surface (alopecia universalis).

Regrowth is tiresomely erratic but the following suggest a poor prognosis.

1 Onset before puberty.

2 Association with atopy or Down's syndrome.

3 Unusually widespread alopecia.

4 Involvement of the scalp margin (ophiasiform type), especially at the nape of the neck.

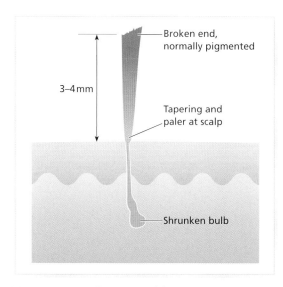

Figure 13.6   An exclamation-mark hair.

Differential diagnosis

Patches are not scaly, in contrast to ringworm, and are usually uninflamed, in contrast to lupus erythematosus and lichen planus. In the hair-pulling habit of children, and in traction alopecia, broken hairs may be seen but true exclamation-mark hairs are absent. Secondary syphilis can also cause a 'moth-eaten' patchy hair loss. A form of scarring alopecia, pseudopelade (see *Scarring alopecia*), can look similar.

Investigations

None are usually needed. The histology of bald skin shows lymphocytes around and in the hair matrix. Syphilis can be excluded with serological tests if necessary. Organ-specific autoantibody screens provide interesting information but do not affect management.

Treatment

A patient with a first or minor attack can be reassured about the prospects for regrowth. Topical corticosteroid creams of high potency can be prescribed, but it is difficult to tell whether the regrowth is spontaneous or results from the use of creams. The use of systemic steroids should be avoided in most cases, but the intradermal injection of 0.2 mL intralesional triamcinolone acetonide (5–10 mg/mL), raising a small bleb within an affected patch, leads to localized tufts of regrowth (Figure 13.7). While not affecting the overall outcome, this may be useful to re-establish eyebrows or to stimulate hope. It works so reliably that some patients come regularly for reinjections into eyebrows or small areas of the scalp. The downside of this treatment is dermal atrophy evident as depressed areas at the sites of injections.

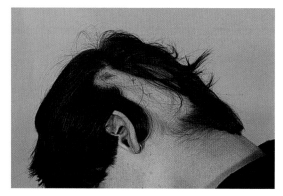

Figure 13.7   Regrowth within a patch of alopecia areata after a triamcinolone injection.

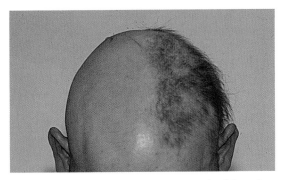

Figure 13.8 A trial of diphencyprone to one side of the scalp caused some regrowth.

Mild irritants, such as 0.1–0.25% dithranol, have been used but with limited success. Ultraviolet radiation or even psoralen with ultraviolet A (PUVA) therapy may help extensive cases, but hair fall often returns when treatment stops. Topical immunotherapy with contact sensitizers (e.g. diphencyprone and squaric acid dibutyl ester) is another promising treatment for patients with extensive disease (Figure 13.8). The efficacy of topical immunosuppressive agents (e.g. tacrolimus) has yet to be proved. Extensive cases should be directed to support groups and given information on wigs and cosmetics.

Androgenetic alopecia (male and female-pattern hair loss)

Cause

Although clearly familial, the exact mode of inheritance has not yet been clarified. The idea of a single autosomal dominant gene, with reduced penetrance in women, now seems less likely than a polygenic type of inheritance. Men seem to have a stronger family history of the disorder than females with pattern hair loss.

Androgen hormones are clearly implicated in the pathogenesis; in particular, androgenetic alopecia is linked to high levels of dihyrotestosterone (DHT) levels. Testosterone is converted to DHT by the enzyme 5α-reductase. DHT is responsible for temporal scalp hair recession, terminal hair growth in the beard, external ears, nostrils and limbs, and acne, In female-pattern hair loss, there may be an increased sensitivity to circulating androgen, as androgen levels are usually within normal limits.

Presentation

The common pattern in men (Figure 13.9) is the loss of hair first from the temples, and then from the crown.

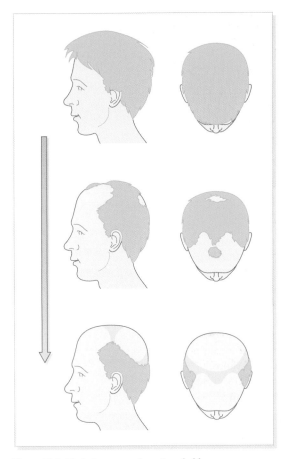

Figure 13.9 Variations on male-pattern baldness.

However, in women the hair loss may be much more diffuse (Figure 13.10), particularly over the crown. In bald areas, terminal hairs are replaced by finer vellus ones.

Clinical course

Hair loss is relentless, tending to follow the family pattern with some losing hair quickly and others more slowly. The diffuse pattern seen in women tends to progress slowly.

Complications

Even minor hair loss may lead to great anxiety and rarely to a monosymptomatic hypochondriasis (p. 336). Bald scalps burn easily in the sun, and may develop multiple actinic keratoses. It has been suggested recently that bald men are more likely to have a heart attack and prostate cancer than those with a full head of hair.

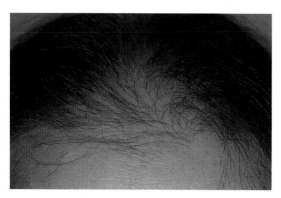

Figure 13.10 Androgenetic alopecia beginning in the frontal area.

Differential diagnosis

The diagnosis is usually obvious in men, but other causes of diffuse hair loss have to be considered in women (Table 13.2).

Investigations

None are usually needed. In women virilization may have to be excluded.

Treatment

Scalp surgery, hair transplants and wigs are welcomed by some. Topical application of minoxidil lotion may slow early hair loss and even stimulate new growth of hair but

---

Table 13.2 Causes of diffuse hair loss.

Telogen effluvium
Endocrine
   hypopituitarism
   hypo- or hyperthyroidism
   hypoparathyroidism
   high androgenic states
Drug-induced
   antimitotic agents (anagen effluvium)
   retinoids
   anticoagulants
   vitamin A excess
   oral contraceptives
Androgenetic
Iron deficiency
Severe chronic illness
Malnutrition
Diffuse type of alopecia areata

---

the results are not dramatic (Formulary 1, p. 409). Small and recently acquired patches respond best. When minoxidil treatment stops, the new hairs fall out after about 3 months. Some women with diffuse type of androgenetic alopecia may benefit from suppressing ovarian androgen production with oral contraceptives or an antiandrogen such as spironolactone.

Finasteride (Propecia, Formulary 2, p. 417), an inhibitor of human type II 5α-reductase, reduces serum and scalp skin levels of DHT in balding men. At the dosage of 1 mg/day, it may increase hair counts and so lead to a noticeable improvement in both frontal and vertex hair thinning. However, the beneficial effects slowly reverse once treatment has stopped. This treatment is not indicated in women or children. Side effects are rare, but include decreased libido, erectile dysfunction and altered prostate-specific antigen levels.

Trichotillomania

This is dealt with on p. 339.

Traction alopecia

Cause

Hair can be pulled out by several procedures intended to beautify, including hot-combing to straighten kinky hair, tight hairstyles such as a pony tail or 'corn rows', and using hair rollers too often or too tightly.

Presentation

The changes are usually seen in girls and young women, particularly those whose hair has always tended to be thin anyway. The pattern of hair loss is determined by the cosmetic procedure in use, hair being lost where there is maximal tug. The term *marginal alopecia* is applied to one common pattern in which hair loss is mainly around the edge of the scalp – at the sides or at the front (Figure 13.11). The bald areas show short broken hairs, folliculitis and, sometimes, scarring.

Clinical course

Patients are often slow to accept that they are responsible for the hair loss, and notoriously slow to alter their cosmetic practices. Even if they do, regrowth is often disappointingly incomplete.

Differential diagnosis

The pattern of hair loss provides the main clue to the diagnosis and, if the possibility of traction alopecia is kept in mind, there is usually no difficulty. The absence

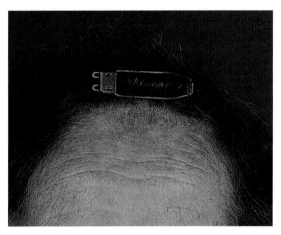

Figure 13.11 Traction alopecia. The rollers she thought would help to disguise her thin hair actually made it worse.

of exclamation-mark hairs distinguishes it from alopecia areata, and of scaling from tinea capitis.

Treatment
Patients have to stop doing whatever is causing their hair loss. Rollers that tug can be replaced by those that only heat.

Patchy hair loss caused by skin disease

Tinea capitis
Inflammation, often with pustulation, occurs mostly after infection with fungi from animals or soil, and the resultant scarring can be severe. The classic scalp ringworm derived from other human beings causes areas of scaling with broken hairs. The subject is covered in more detail on p. 240.

Psoriasis
The rough removal of adherent scales can also remove hairs, but regrowth is the rule.

Scarring alopecia
Hair follicles can be damaged in many ways. If the follicular openings can no longer be seen with a lens, regrowth of hair cannot be expected. In most cases, there is permanent damage to the follicular stem cell region, or the bulge.

Sometimes the cause is obvious: a severe burn, trauma, a carbuncle or an episode of inflammatory scalp ringworm. Discoid lupus erythematosus (p. 129), lichen planus (p. 69) and morphoea (p. 135) can also lead to scarring alopecia. The term *pseudopelade* is applied to a slowly progressive non-inflamed type of scarring which leads to irregular areas of hair loss without any apparent preceding skin disease. If inflammation is present, a biopsy may help to establish the diagnosis. Some cases of long-standing non-scarring alopecia (such as traction alopecia and alopecia areata) can convert to permanent hair loss after decades of involvement.

Central centrifugal cicatricial alopecia

Cause
Central centrifugal cicatricial alopecia (CCCA) is characterized by hair loss with scarring over the vertex of the scalp. The condition is known by many different names in the past, including hot comb alopecia, pseudopelade, follicular degeneration syndrome, and follicular decalvans. While the pathogenesis is multifactorial, hair styling practices including chemical hair relaxer and hot comb use, have been reported in a majority of all female patients presenting with CCCA. However, discontinuation of hair styling practices do not often result in resolution of the disease. Genetically, the curly African hair may be more prone to breakage by these styling methods.

Presentation
CCCA is the most common form of scarring alopecia among black women, often presenting in the third decade of life. Beginning at the vertex of the scalp, the disease gradually spread centrifugally, causing permanent loss of the hair follicles. Pruritus, tenderness and polytrichia (tufted hairs) are common findings. Some patients may note pustules and crusting.

Clinical course
This is chronic and progressive.

Differential diagnosis
Other causes of scarring alopecia affecting the vertex of the scalp (see *Scarring alopecia*) can mimic CCCA. Patients with female pattern hair loss have visible follicular openings. Lichen planopilaris shows characteristic perifollicular erythema and follicular keratosis.

Treatment
As permanent hair loss cannot be reversed, treatment is focused on halting the progression of the disease. Topical and intralesional corticosteroids are often used in combination with oral antibiotics such as doxycycline for their anti-inflammatory properties. Patients should be encouraged to stop damaging hair styling practices.

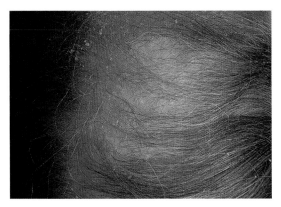

Figure 13.12 Diffuse hair loss causing much anxiety.

Diffuse hair loss

Hair is lost evenly from the whole scalp; this may, or may not, be accompanied by a thinning visible to others (Figure 13.12). Some of the most common causes are listed in Table 13.2, but often a simple explanation cannot be found.

Telogen effluvium

Cause

Telogen effluvium can be triggered by any severe illness, particularly those with bouts of fever or haemorrhage, by childbirth and by severe dieting. All of these synchronize catagen so that, later on, large numbers of hairs are lost at the same time in the telogen phase.

Presentation and course

The diffuse hair fall, 2–3 months after the provoking illness, can be mild or severe. In the latter case Beau's lines (p. 185) may be seen on the nails. Regrowth, not always complete, usually occurs within a few months.

Differential diagnosis

This is from other types of diffuse hair loss (Table 13.2). In androgenetic alopecia in females the onset is gradual in mid adulthood, and hairs remain rather firmly anchored to the scalp. In telogen effluvium the onset is abrupt and follows acute illness, an operation or pregnancy by 1–2 months. Hair fall is prominent and lightly pulling on scalp hairs dislodge many. In diffuse alopecia areata, the hair loss is more patchy, and the onset abrupt with waxing and waning. Shedding may be prominent. Exclamation-mark hairs are often present.

Treatment

This condition is unaffected by therapy, but patients can be reassured that their hair loss will be temporary.

Other causes of diffuse hair loss

The causes mentioned in Table 13.2 should be considered. If no cause is obvious, it is worth checking the haemoglobin, erythrocyte sedimentation rate (ESR), antinuclear antibody, serum iron, ferritin, thyroxine and thyroid-stimulating hormone (TSH) levels. Also consider checking the serum free testosterone and dihydroepiandrosterone sulfate levels in women with menstrual irregularities or hirsutism. Despite these, often no cause for diffuse alopecia can be found.

Rare genetic causes of hypotrichosis

More than 300 genetic conditions exist that have hair abnormalities as one component. The *hypohidrotic ectodermal dysplasias* are a group of rare inherited disorders characterized by sparse hair, scanty sweat glands and poor development of the nails and teeth (Figure 13.13). Heat stroke may follow inadequate sweat production. One type is inherited as an X-linked recessive. The responsible gene for this type (on chromosome Xq12) has recently been shown to encode for a protein (ectodysplasin) involved in the regulation of ectodermal appendage formation. The genes responsible for the dominant or recessive types encode for the ectodysplasin receptor.

In other inherited disorders the hair may be beaded and brittle (*monilethrix*), flattened and twisted (*pili torti*), kinky (*Menkes' syndrome* caused by mutations in a gene encoding for a copper transporting membrane protein), like bamboo (*Netherton's syndrome*, caused by a gene on chromosome 5q32 encoding a serine protease inhibitor),

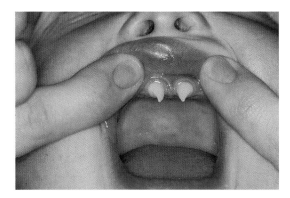

Figure 13.13 The cone-shaped incisors of hypohidrotic ectodermal dysplasia.

partly broken in many places (*trichorrhexis nodosa*) or 'woolly' or 'uncombable'.

Hirsutism and hypertrichosis

Hirsutism is the growth of terminal hair in a woman (Figure 13.14), which is distributed in the pattern normally seen in a man. Hypertrichosis is an excessive growth of terminal hair that does not follow an androgen-induced pattern (Figure 13.15).

Hirsutism

Cause

Some degree of hirsutism may be a racial or familial trait, and minor facial hirsutism is common after the menopause. In addition, some patients without a family background of hirsutism become hirsute in the absence of any demonstrable hormonal cause (idiopathic hirsutism). Some patients with hirsutism will have one of the disorders shown in Figure 13.16, most commonly the polycystic ovarian syndrome.

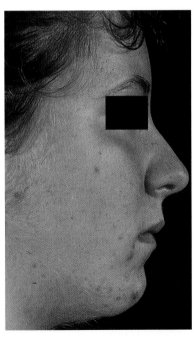

Figure 13.14 Moderate hirsutism caused by polycystic ovaries.

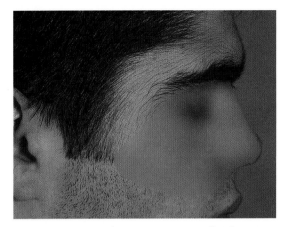

Figure 13.15 Hypertrichosis in a young man of Mediterranean extraction.

Presentation

An excessive growth of hair appears in the beard area, on the chest and shoulder-tips, around the nipples and in the male pattern of pubic hair. Androgenetic alopecia may complete the picture.

Course

Familial, racial or idiopathic hirsutism tends to start at puberty and to worsen with age.

Complications

Virilization causes infertility; psychological disturbances are common.

Investigations

Significant hormonal abnormalities are not usually found in patients with a normal menstrual cycle.

Investigations are needed:

- If hirsutism occurs in childhood;
- If there are other features of virilization, such as clitoromegaly;
- If the hirsutism is of sudden or recent onset; or
- If there is menstrual irregularity or cessation.

Measurement of the serum testosterone, sex hormone binding globulin, dehydroepiandrosterone sulfate, androstenedione and prolactin will help determine the source of excess androgen (i.e. adrenal cortex, ovaries, pituitary). Ovarian ultrasound is useful if polycystic ovaries are suspected.

Treatment (Figure 13.16)

Any underlying disorder must be treated on its merits. Home remedies for minor hirsutism include

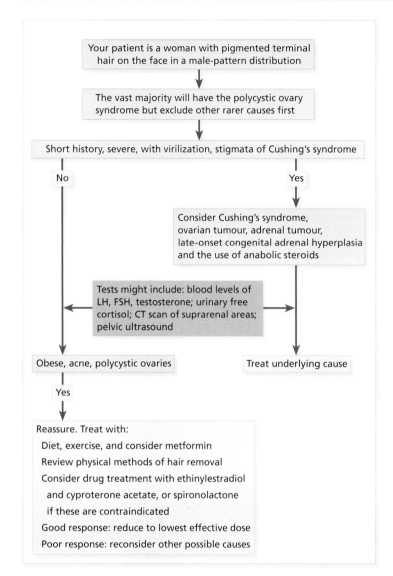

Figure 13.16 An approach to hirsutism. CT, computed tomography; FSH, follicle stimulating hormone; LH, luteinizing hormone.

commercial depilatory creams (often containing a thioglycollate; p. 401), waxing or shaving, or making the appearance less obvious by bleaching; none remove the hair permanently. Plucking should probably be avoided as it can stimulate hair roots into anagen. The abnormally active follicles, if relatively few, can be destroyed by electrolysis. If the hairs are too numerous for this, the excess can be removed by laser (p. 383). Topical therapy with eflornithine, an inhibitor of ornithine decarboxylase, can slow regrowth. Oral antiandrogens (e.g. cyproterone acetate; Dianette, or spironolactone; Formulary 2, p. 417) may sometimes be helpful, but will be needed long-term.

Pregnancy must be avoided during such treatment as it carries the risk of feminizing a male fetus.

Hypertrichosis

The localized type is most commonly seen over melanocytic naevi including Becker's naevi (Figure 13.17). It can also affect the sacral area – as a 'satyr's tuft' – in some patients with spina bifida. Excessive amounts of hair may grow near chronically inflamed joints or under plaster casts. Repeated shaving does not bring on hypertrichosis although occupational pressure may do so (e.g. from carrying weights on the shoulder).

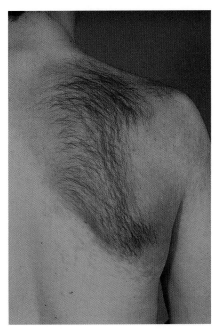

Figure 13.17 A typical Becker's naevus with marked localized hypertrichosis within a patch of hyperpigmentation.

Generalized hypertrichosis is much less common. Some causes are listed in Table 13.3.

Hair cosmetics

Hair can be made more attractive by dyeing, bleaching and waving, but there is often a price to be paid for beauty. Some hair dyes based on paraphenylenediamine are allergens (p. 85). Bleaches can weaken the hair shafts.

Permanent waving solutions reduce disulfide bonds within hair keratin and so allow the hair to be deformed

Table 13.3 Causes of generalized hypertrichosis.

Malnutrition: anorexia nervosa, starvation
Drug-induced (minoxidil, diazoxide, ciclosporin, phenytoin)
Cutaneous porphyrias (p. 316)
Fetal alcohol and fetal phenytoin syndromes
Hypertrichosis lanuginosa (both congenital type and acquired types are very rare – the latter signals an internal malignancy)
Some rare syndromes, for example Cornelia de Lange syndrome (hypertrichosis, microcephaly and mental deficiency) and Hurler's syndrome

before being reset in a new position. The thioglycollates in use to dissolve disulfide bonds are also popular as chemical hair removers. If used incorrectly, either too strong or for too long, or on hair already damaged by excessive bleaching or waving, thioglycollate waving lotions can cause hairs to break off flush with the scalp. This hair loss, which can be severe although temporary, may be accompanied by an irritant dermatitis of the scalp.

> **Learning points**
>
> 1 Full endocrinological assessment is needed for hirsutism plus virilization.
> 2 Significant hormonal abnormalities are rarely found in patients with a normal menstrual cycle.

The nails

The structure of the nail and nail bed is shown in Figure 13.18. The hard keratin of the nail plate is formed in the nail matrix, which lies in an invagination of the epidermis (the nail fold) on the back of the terminal phalanx of each digit. The matrix runs from the proximal end

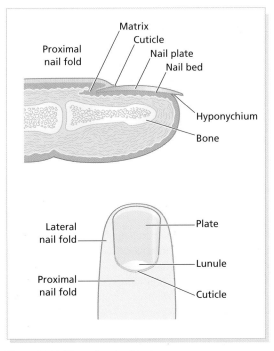

Figure 13.18 The nail and nail bed.

of the floor of the nail fold to the distal margin of the lunule. From this area the nail plate grows forward over the nail bed, ending in a free margin at the tip of the digit. Longitudinal ridges and grooves on the under surface of the nail plate dovetail with similar ones on the upper surface of the nail bed. The nail bed is capable of producing small amounts of keratin which contribute to the nail and which are responsible for the 'false nail' formed when the nail matrix is obliterated by surgery or injury. The cuticle acts as a seal to protect the potential space of the nail fold from chemicals and from infection. The nails provide strength and protection for the terminal phalanx. Their presence helps with fine touch and with the handling of small objects.

The rate at which nails grow varies from person to person: fingernails average 0.5–1.2 mm/week, while toenails grow more slowly. Nails grow faster in the summer, if they are bitten and in youth. They change with ageing from the thin, occasionally spooned, nails of early childhood to the duller, paler and more opaque nails of the very old. Longitudinal ridging and beading are particularly common in the elderly.

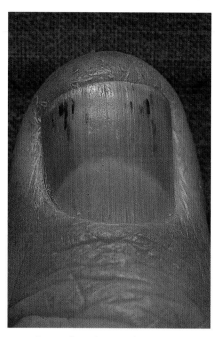

Figure 13.19 Gross splinter haemorrhages caused by trauma.

Effects of trauma

Permanent ridges or splits in the nail plate can follow damage to the nail matrix. Splinter haemorrhages (Figure 13.19), the linear nature of which is determined by longitudinal ridges and grooves in the nail bed, are most commonly seen under the nails of manual workers and are caused by minor trauma. They may also be a feature of psoriasis of the nail and of subacute bacterial endocarditis. Larger subungual haematomas (Figure 13.20) are usually easy to identify but the trauma that caused them may have escaped notice and dark areas of altered blood can raise worries about the presence of a subungual melanoma.

Chronic trauma from sport and from ill-fitting shoes contributes to haemorrhage under the nails of the big toes, to the gross thickening of toenails known as *onychogryphosis* (Figure 13.21) and to ingrowing nails. *Onycholysis*, a separation of the nail plate from the nail bed (Figure 13.22), may be a result of minor trauma although it is also seen in nail psoriasis (see Figure 5.8), phototoxic reactions, repeated immersion in water, after the use of nail hardeners and possibly in thyroid disease. Usually, no cause for it is found. The space created may be colonized by yeasts, or by bacteria such as *Pseudomonas aeruginosa*, which turns it an ugly green colour.

Some nervous habits damage the nails. Bitten nails are short and irregular; some people also bite their cuticles

and the skin around the nails. Viral warts can be seeded rapidly in this way. In the common habit tic nail dystrophy, the cuticle of the thumbnail is the target for picking or rubbing. This repetitive trauma causes a ladder pattern of transverse ridges and grooves to run up the centre of the nail plate called median nail dystrophy (Figure 13.22).

Lamellar splitting (*onychoschizia*) of the distal part of the fingernails, so commonly seen in housewives, has been attributed to repeated wetting and drying (Figure 13.22).

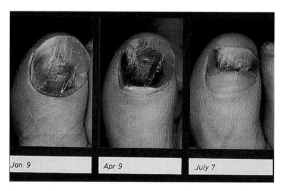

Figure 13.20 A subungual haematoma of the big toe. Although there was no history of trauma we were happy to watch this grow out over 6 months as the appearance was sudden, the colour was right and the nail folds showed no pigment.

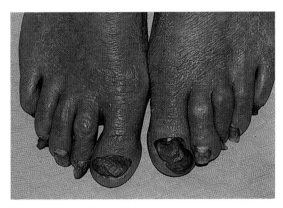

Figure 13.21 Onychogryphosis.

Attempts to beautify nails can lead to contact allergy. Culprits include the acrylate adhesive used with artificial nails and formaldehyde in nail hardeners. In contrast, contact dermatitis caused by allergens in nail polish itself seldom affects the fingers but presents as small itchy eczematous areas where the nail plates rest against the skin during sleep. The eyelids, face and neck are favourite sites.

The nail in systemic disease

The nails can provide useful clues for general physicians.

Clubbing (Figure 13.23) is a bulbous enlargement of the terminal phalanx with an increase in the angle between the nail plate and the proximal fold to over 180° (Figure 13.24). Its association with chronic lung disease and with cyanotic heart disease is well known. Rarely, clubbing may be familial with no underlying cause. The mechanisms involved in its formation are still not known.

Koilonychia, a spooning and thinning of the nail plate, can be physiologic in children. In adults, it indicates iron deficiency (Figure 13.25).

Colour changes: the 'half-and-half' nail, with a white proximal and red or brown distal half, is seen in a minority of patients with chronic renal failure. Whitening of the nail plates (Terry and Muehrcke nails) may be related to hypoalbuminaemia, as in cirrhosis of the liver. In *yellow*

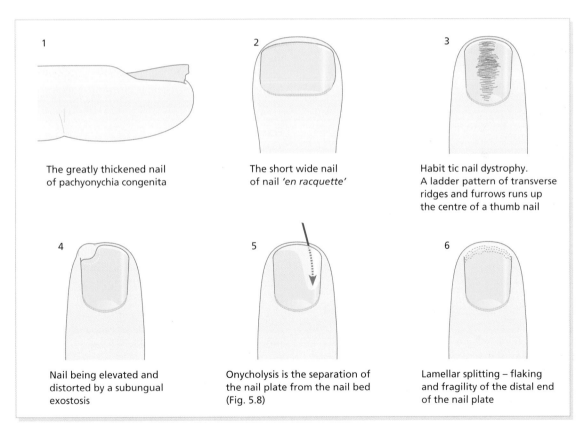

1. The greatly thickened nail of pachyonychia congenita

2. The short wide nail of nail *'en racquette'*

3. Habit tic nail dystrophy. A ladder pattern of transverse ridges and furrows runs up the centre of a thumb nail

4. Nail being elevated and distorted by a subungual exostosis

5. Onycholysis is the separation of the nail plate from the nail bed (Fig. 5.8)

6. Lamellar splitting – flaking and fragility of the distal end of the nail plate

Figure 13.22 Nail plate abnormalities.

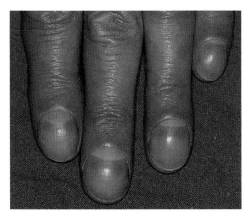

Figure 13.23 In this case severe clubbing was accompanied by hypertrophic pulmonary osteoarthropathy.

nail syndrome (Figure 13.26) the nail changes begin in adult life, against a background of hypoplasia of the lymphatic system. Peripheral lymphoedema is usually present and pleural effusions may occur. All 20 nails grow very slowly and become thickened and greenish-yellow; their surface is smooth but they are over-curved from side to side. Some drugs, notably antimalarials, antibiotics and phenothiazines, can discolour the nails.

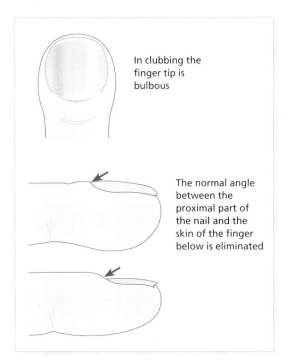

In clubbing the finger tip is bulbous

The normal angle between the proximal part of the nail and the skin of the finger below is eliminated

Figure 13.24 Clubbing.

Beau's lines are transverse grooves which appear synchronously on all nails a few weeks after an acute illness, and which grow steadily out to the free margin (Figure 13.25). These depressions in the nail plate results from a temporary halt in the growth of the nail matrix.

Connective tissue disorders: nail fold telangiectasia or erythema is a useful physical sign in dermatomyositis, systemic sclerosis and systemic lupus erythematosus (Figure 13.27). In dermatomyositis the cuticles become shaggy, and in systemic sclerosis loss of finger pulp leads to overcurvature of the nail plates. Thin nails, with longitudinal ridging and sometimes partial onycholysis, are seen when the peripheral circulation is impaired, as in Raynaud's phenomenon.

Nail changes in the common dermatoses

Psoriasis
Most patients with psoriasis have nail changes at some stage; severe nail involvement is more likely in the presence of arthritis. The best-known nail change is pitting of the surface of the nail plate (see Figure 5.7). Almost as common is psoriasis under the nail plate, showing up as red or brown areas resembling oil spots, often with onycholysis bordered by obvious discoloration (see Figure 5.8). These findings are most often found in the fingernails. Psoriasis in the toenails can be indistinguishable from onychomycosis. There is no effective topical treatment for psoriasis of the nails.

Eczema
Some patients with itchy chronic eczema bring their nails to a high state of polish by scratching. In addition, eczema of the nail folds may lead to a coarse irregularity with transverse ridging of the adjacent nail plates.

Lichen planus
Some 10% of patients with lichen planus have nail changes. Most often this is a reversible thinning of the nail plate with irregular longitudinal grooves and ridges. More severe involvement may lead to pterygium in which the cuticle grows forward over the base of the nail and attaches itself to the nail plate (Figure 13.25). The threat of severe and permanent nail changes can sometimes justify treatment with systemic steroids.

Alopecia areata
The more severe the hair loss, the more likely there is to be nail involvement. A roughness or fine pitting is seen on the surface of the nail plates and the lunulae may appear mottled.

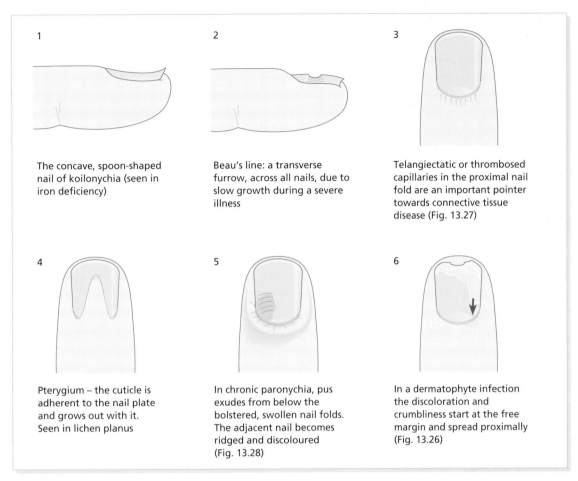

1

The concave, spoon-shaped nail of koilonychia (seen in iron deficiency)

2

Beau's line: a transverse furrow, across all nails, due to slow growth during a severe illness

3

Telangiectatic or thrombosed capillaries in the proximal nail fold are an important pointer towards connective tissue disease (Fig. 13.27)

4

Pterygium – the cuticle is adherent to the nail plate and grows out with it. Seen in lichen planus

5

In chronic paronychia, pus exudes from below the bolstered, swollen nail folds. The adjacent nail becomes ridged and discoloured (Fig. 13.28)

6

In a dermatophyte infection the discoloration and crumbliness start at the free margin and spread proximally (Fig. 13.26)

Figure 13.25 Other nail changes.

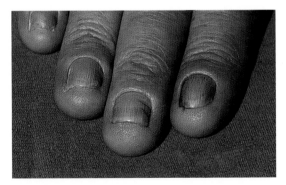

Figure 13.26 The curved slow-growing greenish-yellow nails of the yellow nail syndrome.

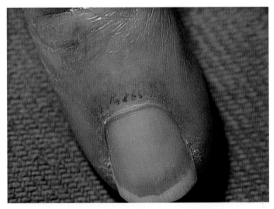

Figure 13.27 Large tortuous capillary loops of the proximal nail fold signal the presence of a connective tissue disorder.

Infections

Acute paronychia

The portal of entry for the organisms concerned, usually staphylococci, is a break in the skin or cuticle as a result of minor trauma. The subsequent acute inflammation, often with the formation of pus in the nail fold or under the nail, requires systemic treatment with flucloxacillin, cephalexin or erythromycin (Formulary 2, p. 410) and appropriate surgical drainage. Recurrent acute paronychia may be related to herpes simplex virus infection.

Chronic paronychia

Cause

A combination of circumstances can allow a mixture of opportunistic pathogens (yeasts, Gram-positive cocci and Gram-negative rods) to colonize the space between the nail fold and nail plate producing a chronic dermatitis. Predisposing factors include a poor peripheral circulation, wet work, working with flour, diabetes, vaginal candidosis and over-vigorous cutting back of the cuticles.

Presentation and course

The nail folds become tender and swollen (Figures 13.25 and 13.28) and small amounts of pus are discharged at intervals. The cuticular seal is damaged and the adjacent nail plate becomes ridged and discoloured. The condition may last for years.

Differential diagnosis

In atypical cases, consider the outside chance of an amelanotic melanoma. Paronychia should not be confused with a dermatophyte infection in which the nail folds are not primarily affected.

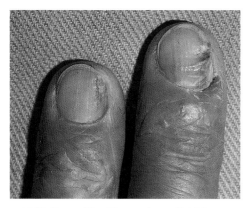

Figure 13.28 Paronychia with secondary nail ridging.

Investigations

Test the urine for sugar, check for vaginal and oral candidosis. Pus should be cultured.

Treatment

Manicuring of the cuticle should cease. Treatment is aimed at both the infective and dermatitic elements of the condition. The hands should be kept as warm and as dry as possible, and the damaged nail folds packed several times a day with an imidazole cream (Formulary 1, p. 404). Highly potent topical corticosteroid creams applied for 3 weeks also help. If there is no response, and swabs confirm that *Candida* is present, a 2-week course of itraconazole should be considered (Formulary 2, p. 414).

Dermatophyte infections (Figures 13.25 and 16.40)

Cause

The common dermatophytes that cause tinea pedis can also invade the nails (p. 240).

Presentation

Toenail infection is common and associated with tinea pedis. The early changes often occur at the free edge of the nail and spread proximally. The nail plate becomes yellow, crumbly and thickened. Usually, only a few nails are infected but occasionally all are. The fingernails are involved less often and the changes, in contrast to those of psoriasis, are usually confined to one hand. Nail infection in patients with HIV infections often involve the proximal subungual skin without distal involvement.

Clinical course

The condition seldom clears spontaneously.

Differential diagnosis

Psoriasis has been mentioned. Yeast and mould infections of the nail plate, much more rare than dermatophyte infections, can look similar. Coexisting tinea pedis favours dermatophyte infection of the nail.

Investigations

The diagnosis is confirmed by microscopic examination of potassium hydroxide treated nail clippings (p. 37). Cultures should be carried out in a mycology laboratory.

Treatment

This is given on p. 242. Remember that most symptom-free fungal infections of the toenails need no treatment at all.

Tumours

Peri-ungual warts are common and stubborn. Cryotherapy must be used carefully to avoid damage to the nail matrix, but is painful.

Peri-ungual fibromas (Figure 24.5), pink or skin-colored papules arising from the nail folds, can be seen in the general population. Multiple periungal fibromas (Koenen tumours) can be seen in patients with tuberous sclerosis, with onset usually in late childhood.

Glomus tumours can occur beneath the nail plate. The small red or bluish lesions are exquisitely painful if touched and when the temperature changes. Treatment is surgical.

Subungual exostoses protrude painfully under the nail plate. Usually secondary to trauma to the terminal phalanx, the bony abnormality can be seen on X-ray and treatment is surgical.

Myxoid cysts (Figure 13.29) occur on the proximal nail folds, usually of the fingers. The smooth domed swelling contains a clear jelly-like material that transilluminates well. A groove may form on the adjacent nail

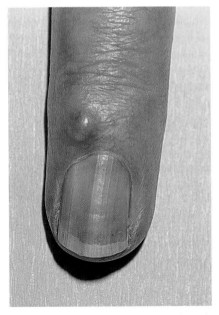

Figure 13.29 Myxoid cyst creating a groove in the nail.

plate. Cryotherapy, injections of triamcinolone and surgical excision all have their advocates.

Malignant melanoma should be suspected in any subungual pigmented lesion, particularly if the pigment spreads to the surrounding skin (Hutchinson's sign). Subungual haematomas may cause confusion but 'grow out' with the nail (Figure 13.20). The risk of misdiagnosis is highest with an amelanotic melanoma, which may mimic chronic paronychia or a pyogenic granuloma.

Some other nail abnormalities

A few people are born with one or more nails missing. In addition, there are many conditions, either inherited or associated with chromosomal abnormalities and usually rare, in which nail changes form a minor part of the clinical picture. Most cannot be dealt with here.

In the rare *nail–patella syndrome*, the thumbnails, and to a lesser extent those of the fingers, are smaller than normal. Rudimentary patellae, renal disease and iliac spines complete the syndrome, which is inherited as an autosomal dominant trait linked with the locus controlling ABO blood groups.

Pachyonychia congenita is also rare and inherited as an autosomal dominant trait. The nails are grossly thickened, especially peripherally, and have a curious triangular profile (Figure 13.21). Hyperkeratosis may occur on areas of friction on the legs and feet.

Permanent loss of the nails may be seen with the dystrophic types of *epidermolysis bullosa* (p. 124).

The *nail 'en racquette'* is a short broad nail (Figure 13.15), usually a thumbnail, which is seen in some 1–2% of the population and inherited as an autosomal dominant trait. The basic abnormality is shortness of the underlying terminal phalanx.

The mouth and genitals

Mucous membranes are covered with a modified stratified squamous epithelium that lacks a stratum corneum. This makes them moist and susceptible to infection, and to conditions not seen elsewhere. In contrast, the skin around them is like that on other body sites, and develops the standard range of skin disorders. It follows that the diagnosis of puzzling mouth or genital changes is often made easier by looking for skin disease elsewhere.

The mouth

The mouth can harbour an enormous range of diseases, affecting each of its component structures. Inflammatory

Table 13.4 Common tongue problems.

Condition	Cause	Treatment
Furred tongue	Hypertrophy of the filiform papillae.	Brush the tongue
Black hairy tongue (Figure 13.30)	Pigmentation and hypertrophy of filiform papillae caused by bacterial overgrowth.	Brush the tongue
Smooth tongue	Nutritional deficiency, sprue, malabsorption.	Vitamins, nutrition
Fissured tongue	Congenital, Down's syndrome, ageing changes.	No treatment needed
Median rhomboid glossitis	Developmental defect and candidiasis. Smoking and dentures worsen.	Topical or oral anticandidal therapy
Geographic tongue (Figure 13.31)	Familial, atopic, psoriasis.	Topical steroids if symptomatic
Varices	Blue compressible blebs of veins.	No treatment needed
Hairy leucoplakia	Epstein–Barr virus infection in patients with HIV/AIDS.	Highly active retroviral therapies (HAART)
Herpetic glossitis	Painful fissures without vesicles.	Aciclovir group (p. 415)
Macroglossia	Developmental, tumours, infections, amyloidosis, thyroid.	Treat the cause
Glossodynia	Trauma, *Candida*, menopause, diabetes, nutritional, dry mouth.	Treat the cause, use tricyclic antidepressants

and infectious disorders of the mouth are usually either red or white – leading to the terms erythroplakia and leucoplakia, respectively. These are descriptive terms but not diagnoses. A biopsy will help sort out the non-dysplastic causes, such as lichen planus and *Candida* infections, from the dysplastic ones that are the precursors of carcinoma.

Some skin diseases cause ulceration in the mouth. These ulcers are accompanied by skin diseases elsewhere on the body, and making a diagnosis there is easier than in the mouth. In other patients with mouth ulcers, the course of the ulcers or erosions, and their size and location in the mouth, provide diagnostic clues. Table 13.4 lists some common tongue problems (Figures 13.30 and 13.31).

Lichen planus

Cause

The cause of oral lichen planus is unknown (p. 69). However, some 40% of patients with symptomatic lichen planus of the mouth have relevant allergies, diagnosable by patch testing. These are usually to metals (especially gold and mercury dental amalgam) and flavourings such as cinnamon, peppermint and spearmint. Lichen planus also results from drug reactions, liver disease and bone marrow transplantation.

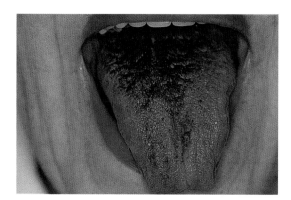

Figure 13.30 Black hairy tongue.

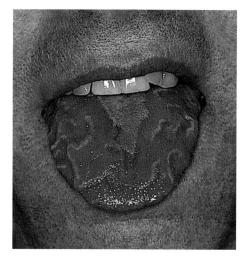

Figure 13.31 Geographic tongue.

Presentation

When a lichen planus-like cutaneous eruption is present, finding lichen planus in the mouth confirms the diagnosis, and vice versa. In the mouth, typically, there is a lace-like whitening of the buccal mucosae called Wickham's striae (see Figure 6.4), but sometimes this laciness is not present. Oral lichen planus can also be red, and can ulcerate. A desquamative gingivitis may occur, in which the mucosa shears off with friction, such as that from brushing the teeth or eating an apple. Desquamative gingivitis can also result from pemphigus or pemphigoid (see *Bullous diseases*). Often oral lichen planus is asymptomatic and more of a curiosity than a problem for the patient.

Course

Oral lichen planus can last for years – even for a lifetime. Asymptomatic lichen planus does not usually progress to the symptomatic form.

Differential diagnosis

In its classic lace-like state, the appearance of oral lichen planus is diagnostic (Figure 6.4). Dysplastic leucoplakias are more likely to be focal, appearing on only a portion of the mucosae, gingivae or lips. They are also more likely to be red and symptomatic, and shown by those who have smoked cigarettes or chewed tobacco. *Candida albicans* infections may occasionally be considered, but their white patches scrape off.

Investigations

A potassium hydroxide (KOH) examination and a culture will rule out candidasis. Biopsy will determine if a white patch is dysplastic or not. The histology of lichen planus, as seen in the skin, may be less typical in the mouth, and may even suggest a dermatitis. Patch testing may be useful as allergic causes can be cured by allergen elimination. Liver function tests, and tests for hepatitis B, hepatitis C and antimitochondrial antibodies are often recommended.

Treatment

If asymptomatic, no treatment is necessary. High potency topical steroids, in gel or ointment bases, are worth a try if the lesions are painful or ulcerated. Newer topical immunomodulators, tacrolimus and pimecrolimus, may be helpful as well (Formulary 1, p. 403). Failing that, a few patients require oral prednisone; they should be referred to a dermatologist or specialist in oral medicine.

Complications

Watch out for carcinoma, even if previous biopsies have shown no dysplasia. The risk is highest in the ulcerative forms, and the overall risk for development of squamous cell carcinoma in oral lichen planus is probably 1–5%. It should be suspected if an area becomes thickened, nodular or ulcerates.

Morsicatio buccarum (cheek chewing)

Repetitive chewing to the buccal mucosa produces the characteristic bilateral shaggy white appearance along the area of the mucosa where the teeth meet. This is asymptomatic and no treatment is needed.

Candidiasis

Cause and presentation

Infections with *Candida albicans* appear suddenly, on the tongue, lips or other mucosae, in the pseudomembranous form (also called thrush; see Figure 16.47). Small lesions are more common than large ones. About 15% of infants develop thrush on the tongue, lips or buccal mucosa. Sometimes, candidiasis appears as red sore patches under dentures, or as angular chelitis (perlèche).

Course

If the candidiasis is a complication of systemic antibiotic therapy, treatment will be curative. Immunosuppressed and denture-wearing patients often have recurrent disease.

Differential diagnosis

Many tongues are coated with desquamated epithelial cells that create a yellow wet powder on their surface. This scapes off easily, and shows no inflammation underneath. Lichen planus, oral hairy leucoplakia and dysplastic leucoplakia may cause confusion.

Investigations

Thrush does not normally occur in healthy adults, in whom the appearance of candidiasis needs more investigation than just a simple diagnosis by appearance, KOH examination or culture. Table 13.5 lists some possible underlying causes.

Treatment

Topical and systemic imidazoles are the treatments of choice. Creams and solutions can be used, but sucking on a clotrimazole troche (Formulary 1, p. 403) three times daily is better. Some patients are best treated with

Table 13.5 Possible causes underlying oral candidiasis in adults.

Antibiotic treatment
HIV infection
Myelodysplastic syndromes
    leukaemia
    lymphoma
    thymoma
Chemotherapy
Inhalation of corticosteroids for asthma
Widespread metastatic malignancy
Vitamin deficiency
Inflammatory bowel disease
Xerostomia
Previous radiation therapy to mouth
Diabetes
Addison's disease
Myasthenia gravis
Dentures
Chronic mucocutaneous candidiasis (on skin and nails
    too; p. 245)

fluconazole, 150 mg once daily for 1–3 days (Formulary 2, p. 414). If an underlying condition is present, this should be identified and treated. Patients with 'denture sore mouth' should scrub their dentures each night with toothpaste and a toothbrush, sleep without dentures and swish a teaspoonful of nystatin solution around the dentureless mouth three times a day (Formulary 1, p. 403).

Contact stomatitis

This underdiagnosed problem usually causes a transient soreness, associated with a diffuse redness of the lips and buccal gingivae. Mouthwashes, hard sweets (candies) and hot pizzas are common causes of the irritant type, whereas cinnamon, vanilla, peppermint, spearmint and dentifrices are the most common causes of allergic contact stomatitis. When local stomatitis or ulcers occur near dental amalgam, metal allergy to gold, copper and mercury should be suspected, but patch testing is needed before recommending that the filling should be removed.

Ulcers

One problem with oral ulcers (as with ulcers elsewhere) is the usual lack of a primary lesion, such as a bulla, papule or plaque. Ulcers are often secondary reactions which rob the clinician of the chance to make a morphological diagnosis. The history, the location of the ulcers within the mouth, their duration and the presence of coexisting nonoral signs or symptoms, especially of the skin, are then all-important clues to the underlying diagnosis.

Bullous diseases

Pemphigus and pemphigoid are most likely (see Chapter 9).

Pemphigus causes large painful long-lasting erosions (see Figure 9.3). The whole mouth can be involved, but more often it affects just the lips, buccal mucosa or tonsillar pillars. Desquamative gingivitis can occur. The ulcers are large, appear without warning and last months. A biopsy may show separation of keratinocytes (acantholysis) and should not be taken from an ulcer, but from normal-appearing mucosa next to an active area. Direct immunofluorescence (biopsy normal mucosa) shows antibody rimming each keratinocyte.

Cicatricial (scarring) pemphigoid affects the mucous membranes predominantly, but occasionally affects the skin too. The eyelid conjunctiva and other mucosae can also be affected; scarring often results (see Figure 9.8). Cicatricial pemphigoid is also a cause of desquamative gingivitis. Biopsy shows a subepidermal bulla, and direct immunofluorescence a linear band of IgG and C3 at the dermal–mucosal junction.

Aphthae

Presentation

These common small oval painful mouth ulcers arise, usually without an obvious cause, most often in 'movable mucosae' such as the gutters of the mouth, tongue or cheek (Figure 13.32). An area of tenderness changes into a small red papule that quickly turns into a grey 2–5 mm painful ulcer with a red halo. Herpetiform aphthae occur

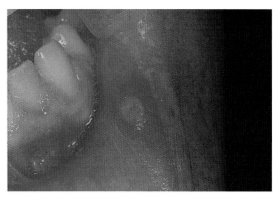

Figure 13.32 Aphthous ulcer of the labial mucosa.

in groups of 2–5 tiny painful ulcers. Major aphthae (peri-adenitis mucosa necrotica) are usually larger than 1 cm across and tend to appear in the back of the mouth.

Course
Small ulcers heal in a week or two; the pain stops within days. Major aphthae may persist for months.

Differential diagnosis
Recurrent herpes simplex infections mimic herpetiform apthae but, in the latter, cultures are negative and blisters are not seen. Behçet's disease causes confusion in patients with major aphthae. In fact, a diagnosis of Behçet's disease is often wrongly made in patients with recurrent aphthae of all sorts, when the patient has some other skin disease or joint pain. Patients with true Behçet's disease should have at least two of these other findings: recurrent genital ulcers, pustular vasculitis of skin, synovitis, uveitis, meningoencephalitis or positive pathergy testing by a physician.

Investigations
Usually none are needed. Occasional associations include Crohn's disease, ulcerative colitis, gluten-sensitive enteropathy, cyclical neutropenia, other neutropenias, HIV infection and deficiencies of iron, vitamin B_{12} or folate.

Treatment
Prevention is best. Trauma, such as aggressive tooth brushing, hard or aggravating foods and stress, should be avoided if relevant. The application of a topical corticosteroid gel, such as fluocinonide, to new lesions may shorten their course. Topical analgesics may provide transient pain relief. In severe or complex cases, consider referral.

Some other oral lumps, bumps and colour changes
• Mucocoeles are collections of mucin following the rupture of a minor salivary gland duct. They are blue-tinted soft translucent nodules, usually of the lips, and arise suddenly without pain.
• Fordyce spots are ectopic sebaceous glands, appearing as pinhead-sized whitish-yellow papules on the vermillion lip and oral mucosa (Figure 13.33). They are quite common and are a variant of normal anatomy.
• Yellow patches in the mouth may suggest pseudoxanthoma elasticum (p. 349).

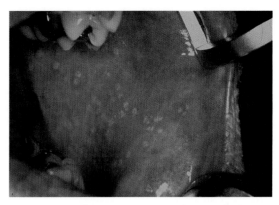

Figure 13.33 Fordyce spots are ectopic sebaceous glands.

• Brown macules on the lips should trigger thoughts about the dominantly inherited Peutz–Jehgers syndrome (see Figure 19.12) and its bowel polyps and tumours.
• Neurofibromas may occur, especially in patients with widespread cutaneous neurofibromatosis.
• Telangiectases may suggest hereditary haemorrhagic telangiectasia. These patients may also have telangiectases in their intestinal tract leading to gastrointestinal bleeding, and arteriovenous fistulae especially in the lungs that may lead to cerebral embolism.
• Venous lakes are blue or black papules on the lips (Figure 13.34). These melanoma-like lesions worry patients and doctors alike, but pressure with a diascope or glass slide causes them to blanch.
• Multiple, somewhat translucent, papules may suggest Cowden's syndrome. These are fibromas. Patients with Cowden's syndrome have facial papules and nodules (tricholemmomas and fibromas), fibrocystic disease of the breasts and a great propensity to develop malignant tumours of the breast, thyroid and other organs.

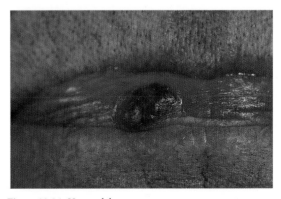

Figure 13.34 Venous lake.

• Multiple mucosal neuromas begining in the first decade of life may be the first sign of multiple endocrine neoplasia syndrome type 2B (MEN 2B). These patients have neuromas affecting mainly the lips, tongue and buccal mucosa. More than 90% of patients with this autosomal dominantly inherited disorder will develop medullary carcinoma of the thyroid, with 75% of them being metastatic at the time of diagnosis. Many also develop phaeochromocytomas.

• Pyogenic granulomas of the gingiva appear as quick-growing red bleeding papules. They are reactive proliferations of blood vessels, and often develop in pregnancy ('pregnancy tumours').

• Fibromas may result from dentures, or from resolving or indolent pyogenic granulomas, but can also appear without reason, usually on the gingiva of adults. Tooth bites may cause fibromas to appear on the tongue and on the buccal mucosae. Cowden's disease (see above) should be considered if multiple lesions are present.

• Warts in the mouth are not uncommon.

• The differential diagnosis of oral papules and nodules also includes lipomas, keloids, giant cell granulomas, granular cell tumours, myxomas, xanthomas, haemangiomas, myomas, neural tumours and a host of uncommon benign growths.

Squamous cell carcinoma (Figure 13.35; see also p. 292)

Cause

Predisposing factors include smoking or chewing tobacco products, and the 'straight-shot' drinking of alcohol. Cancer can also occur in the plaques and ulcers of lichen planus. Lip cancers may be sun-induced. Human papillomavirus types 16 and 18 have been implicated as a cause.

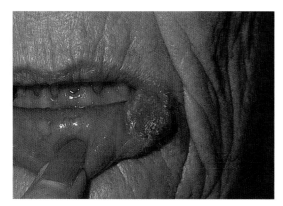

Figure 13.35 Squamous cell carcinoma in a heavy smoker.

Presentation

A thickening or nodule develops, usually on the lower lip, and often in a field of actinic chelitis (rough scaling mucosa from sun damage). Inside the mouth, the tongue is the most common site to be affected, often on its undersurface. The cancer itself appears either as an indurated ulcer with steep edges, or as a diffuse hardness or nodule. Red or white thickened plaques are common precursors, and the cancer may be surrounded by these changes.

Course

Unfortunately, cancer of the mouth often goes undetected. Its symptoms are excused by the patient as aphthous ulcers or denture sores, and its signs are not seen by the physicians who scan the skin. Cancers grow, and squamous cell carcinomas of the mouth are no exception. Plaques and hard areas may ulcerate.

Differential diagnosis

Confusion occurs with ulcerative lichen planus and other causes of white and red patches. Biopsy will differentiate a squamous cell carcinoma from these other conditions.

Treatment

Lip SCC should be treated with Mohs micrographic surgery (p. 371) or by wide local wedge excision through all layers of the lip, with primary repair. Oral surgeons or otolaryngologists usually remove intraoral cancers. Metastatic disease may require radiotherapy or chemotherapy.

Complications

Squamous cell carcinomas (SCC) of the lip caused by sun exposure carry a much better prognosis than the others. SCC of the oral cavity behaves significantly more aggressive than SCC of the skin. Left untreated, oral SCC are prone to metastasize to regional lymph nodes and elsewhere. The overall 5-year survival for stage I–II disease is 80% while stage III–IV is less than 30%. Early detection and aggressive treatment are imperative.

> **Learning points**
>
> 1 Mouths talk, but do not expect one to tell you its diagnosis.
> 2 Leucoplakia is not a diagnosis. Find the cause of your patient's white spots.
> 3 Aphthae are small and heal quickly. Consider pemphigus or another bullous disease if your patient has many, persisting or large erosions in the mouth.
> 4 A mouth ulcer may be cancerous.

The genitals

The genital area is richly supplied with cutaneous nerves. This means that skin disease there makes life more miserable than might be expected from its extent or apparent severity. In addition, patients often feel a special shame when their genitals harbour skin diseases. Skin diseases seen elsewhere may afflict this area, but the patient will often hide them from the examining physician. Many never seek treatment.

Benign conditions

An array of problems can plague the genitals; Table 13.6 lists some of them (Figure 13.36).

Vulvovaginitis

Inflammatory diseases of the vagina often also affect the vulva, but the vagina alone can be affected. Vaginitis causes discharge, odour, painful intercourse and itching or burning sensations. The differential diagnosis includes candidiasis, trichomoniasis, bacterial vaginosis, cytolytic vaginosis and atrophic vaginitis. The diagnosis can be made by the appearance of the discharge both grossly and under the microscope. Most patients with vaginitis obtain

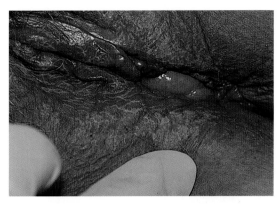

Figure 13.36 White lace-like appearance of vulval lichen planus.

their care from gynaecologists. Swabs for microbiological examination are essential.

Lichen sclerosus (p. 136)

Cause

This is unknown but local conditions have a role. Not only does skin develop the disease after being transplanted into affected areas, but the disease goes away when the grafted skin is returned to a distant site.

Presentation

The affected areas on the vulva, penis (Figure 13.37), perineum and/or perianal skin show well-marginated white thin fragile patches with a crinkled surface. Itching can be severe, especially in women. The fragility of the atrophic areas may lead to purpura and erosions. Scratching can cause lichenification, and diagnostic confusion.

Women are more commonly afflicted than men, but pre-adolescent girls and boys also can develop this problem. In girls, the white patches circling the vulva and anus take on an hourglass shape around the orifices.

Course

As time goes on, scarring occurs. In adult women, the clitoral prepuce may scar over the clitoris, and the vaginal introitus may narrow, preventing enjoyable sexual intercourse. Scarring is rare in girls and boys; treatment may prevent it occurring in adults.

Differential diagnosis

The sharply marginated white patches of vitiligo can afflict the vulva and penis but lack atrophy, and typical

Table 13.6 Benign genital problems.

Pearly penile papules	Pinhead-sized angiofibromas of the glans penis
Fordyce spots	Ectopic sebaceous glands of the glans penis
Angiokeratomas	Red or black papules of scrotum
Balanitis	Many types, but poor hygiene and chronic irritation are common
Warts (condyloma accuminata)	Cauliflower-like growths of moist genital skin (see Chapter 16)
Fixed drug eruptions	Red plaques or ulcers can be localized to the penis (see Chapter 25)
Lichen planus (Figure 13.36)	Look for lesions in the mouth or on the skin to confirm the diagnosis
Psoriasis	Often favours the glans penis
Paget's disease	Intraepithelial adenocarcinoma appearing as a marginated red plaque
Infections	Syphilis, herpes simplex, chancroid, lymphogranuloma venereum

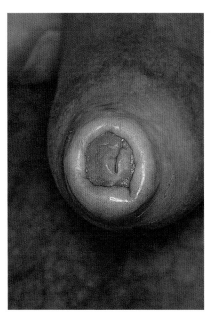

Figure 13.37 Lichen sclerosus of the foreskin, carrying the risk of causing phimosis.

vitiligo may be found elsewhere on the body. Neurodermatitis may be superimposed upon lichen sclerosus after incessant scratching.

Investigations

Biopsy is often unnecessary but the appearances are distinctive. The epidermis is thin, the basal layer shows damage and the papillary dermis contains a homogeneous pink-staining material and lymphocytes.

Treatment

At first sight it might seem unwise to rub potent topical steroids on to atrophic thin occluded skin. Yet, treatment with potent topical steroids not only reduces itch, pain and misery, but also reverses hypopigmentation and atrophy by shutting down its cause. However, atrophy, striae and other complications can develop on untreated adjacent skin, if the medication spreads there. Ointments are preferable to creams. Only small amounts (15 g) should be dispensed. After a course of 8–12 weeks, weaker topical steroids can be used to maintain a remission.

Complications

Scarring can destroy anatomical structures and narrow the vaginal opening. SCC may develop in men as well as women. Any focal thickening needs a biopsy.

Vulval and scrotal pruritus

Cause

Itching of the genital skin is usually caused by skin disease, or by rubbing, sweating, irritation or occlusion. Once started, genital itching seems able to continue on its own.

Presentation

The vulva and scrotum contain nerves that normally transmit pleasurable sensations. However, itching itself is not pleasurable, although scratching is. A torturing itch may be present all day, but more frequently appears or worsens at night. Once scratching has started, it perpetuates itself. The history is of an incessant and embarrassed scratching. Examination may show normal skin, or the tell-tale signs of excoriations and lichenification.

Differential diagnosis

Itch is part of many inflammatory skin diseases. In the groin its most common causes are tinea, *Candida*, erythrasma, atopic dermatitis, psoriasis, pubic lice, intertrigo and irritant or allergic contact dermatitis. However, patients with 'essential' pruritus show no skin changes other than those elicited by scratching. Sometimes the cause is psychogenic, but one should be reluctant to assume that this is the cause. Biopsy rarely helps. Look for clues by hunting for skin disease at other body sites.

Treatment

Low potency topical corticosteroids sometimes help by suppressing secondary inflammation; however, atrophy sometimes quickly occurs, and then the itch is replaced by a burning sensation. A better approach is to eliminate the trigger factors for itch – such as hot baths, tight clothing, rough fabrics, sweating, cool air, the chronic wetness of vaginal secretions, menstrual pads and soaps. Antipruritic creams, such as doxepin cream, pramoxine cream or menthol in a light emollient base, help to abort the itch–scratch–itch cycles. Many patients benefit from systemic antihistamines or tricyclic drugs such as amitriptyline or doxepin.

Complications

Atrophy is common but hard to see. Lichenification creates leathery thickenings, marked with grooves resembling fissures.

Dermatoses

The skin of the groins and genitalia is susceptible to many inflammatory skin diseases. They are listed in Table 13.7, but discussed in other chapters.

Squamous cell carcinoma

Cause

Human papilloma viruses, especially HPV types 6, 11, 16 and 18, often play a part. These are sexually transmitted, so the risk of carcinoma of the vulva or penis is greatest in those who have had many sexual partners. SCC of the glans penis is especially common in the uncircumcised. Smegma can incite inflammation leading to both phimosis and carcinoma. Exposure to tar also predisposes to scrotal carcinoma. Other predisposing factors are immunosuppression, lichen sclerosus and, possibly, lichen planus. Cancer can also develop from bowenoid papulosis – growths on the penis that resemble dark seborrhoeic keratoses clinically, and Bowen's disease histologically. The female equivalent is vulvar intraepithelial neoplasia.

Table 13.7 Nine common groin dermatoses.

Condition	Clinical comments
Tinea cruris	Involves the groin but seldom the scrotum
Candidiasis	Beefy red with satellite papules and pustules
Erythrasma	Brown patches of the upper thighs
Irritant contact dermatitis	Burning sensations may predominate
Allergic contact dermatitis	The scrotum may be oedematous
Inverse psoriasis	Beefy red marginated plaques extend up the gluteal fold
Seborrhoeic dermatitis	Look at the scalp for disease there, to confirm the diagnosis
Neurodermatitis	It feels wonderful to scratch an itchy groin
Intertrigo	Skin breaks down from maceration

Presentation

In men, a glistening irregular red moist patch (Bowen's disease and/or erythroplasia of Queyrat) develops on an uncircumcised penis, either on the glans or on the inner prepuce. Maceration may make it look white until evaporation reveals its true colour. It enlarges slowly, and invasion and tumour formation may not occur for years in immunocompetent men. In women, the precursor lesion is often Bowen's disease presenting as a sharply marginated, very slowly growing, mildly hyperkeratotic or slightly scaling, oddly shaped red patch or plaque that is usually a single lesion on one labia or in the perineum. This may become huge (up to 10 cm diameter). Sometimes, cancer of the penis or labia resembles a large wart destroying the underlying tissue. Biopsy confirms the diagnosis.

Course

Eventually the precursor lesions become frankly invasive and capable of metastasizing. Invasive carcinomas present either as bleeding ulcerated indurated plaques or as tumorous nodules.

Treatment

Mohs' micrographic surgery (p. 371) is probably the best treatment for small and minimally invasive carcinomas, but partial penectomy is indicated if the tumour is large. Precursor lesions such as warts, bowenoid papulosis, vulvar intraepithelial neoplasia and Bowen's disease can be destroyed with laser surgery (p. 383) or cryotherapy (p. 369), although recurrence is common. In some patients with minimally invasive carcinomas, topical applications of the cytokine inducer imiquimod cream (Formulary 1, p. 405) or the chemotherapeutic 5-fluorouracil cream (Formulary 1, p. 408) can be curative. It is hoped that immunization with the new HPV vaccine will prevent infections with the oncogenic wart viruses and relegate genital SCC to the history books.

Further reading

Baran R, Dawber RPR, de Berker DAR, Haneke E, Tosti A. (2001) *Baran and Dawber's Diseases of the Nails and their Management*, 3rd edition. Blackwell Science, Oxford.

Bruce AJ, Rogers RS. (2004) Oral manifestations of sexually transmitted diseases. *Clinical Dermatology* **22**, 520–527. Review.

Edwards L. (2004) *Genital Dermatology Atlas 2004.* Lippincott Williams & Wilkins, Philadelphia.

Hordinsky MK, Sawaya ME, Scher RK. (2000) *Atlas of the Hair and Nails.* Churchill-Livingstone, Philadelphia.

Lynch PJ, Edwards L. (1994) *Genital Dermatology.* Churchill Livingstone, Edinburgh.

MacDonald Hull SP, Wood ML, Hutchinson PE, Sladden M, Messenger AG. (2003) Guidelines for the management of alopecia areata. *British Journal of Dermatology* **149**, 692–699.

Margesson LJ. (2006) Vulvar disease pearls. *Dermatologic Clinics* **24**, 145–155, v. Review.

Ridley CM, Oriel JD, Robinson A. (2000) *Vulval Disease.* Arnold, London.

Scully C. (2006) Clinical practice. Aphthous ulceration. *New England Journal of Medicine* **355**, 165–172. Review.

Summers P, Kyei A, Bergfeld W. (2011) Central centrifugal cicatricial alopecia: an approach to diagnosis and management. *International Journal of Dermatology* **50**, 1457–1464.

14 Racial Skin Differences

Historical views on racial classification have been largely superseded by the understanding that biological variation does not fall into well-demarcated categories, but is a continuum. Greater genetic variance is found between individuals within traditionally described 'races' than between races.

The most obvious difference in the appearance of humans around the world is skin colour. Evolution favoured a dark skin in those exposed to high amounts of sunlight, thereby protecting the skin from damaging ultraviolet rays. It favoured a lighter skin in those living further from the equator to promote the production of vitamin D. These two competing evolutionary pressures favour a range of skin colours dependent on different UV exposure. This has been confirmed by studying latitude and skin colour as measured by reflectance spectrophotometry (Table 14.1). Dark skin differs from light skin not only in its colour, but also in its structure and function.

No colour defines normal skin and the same skin diseases occur in all parts of the world. Because of both genetic and environmental differences, skin diseases in those with pigmented skin often differ from those with non-pigmented skin in their incidence, prevalence, appearance and behaviour. They also differ in the types of cosmetic impairment they produce. For example, an acne papule in a white person can cause a transient mild tan or pink colour after the inflammation subsides, but the same papule may produce a long-lasting black macule in an African with darker skin.

Skin types

For the most part, melanin determines the colour of the skin. Other determinants that modify colour are capillary blood flow, carotene, lycopene, dermal collagen and the amounts of absorbed or reflected colours of light. As discussed in detail in Chapter 2, each melanocyte supplies melanin to about 30 nearby keratinocytes and it is the type, amount and distribution of melanin in keratinocytes that determines the colour of the skin. Tyrosinase in melanosomes converts tyrosine to dopa and then dopa to dopaquinone. This generates eumelanin, which is a dark brown–black colour. Eumelanin is plentiful in the dark skin of Africans and East Indians. Pheomelanin is yellow–red and forms when dopaquinone combines with cysteine or glutathione (p. 268). It is more plentiful in freckles in the light skin of Celtic populations in northern Europe.

As people of the same race may have a darker or lighter skin, dermatologists use skin typing numbers to grade baseline pigmentation. These skin types range from the pale, white, sun burning skin of type I individuals to the dark brown or black, never sun burning skin of type VI individuals. Skin types are assigned by criteria listed in Table 18.1).

Racial differences in structure and function

Despite obvious differences in colour, the skin of the various races is remarkably similar in structure and function. However, the epidermis is often thicker in dark skin, perhaps because it is less photodamaged. The stratum corneum of African skin may be more compact and contain higher concentrations of lipids. Functional differences in sweating may be ascribed to acclimatization and climate.

Fibroblasts are larger and more numerous in black than in white skin and the collagen bundles are finer and stacked more closely together. They may also be more active. This, combined with the decreased collagenase activity of black skin, predisposes it to form keloids.

African hair is more likely to be spiral in type, rather than straight, wavy or helical. African hair shafts tend to be more elliptical and hair follicles more curved. Asian hair has the largest cross-sectional area, while hair of

Table 14.1 Skin colour (measured by reflectance at 685nm) and latitude. Lower numbers represent darker skin. Adapted from Jablonski and Chaplin, *Journal of Human Evolution* (2000).

	Skin colour	Approximate Latitude
Kenya	32	0° (Equator)
Papua New Guinea (Goroka)	33	6°S
Ethiopian Highlands	34	8°N
South Africa (San)	44	22°S
Libya (Fezzan)	44	24°N
South Africa	51	32°S
Northern England	67	54°N
Greenland (dietary Vitamin D)	56	60°N

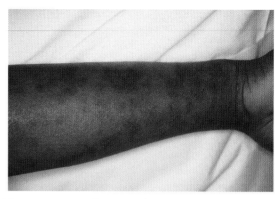

Figure 14.1 Post-inflammatory hyperpigmentation. Inflammation often stimulates pigment cells to produce excessive melanin, so that previously inflamed areas are marked long afterwards with dark patches.

western Europeans has the smallest. Native Americans and Mayan Indians have hair with large round cross-sections.

Darker skin seems more resistant to irritation, but this may be because erythema is difficult to see in dark skin, so visual measures of irritation falsely under-estimate the degree of inflammation. Chemicals penetrate black skin at about the same rate as they penetrate white skin so skin irritants produce comparable irritation if this is measured with surrogate markers such as the rate of transepidermal water loss across irritated skin.

Racially dependent variations in skin conditions

Inflammatory conditions

Common inflammatory conditions may present differently in darker skinned individuals. Erythema is difficult to appreciate in black skin; the overlying pigmentation masks the erythema to give a purplish hue. Pigment alteration may dominate the picture. Inflammation often leaves either dark or light spots; in other words, either it increases melanocyte activity or it increases epidermal turnover so that melanocytes inject less pigment into the surrounding keratinocytes. Although these areas are not scars, patients often refer to them as such and, like scars, they can be unsightly and persistent (Figure 14.1).

Acne

Acne in darker skinned patients causes hyperpigmented macules when papules and pustules resolve. Like the acne itself, these marks are hard to hide and the facial appearance worsens progressively as they accumulate. For this reason, acne in coloured skin calls for more aggressive treatment, but, unfortunately, irritation from acne treatments can also induce hyperpigmentation. Less irritating retinoids such as adapalene (Formulary 1, p. 405) are often preferred and lower concentration in a cream vehicle is more tolerable. Systemic antibiotics should be prescribed earlier in the course of treatment. Azelaic acid preparations (Formulary 1, pp. 399 and 406) lighten the skin while opening comedones and reducing papule counts, so agents containing it are useful for mild cases.

Eczema

Atopic dermatitis may be severe, especially in Asians. Eyelid dermatitis is particularly common and resists the usual treatments. In African patients, eczema has a tendency to surround and involve hair follicles, leading to evenly spaced skin-coloured papules resembling goose flesh. If accompanied by itching, this appearance should suggest eczema in black skin rather than other forms of folliculitis.

Lichen nitidus

Lichen nitidus occurs most commonly in black skin. Pinhead-sized uniformly distributed, shiny flat-topped skin-coloured papules occur on the genitals, abdomen or flexor surfaces of the extremities. The lesions do not itch. Skin biopsy establishes the diagnosis. No treatment is necessary; the disease is asymptomatic and goes away after 2–3 months.

Lichen planus

Lichen planus, classically described as flat-topped papules with a violaceous colour (p. 69), is darker in appearance in black skin. Any inflammation can leave dark spots, but in darker races these are especially prominent and persistent in diseases that damage basal melanocytes and lead to pigmentary incontinence, such as lichen planus, erythema dyschromicum perstans (p. 200) and erythema multiforme (p. 105).

Pityriasis alba

Presentation

Pityriasis alba appears as poorly marginated, light patches on pigmented skin (Figure 19.6). Although it occurs in skin types I and II, it is far more easily seen in darker skin types as the contrast is greater. Sometimes there is fine superficial scaling – hence the term pityriasis. Many patients are children with atopic dermatitis elsewhere. Examination under Wood's light highlights the pigmentary abnormality. Other provokers of pityriasis alba are bites, sunburn (even among those who are dark skinned), mechanical irritation from scrubbing, or other forms of eczematous dermatitis.

Course

The higher the skin type number, the more resistant this disorder is to treatment. Most children with the disease improve at puberty.

Differential diagnosis

In vitiligo (p. 298) the spots are much whiter, much more sharply marginated and always without scaling (Figure 14.2). Pityriasis versicolor (p. 245) is also more sharply marginated and is usually scaly (Figure 16.49). Potassium hydroxide (KOH) examination of scraping from these scales should be carried out if there is doubt. Sarcoidosis and leprosy should also be kept in mind.

Treatment

If mild eczema is the provoking factor, treatment with a weak corticosteroid such as hydrocortisone 0.5 or 1% or a cream containing a calcineurin inhibitor such as pimecrolimus is often prescribed. However, the pigmentary abnormality will take months to improve. Syndets (synthetic balanced detergents, Formulary 1, p. 398) can be used to wash the face as they are often less irritating than alkaline soaps. Moisturizers can be applied twice daily and after face washing. Tanning does not help; too often it accentuates the contrast.

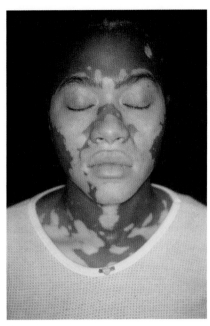

Figure 14.2 Vitiligo. Note the complete loss of pigment and the mirror-like symmetry.

Other considerations

Pityriasis rosea (p. 68) tends to be itchier in blacks and to leave long-standing black macules of post-inflammatory hyperpigmentation. For that reason, systemic steroids are sometimes given (do not forget to rule out syphilis!).

Cutaneous T-cell lymphoma occurs about twice as often in Africans than Caucasians. Persisting pruritic hypopigmented patches may prompt biopsy.

Sarcoidosis (p. 313) is up to 18 times more common in blacks than in whites. Its skin manifestations include erythema nodosum, widespread non-scaling papules, flesh coloured or blue–red nodules on the trunk, bulbous purple nodules and plaques on the face or ears (lupus pernio), inflammation in scars (scar sarcoid), soft swellings on the cheeks with overlying telangiectases (angiolupoid sarcoid) and lesions resembling psoriasis or ichthyosis. Sarcoidosis imitates many skin diseases, but biopsy will show its typical granulomas.

Post-inflammatory hyperpigmentation and hypopigmentation

Patients with darker skin types are more prone to post-inflammatory pigment alteration. This can be a result of their underlying inflammatory disease, but can also occur from iatrogenic effects during treatment. Retinoids have the potential to be irritating, promoting inflammation and hyperpigmentation. Aggressive laser treatments in skin of colour can cause hyperpigmentation. Warts, skin tags and seborrhoeic keratoses treated with cryotherapy can result in hypopigmentation.

Treatment for hyperpigmentation is two-fold. First, the primary disease should be suppressed or cured. Secondly, the darker spots can be treated with a bleaching agent such as 4% hydroquinone cream (Formulary 1, p. 399). Proprietary creams containing hydroquinone plus a retinoid, a glucocorticosteroid, or all three are available. Again care has to be taken not to irritate the skin with treatments designed to lighten it. Hydroquinone in concentrations greater than 4% can be compounded but carries a risk of inducing irreversible exogenous pigmentation ochronosis. This darkens the skin and prompts applications of even more hydroquinone.

Areas of skin with inflammation or an increased epidermal turnover can leave light spots. These are not completely depigmented and so can be distinguished from vitiligo by their appearance, as well as by their history. Few treatments exist for hypopigmentation. Use of excimer and fractionated laser show modest results at best. Fortunately, hypopigmentation generally resolves with time.

Pigmentary conditions

Voigt line
About two-thirds of Africans have a 'demarcation line', also called Voigt line or Futcher line, running down the ventral sides of their arms and forearms, and often also on their thighs. These lines are normal; they signify no disease and need no treatment. Most Africans also have a line of a different shade about 1 cm in width running from the umbilicus to the pubis. If dark, this line is called a 'linea nigra': if light, it is a 'linea alba'.

Dermatosis papulosa nigrans
Africans are prone to develop small black seborrhoeic keratoses on their faces (Figure 14.3). Although these are harmless, patients dislike them. Unfortunately, attempts to remove them with cryosurgery, electrosurgery, acids or even lasers can leave white or brown macules that are even more unsightly.

Melasma
Melasma (p. 275) can be severe in pigmented skin and challenging to treat. At least half of Hispanic women develop melasma during pregnancy. Patients can apply creams containing up to 4% hydroquinone. Sun protec-

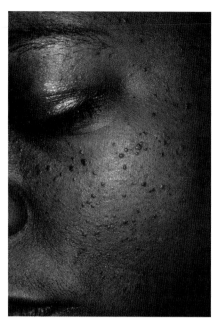

Figure 14.3 Dermatosis papulosa nigra. These small facial seborrhoeic keratoses commonly occur on the faces of Africans. Removing them may leave unsatisfactory white scars.

tion is essential. Because they are so seldom sunburned, many black patients do not apply sunscreens regularly and may need special instructions.

Erythema dyschromicum perstans
This is a chronic progressive disorder of unknown cause. Some call it the 'ashy dermatosis' because of its distinctive slate-grey colour. Most patients are Hispanic or Asian, but the disorder can occur in other people with darker skins.

Presentation and course
Many slate-grey, usually asymptomatic, patches develop on the trunk and extremities. They may cover large areas of the body. The scalp, palms, soles and mucous membranes are spared. Biopsy shows pigmentary incontinence, with melanin packed into dermal histiocytes. Pigmentation is chronic, as the word 'perstans' suggests.

Differential diagnosis
Post-inflammatory hyperpigmentation is hard to disregard. In fact, sometimes slightly raised, subtle pink smooth plaques arise before pigment changes become evident at the sites. Fixed drug reactions (p. 355) are slate-grey between their active phases, but arise from obvious urticaria-like wheals and are associated with taking

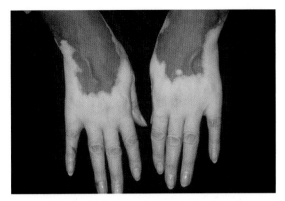

Figure 14.4 Vitiligo. If just on the hands, it may have been set off by depigmenting chemicals.

a drug. Photodermatoses (p. 260), some reactions to tick bites and urticaria pigmentosa (p. 305) may show grey or brown patches too.

Treatment
There is no effective treatment other than cosmetic cover-up. Sun tanning may mask lesions by darkening the skin around and over them.

Leprosy (Hansen's disease)
This is discussed in Chapter 16. Patients with tuberculoid and borderline tuberculoid leprosy often present with lighter patches, sometimes with a subtle erythema at the edges (see Figure 16.10). Palpate for nerve enlargement, test the skin for pinprick anaesthesia or stain skin biopsy sections for mycobacteria (may be hard to find organisms in tuberculoid forms). Asians seem especially prone to leprosy.

Vitiligo
This disorder is discussed in Chapter 19. It can occur in any skin type, but is especially disfiguring in those with a dark skin (Figures 14.4 and 14.5). Furthermore, many cultures assume that patients with depigmented areas of skin carry leprosy and therefore those with vitiligo may be thrown out of society, for example into an 'untouchable' class. Vitiliginous skin is prone to sunburn.

Idiopathic guttate hypomelanosis
While this can be seen in all skin types, idiopathic guttate hypomelanosis is more prominent in patients with skin types V and VI. Lesions are characterized by small discrete 1–2 mm hypopigmented macules, usually on the limbs, and progress with age.

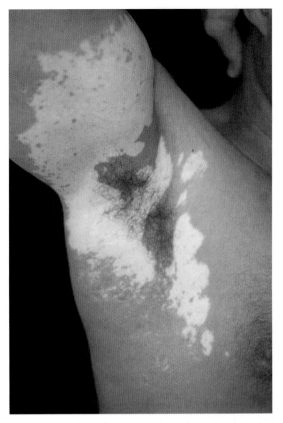

Figure 14.5 Vitiligo. The pigmented macules in the porcelain-white patches are areas where pigment cells have migrated to the skin surface from hair follicles. Phototherapy regimens work by encouraging this.

Naevus and melanoma

As might be predicted, individuals with a dark skin are less likely to develop non-melanoma skin cancers (p. 289). Melanin in the skin confers natural protection against ultraviolet radiation. Basal cell carcinomas are rare, but sometimes occur on sun-exposed areas. Other risk factors are albinism, ulcers, Naevus Sebaceus (p. 286), prior radiation exposure, traumas, immunosuppression and scars. Squamous cell carcinomas are more common and usually arise in areas of chronic inflammation such as scars, ulcers, discoid lupus erythematosus or draining sinus tracts. In Africans and Asians, basal cell carcinomas tend to be pigmented ('black pearly' appearance, Figure 20.30).

In Hispanic, Asian and black people, melanomas (p. 294) tend to develop on non-sun-exposed skin, such as that on the soles, palms, mouth, nail bed or nail matrix. About 90% of black people have at least one mole and usually these are on the extremities. The incidence of melanomas on the soles of black-skinned patients approaches the incidence of melanomas on the soles of others, but melanomas of the sole make up more than 50% of all melanomas of blacks, compared with 5% in whites. Most melanomas in blacks are of the acral lentiginous type. They are sharply marginated, irregular brown macules or patches. Melanomas in black patients tend to be thicker tumours at the time of diagnosis and thus have an overall poorer prognosis and higher mortality than melanomas in white patients. The same is true to a lesser extent for Hawaiians, Hispanics and Asians.

Melanonychia

Discrete longitudinal pigmented streaks called melanonychia are commonly found in the nails of patients with darker skin types. Generally, the finding of these does not cause the concern for melanoma that arises when these are seen in whites. Yet, melanomas around the nails are not uncommon in persons with skin types V and VI. When they occur, they are often misdiagnosed as paronychia or subungual haematomas, or ignored until at an advanced stage. Hutchinson's sign is an increased pigmentation of skin of the proximal nail fold in association with a subungual melanoma (Figure 14.6). Unfortunately, this sign

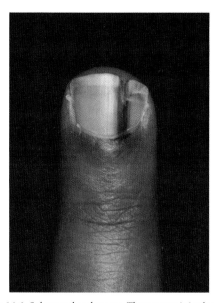

Figure 14.6 Subungual melanoma. The tumour is in the proximal nail fold and has caused a longitudinal band of pigment and a groove in the nail plate. Note the pigmentation of the proximal nail fold (positive Hutchinson's sign).

is not always present in whites or in blacks with nearby melanomas. Other clues suggesting melanoma as origin of longitudinal melanonycia are width greater than 3 mm, variable pigmentation, rapid increase in size and the presence of just a single streak. Nail bed or nail matrix biopsy should be performed if there is diagnostic doubt.

Naevus of Ota and naevus of Ito

Both are forms of dermal melanosis, usually arising at birth. Naevus of Ota refers to the slate-grey pigmentation usually unilateral on the peri-orbital area. It is more common in Asian females. Naevus of Ito occurs around the neck and shoulder regions.

Mongolian spots

Mongolian spots (Figure 15.1) arise from dermal melanocytic naevi. These slate-grey to slightly blue patches are found among the majority of black and Asian babies, often on the lower back and sacral region.

Keratodermas

Keratodermas are more common on the dorsum of the hands and feet in black patients. They may also have crateriform keratotic papules along the borders of the hands and feet and keratotic pits (keratosis punctata) in their palmar creases.

Infections

People with pigmented skin acquire the same infections as other people, yet their cutaneous manifestations and prognosis may be different. Post-inflammatory pigment changes are common after many infections, including impetigo, herpes simples, tineas and pityriasis versicolor.

Tinea capitis (see p. 240)

Cause

For some reason, the scalps and hairs of black children are especially prone to infection with *Trichophyton tonsurans*. This fungus invades the hair shaft as well as the stratum corneum. It is transferred from person to person by direct contact, or via contaminated fomites such as brushes, combs, barber's instruments and pillows.

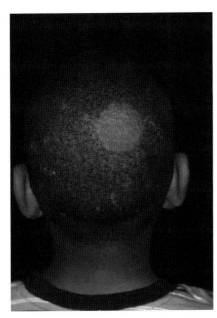

Figure 14.7 Tinea capitis. This is the seborrhoeic form where inflammation is slight and hair loss and scaling prevail. Culture scale and short hairs for fungus.

Presentation and course

Presentations vary, depending upon the amount of cell-mediated immunity. Inflammation is usually mild and the disorder mimics seborrhoeic dermatitis. Fine scaling covers some or all of the hair-bearing areas of scalp (Figure 14.7). In some patients, the fungus weakens the hair shaft, so that it breaks off at the surface of the scalp – the remaining proximal hair appearing as 1–3 mm long black dots (*black dot ringworm*). A patchy alopecia develops in these patients. If host resistance is greater, discernable inflammation may create pink plaques or follicular pustules. Cervical lymph nodes may then enlarge. Kerions from *T. tonsurans* (see Figure 16.42) are rare. Adults seem resistant to infection, perhaps because of the antifungal effects of sebum. Untreated infections persist and organisms can be spread to others.

Differential diagnosis

The disorder is so common that seborrhoeic dermatitis of the scalp in a black child aged 4–7 years is likely to be tinea capitis until proved otherwise. Although arthroconidia or hyphae can be seen inside the hair on KOH mounts, the presence of many other pigment granules, bubble-like abnormalities, superimposed scales and hair accretions often fools the non-cognoscenti. The organism does not fluoresce, so examination with a Wood's light is not helpful except to rule out infecting fluorescent fungi such as *Microsporum canis*. The diagnosis is best made by culture of the hair and scales on Sabouraud's agar containing the antibiotic cycloheximide to prevent overgrowth of bacteria. Some paediatricians scrub the scalp with a new toothbrush or wet cotton applicator and then brush the acquired scale and hair into the culture dish (plucked hairs should not be cultured because they often break off at the point of infection, leaving uninfected hairs on the culture medium).

Other hair breakage syndromes can mimic tinea capitis with patchy alopecia. This is especially true of hair that has been straightened, as the chemicals used to do this weaken the hair bonds. Traction alopecia (p. 176), trichotillomania and other alopecias may also be considered, but these seldom have associated scalp scaling. When the infection is accompanied by inflammation, traction alopecia, bacterial folliculitis, chemical folliculitis and 'pomade acne' from oils may be considered. If kerions develop, they are often misdiagnosed as bacterial abscesses. Think too of discoid lupus erythematosus and lichen planopilaris in atypical patients with scarring.

As the disease occasionally occurs in neonates, infants and adults, the disorder may then suggest other causes of scaling scalps such as cradle cap, psoriasis and dandruff. 'Dry scalp' in adults may be tinea, but in black adults 'dry scalp' more commonly results from alcohol in hair care products.

Treatment

Most clinicians practising in endemic areas start treatment without waiting for culture results. This reduces time lost from school, scarring and the potential to infect others. Oral treatment is essential as the infecting organism invades the hair follicles where they are not reached by topical agents. Microsize griseofulvin is the oral antifungal of choice. It is given at a daily dose of 20–25 mg/kg until cultures are negative, which is often 6–8 weeks. Gastrointestinal upset, vomiting and headaches are the most common side effects. Itraconazole, fluconazole and terbinafine are effective too.

As part of the treatment, children should use a shampoo that inhibits the growth of fungal spores. These include shampoos containing selenium sulfide, zinc pyrithione and ketoconazole. Otherwise, spores in the distal part of hairs may reinfect the child or infect other children. Some experts suggest that family members should use these shampoos too.

Hair and scalp

Pseudofolliculitis barbae ('hair bumps')

This is common in Africans and is related to the curliness of their hair. The hair either exits the follicle below the skin surface or curls around and 'ingrows' into the dermis, where it elicits a foreign body reaction.

Presentation

The patient is usually a black male, but black women and persons of other colours develop this too. Often, the person is unaffected, or only minimally affected, until he or she shaves. Shortly thereafter, papules and pustules develop at the shave site, most typically in the beard area (Figure 14.8). Comedones are not seen. Sometimes, inflammatory nodules develop; often a hair can be found curled up within them.

Course

Long hair simply does not ingrow. If shaving stops, the number of inflammatory lesions lessens. If shaving is resumed, the process recurs. Individual lesions resolve, often leaving scars or hyperpigmented macules. Long-standing cases may have scars and scar-distorted follicles that are even more prone to inflammation. Hairs sometimes grow sideways.

Differential diagnosis

Acne vulgaris can mimic this disorder, as both occur on the face and neck. Acne is associated with comedones and with papules and pustules on non-hair-bearing areas such as the forehead and temples. Darker skinned individuals tend to use oily cosmetics to produce a desirable sheen on

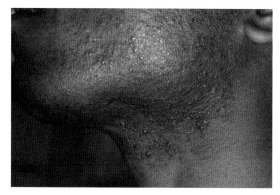

Figure 14.8 Pseudofolliculitis barbae (shaving bumps). These are caused by ingrown hairs.

their faces and sometimes these can produce acne cosmetica (p. 157).

Treatment

It is easy to advise patients to stop shaving, but they may not want a beard. A compromise lets the hair grow slightly longer than the length provided by a close shave. Special electric razors are widely available. They cut the hair above the skin surface to prevent ingrowth from below and depend on daily shaving to prevent the ingrowth from above. Some find that daily aggressive rubs with a washcloth dislodge early ingrown hairs. Others prefer to dissolve hair with chemical depilatories. These leave a blunt edge on the hair end, rather than the spear-like point left by razors. Care must be taken with these chemicals as irritation can cause post-inflammatory hyperpigmentation. Epilation is generally not recommended because curved follicles are more difficult to ablate with a needle and the resultant hyperpigmentation is not desirable. Laser treatment is a safe and effective solution for long-term hair removal in darker skin types, but longer wavelength and adequate epidermal cooling must be used to prevent epidermal damage during treatments (p. 382). Some doctors prescribe topical retinoids and systemic antibiotics, but the rationale and efficacy of this is questionable. Hot compresses and topical steroids may reduce inflammation.

Dissecting folliculitis

Bacteria can also cause boggy, inflamed scalps in African-Americans. The scalp is tender, hair loss is common, and pressure on the boggy scalp causes pus to exude from sinus tract openings both nearby and far away. Some patients have manifestations of the follicular occlusion tetrad comprising acne conglobata (p. 157), hidradenitis suppurativa (p. 170) and pilonidal disease. Bacterial culture is usually negative, although a superinfection may complicate the disease. Treatment includes long-term antibiotics for their anti-inflammatory properties, systemic steroids and isotretinoin. Scarring and keloid formation often follows.

Alopecia (hair loss)

The hair of most Africans is curly. This makes it difficult to brush, comb, wash and set, because it tends to form knots. As a consequence, most Africans do not shampoo their hair daily or even weekly. This can lead to seborrhoeic dermatitis and an itchy scalp. Therapeutic shampoos often cannot be used frequently enough. Instead, patients apply topical antifungal agents and corticosteroid solutions, lotions and foams.

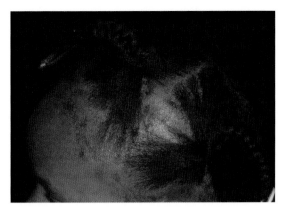

Figure 14.9 Traction alopecia. The tight braids have caused hair loss.

Hair loss in black patients can be caused by hair breakage, traction alopecia (p. 177) and central centrifugal cicatricial alopecia (p. 178). Follicular degeneration syndrome or central centrifugal scarring alopecia is characterized by hair loss with scarring over the vertex of the scalp. It is more common in Afro-Caribbean women. While the pathogenesis is multifactorial, hair styling practices may play a part.

Patients with curly hair often try to straighten it by using 'hair relaxers', or to create permanent waves through chemical treatments. These work by dissolving disulfide bonds and then reforming them after the hair is styled. Not all bonds reform, so chemically treated hair is weaker. Broken hairs and patchy hair loss are therefore common. 'Texturizers' use these chemicals too, in weaker concentrations, to 'loosen' a curl and make it more manageable and straighter. Thermal hairstyling depends upon high temperatures delivered to styled hair by curling irons, flat irons and hot combs. These can damage hair.

Traction on hair can cause alopecia (traction alopecia; p. 177). In Africans this often follows vigorous combing, brushing, using fork-like 'Afro picks' and styling into tight pony tails, tight braids, microbraids, twists, or 'corn rows' that pull on hair (Figure 14.9). Hair curlers and hairpiece wigs or extenders woven into the natural hair can also produce traction leading to hair loss.

Keloids

Keloids are thick scars. Some cultures intentionally provoke keloids as a decoration similar to a tattoo. Men and women develop them equally easily, although earlobe

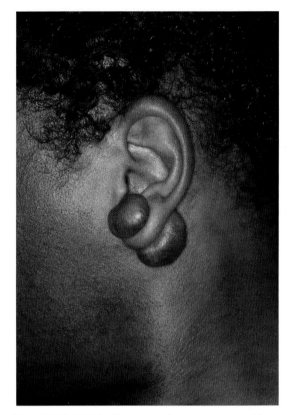

Figure 14.10 Keloids. These arose after ears were pierced for jewelry.

piercing gives the current edge to women (Figure 14.10). Black patients develop keloids much more often than people with type I skin. Chinese patients are slightly more prone to keloids too.

Cause

Keloids usually follow trauma although some can appear spontaneously. A typical patient is 10–30 years old and develops a thickening of skin at the site of a previous wound or surgery (Figure 14.11). The injury may be major or trivial. Keloids occur after burns, bites, piercings, surgery, acne pustules, vaccinations and even tattooing. Acne keloidalis nuchae occurs almost exclusively in blacks as small skin-coloured hard discrete and agminated papules at the nape of the neck associated with hair loss there. The provoking factor is assumed to be the inflammation of pseudofolliculitis (see *Pseudofolliculitis barbae*, p. 203). Surgeons must consider the increased risk of keloid formation and counsel patients appropriately

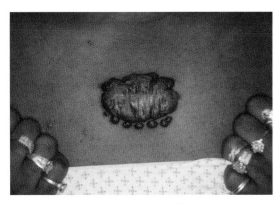

Figure 14.11 Post-surgical keloid. Small keloids even developed where the skin was pierced by sutures used to close the excision site.

regarding the risk, especially in keloid-prone areas of skin such as the upper chest, upper back and shoulders.

Fibroblasts in keloids produce more collagen and tend to proliferate more than normal fibroblasts, perhaps because of the stimulating effect of transforming growth factor β.

Presentation

Itching or pain is common. Keloids commonly erupt on the shoulders, upper chest, upper back, upper arms and earlobes. As opposed to hypertrophic scars, keloids often do not develop until weeks, months or years after the injury. They extend beyond the confines of the original wound and seem to invade the surrounding skin rather than expand locally.

Course

Keloids may enlarge and over decades may regress. Some are self-perpetuating, especially on the chest where they can become larger, harder, trabeculated, itching and deforming thick scars.

Treatment

Treatment is complicated by the tendency of keloids to regrow after their removal. Intralesional injection of corticosteroids, such as triamcinolone acetonide at a concentration of at least 10–20 mg, soften the keloid after repeated treatments and also decrease the intensity of pain and itch. Excision is frequently followed by regrowth unless the surgical wound is injected with corticosteroids or X-irradiated monthly for several months. Silicone gel dressings applied continuously to the wound site may

also prevent recurrence. Although cryotherapy with liquid nitrogen flattens a small number of keloids, it is often contraindicated in deeply pigmented individuals because it destroys pigment cells, leaving whiter skin at the sites treated.

Cultural practices

Different societies decorate their skins in different ways. Some practice rituals that scar or mark the skin. These may surprise physicians from other cultures. In addition, cultural practices can be associated with specific skin diseases in certain ethnic groups. Pomade acne secondary to comedogenic grooming products used on the scalp and forehead is seem primarily in black and Hispanic population. Capsaicin hand dermatitis can be seen in the Hispanic population who handle chile peppers barehanded and use them as condiments. Certain Asian populations may practice coining, cupping or moxibustion. Coining produces linear petechiae and ecchymoses after a coin or other instrument is rubbed hard against oil-coated skin. Cupping produces petechiae in perfect circles after suction has been created inside a bell-like device attached to skin. Asian and African societies sometimes burn the skin (moxibustion) to treat various maladies including eczemas. One must keep these 'cultural treatments' in mind before accusing a parent of child abuse.

Learning points

1 Rashes may be difficult to appreciate in darker skin individuals. Appropriate diagnosis and treatment are necessary to prevent the frequently associated post-inflammatory hyper- or hypopigmentation.
2 Cryotherapy may leave dark skin white.
3 Fungus may lurk in the dandruff-like scale of black children.
4 Take cultural differences into account when prescribing treatment.

Further reading

Gloster HM, Neal K. (2006) Skin cancer in skin or color. *Journal of the American Academy of Dermatology* **55**, 741–760.
Halder RM, Nootheti PK. (2003) Ethnic skin disorders overview. *Journal of the American Academy of Dermatology* **48**, S143–S148.

Nordlund JJ, Ortonne JP, Cesstari T, Grimes P, Chan H. (2006) Confusions about color: formatting a more precise lexicon for pigmentation, pigmentary disorders, and abnormalities of 'chromatics'. *Journal of the American Academy of Dermatology* **54** (Suppl 2), 291–297.

Rendon M, Berneburg M, Arellano I, Picardo M. (2006) Treatment of melasma. *Journal of the American Academy of Dermatology* **12** (Suppl 2), 272–280.

Shaffer JJ, Taylor SC, Cook-Bolden F. (2002) Keloidal scars: a review with critical look at therapeutic options. *Journal of the American Academy of Dermatology* **46** (Suppl Understanding), 63–97.

Taylor SC. (2002) Skin of color: biology, structure, function, and implications for dermatologic disease. *Journal of the American Academy of Dermatology* **46** (Suppl Understanding), 41–62.

Taylor SC, Burgess CM, Callendar VD, *et al.* (2006) Postinflammatory hyperpigmentation: evolving combination strategies. *Cutis* **78**, 6–19.

15 The Skin at Different Ages

Shakespeare knew how the skin changes with age: from the shining morning face of youth to the dry hand, yellow cheek and white beard of old age. In this chapter, we bring together the skin conditions encountered in different age groups, and add two more to Shakespeare's seven ages – those of the fetus and the pregnant woman.

Fetal skin

In utero, the skin remains one cell thick until weeks 4–6, when two layers can be seen; by weeks 8–11, there are three layers. Hair follicles start to appear at about 9 weeks, as do nails. Sebaceous glands arrive by 14 weeks, and pigmentation by months 4–6. Free nerve endings begin to develop in the skin at about 7 weeks but the central connections required for a fetus to appreciate pain are not complete until weeks 23–25.

Some families are at high risk of having a child with an intolerable genetic skin disorder. Prenatal diagnosis coupled with genetic counselling is then required, as early as possible so that selective termination is easy and safe. In the past, a fetal skin biopsy was sometimes taken under ultrasound guidance to help such families. However, this technique cannot be undertaken before 15 weeks' gestation and has gradually been superseded by DNA-based diagnostic screening of amniotic fluid cells (at 12–15 weeks) or chorionic villi samples (at 10–12 weeks). This type of testing has been used for conditions such as epidermolysis bullosa (p. 122; see Figure 9.13), severe ichthyoses including harlequin fetus (p. 47) and oculocutaneous albinism (p. 270). Pre-implantation diagnosis is gradually replacing prenatal diagnosis for couples known to be at high risk of severe Mendelian disorders, or structural chromosomal abnormalities. *In vitro* fertilization is carried out, and then the embryo biopsied and examined for the abnormality in question by fluorescence *in situ* hybridization, or by polymerase chain reaction (PCR). An embryo free of disease can then be re-implanted, removing the need for selective termination.

Infancy (the first year of life)

At birth, the skin is covered, wholly or partly, with a whitish slimy layer, the vernix caseosa. This comes off over the first few days, although some think that cradle cap (scaling of the scalp during the first weeks of life) is a result of its localized persistence.

An infant's skin is often mottled at birth (cutis marmorata) and peripheral cyanosis is common, as is a generalized erythema lasting for a day or two. The term harlequin skin change refers to an appearance seen in a few babies when they lie on their side; the uppermost part of their body becomes pale and is sharply demarcated from a redder lower half.

Preterm infants may be covered with fine lanugo hairs. In full-term babies there is usually some loss of scalp hair over the first few weeks. Multiple milia (tiny white epidermal cysts) are seen in about half of all babies. The tiny yellowish papules on the face of many babies are sebaceous glands that have hypertrophied under the influence of maternal androgens that have passed via the placenta. Neonatal acne (p. 158) may have the same trigger.

Rarely, maternal autoantibodies pass through the placenta. The child of a mother with subacute lupus erythematosus (p. 129) and anti Ro (SS-A) antibodies, for example, may develop an elevated, often annular, erythema (neonatal lupus erythematosus). This clears over the first few months, but may be associated with congenital heart block.

Other important changes seen at birth include those caused by underlying genetic disorders. A collodion baby (p. 47), for example, whose shiny smooth skin looks almost as though it has been painted with collodion, may have an underlying non-bullous ichthyosiform

Clinical Dermatology, Fifth Edition. Richard B. Weller, Hamish J.A. Hunter and Margaret W. Mann.
© 2015 John Wiley & Sons, Ltd. Published 2015 by John Wiley & Sons, Ltd.

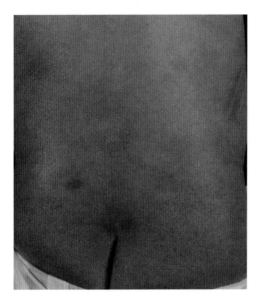

Figure 15.1 Mongolian spot.

erythroderma (see Figure 9.13 or lamellar ichthyosis (p. 47). Incontinentia pigmenti (p. 348) is in its linear vesicular stage at birth. In the severe junctional type of epidermolysis bullosa (p. 124), the newborn child has a mixture of large raw areas and flaccid blisters. In contrast, in tuberous sclerosis (p. 345), tiny white patches may be the only manifestation at birth.

Common birthmarks include congenital melanocytic naevi (p. 282), Mongolian spots (Figure 15.1) and haemangiomas (portwine stains, p. 302; salmon patches, p. 302). Capillary cavernous haemangiomas (strawberry naevi) appear within a few weeks of birth and then tend to regress slowly over the next few years (p. 303).

The stratum corneum is fully formed at birth, and so barrier function is normal except in premature babies. Nevertheless, newborn skin tolerates irritants poorly. Primary irritant reactions are common after prolonged contact with faeces and urine in the napkin and peri-anal areas, although severe napkin (diaper) dermatitis has become much less common since the introduction of disposable napkins (p. 83). True allergic contact eczema is rare in infancy. Atopic eczema (p. 87) commonly starts before the age of 6 months, often appearing on the face with a patchy non-specific distribution elsewhere.

There is large surface area to body weight ratio in babies and the risk of side effects from absorption of topically applied medications (e.g. topical corticosteroids and scabicides) is increased.

Sadly, practitioners may see signs suggestive of physical abuse. Contusions, abrasions, lacerations, burns and scalds, associated with broken bones or other evidence of trauma are classic features of the battered baby, but the signs may be more subtle. In any event, disorders responsible for the blisters and raw areas, such as epidermolysis bullosa (p. 122) or for bruising (Table 11.7), such as a coagulation or platelet defect, must be excluded.

Childhood

Parents soon learn that nurseries and schools are mixed blessings for health. Snuffles, coughs and colds are usually considered an inevitable part of the growing-up process and essential for the development of an effective immune system. But exposure and close contact at school also bring a host of skin infections and infestations; for example impetigo (p. 215), warts (p. 227), molluscum contagiosum (p. 234), head lice (p. 249) and scabies (p. 253). Such unwelcome guests are seldom accepted passively by mothers who require full explanations to lessen blame.

Atopic dermatitis (p. 87) is common in children, with a 1-year period prevalence of 8% in 2- to 11-year-old children in Scotland. Even before the advent of corticosteroid treatment, retarded growth in children with atopic dermatitis was well recognized. It is thought to be caused by a decreased frequency and size of growth hormone pulses during sleep which is presumably interrupted by scratching. Nevertheless, the amount of corticosteroids prescribed in this age group should be carefully monitored (p. 364), just as with children with asthma, as these drugs retard growth.

Both boys and girls may be seen by family doctors with symptoms and signs that might indicate sexual abuse. Vulval and peri-anal soreness and inflammation for which no other cause, especially threadworms, can be found should be considered suspicious. Anogenital warts (p. 228) should also ring alarm bells although some are innocently acquired. The situation is usually more clear-cut if a sexually transmitted disease such as gonorrhoea, herpes simplex or even HIV infection is found. Suspicion is increased if there is delay in seeking medical help, if the accompanying person's explanation for the appearance is not compatible with the signs and if the child discloses the cause. Again, it is important to note, as with battered babies, that skin conditions such as psoriasis (p. 56), lichen sclerosus (p. 193; Figure 15.2) and Crohn's disease in childhood can be mistaken for evidence of sexual abuse. Of course, this is a highly charged area

Figure 15.2 Lichen sclerosus.

and the diagnosis of sexual abuse, just as non-accidental injury, should be a multidisciplinary exercise involving paediatricians, family doctors, dermatologists and social workers.

Trichotillomania or hair-pulling habit in children is described on p. 339.

Adolescence

A sudden increase in androgen and oestrogen levels leads to sexual maturation. The skin changes of adolescence therefore include the appearance of pubic, facial and axillary hair, and increasing activity of the sebaceous glands. The adolescent growth spurt can be vigorous enough to cause stretch marks (Figure 15.3), or retarded by the presence of severe atopic eczema (p. 87).

The skin disorders of adolescents often operate against a background of social and examination stress. Personal

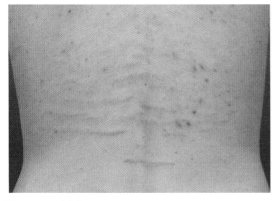

Figure 15.3 Adolescent striae.

appearance has become important, so that minor skin conditions can have a disproportionate effect on quality of life. Even a mild greasiness of the skin and hair can cause much embarrassment, worsened by the presence of acne (p. 156) – which itself may be subjected to regular picking – and/or seborrhoeic dermatitis (p. 92). Smelly armpits and heavy eccrine sweating of the palms (p. 167) can have the same effect. Neurotic excoriations (p. 338) and other forms of dermatitis artefacta (p. 336) are also triggered by stress.

Sexual awakening leads to close contact with others and so to a high incidence of infections and infestations, such as scabies (p. 253). Cosmetics and jewellery become popular, and can lead to contact allergy to materials such as nickel (p. 84), especially if skin piercing is involved.

Young adults

The quest for independence and work usually precedes the hunt for a social partner. Whichever comes first, personal appearance assumes even more importance with early male-pattern baldness (p. 182) and hirsutism (p. 186) becoming reasons for consultation. Stubborn acne causes increasing depression and management (p. 160) is both tricky and time-consuming.

Many women notice changes in their skin and hair during the menstrual cycle. These range from the development of a few acne spots in the premenstrual phase to textural (greasy or dry) changes. Premenstrual exacerbations of psoriasis, rosacea, atopic dermatitis, recurrent oral aphthous ulcers and herpes simplex are also well recognized. Autoimmune progesterone dermatitis is the name given to various reaction patterns in the skin that occur regularly in the premenstrual period. They include eczema, urticaria, erythema multiforme and dermatitis herpetiformis. Exogenous challenge with progesterone reproduces the picture.

Finally, there is the problem of selecting the right job. Young adults with atopic eczema, for example, or psoriasis on their hands, will react badly to contact with irritants (p. 83), and so should avoid jobs in catering, engineering or hairdressing.

Pregnancy

Some of the many skin changes that may occur during pregnancy are listed below.

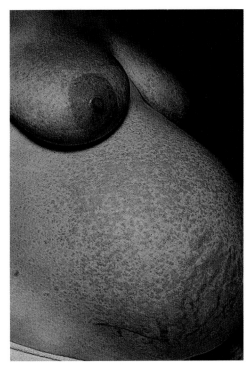

Figure 15.4 Polymorphic eruption of pregnancy with stretch marks. Widespread urticated papules.

• *Pigmentation*: the skin tends to darken generally. This is most obvious on the nipples, genitalia and in the midline of the lower abdomen (the linea nigra). Chloasma (p. 275) – an irregular pigmentation of the face – is common.
• *Skin tags* (p. 281).
• *Vascular changes*: these include oestrogen-induced spider naevi and palmar erythema. Varicose veins may become troublesome.
• *Stretch marks* (Figure 15.4): these are common on the abdomen. After childbirth they change from red lines to permanent silvery ones.
• *Decreased cell-mediated immunity*: this may lead to candidal and other infections. Genital and perianal warts may be luxuriant but should not be treated with podophyllin.
• *Itching* with no obvious skin cause is common in the third trimester and may be caused by cholestasis.
• *Pre-existing skin diseases* react unpredictably to pregnancy. Usually, atopic eczema, psoriasis and acne tend to improve.

Skin disorders specific to pregnancy include the following:
• *Polymorphic eruption of pregnancy* (Figure 15.4): itchy red urticarial papules and plaques or vesicles appear, usually in the third trimester, mainly on the abdomen and tending to follow the lines of stretch marks. They clear when, or soon after, the baby is born. The rash carries no risk of damaging the baby.
• *Prurigo of pregnancy*: many itchy and scratched papules come up, often at about 25 weeks. They too tend to clear, although more slowly, after childbirth, but may come back in subsequent pregnancies. Again, the baby is unharmed.
• *Pemphigoid gestationis* (p. 118): is a rare disorder, related to pemphigoid (p. 124), with autoantibodies directed against the same targets. Erythematous urticarial papules, plaques and bullae appear, especially around the umbilicus. It may occur at any time in the pregnancy (including the post-partum period) and recur in subsequent pregnancies. The baby may be born prematurely and be of low birth weight.

Middle age

As far as the skin goes, the most consistent and distressing middle age crisis is menopausal flushing or 'hot flushes' (p. 142): a sudden feeling of intense heat, discomfort and sweating, accompanied by blotchy erythema on the face, neck, upper chest and breasts that lasts for 3–5 minutes. Some women also develop palpitations, headaches and nausea. Hormone replacement therapy with oestrogens is the most effective treatment.

Keratoderma climactericum (p. 50), most commonly seen in middle aged women around the menopause, may also occur in men and women of other ages, many of whom are obese.

Male-pattern baldness (androgenetic alopecia; p. 175) is becoming more prevalent and occurring at an earlier age than 50 years ago. The burgeoning number of hair clinics are testimony to the fact that many men do not suffer this indignity lightly. Androgenetic alopecia in women, much more common than generally thought, usually causes a more diffuse hair loss, especially over the crown.

Whereas the prevalence of atopic eczema declines sharply in middle age, the discoid and asteatotic types (pp. 93, 96) appear.

Old age

Shakespeare's 'last scene of all' does not single out the skin, because it perhaps puts up with the ravages of time better

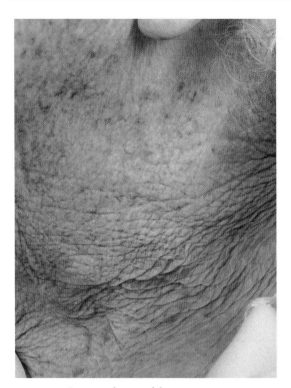

Figure 15.5 Cosmetic changes of skin ageing.

than the eyes and the teeth. But the skin is certainly not exempt from problems in old age.

Ageing changes in skin are caused by intrinsic factors, which are genetically determined, and extrinsic environmental factors of which the most important are UV exposure and cigarette smoking (Figure 15.5; Table 15.1).

Table 15.1 Cosmetic changes of old age (see Chapter 22).

Atrophy, sagging and wrinkling (Figure 15.5)
Coarse wrinkling of facial skin as a result of long-term
    cigarette smoking
Dryness
Photodamage (exposed skin only) including elastosis,
    cutis rhomboidalis nuchae and irregular
    pigmentation
Senile/solar lentigines ('liver spots'; p. 274)
Hair loss and greying of hair (as a result of loss of
    pigment in the hair shaft, secondary to depletion of
    melanocytes in the hair bulb and outer root sheath)
Slowed nail growth

Table 15.2 Skin conditions common in old age

Xerosis/asteatotic eczema (p. 96)/senile pruritus
    (p. 320)
Seborrhoeic keratoses (p. 278)
Precancerous lesions (e.g. actinic keratoses; p. 287)
Skin cancers (see Chapter 20)
Hirsutism (p. 179)
Pemphigoid (p. 117)
Shingles with post-herpetic neuralgia (p. 232)
Actinic reticuloid (p. 262)
Slow healing of leg ulcers (p. 147) and pressure sores
    (p. 145)
Scabies in homes for the elderly (p. 253)

In addition, immune responses are relatively defective in aged skin leading to an increased incidence in cutaneous infections and also skin cancers (Table 15.2). The normal intrinsic process of ageing leads to a gradually thinned epidermis, reduced pigmentation and fine wrinkles caused by an age-dependent reduction in dermal matrix and elasticity. The accumulation of a lifetime of sunlight exposure and cigarette smoking produce the more marked changes of extrinsic ageing. Both factors lead to a marked reduction in dermal collagen and disordered arrangement of the remaining collagen fibres and elastic tissue which cause the deeper wrinkles and sagging of sun aged skin. In the epidermis, variations in pigmentation (dyschromia), keratoses and wrinkling give the typical 'leathery' appearance of extrinsically aged skin. Skin type is a major determinant of the degree to which photoageing affects the skin, with Africans and Asians showing far less changes than Caucasians.

> **Learning points**
>
> 1 Most skin diseases vary in prevalence at different times of life.
> 2 Ageing of skin can be chronological alone, or additionally a result of environmental factors.

Further reading

Black M, Ambros-Rudolph C, Edwards L, Lynch P. (2008) *Obstetric and Gynecologic Dermatology*, 3rd edition. Mosby, London.

Eichenfield LF, Frieden IJ, Esterly NB. (2001) *Textbook of Neonatal Dermatology*. Elsevier Saunders, Philadelphia.

Farage MA, Miller KW, Elsner P, Maibach HI. (2008) Intrinsic and extrinsic factors in skin ageing: a review. *International Journal of Cosmetic Science* **30**, 87–95.

Harper J, Oranje A, Prose N. (2005) *Textbook of Pediatric Dermatology*, 2nd edition. Blackwell Publishing, Oxford.

Vukmanovic-Stejic M, Rustin MH, Nikolich-Zugich J, Akbar AN. (2011) Immune responses in the skin in old age. *Current Opinion in Immunology* **23**, 525–531.

16 Infections

Bacterial infections

The resident flora of the skin

The surface of the skin teems with micro-organisms, which are most numerous in moist hairy areas, and areas rich in sebaceous glands. The move away from culture-based approaches to genomic characterization has revealed that the skin microbiome is greatly more diverse than we had previously thought and generally exists in a delicate balance with their human host. Organisms are found, in clusters, in irregularities in the stratum corneum and within the hair follicles. The resident flora is a mixture of harmless and poorly classified staphylococci, micrococci and diphtheroids. *Staphylococcus epidermidis* and aerobic diphtheroids predominate on the surface, and anaerobic diphtheroids (Propionibacteria sp.) deep in the hair follicles. As a general rule, Gram-positive species such as *Staphylococcus epidermidis*, *Corynebacteria*, *Staphylococcus aureus* and *Streptococcus pyogenes* colonize the skin above the waist, while Gram-negative bacteria such as Enterobacteriaceae and Enterococci are additionally found below the waist. Several species of lipophilic yeasts also exist on the skin. The proportion of the different organisms varies from person to person but, once established, an individual's skin flora tends to remain stable and helps to defend the skin against outside pathogens by bacterial interference or antibiotic production. Nevertheless, overgrowth of skin diphtheroids can itself lead to clinical problems. The role of Propionibacteria in the pathogenesis of acne is discussed on p. 157. Overgrowth of aerobic diphtheroids causes the following conditions.

Trichomycosis axillaris

The axillary hairs become beaded with concretions, usually yellow, made up of colonies of commensal diphtheroids. Clothing becomes stained in the armpits. Topical antibiotic ointments, or shaving, will clear the condi-

tion, and frequent washing with antibacterial soaps will keep it clear.

Pitted keratolysis

The combination of unusually sweaty feet and occlusive shoes encourages the growth of diphtheroid organisms that can digest keratin. The result is a cribriform pattern of fine punched-out depressions on the plantar surface (Figure 16.1), coupled with an unpleasant smell (of methanethiol). Fusidic acid or mupirocin ointment is usually effective, and antiperspirants (Formulary 1, p. 400) can also help. Occlusive footwear should be replaced by sandals and cotton socks if possible.

Erythrasma

Some diphtheroid members of the skin flora produce porphyrins when grown in a suitable medium. Overgrowth of these strains is sometimes the cause of symptom-free macular wrinkled, slightly scaly, pink, brown or macerated white areas, most often found in the armpits or groins, or between the toes. In diabetics, larger areas of the trunk may be involved. Diagnosis is helped by the fact that the porphyrins produced by these diptheroids fluoresce coral pink with Wood's light. Topical fusidic acid or azoles will clear the condition.

Staphylococcal infections

Staphylococcus aureus is not part of the resident flora of the skin other than in a minority who carry it in their nostrils, perineum or armpits. Carriage rates vary with age. Nasal carriage is almost invariable in babies born in hospital, becomes less frequent during infancy, and rises again during the school years to the adult level of roughly 30%. Rather fewer carry the organism in the armpits or groin. Staphylococci can also multiply on areas of diseased skin such as eczema, often without causing obvious sepsis. A minor breach in the skin's defences is probably necessary for a frank staphylococcal infection

Clinical Dermatology, Fifth Edition. Richard B. Weller, Hamish J.A. Hunter and Margaret W. Mann.
© 2015 John Wiley & Sons, Ltd. Published 2015 by John Wiley & Sons, Ltd.

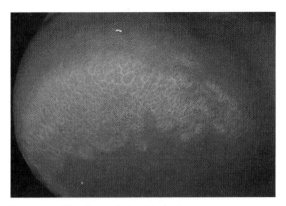

Figure 16.1 Pitted keratolysis of the heel.

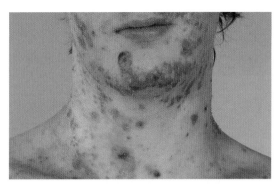

Figure 16.2 Impetigo on an uncommon site showing erosions, crusting and rupture blisters.

to establish itself; some strains are particularly likely to cause skin sepsis. Of concern is the rise in incidence of methicillin-resistant *Staphylococcus aureus* (MRSA) in the community and in hospitalized patients. This can result in abscesses and furunculosis as well as other infections. Prevention of emerging resistant strains is with a combination of scrupulous hygiene, patient isolation, antiseptic agents and restriction of antibiotics.

Impetigo

Cause
Impetigo may be caused by staphylococci, streptococci, or by both together. It is the most common skin infection of children and occurs particularly in tropical or subtropical regions, or during summer months in the nothern hemisphere. As a useful rule of thumb, the bullous type is usually caused by *Staphylococcus aureus*, whereas the crusted ulcerated type is caused by β-haemolytic strains of streptococci. Both are highly contagious. Exfoliative toxins produced by *S. aureus* cleave the cell adhesion molecule desmoglein 1 (p. 8). If the toxin is localized this produces the blisters of bullous impetigo, but if generalized leads to more widespread blistering as in the staphylococcal scalded skin syndrome.

Presentation
A thin-walled flaccid clear blister forms on non-follicular skin, and may become pustular before rupturing to leave an extending area of exudation and yellowish varnish-like crusting (Figure 16.2). Lesions are often multiple, particularly around the face. The lesions may be more obviously bullous in infants. Superficial infection of the hair follicles (superficial folliculitis) with pus in the epidermis is also common.

Course
The condition can spread rapidly through a family or class. It tends to clear even without treatment.

Complications
Streptococcal impetigo can trigger an acute glomerulonephritis.

Differential diagnosis
Herpes simplex may become impetiginized, as may eczema. Always think of a possible underlying cause such as this. Recurrent impetigo of the head and neck, for example, should prompt a search for scalp lice.

Investigation and treatment
The diagnosis is usually made on clinical grounds. Gram stains can be done or swabs can be taken and sent to the laboratory for culture, but treatment must not be held up until the results are available. Systemic antibiotics (such as flucloxacillin, erythromycin or cefalexin) are needed for severe cases or if a nephritogenic strain of streptococcus is suspected (penicillin V). For minor cases the removal of crusts by compressing them and application of a topical antibiotic such as neomycin, fusidic acid (not available in the United States), mupirocin or bacitracin will suffice (Formulary 1, p. 404).

Ecthyma
This term describes ulcers forming under a crusted surface infection. The site may have been that of an insect bite or of neglected minor trauma. The bacterial pathogens and their treatment are similar to those of impetigo. Whereas in impetigo the erosion is at the stratum corneum, in ecthyma the ulcer is full thickness, and thus heals with scarring.

Furunculosis (boils)

Cause
A furuncle is an acute pustular infection of a hair follicle, usually with *Staphylococcus aureus*. Infection spreads to the deep dermis, where small abscesses may form. Adolescent boys are especially susceptible to them.

Presentation and course
A tender red nodule enlarges, and later may discharge pus and its central 'core' before healing to leave a scar. Fever and enlarged draining nodes are rare. Most patients have one or two boils only, and then clear. The sudden appearance of many furuncles suggests a virulent staphlococcus including strains of community-aquired MRSA, or staphylococci expressing Panton–Valentine leucocidin toxin. A few unfortunate persons suffer from a tiresome sequence of boils (chronic furunculosis; Figure 16.3), often due to susceptibilty of follicles or colonization of nares or groins with pathogenic bacteria. Immunodeficiency is rarely the problem.

Complications
Cavernous sinus thrombosis is an unusual complication of boils on the central face. Septicaemia may occur but is rare.

Differential diagnosis
The diagnosis is straightforward but hidradenitis suppurativa (p. 169) should be considered if only the groin and axillae are involved.

Investigations in chronic furunculosis
- General examination: look for underlying skin disease (e.g. scabies, pediculosis, eczema).
- Test the urine for sugar. Full blood count.
- Culture swabs from lesions and carrier sites (nostrils, perineum) of the patient and immediate family. Test both to identify the organism and to evaluate sensitivity to various antibiotics.
- Immunological evaluation only if the patient has recurrent or unusual internal infections too.

Treatment
- Acute episodes will respond to simple incision and drainage. An appropriate systemic antibiotic is needed when many furuncles are erupting, when fever is present, or when the patient is immunosuppressed.
- In recurrent furunculosis, treat carrier sites such as the nose twice daily for the first 5 days of each month with an appropriate topical antiseptic or antibiotic (e.g. mupirocin cream or fusidic acid ointment) to try to eliminate

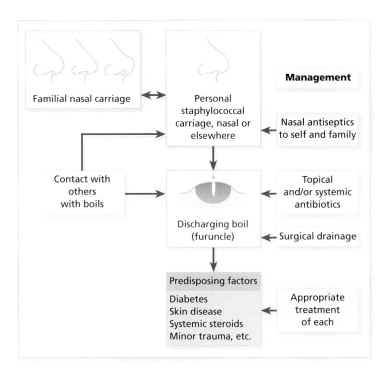

Figure 16.3 Chronic furunculosis.

staphylococcal carriage. A 10-day course of rifampicin may also help eradicate carriage. Treat family carriers in the same way.

• In stubborn chronic cases long-term treatment with sequential topical and systemic antibiotics chosen to cover organism's proven sensitivities will be needed.
• Daily bath using an antiseptic soap.
• Improve hygiene and nutritional state, if faulty.

Carbuncle

A group of adjacent hair follicles becomes deeply infected with *Staphylococcus aureus*, leading to a swollen painful suppurating area discharging pus from several points. The pain and systemic upset are greater than those of a boil. Diabetes must be excluded. Treatment needs both topical and systemic antibiotics. Incision and drainage has been shown to speed up healing, although it is not always easy when there are multiple deep pus-filled pockets. Consider the possibility of a fungal kerion (p. 241) in unresponsive carbuncles.

Scalded skin syndrome

In this condition the skin changes resemble a scald. Erythema and tenderness are followed by the loosening of large areas of overlying epidermis (Figure 16.4). In children the condition is usually caused by a toxin produced by staphylococcal infection elsewhere (e.g. impetigo or conjunctivitis). Organisms in what may be only a minor local infection release exfoliative toxins that cleave the

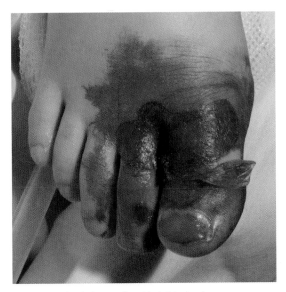

Figure 16.4 Staphylococcal scalded skin syndrome.

superficial skin adhesion molecule desmoglein 1 (p. 8) to disrupt adhesion high in the epidermis, causing the stratum corneum to slough off. With systemic antibiotics the outlook is good. The disorder affects children and patients with renal failure; most adults have antibodies to the toxin, and therefore are protected. In adults with widespread exfoliation, consider toxic epidermal necrolysis, which is usually drug-induced. The damage to the epidermis in toxic epidermal necrolysis is full thickness, and a skin biopsy will distinguish it from the scalded skin syndrome (p. 121).

Toxic shock syndrome

Bacterial toxins are also responsible for this condition, in which fever, a rash – usually a widespread erythema – and sometimes circulatory collapse are followed a week or two later by characteristic desquamation, most marked on the fingers and hands. Many cases have followed staphylococcal overgrowth in the vagina of women using tampons, although group A streptococci can also be responsible. The bacterial toxins act as superantigens, directly stimulating T cells and causing massive cytokine release. Systemic antibiotics and irrigation of the infected site are needed. Intravenous immunoglobulin may neutralize superantigen and reduce tissue damage.

Learning points

1 Look for head lice in the patient with recurrent impetigo of the head and neck.
2 The skin changes of the scalded skin syndrome, and of the toxic shock syndrome, are caused by staphylococcal exotoxins. Look for the primary infection elsewhere.

Streptococcal infections

Erysipelas

Erysipelas is an acute infection of the dermis or hypodermis. The first warning of an attack is often malaise, shivering and a fever. After a few hours the affected area of skin becomes red, and the eruption spreads with a well-defined advancing edge. Blisters may develop on the red plaques (Figure 16.5). Untreated, the condition can even be fatal, but it responds rapidly to systemic penicillin, sometimes given intravenously. The causative streptococci usually gain their entry through a split in the skin (e.g. between the toes or under an ear lobe).

Treatment of erysipelas should include antibiotics active against streptococci, usually penicillin. The choice

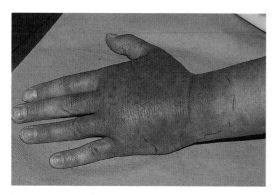

Figure 16.5 Erysipelas – note sharp spreading edge, here demarcated with a ballpoint pen.

of oral or parenteral route is dictated by the severity of the infection. Recurrence occurs in up to 20% of erysipelas patients.

Learning points

1 Unlike lightning, erysipelas often strikes in the same place twice.
2 Shivering and malaise precede the rash – and that is when the penicillin should be given.
3 Recurrent bouts may need long-term prophylactic penicillin.

Cellulitis

This inflammation of the skin occurs at a deeper level than erysipelas. The subcutaneous tissues are involved; and the area is more raised and swollen, and the erythema less marginated than in erysipelas. Cellulitis often follows an injury and favours areas of hypostatic oedema. Streptococci, staphylococci, or other organisms may be the cause. Treatment is elevation, rest – sometimes in hospital – and systemic antibiotics, sometimes given intravenously and active against both staphylococci and streptococci. A combination of a macrolide with a streptogramin may be more effective than penicillins.

Toe web intertrigo and lymphoedema are risk factors for the development of both erysipelas and cellulitis, which in turn predispose patients to persistent lymphoedema. It is important to treat these underlying factors as well as the bacterial infection to reduce the risks of recurrence.

Necrotizing fasciitis

A mixture of pathogens, usually including streptococci and anaerobes, is responsible for this rare condition, which is a surgical emergency. Diabetics and post-surgical patients are predisposed. At first the infection resembles a dusky, often painful, cellulitis, but it quickly turns into an extending necrosis of the skin and subcutaneous tissues. Classically, the central area of skin involvement becomes anaesthetic due to cutaneous nerve damage. Hyponatraemia is often present and in a septic patient with clinical signs of soft tissue infection should arouse the doctor's suspicions. A deep 'stab' incision biopsy through the skin into the fascia may be necessary to establish the diagnosis and to obtain material for bacteriological culture. Computed tomography, or a magnetic resonance imaging (MRI) scan may help to establish how far the infection has spread. The prognosis is often poor despite early wide surgical debridement and prompt intravenous antibiotic administration, even when given before the bacteriological results are available.

Erysipeloid

It is convenient to mention this here, but the causative organism is *Erysipelothrix rhusiopathiae.* and not a streptococcus. This Gram-positive rod infects a wide range of animals, birds and fish. In humans, infections are most common in butchers, fishmongers and cooks, the organisms penetrating the skin after a prick from an infected bone. The disease has become less common with improvements in the animal handling industry. Infections are usually mild, and localized to the area around the inoculation site. The swollen purple area spreads slowly with a clear-cut advancing edge. With penicillin the condition clears quickly; without it, resolution takes several weeks.

Cat-scratch disease

The infective agent is the bacillus *Bartonella (Rochalimea) henselae.* A few days after a cat bite or scratch, a reddish granulomatous papule appears at the site of inoculation. Tender regional lymphadenopathy follows some weeks later, and lasts for several weeks, often being accompanied by a mild fever. The glands may discharge before settling spontaneously. There is no specific treatment. In immunosuppressed patients, most commonly those with HIV, *Bartonella henselae* causes bacillary angiomatosis (p. 237).

Meningococcal infection

Neisseria meningitides is a Gram-negative coccus that commonly colonizes the upper respiratory tract. Usually, it is only responsible for local infections such as conjunctivitis, but for unknown reasons it may rarely become invasive and cause a severe and life-threatening disease. Meningitis and septicaemia are not always easy to recognize in their early stages when their symptoms can be very similar to common illnesses such as influenza. The signs and symptoms do not appear in any order and some may not appear at all. Acute meningococcal septicaemia can present as a fulminating disease with septic shock and meningitis or more non-specifically with rigors, leg pain, headache, stiff neck, vomiting and pallor. A haemorrhagic rash with petechiae and then purpura (with no blanching or change on diascopy), found mainly on the trunk and limbs, is characteristic. An unwell feverish child with these skin signs should considered highly likely to have meningococcal disease. Diagnosis is confirmed by the isolation of *N. meningitidis* from blood or cerebrospinal fluid, but treatment with high dose intravenous benzyl-penicillin should be started as soon as the diagnosis is suspected. Rifampicin prophylaxis can be used for close contacts. Trust your instincts, if you suspect meningitis or septicaemia and seek hospital help immediately.

Learning point

Trust your instincts, if you suspect meningitis or septicaemia and seek hospital help **immediately**.

Spirochaetal infections

Syphilis

Cause

Infection with the causative organism, *Treponema pallidum*, may be congenital, acquired through transfusion with contaminated blood or by accidental inoculation. The most important route, however, is through sexual contact with an infected partner, and the incidence is currently rising, with concurrent HIV infection.

Presentation

Congenital syphilis. If there is a high standard of antenatal care and testing, syphilis in the mother will be detected and treated during pregnancy, and congenital syphilis will be rare. Otherwise, stillbirth is a common outcome, although some children with congenital syphilis may develop the stigmata of the disease only in late childhood.

Acquired syphilis. The features of the different stages are given in Figure 16.6. After an incubation period (9–90 days), a primary chancre develops at the site of inoculation. Often this is genital, but oral and anal chancres are not uncommon. A typical chancre is a painless button-like

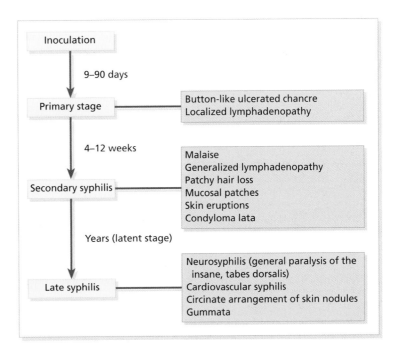

Figure 16.6 The stages of syphilis.

ulcer of up to 1 cm in diameter accompanied by local lymphadenopathy. Untreated it lasts about 6 weeks and then clears leaving an inconspicuous scar.

The secondary stage may be reached while the chancre is still subsiding. Systemic symptoms and a generalized lymphadenopathy usher in eruptions that at first are macules and inconspicuous, and later papules and more obvious. Lesions are distributed symmetrically and are of a coppery ham colour. Sometimes they resemble pityriasis rosea or guttate psoriasis. Classically, there are obvious lesions on the palms and soles. Annular lesions are not uncommon. Condyloma lata are moist papules in the genital and anal areas. Other signs include a 'moth-eaten' alopecia and mucous patches in the mouth.

The skin lesions of late syphilis may be nodules that spread peripherally and clear centrally, leaving a serpiginous outline. Gummas are granulomatous areas; in the skin they quickly break down to leave punched-out ulcers that heal poorly, leaving papery white scars.

Clinical course

Even if left untreated, most of those who contract syphilis have no further problems after the secondary stage has passed. Others develop the cutaneous or systemic manifestations of late syphilis such as gummas and dementia.

Differential diagnosis

The skin changes of syphilis can mimic many other skin diseases. Always consider the following.
1 *Chancre:* chancroid (multiple and painful), herpes simplex, anal fissure, cervical erosions.
2 *Secondary syphilis:*
  • Eruption: measles, rubella, drug eruptions, pityriasis rosea, lichen planus, psoriasis;
  • Condylomas: genital warts, haemorrhoids;
  • Oral lesions: aphthous ulcers, candidiasis;
  • Alopecia: tinea, trichotillomania, traction alopecia.
3 *Late syphilis:* bromide and iodide reactions, other granulomas, erythema induratum.

Investigations

The diagnosis of syphilis in its infectious (primary and secondary) stages has traditionally been confirmed using dark field microscopy to show up spirochaetes in smears from chancres, oral lesions or moist areas in a secondary eruption.

Serological tests for syphilis become positive only some 5–6 weeks after infection (usually a week or two after the appearance of the chancre). The non-treponemal (rapid

plasma reagin (RPR) and Venereal Disease Research Laboratory (VDRL)) tests are 78–86% sensitive in primary and 100% sensitive in secondary syphilis, but may produce false positive results. Positive results are thus confirmed with more specific treponemal tests such as the fluorescent treponemal antibody/absorption (FTA/ABS) and *T. pallidum* particle agglutination (TPPA) tests, although HIV infection may cause false negative results. Serological tests may not become negative after treatment if an infection has been present for more than a few months and thus cannot be relied on to differentiate between and active and successfully treated infections.

Patients with syphilis should be screened for concurrent sexually transmitted infections, including gonorrhoea and HIV.

Treatment

This should follow the current national recommendations (see www.guidelines.gov) Penicillin is still the treatment of choice. Procaine penicillin is given parenterally for 10 days in early syphilis and 17 days in late stage disease or in early syphilis with neurological involvement. Benzithine penicillin can be given as a single intramuscular dose in primary or secondary syphilis. Doxycycline for 14 days or azithromycin for 10 days are alternatives for those with penicillin allergy. Patients with concomitant HIV infection need longer treatment and higher doses. Lumbar puncture is indicated in later stages as a guide to treatment. The use of long-acting penicillin injections overcomes the ever-present danger of poor compliance with oral treatment. Every effort must be made to trace and treat infected contacts.

Learning points

1 Syphilis is still around. Remember that today's general was yesterday's lieutenant.
2 It is still worth checking for syphilis in perplexing rashes.

Yaws

Yaws is distributed widely across the poorer parts of the tropics. The spirochaete, *Treponema pallidum* ssp. *pertenue*, gains its entry through skin abrasions. After an incubation period of up to 6 months, the primary lesion, a crusting and ulcerated papule known as the 'mother yaw', develops at the site of inoculation; later it may enlarge to an exuberant raspberry-like swelling which lasts for several months before healing to leave an atrophic pale scar. In the secondary stage, other lesions may develop in any area but do so especially around the orifices. They are not unlike the primary lesion but are smaller and more numerous ('daughter yaws'). Hyperkeratotic plaques may appear on the palms and soles. The tertiary stage is characterized by ulcerated gummatous skin lesions, hyperkeratosis of the palms and soles, and a painful periostitis that distorts the long bones. Serological tests for syphilis are positive. Treatment is with penicillin.

Lyme disease

The spirochaete *Borrelia burgdorferi* is responsible for this condition, named after the town in the United States where it was first recognized. It is transmitted to humans by ticks of the genus *Ixodes*, commonly harboured by deer. Ticks need to remain attached to the skin for 1 or 2 days to be able to effectively pass the infection on. The site of the tick bite becomes the centre of a slowly expanding erythematous ring (*erythema migrans*; Figure 16.7). Later, many annular non-scaly plaques may develop. In the United States, a few of those affected develop arthritis and heart disease, both of which are less common in European cases. Other internal complications include meningitis and cranial nerve palsies. Treated early, the condition clears well with a 21-day course of oral amoxicillin or doxycycline: patients affected systemically need longer courses of parenteral antibiotics. Infection may be confirmed by serology, although this is usually negative in the first few weeks after inoculation and individuals living in endemic areas can have positive serologic tests, probably as a result of minor infection that resolved spontaneously. Serial testing can sometimes help to sort this out in patients with atypical rash.

Other infections

Cutaneous anthrax

This condition is usually acquired through contact with infected livestock or animal products such as wool or bristles. Previously rare in industrialized countries, its importance increased after the infectious agent was used in the United States for a bioterrorism attack.

Anthrax has two main clinical variants: the often fatal inhalational anthrax, which is outside the scope of this book; and cutaneous anthrax. The incubation period of the latter is usually 2–5 days. A skin lesion then appears on an exposed part, often in association with a variable degree of cutaneous oedema, which can sometimes be massive, especially on the face. Within a day or two, the original small painless papule shows vesicles that quickly coalesce into a larger single blister. This ruptures to form an ulcer with a central dark eschar, which falls off after 1–2 weeks leaving a scar. The skin lesions are often accompanied by fever, headache, myalgia and regional lymphadenopathy. The mortality rate for untreated cutaneous anthrax is up to 20%; with appropriate antibiotic treatment, this falls to less than 1%.

Cultures of material taken from the vesicle may be positive in 12–48 hours; a Gram stain will show Gram-positive bacilli, occurring singly or in short chains. Quicker results may be obtained by a direct fluorescence antibody test, or by an enzyme-linked immunoabsorbant assay (ELISA) – both of which are currently available only at reference laboratories. Before the results are available, it is wise to assume that the organism is penicillin- and tetracycline-resistant, and to start treatment with ciprofloxacin at 400 mg intravenously every 12 hours or, for milder cases, ciprofloxacin 500 mg orally every 12 hours. The latter dose is suitable for prophylactic use in those who are known to have been exposed to spores. A switch to an alternative regimen can be made once the antibiotic sensitivity of the organism has been established. At present, anthrax vaccine is in short supply; it requires six injections over 18 months, with subsequent boosters, to prevent anthrax. The spores of *Bacillus anthracis*, the causative organism, are highly resistant to physical and chemical agents.

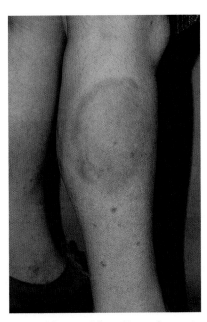

Figure 16.7 A tick bite was followed by erythema migrans.

Gonococcal septicaemia

Skin lesions are important clues to the diagnosis of this condition, in which the symptoms and signs of classic gonorrhoea are usually absent. The patient, usually a menstruating woman with recurring fever and joint pains, develops sparse crops of skin lesions, usually around the hands and feet. The grey, often haemorrhagic, vesicopustules are characteristic. Rather similar lesions are seen in chronic meningococcal septicaemia.

Mycobacterial infections

Tuberculosis

Most infections in the United Kingdom are caused by *Mycobacterium tuberculosis*. *Mycobacterium bovis* infection, endemic in cattle, can be spread to humans by milk, but human infection with this organism is now rare in countries where cattle have been vaccinated against tuberculosis and the milk is pasteurized. The steady decline of tuberculosis in developed countries has been reversed in some areas where AIDS is especially prevalent. Dormant tuberculosis of the skin can also be reactivated by systemic corticosteroids, immunosuppressants and anti-tumour necrosis factor biological agents.

Inoculation tuberculosis

Inocculation into skin causes a wart-like lesion at the site. Systemic spread to the skin (lupus vulgaris; Figure 16.8) can follow from an underlying infected lymph node or from a pulmonary lesion. Lesions occur most often around the head and neck. A reddish-brown scaly plaque slowly enlarges, and can damage deeper tissues such as cartilage, leading to ugly mutilation. Scarring and contractures may follow.

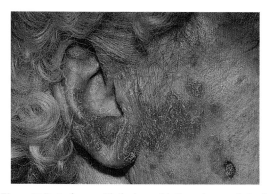

Figure 16.8 A plaque with the brownish tinge characteristic of lupus vulgaris. Diascopy was positive.

Diascopy (p. 36) shows up the characteristic brownish 'apple jelly' nodules. The clinical diagnosis should be confirmed by a biopsy.

Scrofuloderma

The skin overlying a tuberculous lymph node or joint may become involved in the process. The subsequent mixture of lesions (irregular puckered scars, fistulae and abscesses) is most commonly seen in the neck.

Tuberculides

A number of granulomatous skin eruptions have, in the past, been attributed to a reaction to internal foci of tuberculosis. Of these, the best authenticated – by finding mycobacterial DNA by polymerase chain reaction (PCR) – are the *papulonecrotic tuberculides* – recurring crops of firm dusky papules, which may ulcerate, favouring the points of the knees and elbows. Most tuberculosis-like granulomas of the face are forms of granulomatous rosacea.

Erythema induratum (Bazin's disease)

In erythema induratum, deep purplish ulcerating nodules occur on the backs of the lower legs, usually in women with a poor 'chilblain' type of circulation. Sometimes, this is associated with a tuberculous focus elsewhere. Erythema nodosum (p. 107) may also be the result of tuberculosis elsewhere.

Investigations

Biopsy for:
- Microscopy (tuberculoid granulomas);
- Bacteriological culture; and
- Detection of mycobacterial DNA by PCR.
- Mantoux test.
- Chest X-ray

Treatment

The treatment of all types of cutaneous tuberculosis should be with a full course of a standard multidrug anti-tuberculosis regimen. There is no longer any excuse for the use of one drug alone.

Prevention

Outbreaks of pulmonary tuberculosis are reminders that this disease has not yet been conquered and that vigilance is important. Bacillus Calmette–Guérin (BCG) vaccination of schoolchildren, immunization of cattle and pasteurization of milk remain the most effective protective measures.

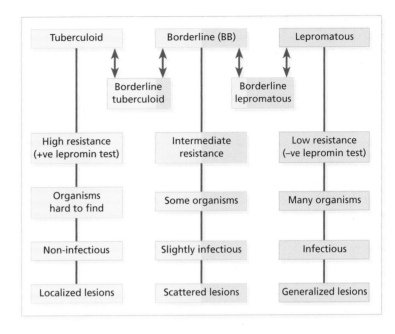

Figure 16.9 The spectrum of leprosy: tuberculoid to lepromatous.

Leprosy

Cause

Mycobacterium leprae was discovered by Hansen in 1873, but has still not been cultured *in vitro*, although it can be made to grow in some animals (e.g. armadillos, mouse foot-pads). In humans, the main route of infection is through nasal droplets from cases of lepromatous leprosy.

Epidemiology

Leprosy is present in around 120 countries worldwide, particularly in the tropics and subtropics with hotspots in central Africa, parts of Asia and Brazil. The World Health Organization's aim to eliminate (i.e. have less than 1 registered case per 10 000 population) the disease worldwide by 2000 has not been met, but the incidence is slowly falling, and less than a quarter of a million new diagnoses are made each year. The incubation period is usually 3–5 years, although it can be up to 20 years.

Presentation

The range of clinical manifestations and complications depends upon the immune response of the patient (Figure 16.9). Those with a strong cell-mediated immune response develop a paucibacillary tuberculoid type (Figure 16.10) and those with a poor response a multibacillary lepromatous type. Lymphocytic infiltration leads to earlier nerve thickening and damage in the tuber-

culoid than lepromatous disease (Figure 16.11). A few hypopigmented, discrete macules are found. Widespread haematogenous spread occurs in lepromatous leprosy. Some patients develop macular lepromatous leprosy with widespread hypopigmented macules. In the nodular form of lepromatous leprosy, patients develop nodules, loss of

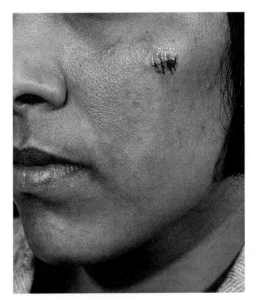

Figure 16.10 Tuberculoid leprosy: subtle depigmentation with a palpable erythematous rim at the upper edge.

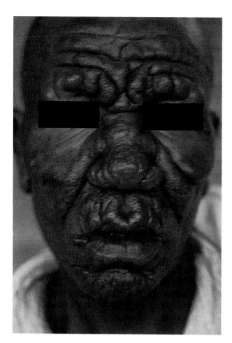

Figure 16.11 The 'leonine' facies of lepromatous leprosy.

eyebrows and the corrugated facial appearance known as leonine facies. Between the extremes lies a spectrum of reactions classified as 'borderline'. Those most like the tuberculoid type are known as borderline tuberculoid (BT) and those nearest to the lepromatous type as borderline lepromatous (BL). The clinical differences between the two polar types are given in Figure 16.12.

Differential diagnosis

Tuberculoid leprosy. Consider the following – in none of which is there any loss of sensation.
• Vitiligo (p. 271) – loss of pigment is usually complete.
• Pityriasis versicolor (p. 245) – scrapings show mycelia and spores.
• Pityriasis alba – a common cause of scaly hypopigmented areas on the cheeks of children.
• Post-inflammatory depigmentation of any cause.
• Sarcoidosis, granuloma annulare, necrobiosis lipoidica.

Lepromatous leprosy. Widespread leishmaniasis can closely simulate lepromatous leprosy. The nodules seen in neurofibromatosis and mycosis fungoides, and multiple sebaceous cysts, can cause confusion, as can the acral deformities seen in yaws and systemic sclerosis. Leprosy is a great imitator.

Diagnosis

In endemic countries, diagnosis is based on the clinical findings of typical skin lesions of leprosy in association with anaesthetic patches and possibly thickened nerves with demonstrable loss of function, combined with positive slit skin smears. Histology from a skin or nerve biopsy and PCR examination for *M. leprae* DNA in biopsy material can help the diagnosis, but these investigations are not often available in resource-poor countries, where leprosy mostly occurs.

Slit skin smears are taken from six sites at cool parts of the body (e.g. ear lobes, buttocks, forehead). Cuts are made 5 mm long by 3 mm deep, and scraped with the scalpel blade sideways. The scrapings are stained with a modified Ziehl–Neelsen stain, and the number of bacteria counted to determine whether the patient has multibacillary or paucibacillary leprosy.

Lepromin testing is of no use in the diagnosis of leprosy but, once the diagnosis has been made, it will help in deciding which type of disease is present (positive in tuberculoid type).

Treatment

The development of resistance to single agent treatment with dapsone means that multidrug therapy (MDT) is now offered free to all patients with leprosy by the World Health Organization. Patients with multibacillary leprosy are treated with 12 months of rifampicin, dapsone and clofazimine. Those with paucibacillary disease receive 6 months of rifampicin and dapsone. A brief period of isolation is needed only for patients with infectious lepromatous leprosy; with treatment they quickly become non-infectious and can return to the community. However, their management should remain in the hands of physicians with a special interest in the disease. Treating lepra reactions and reducing nerve damage is an important part of leprosy treatment as is teaching patients to cope with the results of nerve damage and anaesthesia.

Special care is needed with the two types of lepra reaction that can occur during treatment:
• Type 1 (reversal) reactions are delayed-type hypersensitivity reactions which are seen mainly in borderline tuberculoid disease (Figure 16.13). Lesions become red and angry, and pain and paralysis follow neural inflammation. Treatment is with analgesics such as aspirin and paracetamol and reducing courses of oral steroids. Treatment for the underlying leprosy should be continued and the limbs splinted if necessary to prevent further damage.

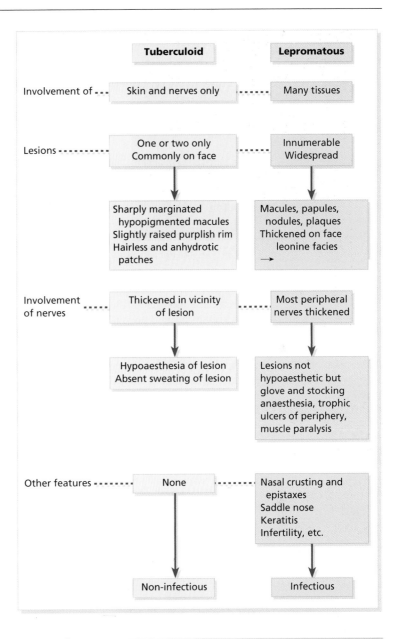

Figure 16.12 Tuberculoid and lepromatous leprosy.

• Type 2 reactions (erythema nodosum leprosum) are common in lepromatous leprosy and include erythema nodosum, nerve palsies, lymphadenopathy, arthritis, iridocyclitis, epididymo-orchitis and proteinuria. They are treated with the drugs used for type 1 reactions, and also with increased doses of clofazimine and with thalidomide.

The household contacts of lepromatous patients are at risk of developing leprosy and should be followed up. Child contacts may benefit from prophylactic therapy and BCG inoculation.

Other mycobacterial infections

Mycobacteria are widespread in nature, living as environmental saprophytes. Some can infect humans.

Mycobacterium marinum

Mycobacterium marinum lives in water. Human infections have occurred in epidemics centred on infected swimming pools. Another route of infection is through

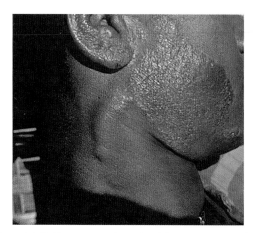

Figure 16.13 Type 1 reversal reaction. The posterior auricular nerve is grossly swollen.

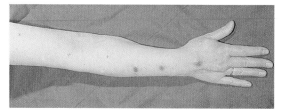

Figure 16.15 The sporotrichoid spread of an atypical mycobacterial infection.

minor skin breaches in those who clean out tropical fish tanks (Figure 16.14). After a 3-week incubation period, an indolent abscess or ulcerated nodule forms at the site of inoculation; later nodules may develop along the draining lymphatics (sporotrichoid spread; Figures 16.15 and p. 247). The lesions heal spontaneously, but slowly. Resolution may be speeded by an 8-week course of co-trimoxazole or minocycline. Should these fail, rifampicin in combination with ethambutol is worth a trial.

Mycobacterium ulcerans

Infections are confined to certain humid tropical areas where the organism lives on the vegetation, and are most common in Uganda (Buruli ulcers). The necrotic spreading ulcers, with their undermined edges, are usually found on the legs. Drug therapy is often disappointing and the

treatment of choice is probably the surgical removal of infected tissue.

Leishmaniasis

Leishmania organisms are protozoa whose life cycle includes stages in phlebotomus flies, from which they are transmitted to humans as the sandflies feed from the superficial vascular plexus. In the dermis the promastigotes infect macrophages, and the success or otherwise of the immune response to this determines whether disease develops, and how extensive it is. Different species, in different geographical areas, have different mammalian reservoirs and cause different clinical pictures. Children are mostly affected and primary disease usually affects skin of exposed sites such as the face.

• *Leishmania tropica* is found around the Mediterranean coast and in southern Asia; it causes chronically discharging skin nodules (oriental sores; Figure 16.16). It can persist as leishmaniasis recidivans.

• *Leishmania major* occurs in the Middle East, northern India and north Africa. After an incubation period of several weeks, a nodule forms at the site of infection, which crusts, ulcerates and then heals with scarring over several months.

• *Leishmania aethiopica* occurs in the horn of Africa. It causes localized cutaneous leishmaniasis, but can also cause the destructive mucocutaneous disease and also

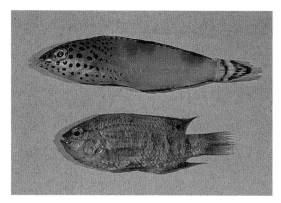

Figure 16.14 Dead tropical fish picked out of the tank by the patient shown in Figure 16.15.

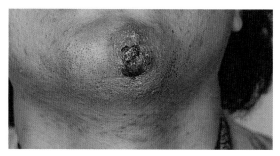

Figure 16.16 Leishmaniasis acquired in the Middle East.

diffuse cutaneous leishmaniasis, in which slow spead of heavily infected cutaneous nodules occurs.

• *Leishmania donovani* causes kala azar, a disease characterized by fever, hepatosplenomegaly and anaemia. The skin may show an irregular darkening, particularly on the face and hands.

• *Leishmania mexicana* and *braziliensis* are found in Central and South America. They also cause deep sores, but up to 40% of those infected with *L. braziliensis* develop 'episodic' destructive metastatic lesions in the mucosa of the nose or month.

Diagnosis

This is confirmed by:

• Histology – amastigote parasites, granulomatous reaction;
• Slit skin smears (as for leprosy) – amastigote parasites;
• Culture; and
• PCR tests.

Treatment

The aims of treatment are to accerate healing, and thus avoid disfiguring scars, and in New World leishmaniasis and *L. aethiopica* to prevent metastatic spread to the oropharynx which would result in mucocutaneous disease. Single nodules often resolve spontaneously and may not need treatment. Destructive measures, including cryotherapy, are sometimes used for localized skin lesions as are intralesional antimony compounds.

Intravenous antimony compounds are still the treatment of choice for most types of leishmaniasis (e.g. sodium stibogluconate or meglumine antimoniate; Formulary 2, p. 415) with regular blood tests and electrocardiographic monitoring.

Viral infections

The viral infections dealt with here are those that are commonly seen in dermatology clinics. A textbook of infectious diseases should be consulted for details of systemic viral infections, many of which, like measles and German measles, have their own specific rashes.

Viral warts

Most people will have a wart at some time in their lives. Their prevalence is highest in childhood, and they affect an estimated 4–5% of schoolchildren in the United Kingdom.

Cause

Warts are caused by the human papilloma virus (HPV), which has still not been cultured *in vitro*. Nevertheless, more than 70 'types' of the virus are now recognized by DNA sequencing; each has its own range of clinical manifestations. HPV-1, 2 and 4, for example, are found in common warts, whereas HPV-3 is found in plane warts, and HPV-6, 11, 16 and 18 are most common in genital warts. Infections occur when wart virus in skin scales comes into contact with breaches in the skin or mucous membranes or when immunity is suppressed and dormant viruses escape from their resting place in the outer root sheaths of hairs.

Presentation

Warts adopt a variety of patterns (Figure 16.17), some of which are described here.

Common warts (Figures 16.18 and 16.19). The first sign is a smooth skin-coloured papule, often more easily felt than seen. As the lesion enlarges, its irregular hyperkeratotic surface and vertical shoulders give it the classic 'warty' appearance. Common warts usually occur on the hands but are also often on the face and genitals. They are more often multiple than single. Pain is rare.

Plantar warts. These have a rough surface, which protrudes only slightly from the skin and is surrounded by

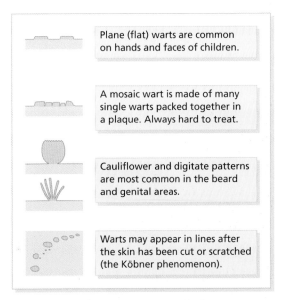

Plane (flat) warts are common on hands and faces of children.

A mosaic wart is made of many single warts packed together in a plaque. Always hard to treat.

Cauliflower and digitate patterns are most common in the beard and genital areas.

Warts may appear in lines after the skin has been cut or scratched (the Köbner phenomenon).

Figure 16.17 Viral warts – variations on the theme.

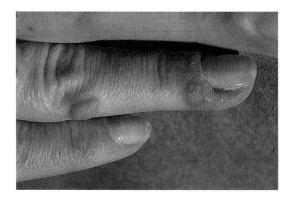

Figure 16.18 Typical common warts on the fingers.

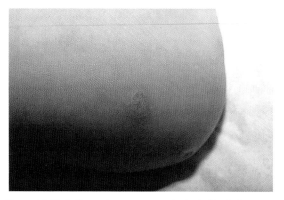

Figure 16.20 Solitary plantar wart on the heel. (Dr E.C. Benton. Reproduced with permission of Dr E.C. Benton.)

a horny collar (Figure 16.20). On paring, the presence of bleeding capillary loops allows plantar warts to be distinguished from corns. Often multiple, plantar warts can be painful.

Mosaic warts (Figure 16.21). These rough marginated plaques are made up of many small tightly packed but discrete individual warts. They are most common on the soles but are also seen on palms and around fingernails. Usually, they are not painful.

Plane warts (Figure 16.22). These smooth flat-topped papules are most common on the face and brow, on the backs of the hands, and on the shaven legs of women. Usually skin-coloured or light brown, they become inflamed as a result of an immunological reaction, just before they resolve spontaneously. Lesions are multiple, painless and, like common warts, are sometimes arranged along a scratch line.

Facial warts. These are most common in the beard area of adult males and are spread by shaving. A digitate appearance is common. Lesions are often ugly but are painless.

Anogenital warts (condyloma acuminata) (Figure 16.23). Papillomatous cauliflower-like lesions, with a moist macerated vascular surface, can appear anywhere in this area. They may coalesce to form huge fungating plagues causing discomfort and irritation. The vaginal and anorectal mucosae may be affected. The presence of anogenital warts in children raises the spectre of sexual abuse, but is usually caused by autoinoculation from common warts elsewhere.

Course

Warts resolve spontaneously in the healthy as the immune response overcomes the infection. This happens within

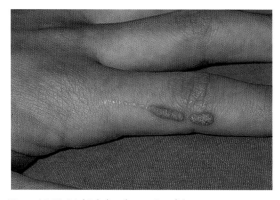

Figure 16.19 Multiple hand warts in a fishmonger.

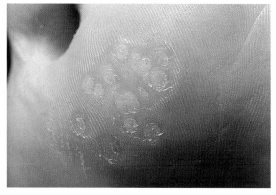

Figure 16.21 Group of warts under the forefoot pared to show mosaic pattern.

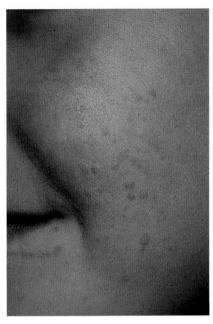

Figure 16.22 Plane warts resolving with inflammation.

6 months in some 30% of patients, and within 2 years in 65%. Such spontaneous resolution, sometimes heralded by a punctate blackening caused by capillary thrombosis (Figure 16.24), leaves no trace. Mosaic warts are notoriously slow to resolve and often resist all treatments. Warts persist and spread in immunocompromised patients (e.g. those on immunosuppressive therapy or with lymphoreticular disease). Seventy per cent of renal allograft recipients will have warts 5 years after transplantation.

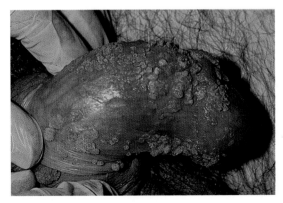

Figure 16.23 Multiple penile warts in an immunosuppressed patient.

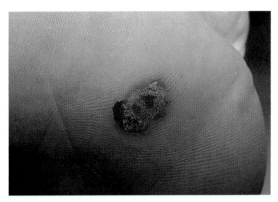

Figure 16.24 Spontaneous resolution of a group of plantar warts. The blackness is caused by capillary thrombosis.

Complications
1 Some plantar warts are very painful.
2 Epidermodysplasia verruciformis is a rare inherited disorder in which there is a universal wart infection, usually with HPV of unusual types. An impairment of cell-mediated immunity (p. 25) is commonly found and ensuing carcinomatous change frequently occurs.
3 Malignant change is otherwise rare, although infection with HPV types 16 and 18 predisposes to cervical carcinoma. HPV infections in immunocompromised patients (e.g. renal allograft recipients) have also been linked with skin cancer, especially on light-exposed areas.

Differential diagnosis
Most warts are easily recognized. The following must be ruled out.
• *Molluscum contagiosum* (p. 234) are smooth, dome-shaped and pearly, with central umbilication.
• *Plantar corns* are found on pressure areas; there is no capillary bleeding on paring. They have a central keratotic core and are painful.
• *Granuloma annulare* lesions (p. 312) have a smooth surface, as the lesions are dermal, and their outline is often annular.
• *Condyloma lata* are seen in syphilis. They are rare but should not be confused with condyloma acuminata (warts). The lesions are flatter, greyer and less well defined. If in doubt, look for other signs of secondary syphilis (p. 220) and carry out serological tests.
• *Amelanotic melanomas, squamous cell carcinomas and other epithelial malignancies* can present as verrucose nodules – those in patients over the age of 40 years should be examined with special care as mistakes have been made in the past.

Treatment

Many warts give no trouble, need no treatment and go away by themselves. Otherwise, treatment will depend on the type of wart. In general terms, destruction by cryotherapy is less likely to cause scars than excision or electrosurgery.

Palmoplantar warts

Regression of warts and prevention of their recurrence depends on establishment of cell-mediated immunity. Both induction of immunity and elicitation of cytotoxic responses are hindered by the insulation of wart virus in relatively inaccessible upper epidermis. Irritating the warts or 'blowing them up' with cryotherapy helps induce immunity by bringing wart virus and immune cells together.

For now, home treatment is best, with one of the many wart paints or plasters now available (Formulary 1, p. 401). Most contain salicylic acid (12–20%). The success rate is good if the patient is prepared to persist with regular treatment. Paints should be applied once daily, after moistening the warts in hot water for at least 5 minutes. After drying, dead tissue and old paint are removed with an emery board or pumice stone. Enough paint to cover the surface of the wart, but not the surrounding skin, is applied and allowed to dry. Warts on the plantar surface should be covered with plasters although this is not necessary elsewhere. Side effects are rare if these instructions are followed. Wart paints should not be applied to facial or anogenital skin, or to patients with adjacent eczema.

If no progress is being made after the regular and correct use of a salicylic acid wart paint for 12 weeks, then a paint containing formaldehyde or glutaraldehyde is worth trying. A useful way of dealing with multiple small plantar warts is for the area to be soaked for 10 minutes each night in a 4% formalin solution, although a few patients become allergic to this.

Cryotherapy with liquid nitrogen (at −196°C) is more effective than the less cold, dry ice or dimethyl ether/propane techniques. However, it is painful. The wart is sprayed with liquid nitrogen until a small frozen halo appears in the surrounding normal skin (Figure 16.25). The use of two freeze–thaw cycles increases the clearance rate of plantar warts but not of hand warts. If further treatments are necessary, the optimal interval is 3 weeks. The cure rate is higher if plantar warts are pared before they are frozen, but this makes no difference to warts elsewhere. If there has been no improvement after four or five treatments there is little to be gained from further freezings.

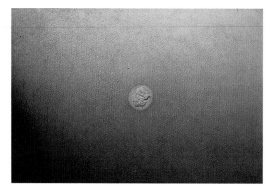

Figure 16.25 A wart treated with cryotherapy: area includes a small frozen halo of normal surrounding skin.

A few minutes tuition from a dermatologist will help practitioners wishing to start cryotherapy. Blisters should not be provoked intentionally, but occur from time to time, and will not alarm patients who have been forewarned.

Anogenital warts

Two vaccines, a bivalent one against the high risk HPV-16 and 18 and a quadrivalent vaccine which is also effective against HPV-6 and 11 are now available. These are now part of the standard vaccination protocol for young women in many countries and have resulted in a marked fall in new cases of anogenital warts. More importantly, rates of cervical cancer should also fall with the removal of the main risk factor for this devastating disease.

Women with anogenital warts, or who are the partners of men with anogenital warts, should have their cervical cytology checked regularly as the wart virus can cause cervical cancer.

The focus has shifted towards self-treatment using podophyllotoxin (0.5% solution or 0.15% cream) or imiquimod (5% cream). Both are irritants and should be used carefully according to the manufacturer's instructions. Imiquimod is an immune response modifier that induces keratinocytes to produce cytokines, leading to wart regression, and may help to build cell-mediated immunity for long-lasting protection. It is applied as a thin layer three times weekly and washed off with a mild soap 6–10 hours after application. Podophyllin paint (15%) is used much less often now. It should be applied carefully to the warts and allowed to dry before powdering with talcum. On the first occasion it should be washed off with soap and water after 2 hours but, if there has been little discomfort, this can be increased stepwise to 6 hours.

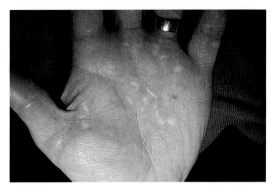

Figure 16.26 Multiple scars following the injudicious surgical treatment of warts.

Treatment is best carried out weekly by a doctor or nurse, but not by the patient. Podophyllin must not be used in pregnancy. Cryotherapy, electrosurgery and laser treatment are all effective treatments in the clinic.

Facial common warts
These are best treated with electrocautery or a hyfrecator but also surrender to careful cryotherapy. Scarring is an unwanted complication. Shaving, if essential, should be with a brushless foam and a disposable razor.

Plane warts
On the face these are best left untreated and the patient or parent can be reasonably assured that spontaneous resolution will occur. When treatment is demanded, the use of a wart paint, tretinoin gel or imiquimod cream is reasonable. Gentle cryotherapy of just a few warts may help to induce immunity.

Solitary, stubborn or painful warts
These can be removed under local anaesthetic with a curette, although cure is not assured with this or any other method, and a scar often follows. Surgical excision is never justifiable (Figure 16.26). Bleomycin can also be injected into such warts with success but this treatment should only be undertaken by a specialist.

Learning points

1 Do not hurt children by using cryotherapy without a good trial of a wart paint first.
2 Treat most common warts with a wart paint for 12 weeks before referring.
3 Do not leave scars; nature does not.
4 Avoid podophyllin during pregnancy.
5 Do not miss an amelanotic malignant melanoma.

Varicella (chickenpox)

Cause
The herpes virus varicella-zoster is spread by the respiratory route; its incubation period is about 14 days.

Presentation and course
Slight malaise is followed by the development of papules, which turn rapidly into clear vesicles on a pink base ('dew drops on a rose petal'). Vesicles soon become pustules and then umbilicate. Over the next few days the lesions crust and then clear, sometimes leaving white depressed scars. Lesions appear in crops, are often itchy and are most profuse on the trunk and least profuse on the periphery of the limbs (centripetal). Second attacks are rare. Varicella can be fatal in those who are immunologically compromised.

Complications
• Pneumonitis, with pulmonary opacities on X-ray.
• Secondary infection of skin lesions.
• Haemorrhagic or lethal chickenpox in patients with leukaemia and other immunocompromised children and adults.
• Scarring.

Differential diagnosis
Smallpox, mainly centrifugal anyway, has been universally eradicated, and the diagnosis of chickenpox is seldom in doubt.

Investigations
None are usually needed. The Tzanck smear (p. 38) is positive.

Treatment
Aciclovir, famciclovir and valaciclovir (Formulary 2, p. 415) should be reserved for severe attacks and for immunocompromised patients; for the latter, prophylactic aciclovir can also be used to prevent disease if given within a day or two of exposure. In mild attacks, calamine lotion topically is all that is required. A live attenuated vaccine is now available, and being more widely used. It is not universally effective and should not be given to patients with immunodeficiencies, therapeutic immunosuppression, or blood dyscrasias who might not be able to resist even the attenuated organism.

Herpes zoster

Cause
Shingles too is caused by the herpes virus varicella-zoster. An attack is a result of the reactivation, usually for no

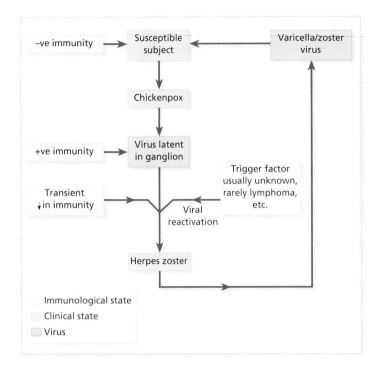

Figure 16.27 Zoster–varicella relationships.

obvious reason, of virus that has remained dormant in a sensory root ganglion since an earlier episode of chickenpox (varicella). The incidence of shingles is highest in old age, and in conditions such as Hodgkin's disease, AIDS and leukaemia, which weaken normal defence mechanisms. Shingles does not occur in epidemics; its clinical manifestations are caused by virus acquired in the past. However, patients with zoster can transmit the virus to others in whom it will cause chickenpox (Figure 16.27).

Presentation and course

Attacks usually start with a burning pain, soon followed by erythema and grouped, sometimes blood-filled, vesicles scattered over a dermatome. The clear vesicles quickly become purulent, and over the space of a few days burst and crust. Scabs usually separate in 2–3 weeks, sometimes leaving depressed depigmented scars.

Zoster is characteristically unilateral (Figure 16.28). It may affect more than one adjacent dermatome. The thoracic segments and the ophthalmic division of the trigeminal nerve are involved disproportionately often.

It is not uncommon for a few pock-like lesions to be found outside the main segment of involvement, but a generalized chickenpox-like eruption accompanying segmental zoster should raise suspicions of an underlying immunocompromised state or malignancy, particularly if the lesions are unusually haemorrhagic or necrotic.

Complications

- Secondary bacterial infection is common.
- Motor nerve involvement is uncommon, but has led to paralysis of ocular muscles, the facial muscles, the diaphragm and the bladder.
- Zoster of the ophthalmic division of the trigeminal nerve can lead to corneal ulcers and scarring. A good

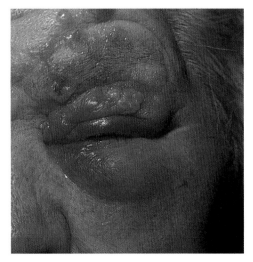

Figure 16.28 Herpes zoster of the left ophthalmic division of the trigeminal nerve. No nasociliary involvement (see text); this is reassuring.

clinical clue here is involvement of the nasociliary branch (vesicles grouped on the side of the nose).

• Persistent neuralgic pain, after the acute episode is over, is most common in the elderly.

Differential diagnosis

Occasionally, before the rash has appeared, the initial pain is taken for an emergency such as acute appendicitis or myocardial infarction. An early painful red plaque may suggest cellulitis until other plaques in the dermatome appear or until vesicles develop on their tops. Otherwise, the dermatomal distribution and the pain allow zoster to be distinguished easily from herpes simplex, eczema and impetigo.

Investigations

Cultures are of little help as they take 5–7 days, and are only positive in 70% of cases. Biopsy or Tzanck smears show multinucleated giant cells and a ballooning degeneration of keratinocytes, indicative of a herpes infection. Any clinical suspicions about underlying conditions, such as Hodgkin's disease, chronic lymphatic leukaemia or AIDS, require further investigation.

Treatment

Systemic treatment should be given to all patients if diagnosed in the early stages of the disease. It is essential that this treatment should start within the first 5 days of an attack. Famciclovir and valaciclovir are as effective as aciclovir (Formulary 2, p. 415) and more reliably absorbed; they depend on virus-specific thymidine kinase for their antiviral activity. All three drugs are safe, and using them early cuts down the chance of getting post-herpetic neuralgia, particularly in the elderly.

If diagnosed late in the course of the disease, systemic treatment is not likely to be effective and treatment should be supportive with rest, analgesics and bland applications such as calamine. Secondary bacterial infection should be treated appropriately.

A trial of systemic carbamazepine, gabapentin or amitriptyline, or 4 weeks of topical capsaicin cream (Formulary 1, p. 409), despite the burning sensation it sometimes causes, may be worthwhile for established post-herpetic neuralgia.

Prevention may be better than cure. Vaccination of elderly patients with a live attenuated vaccine to the varicella zoster virus has been shown to reduce the incidence of both herpes zoster and post-herpetic neuralgia, but the place for this treatment has not yet been established.

> **Learning points**
>
> 1 Post-herpetic neuralgia affects the elderly rather than the young.
> 2 Systemic antivirals works best if given early in the course of the disease.
> 3 Look for an underlying cause when there is dissemination outside the main affected dermatomes.

Herpes simplex

Cause

Herpesvirus hominis is the cause of herpes simplex. The virus is ubiquitous and carriers continue to shed virus particles in their saliva or tears. It has been separated into two types. The lesions caused by type II virus occur mainly on the genitals, while those of type I are usually extragenital; however, this distinction is not absolute.

The route of infection is through mucous membranes or abraded skin. After the episode associated with the primary infection, the virus may become latent, possibly within nerve ganglia, but still capable of giving rise to recurrent bouts of vesication (recrudescences).

Presentation

Primary infection

The most common recognizable manifestation of a primary type I infection in children is an acute gingivostomatitis accompanied by malaise, headache, fever and enlarged cervical nodes. Vesicles, soon turning into ulcers, can be seen scattered over the lips and mucous membranes. The illness lasts about 2 weeks.

Primary type II virus infections, usually transmitted sexually, cause multiple and painful genital or peri-anal blisters which rapidly ulcerate.

The virus can also be inoculated directly into the skin (e.g. during wrestling). A herpetic whitlow is one example of this direct inoculation. The uncomfortable pus-filled blisters on a fingertip are seen most often in medical personnel attending patients with unsuspected herpes simplex infections.

Recurrent (recrudescent) infections

These strike in roughly the same place each time. They may be precipitated by respiratory tract infections (cold sores), ultraviolet radiation, menstruation or even stress. Common sites include the face (Figure 16.29) and lips (type I), and the genitals (type II), but lesions can occur anywhere. Tingling, burning or even pain is followed within a few hours by the development of erythema and

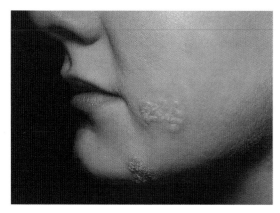

Figure 16.29 The grouped vesicles of herpes simplex, here provoked by sunlight. Those in the lower group are beginning to crust.

clusters of tense vesicles. Crusting occurs within 24–48 hours and the whole episode lasts about 12 days.

Complications

• Herpes encephalitis or meningitis can occur without any cutaneous clues.
• Disseminated herpes simplex: widespread vesicles may be part of a severe illness in newborns, debilitated children or immunosuppressed adults.
• Eczema herpeticum: patients with atopic eczema are particularly susceptible to widespread cutaneous herpes simplex infections. Those looking after patients with atopic eczema should stay away if they have cold sores.
• Herpes simplex can cause recurrent dendritic ulcers leading to corneal scarring.
• In some patients, recurrent herpes simplex infections are regularly followed by erythema multiforme (p. 105).

Investigations

None are usually needed. Doubts over the diagnosis can be dispelled by culturing the virus from vesicle fluid. Antibody titres rise with primary, but not with recurrent infections.

Treatment

'Old-fashioned' remedies suffice for occasional mild recurrent attacks; sun block may cut down their frequency. Dabbing with surgical spirit is helpful, and secondary bacterial infection can be reduced by topical bacitracin, mupirocin, framycetin or fusidic acid. Aciclovir cream, applied five or six times a day for the first 4 days of the episode may cut down the length of attacks. More

effective still is oral aciclovir (Formulary 2, p. 415), 200 mg five times daily for 5 days, although this is is usually reserved for those with widespread or systemic involvement. Famciclovir and valaciclovir are metabolized by the body into aciclovir and are as effective as aciclovir, having the additional advantage of better absorbtion and fewer doses per day.

Recurrences in the immunocompromised can usually be prevented by long-term treatment at a lower dosage.

Molluscum contagiosum

Cause

This common pox virus infection can be spread by direct contact (e.g. sexually or by sharing a towel at the swimming bath).

Presentation and course

The incubation period ranges from 2 to 6 weeks. Often several members of one family are affected. Individual lesions are shiny, white or pink, and hemispherical; they grow slowly up to 0.5 cm in diameter. A central punctum, which may contain a cheesy core, gives the lesions their characteristic umbilicated look.

On close inspection a mosaic appearance may be seen. Multiple lesions are common (Figure 16.30) and their distribution depends on the mode of infection. Atopic individuals and the immunocompromised are prone to especially extensive infections, spread by scratching and the use of topical steroids.

Untreated lesions usually clear in 6–9 months, often after a brief local inflammation. Large solitary lesions may take longer. Some leave depressed scars.

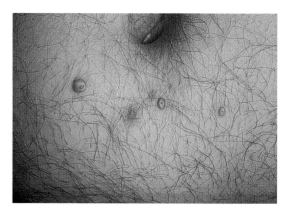

Figure 16.30 An umbilicus surrounded by umbilicated papules of molluscum contagiosum.

Complications

Eczematous patches often appear around mollusca. Traumatized or overtreated lesions may become secondarily infected.

Differential diagnosis

Inflamed lesions can simulate a boil. Large solitary lesions in adults can be confused with a keratocanthoma (p. 293), an intradermal naevus (p. 284) or even a cystic basal cell carcinoma (p. 289). Confusion with warts should not arise as these have a rough surface and no central pore.

Investigations

None are usually needed, but the diagnosis can be confirmed by looking under the microscope for large swollen epidermal cells, easily seen in unstained preparations of debris expressed from a lesion. Extensive mollusa of the beard area may suggest need for HIV testing.

Treatment

Many simple destructive measures cause inflammation and then resolution. They include squeezing out the lesions with forceps, piercing them with an orange stick (preferably without phenol), and curettage. Liquid nitrogen, wart paints and topical imiquimod may also be helpful.

These measures are fine for adults, but young children dislike them and as mollusca are self-limiting, doing nothing is often the best option. Sometimes a local anaesthetic cream (EMLA; see Formulary 1, p. 409), under polythene occlusion for an hour, will help children to tolerate more attacking treatment. Sparse eyelid lesions can be left alone but patients with numerous lesions may need to be referred to an ophthalmologist for curettage. Common sense measures help to limit spread within the family.

Learning points

1 If you cannot tell mollusca from warts, buy a lens.
2 Do not hurt young children with mollusca. You will not be able to get near them next time something more serious goes wrong.

Orf

Cause

Contagious pustular dermatitis is common in lambs. Its cause is a parapox virus that can be transmitted to those handling infected animals. The condition is therefore most commonly seen on the hands of shepherds, of their

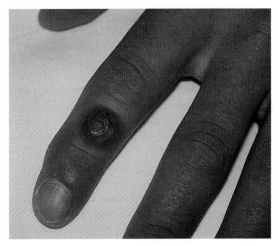

Figure 16.31 The pseudopustular nodule of orf.

wives who bottle-feed lambs, and of butchers, vets and meat porters.

Presentation and course

The incubation period is 5–6 days. Lesions, which may be single or multiple, start as small firm papules that change into flat-topped apparently pustular nodules with a violaceous and erythematous surround (Figure 16.31). The condition clears up spontaneously in about a month.

Complications

• Lymphadenitis and malaise are common.
• Erythema multiforme.
• 'Giant' lesions can appear in the immunosuppressed.

Differential diagnosis

Diagnosis is usually simple if contact with sheep is recognized. Milker's nodules, a pox virus infection acquired from cow's udders, can look like orf, as can staphylococcal furuncles.

Investigations

None are usually needed. If there is any doubt, the diagnosis can be confirmed by the distinctive electron microscopic appearance of the virus obtained from crusts.

Treatment

A topical antibiotic helps to prevent secondary infection; otherwise no active therapy is needed.

Acquired immunodeficiency syndrome (AIDS)

The human immunodeficiency virus (HIV) can be acquired from contaminated body fluids, particularly semen and blood. In the United Kingdom and the United

States, most cases have been homosexual or bisexual men; in much of Africa, on the other hand, the disease is most often spread heterosexually. Intravenous drug abusers who share contaminated needles and syringes are also at high risk. Up to half of babies born to infected mothers can be infected transplacentally, but this reduces to less than 2% with the use of maternal antiretroviral therapy, elective caesarian section and avoidance of breastfeeding.

Around 33 million people arround the world were living with HIV in 2010, the majority of these in sub-Saharan Africa. The good news is that education and the more widespread us of highly active antiretroviral treatment (HAART) has led to a fall in new infections, and in AIDS-related deaths since the turn of the millennium. Nonetheless, the number of new cases each year exceeds the number of people starting HAART worldwide, and in some areas of eastern Europe and central Asia there are expanding, concentrated epidemics. Heterosexual transmission now accounts for 25–30% of new cases in Europe and the United States. Each year around 2.7 million people are newly infected with HIV worldwide and 1.8 million die from it.

Pathogenesis

The human immunodeficiency viruses, HIV-1 and HIV-2 (mainly in West Africa), are RNA retroviruses containing reverse transcriptase enzymes, which allow the viral DNA copy to be incorporated into the chromosomes of the host cell. Their main target is a subset of T lymphocytes (helper/inducer cells) that express glycoprotein CD4 molecules on their surface (p. 18). These bind to the surface envelope of the HIV. Viral replication within the helper/inducer cells kills them, and their depletion leads to the loss of cell-mediated immunity so characteristic of HIV infection. A variety of opportunistic infections may then follow.

Course

The original infection may be asymptomatic, or followed by a glandular fever-like illness at the time of seroconversion. After a variable latent phase, which may last several years, a persistent generalized lymphadenopathy develops. The term AIDS-related complex refers to the next stage, in which many of the symptoms of AIDS (e.g. fever, weight-loss, fatigue or diarrhoea) may be present without the opportunistic infections or tumours characteristic of full-blown AIDS. Not all of those infected with HIV will develop AIDS but, for those who do, the average time from infection to the onset of AIDS is about 10 years with-

out treatment. Once AIDS develops, if untreated, about half will die within 1 year and three-quarters within 4 years. The use of HAART has led to marked reductions in the rates of illness and death in HIV infected individuals, and a life expectancy following diagnosis now measured in decades.

Skin changes in AIDS

Skin conditions are often the first clue to the presence of AIDS and can either present as more florid examples of conditions found in the HIV negative population or alternatively as conditions specific to HIV infected individuals. The following conditions are important.

1 *Kaposi's sarcoma* (Figures 16.32–16.34) is caused by human herpesvirus 8 and is the most common HIV-associated malignancy, although the incidence has dropped markedly since the introduction of antiretroviral therapy. The lesions of classic Kaposi's sarcoma are multiple purplish patches or nodules. In AIDS the lesions may be atypical, sometimes looking like bruises or pyogenic granulomata (p. 304). The diagnosis can easily be missed and the mouth must always be examined.

2 *Seborrhoeic eczema and folliculitis* (Figure 16.35) are seen in at least 50% of patients, often starting at an early stage of immunosuppression. The underlying cause may

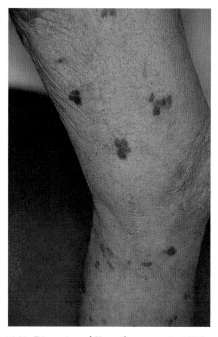

Figure 16.32 Disseminated Kaposi's sarcoma in AIDS.

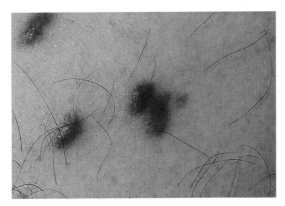

Figure 16.33 Kaposi's sarcoma in AIDS.

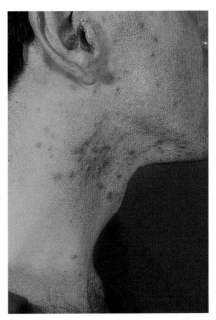

Figure 16.35 Seborrhoeic dermatitis (otitis externa) and seborrhoeic folliculitis in HIV disease.

be an overgrowth of *Pityrosporum* yeasts. An itchy folliculitis of the head, neck and trunk, and an eosinophilic folliculitis, have also been described.

3 *Skin infections* – florid, unusually extensive or atypical examples of common infections may be seen with one or more of the following: herpes simplex, herpes zoster, molluscum contagiosum, oral and cutaneous *Candida*, tinea, scabies and staphylococci. Facial and perianal warts are common. Hairy leucoplakia (Figure 16.36), often on the sides of the tongue, may be caused by proliferation of the Epstein–Barr virus. Bacillary angiomatosis may look like Kaposi's sarcoma and is caused by the bacillus that causes cat-scratch fever (*Bartonella henselae*). Syphilis can coexist with AIDS, as can mycobacterial infections.

4 *Other manifestations* – dry skin is common in AIDS, so is pruritus. Psoriasis may start or worsen with AIDS. Diffuse alopecia is not uncommon. Eosinophilic folliculitis is a non-infectious condition characterized by pruritic follicular papules, usually on the upper trunk and peripheral eosinophilia. It is found in about 10% of HIV patients, and is helped by UVB phototherapy.

5 *Drug eruptions* are around 10 times more common in HIV patients than the non-HIV population. As the drugs used in HAART themselves commonly cause rashes, this is probably the most common reason for dermatological referral now. Morbilliform and urticarial rashes are the most common eruptions, but both Stevens–Johnson

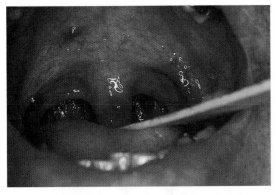

Figure 16.34 Kaposi's sarcoma of hard palate, anterior fauces and uvula in AIDS.

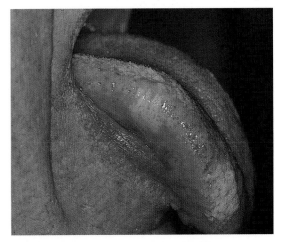

Figure 16.36 Hairy leucoplakia on the side of the tongue.

syndrome (SJS) and toxic epidermal necrolysis also occur. Identifying the causative drug is difficult, as multiple drug therapy underlies HAART and the number of drugs available is constantly evolving. As a starting point, however, non-nucleoside reverse transcriptase inhibitors commonly cause morbilliform rashes, while the protease inhibitors amprenavir, darunavir and indinavir are most likely to cause SJS. Drug reaction with eosinophilia and systemic symptoms (DRESS) can be caused by abacavir or nevirapine.

Around one-quarter of HIV patients who have been immunosuppressed will develop the immune reconstitution inflammatory syndrome (IRIS) after initiation of HAART. Recovery of the immune system leads to marked reactions to latent infections, most commonly mycobacterial or one of the human herpes viruses.

Management

The clinical diagnosis of HIV infection is confirmed by a positive blood test for antibodies to the virus. Sexual contacts of infected individuals should be traced.

Modern drugs for HIV infections increase life expectancy, but are not 'cures' in the usual sense. They reduce the viral load but are expensive and sometimes toxic. Guidelines on how to use them change constantly, and so the drug treatment of HIV infections should be directed by specialists in the field, who will monitor the plasma viral load and CD4 count regularly (Table 16.1). Antiretroviral drugs fall into a number of classes: nucleoside reverse transcriptase inhibitors (NRTIs), nucleotide reverse transcriptase inhibitor, non-nucleoside reverse transcriptase inhibitors (NNRTIs), protease inhibitors (PIs), fusion inhibitor, chemokine receptor 5 (CCR5) inhibitor and integrase inhibitors. Treatment is usually with a combination of three of these drugs from two or more classes and aims to restore CD4 T-cell counts to normal levels, and to suppress HIV viral load to below the detection limits of commercial assays. Difficult decisions to be made include the timing of treatment – the benefits of starting early have to be balanced against the risk of toxicity – and choosing the right drug combination of HAART, but generally it is started when CD4 counts fall below 350 cell/μL. The regimen will be changed if there is clinical or virological deterioration, or if the patient becomes pregnant.

Treatment otherwise is symptomatic and varies according to the type of opportunistic infection detected. Educating the public to avoid risky behaviour, such as unprotected sexual intercourse, is still hugely important.

Mucocutaneous lymph node syndrome (Kawasaki's disease)

This acute systemic vasculitis involving medium-sized vessels may be caused by a recent parvovirus infection. The disease affects young children whose erythema, although often generalized, becomes most marked in a glove and stocking distribution; it may be associated with indurated oedema of the palms and soles. Peeling around the fingers and toes is one obvious feature but is not seen at the start. Bilateral conjunctival injection and erythema of the lips, buccal mucosa and tongue ('strawberry tongue') are common.

The episode is accompanied by fever and usually resolves within 2 weeks. Despite its name, not all patients have lymphadenopathy. The danger of this condition lies in the risk of developing pancarditis and coronary artery vasculitis leading on to aneurysms or dilatation. The pathology is close to that of polyarteritis nodosa. Aspirin and intravenous gammaglobulin are the mainstay of treatment; both should be given early in the disease and reduce the risk of coronary artery involvement.

Gianotti–Crosti syndrome

This is a rather uncommon reaction to an infection with hepatitis B virus in childhood. Small reddish papules erupt bilaterally over the limbs and face, and fade over the course of a few weeks. Jaundice is uncommon, although tests of liver function give abnormal results.

Herpangina

This is an acute infectious illness, caused by group A Coxsackie viruses. The patient is usually a child with a fever, and a severe sore throat covered in many small vesicles, which rapidly become superficial ulcers. Episodes resolve in about a week.

Table 16.1 Recommendations for starting highly active antiretroviral treatment (HAART) in the adult.

Disease stage	Decision
Symptomatic	Treat
Asymptomatic	
CD4 <200 × 10^6/L	Treat
CD4 200–350 × 10^6/L	Treatment generally offered
CD4 >350 × 10^6/L	Defer treatment unless high viral load

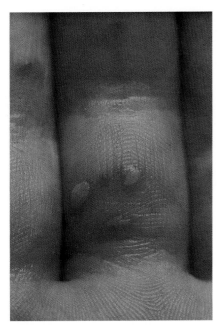

Figure 16.37 The typical vesicles of hand, foot and mouth disease.

Hand, foot and mouth disease

This is usually caused by coxsackie A16. Minor epidemics occur in institutions. The oral vesicles are larger and fewer than those of herpangina. The hand and foot lesions are small greyish vesicles with a narrow rim of redness around (Figure 16.37). The condition settles within a few days.

Measles

An incubation period of 10 days is followed by fever, conjunctival injection, photophobia and upper respiratory tract catarrh. Koplik's spots (pinhead-sized white spots with a bright red margin) are seen at this stage on the buccal mucosa. The characteristic 'net-like' rash starts after a few days, on the brow and behind the ears, and soon becomes extensive before fading with much desquamation. Prevention is by immunization with the combined MMR (measles/mumps/rubella) vaccine.

Rubella

After an incubation period of about 18 days, lymphadenopathy occurs a few days before the evanescent pink macular rash, which fades, first on the trunk, over the course of a few days. Rubella during the first trimester of pregnancy carries a risk of damage to the unborn child.

Prevention is by immunization with the combined MMR vaccine.

Erythema infectiosum (fifth disease)

This is caused by the human parvovirus B19 and occurs in outbreaks, often in the spring. A slapped cheek erythema is quickly followed by a reticulate erythema of the shoulders. The affected child feels well, and the rash clears over the course of a few days. Other features, sometimes not accompanied by a rash, include transient anaemia and arthritis.

Fungal infections

Dermatophyte infections (ringworm)

Cause

Three genera of dermatophyte fungi cause tinea infections (ringworm).
- *Trichophyton*: skin, hair and nail infections.
- *Microsporum*: skin and hair.
- *Epidermophyton*: skin and nails.

Dermatophytes invade keratin only, and the inflammation they cause is due to metabolic products of the fungus or to delayed hypersensitivity. In general, zoophilic fungi (those transmitted to humans by animals) cause a more severe inflammation than anthropophilic ones (spread from person to person).

Presentation and course

This depends upon the site and on the strain of fungus involved.

Tinea pedis (athlete's foot)

This is the most common type of fungal infection in humans. The sharing of wash places (e.g. in showers) and of swimming pools, predisposes to infection; occlusive footwear encourages relapses.

Most cases are caused by one of three organisms: *Trichophyton rubrum* (the most common and the most stubborn), *Trichophyton mentagrophytes* var. *interdigitale* and *Epidermophyton floccosum*.

There are three common clinical patterns.
1 Soggy interdigital scaling, particularly in the fourth and fifth interspace (all three organisms; Figure 16.38).
2 A diffuse dry scaling of the soles (usually *T. rubrum*; Figure 16.39).
3 Recurrent episodes of vesication (usually *T. mentagrophytes* var. *interdigitale* or *E. floccosum*).

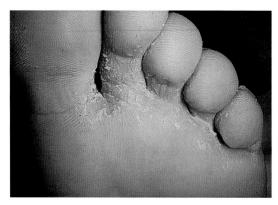

Figure 16.38 Tinea pedis. Scaly area spreading to the sole from the toe webs.

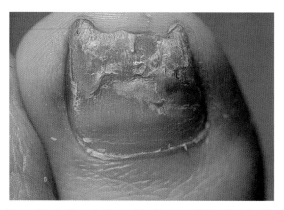

Figure 16.40 Chronic tinea of the big toe nail. Starting distally, the thickness and discoloration are spreading proximally.

Tinea of the nails

Toenail infection is usually associated with tinea pedis. The initial changes occur at the free edge of the nail, which becomes yellow and crumbly (Figure 16.40). Subungual hyperkeratosis, separation of the nail from its bed, and thickening may then follow. Usually only a few nails are infected but rarely all are. Fingernail lesions are similar, but less common, and are seldom seen without a chronic *T. rubrum* infection of the skin of the same hand.

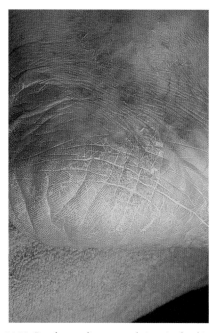

Figure 16.39 Powdery scaling, most obvious in the skin creases, caused by a *Trychophyton rubrum* infection.

Tinea of the hands

This is usually asymmetrical and associated with tinea pedis and unilateral onychomycosis. *T. rubrum* may cause a barely perceptible erythema of one palm with a characteristic powdery scale in the creases.

Tinea of the groin

This is common and affects men more often than women. The eruption is sometimes unilateral or asymmetrical. The upper inner thigh is involved and lesions expand slowly to form sharply demarcated plaques with peripheral scaling (Figure 16.41). In contrast to candidiasis of the groin area, the scrotum is usually spared. A few vesicles or pustules may be seen within the lesions. The organisms are the same as those causing tinea pedis.

Tinea of the trunk and limbs

Tinea corporis is characterized by plaques with scaling and erythema, most pronounced at the periphery. A few small vesicles and pustules may be seen within them. The lesions expand slowly and healing in the centre leaves a typical ring-like pattern. In some patients the fungus elicits almost no inflammation, in which case the infection is a marginated patch of rough scaling skin.

Tinea of the scalp (tinea capitis)

This is usually a disease of children. The causative organism varies from country to country. Fungi coming from human sources (anthropophilic organisms) cause bald and scaly areas, with minimal inflammation and hairs broken off 3–4 mm from the scalp.

Fungi coming from animal sources (zoophilic fungi) induce a more intense inflammation than those spread from person to person. In ringworm acquired from cattle, for example, the boggy swelling, with inflammation,

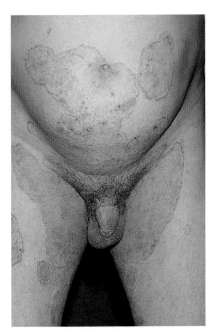

Figure 16.41 A very gross example of tinea of the groin. The *T. rubrum* infection has spread on to the abdomen and thighs, aided by the use of topical steroids.

pustulation and lymphadenopathy, is often so fierce that a bacterial infection is suspected; such a lesion is called a kerion and the hair loss associated with it may be permanent.

Tinea of the beard area is usually caused by zoophilic species and shows the same features (Figure 16.42). In favus, caused by *Trichophyton schoenleini*, the picture is dominated by foul-smelling yellowish crusts surrounding many scalp hairs, and sometimes leading to scarring alopecia.

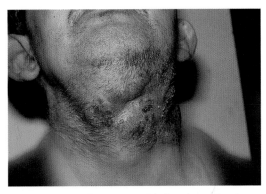

Figure 16.42 Animal ringworm of the beard area showing boggy inamed swellings (kerion).

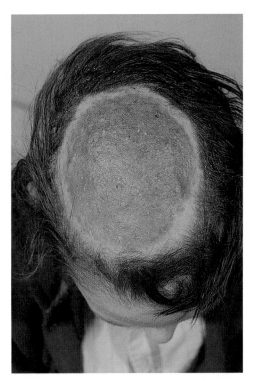

Figure 16.43 Animal ringworm of a child's scalp: not truly a kerion as flat and non-pustular.

Complications

1 Fierce animal ringworm of the scalp (Figure 16.43) can lead to a permanent scarring alopecia.
2 A florid fungal infection anywhere can induce vesication on the sides of the fingers and palms (a trichophytide).
3 Epidemics of ringworm occur in schools.
4 The usual appearance of a fungal infection can be masked by mistreatment with topical steroids (tinea incognito; Figure 16.44).

Differential diagnosis

This varies with the site. Some of the more common problems are listed in Table 16.2.

Investigations

The microscopic examination of a skin scraping, nail clipping or plucked hair is a simple procedure. The scraping should be taken from the scaly margin of a lesion, with a small curette or a scalpel blade, and clippings or scrapings from the most crumbly part of a nail. Broken hairs should be plucked with tweezers. Specimens are cleared in potassium hydroxide (p. 37). Branching hyphae can

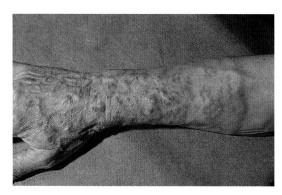

Figure 16.44 Tinea incognito. Topical steroid applications have thinned the skin and altered much of the morphology. A recognizable active spreading edge is still visible.

easily be seen (see Figure 3.7) using a scanning (×10) or low-power (×25) objective lens, with the iris diaphragm almost closed and the condenser racked down. Hyphae may also be seen within a cleared hair shaft, or spores may be noted around it.

Cultures should be carried out in a mycology or bacteriology laboratory. Transport medium is not necessary, and specimens can be sent in folded black paper or a dry Petri dish. The report may take as long as a month; microscopy is much quicker.

Wood's light (ultraviolet light) examination of the scalp usually reveals a green fluorescence of the hairs in *Microsporum audouini* and *M. canis* infections. The technique is useful for screening children in institutions where outbreaks of tinea capitis still sometimes occur, but the most common fungi causing tinea capitis (e.g. *Trichophyton tonsurans*) do not fluoresce.

Table 16.2 Common problems in the differential diagnosis of dermatophyte infections.

Area	Differential diagnosis
Scalp	Alopecia areata, psoriasis, seborrhoeic eczema, carbuncle, abscess, trichotillomania
Feet	Erythrasma, interdigital intertrigo, eczema
Trunk	Discoid eczema, psoriasis, candidiasis, pityriasis rosea
Groin	Candidiasis, erythrasma, intertrigo, irritant and allergic contact dermatitis, psoriasis, neurodermatitis
Nails	Psoriasis, paronychia, trauma, ageing changes
Hand	Chronic eczema, granuloma annulare, xerosis, dyshidrotic eczema

Treatment

Local

This is all that is needed for minor skin infections. The more recent imidazole preparations (e.g. miconazole and clotrimazole) and the allylamines such as terbinafine (Formulary 1, p. 404) have largely superseded time-honoured remedies such as benzoic acid ointment (Whitfield's ointment) and tolnaftate. They should be applied twice daily. Magenta paint (Castellani's paint), although highly coloured, is helpful for exudative or macerated areas in body folds or toe webs. Occasional dusting with an antifungal powder is useful to prevent relapses.

Topical nail preparations. Many patients now prefer to avoid systemic treatment. For them a nail lacquer containing amorolfine is worth a trial. It should be applied once or twice a week for 6 months; it is effective against stubborn moulds such as *Hendersonula* and *Scopulariopsis*. Ciclopirox is an alternative topical treatment available in the United States. Both amorolfine and tioconazole nail solutions (Formulary 1, p. 404) can be used as adjuncts to systemic therapy (see below).

Systemic

This is needed for tinea of the scalp or of the nails, and for widespread or chronic infections of the skin that have not responded to local measures.

Terbinafine (Formulary 2, p. 413) has now largely superceded griseofulvin. It acts by inhibiting fungal squalene epoxidase and does not interact with the cytochrome P-450 system. It is fungicidal and so cures chronic dermatophyte infections more quickly and more reliably than griseofulvin. For tinea capitis in children caused by *Trychophyton* species for example, a 4-week course of terbinafine is as effective as an 8-week course of griseofulvin. Cure rates of 70–90% can be expected for infected fingernails after a 6-week course of terbinafine, and for infected toenails after a 3-month course. It is not effective in pityriasis versicolor or *Candida* infections.

Itraconazole (Formulary 2, p. 414) is now preferred to ketoconazole, which occasionally damages the liver, and is a reasonable alternative to terbinafine if this is contraindicated. It is effective in tinea corporis, cruris and pedis; and also in nail infections. Fungistatic rather than fungicidal, it interferes with the cytochrome P-450 system, so a review of any other medication being taken is needed before a prescription is issued. Its wide spectrum makes it useful also in pityriasis versicolor and candidiasis.

Griseofulvin (Formulary 2, p. 413) was for many years the drug of choice for chronic dermatophyte infections,

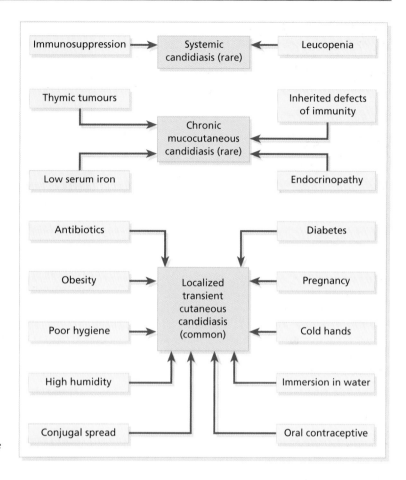

Figure 16.45 Factors predisposing to the different types of candidiasis.

but is now largely reserved for the treatment of tinea capitis. It has proved to be a safe drug, but treatment may have to be stopped because of persistent headache, nausea, vomiting or skin eruptions. The drug should not be given in pregnancy or to patients with liver failure or porphyria. It interacts with coumarin anticoagulants, the dosage of which may have to be increased. In children it remains the treatment of choice for tinea capitis caused by *Trichophyton* and *Microsporum* infections and should be used for 6–8 weeks continually.

Learning points

1 Do not prescribe terbinafine or itraconazole for psoriasis of the nails or chronic paronychia. Get mycological proof first.
2 Your patient's asymmetrical 'eczema' is spreading despite local steroids – think of a dermatophyte infection.
3 Consider tinea in acute inflammatory and purulent reactions of the scalp and beard.

Candidiasis

Cause
Candida albicans is a classic opportunistic pathogen. Even in transient and trivial local infections in the apparently fit, one or more predisposing factors such as obesity, moisture and maceration, immobility, diabetes, pregnancy, the use of broad-spectrum antibiotics or perhaps the use of the contraceptive pill, will often be found to be playing some part. Opportunism is even more obvious in the overwhelming systemic infections of the immunocompromised (Figure 16.45).

Presentation
This varies with the site (Figure 16.46).

Oral candidiasis (see also Chapter 13)
One or more whitish adherent plaques (like bread sauce) appear on the mucous membranes. If wiped off they leave an erythematous base. Under dentures, candidiasis will

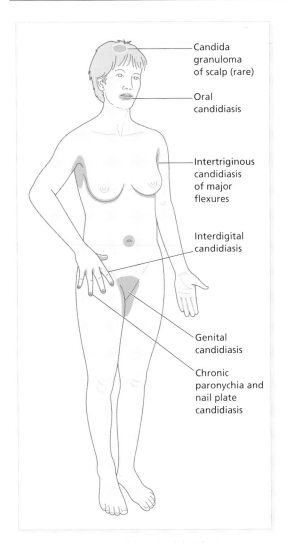

Figure 16.46 Sites susceptible to *Candida* infection.

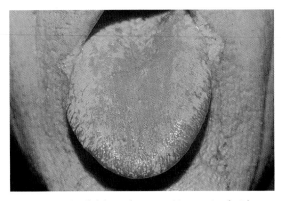

Figure 16.47 Candidal angular stomatitis associated with severe candidiasis of the tongue.

produce sore red areas. Angular stomatitis, usually in denture wearers (Figure 16.47), may be candidal.

Candidal intertrigo
A moist glazed area of erythema and maceration appears in a body fold; the edge shows soggy scaling and outlying satellite papulo-pustules. These changes are most common under the breasts, and in the armpits and groin, but can also occur between the fingers of those whose hands are often in water.

Genital candidiasis
Most commonly presents as a sore itchy vulvovaginitis, with white curdy plaques adherent to the inflamed mucous membranes, and a whitish discharge. The eruption may extend to the groin folds. Conjugal spread is common; in males similar changes occur under the foreskin (Figure 16.48) and in the groin.

Diabetes, pregnancy and antibiotic therapy are common predisposing factors.

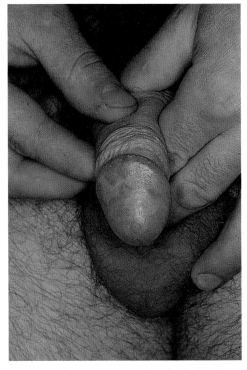

Figure 16.48 Pink circinate areas with only a little scaling. Consider Reiter's syndrome or candidiasis.

Paronychia

Acute paronychia is usually bacterial, but in chronic paronychia *Candida* may be the sole pathogen, or be found with other opportunists such as *Proteus* or *Pseudomonas sp.* The proximal and sometimes the lateral nail folds of one or more fingers become bolstered and red (see Figure 13.28). The cuticles are lost and small amounts of pus can be expressed. The adjacent nail plate becomes ridged and discoloured. Predisposing factors include wet work, poor peripheral circulation and vulval candidiasis.

Chronic mucocutaneous candidiasis

Persistent candidiasis, affecting most or all of the areas described above, can start in infancy. Sometimes the nail plates as well as the nail folds are involved. *Candida* granulomas may appear on the scalp. Several different forms have been described including those with autosomal recessive and dominant inheritance patterns. In the *Candida* endocrinopathy syndrome, chronic candidiasis occurs with one or more endocrine defects, the most common of which are hypoparathyroidism, and Addison's disease. A few late-onset cases have underlying thymic tumours.

Systemic candidiasis

This is seen against a background of severe illness, leucopenia and immunosuppression. The skin lesions are firm red nodules, which can be shown by biopsy to contain yeasts and pseudohyphae.

Investigations

Swabs from suspected areas should be sent for culture. The urine can be tested for sugar. In chronic mucocutaneous candidiasis, a detailed immunological work-up will be needed, focusing on troubles associated with cell-mediated immunity.

Treatment

Predisposing factors should be sought and eliminated (e.g. denture hygiene may be important). Infected skin folds should be separated and kept dry. Those with chronic paronychia should keep their hands warm and dry.

Amphotericin, nystatin and the imidazole group of compounds are all effective topically. For the mouth, these are available as oral suspensions, lozenges and oral gels (Formulary 1, p. 403). False teeth should be removed at night, washed and steeped in antiseptic or a nystatin solution. For other areas of candidiasis, creams, ointment and pessaries are available (Formulary 1, p. 404). Magenta paint is also a useful but messy remedy for the skin flexures. In chronic paronychia, the nail folds can be packed with an imidazole cream or drenched in an imidazole solution several times a day. Genital candidiasis responds well to a single day's treatment with either itraconazole and fluconazole (Formulary 2, p. 414). Both are also valuable for recurrent oral candidiasis of the immunocompromised, and for the various types of chronic mucocutaneous candidiasis.

Learning points

1 Something else is often amiss in patients with cutaneous candidiasis
2 Remember that terbinafine has no action against *Candida*.
3 This is not a dermatophyte infection, so do not try griseofulvin or terbinafine.
4 Patients think the treatment has not worked if their pale patches do not disappear straight away – warn them about this in advance.

Pityriasis versicolor

Cause

The old name, tinea versicolor, should be dropped as the disorder is caused by commensal yeasts (*Pityrosporum orbiculare*) and not by dermatophyte fungi. Overgrowth of these yeasts, particularly in hot humid conditions, is responsible for the clinical lesions.

Carboxylic acids released by the organisms inhibit the increase in pigment production by melanocytes that occurs normally after exposure to sunlight. The term 'versicolor' refers to the way in which the superficial scaly patches, fawn or pink on non-tanned skin (Figure 16.49), become paler than the surrounding skin after exposure to sunlight (Figure 16.50). The condition should be regarded as non-infectious.

Presentation and course

The fawn or depigmented areas, with their slightly branny scaling and fine wrinkling, look ugly. Otherwise they are symptom-free or only slightly itchy. Lesions are most common on the upper trunk but can become widespread. Untreated lesions persist, and depigmented areas, even after adequate treatment, are slow to regain their former colour. Recurrences are common.

Differential diagnosis

In vitiligo (p. 271), the border is clearly defined, scaling is absent, lesions are larger, the limbs and face are often

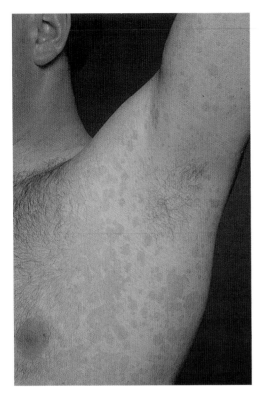

Figure 16.49 Pityriasis versicolor: fawn areas stand out against the untanned background.

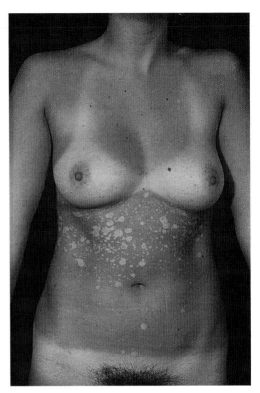

Figure 16.50 This patient's holiday was spoilt by versicolor ruining her expensive tan.

affected, and depigmentation is more complete; however, it may sometimes be hard to distinguish vitiligo from the pale non-scaly areas of treated versicolor. Seborrhoeic eczema of the trunk tends to be more erythematous, and is often confined to the presternal or interscapular areas. Pityriasis alba often affects the cheeks. Pityriasis rosea, tinea corporis, secondary syphilis, leprosy and erythrasma seldom cause real confusion.

Investigations

Scrapings, prepared and examined as for a dermatophyte infection (p. 37), show a mixture of short branched hyphae and spores (a 'spaghetti and meatballs' appearance). Culture is not helpful because the organism does not grow on Sabouroud's medium.

Treatment

A topical preparation of one of the imidazole group of antifungal drugs (Formulary 1, p. 404) can be applied at night to all affected areas for 2–4 weeks. Equally effective and cheaper, but messier and more irritant, is a 2.5% sele-nium sulfide mixture in a detergent base (Selsun shampoo). This should be lathered on to the patches after an evening bath, and allowed to dry. Next morning it should be washed off. Three applications at weekly intervals are adequate. A shampoo containing ketoconazole is now available (Formulary 1, p. 398) and is less messy but just as effective as the selenium ones. Alternatively, selenium sulfide lotion (United States) can be applied for 10 minutes, rinsed off and re-applied daily for 1 week. For widespread or stubborn infections systemic itraconazole (200 mg/day for 7 days), fluconazole or ketoconazole may be curative, but interactions with other drugs must be avoided (Formulary 2, p. 414). Recurrence is common after any treatment.

Deep fungal infections

Subcutaneous mycoses are caused by inoculation of naturally occurring fungi to the deeper tissues by a penetrating injury. They mostly occur in tropical countries and treatment is generally unsatisfactory. Diagnosis is confirmed by histopathology, or culture and KOH examination of pus and exudate from affected sites.

Sporotrichosis

The causative fungus, *Sporotrichum schencki*, lives saprophytically in soil or on wood in warm humid countries.

Infection is through a wound, where later a lesion like an indolent nodule arises. Later still, nodules appear in succession along the draining lymphatics (Figure 16.15). Itraconazole (100–200 mg/day for 3–6 months) or terbinafine (250 mg/day) are the treatments of choice. Potassium iodide is also effective and much cheaper.

Mycetoma (Madura foot)

This is a disease of the tropics and subtropics and involves various species of fungus or actinomycetes. They gain access to the subcutaneous tissues, usually of the feet or legs, via a penetrating wound. The area becomes lumpy and distorted, later enlarging and developing multiple sinuses. Pus exuding from these shows tiny diagnostic granules. Surgery may be a valuable alternative to the often poor results of medical treatment, which is with systemic antibiotics or antifungal drugs, depending on the organism isolated.

Chromoblastomycosis

A range of pigmented fungi cause this infection of skin and subcutaneous tissues, characterized by indolent warty nodules and plaques. It most commonly occurs on the feet and legs of poor farmers and histology is of a foreign body granuloma. The condition occurs throughout the Americas, India, southern Africa, and also occasionally in Australia and northern Europe. Treatment is usually with antifungal medication, but is dependent on the causative organism

Histoplasmosis

Histoplasma capsulatum is found in soil and in the droppings of some animals (e.g. bats). Airborne spores are inhaled and cause lung lesions, which are in many ways like those of tuberculosis. Later, granulomatous skin lesions may appear, particularly in the immunocompromised. Amphotericin B or itraconazole, given systemically, is often helpful.

Coccidioidomycosis

The causative organism, *Coccidioides immitis*, is present in the soil in arid areas in the United States. Its spores are inhaled, and the pulmonary infection may be accompanied by a fever and plaques. As cell-mediated immunity develops, erythema nodosum (p. 107) may be seen. In a few patients the infection becomes disseminated, with ulcers or deep abscesses in the skin. Treatment is usually not needed; the disorder is typically self-limiting. Fluconazole, is used for progressing cavitations of the lungs, for the immunosuppressed and for severe cases.

Blastomycosis

Infections with *Blastomyces dermatitidis* are virtually confined to rural areas of the United States. Rarely, the organism is inoculated into the skin; more often it is inhaled and then spreads systemically from the pulmonary focus to other organs including the skin. There the lesions are wart-like hyperkeratotic nodules, which spread peripherally with a verrucose edge, suggesting squamous cell carcinomas. They tend to clear and scar centrally. Treatment is with systemic amphotericin B or itraconazole.

Actinomycosis

The causative organism, *Actinomyces israeli*, is bacterial but traditionally considered with the fungi. It has long branching hyphae and is part of the normal flora of the mouth and bowel. In actinomycosis, a lumpy induration and scarring coexist with multiple sinuses discharging pus containing 'sulfur granules', made up of tangled filaments. Favourite sites are the jaw, and the chest and abdominal walls. Long-term penicillin is the treatment of choice.

Further reading

Angus J, Langan SM, Stanway A, Leach IH, Littlewood SM, English JS. (2006) The many faces of secondary syphilis: a re-emergence of an old disease. *Clinical and Experimental Dermatology* **31**, 741–745.

Bath-Hextall FJ, Birnie AJ, Ravenscroft JC, Williams HC. (2010) Interventions to reduce *Staphylococcus aureus* in the management of atopic eczema: an updated Cochrane Review. *British Journal of Dermatology* **163**, 12–26.

Bernard P. (2008) Management of common bacterial infections of the skin. *Current Opinion in Infectious Diseases* **21**, 122–128.

British HIV Association with links to current HIV treatment guidelines. www.bhiva.org (accessed 28 June 2014).

Graham SM. (2011) Treatment of paediatric TB: Revised WHO Guidelines. *Paediatric Respiratory Reviews* **12**, 22–26.

Grice EA, Segre JA. (2011) The skin microbiome. *Nature Reviews: Microbiology* **9**, 244–253.

Hart CA, Thomson AP. (2006) Meningococcal disease and its management in children. *British Medical Journal* **333**, 685–690.

Higgins EM, Fuller LC, Smith CH. (2000) Guidelines for the management of tinea capitis. *British Journal of Dermatology* **143**, 53–58.

Lappin E, Ferguson AJ. (2009) Gram-positive toxic shock syndromes. *Lancet Infectious Diseases* **9**, 281–290.

Marques AR. (2010) Lyme disease: a review. *Current Allergy and Asthma Reports* **10**, 13–20.

Roberts DT, Taylor WD, Boyle J. (2003) Guidelines for treatment of onychomycosis. *British Journal of Dermatology* **148**, 402–410.

Silversides JA, Lappin E, Ferguson AJ. (2010) Staphylococcal toxic shock syndrome: mechanisms and management. *Current Infectious Disease Reports* **12**, 392–400.

Sterling JC, Handfield-Jones S, Hudson P. (2001) Guidelines for the treatment of cutaneous warts. *British Journal of Dermatology* **144**, 4–11.

Sultan HY, Boyle AA, Sheppard N. (2012) Necrotising fasciitis. *British Medical Journal* **345**, e4274.

Veraldi S, Girgenti V, Dassoni F, Gianotti R. (2009) Erysipeloid: a review. *Clinical and Experimental Dermatology* **34**, 859–862.

17 Infestations

Infestation, the presence of animal parasites on or in the body, is common in tropical countries and less so in temperate ones. Infestations fall into two main groups:
1 Those caused by arthropods; and
2 Those caused by worms.

Arthropods

Table 17.1 lists some of the ways in which arthropods affect the skin. Only a few can be discussed here.

Lice infestations (pediculosis)

Lice are flattened wingless insects that suck blood. Their eggs, attached to hairs or clothing, are known as nits. The main feature of all lice infestations is severe itching, followed by scratching and secondary infection.

Two species are obligate parasites in humans: *Pediculus humanus* (with its two varieties *P. humanus capitis*, the head louse, and *P. humanus corporis*, the body louse) and *Phthirus pubis* (the pubic louse).

Head lice

Cause

Head lice are still common: up to 10% of children have them (Figure 17.1), even in the smartest schools. Many of these children have few or no symptoms. Infestations peak between the ages of 4 and 11, and are more common in girls than boys. A typical infested scalp will carry about 10 adult lice, which measure some 1–3 mm in length and are greyish, and often rather hard to find. An adult female louse lives for about 1 month and during that time lays 5–10 eggs per day. These egg cases (nits) can be seen easily enough, firmly stuck to the hair shafts. Spread from person to person is achieved by head-to-head contact, and perhaps by shared combs or hats.

Presentation and course

The main symptom is itching, although this may take several months to develop after the first infestation. Subsequent infestations produce itching more rapidly, suggesting that this is due to a delayed-type hypersensitivity reaction. At first the itching is mainly around the sides and back of the scalp; later it spreads generally over the scalp. Scratching and secondary infection soon follow and, in heavy infestations, the hair becomes matted and smelly. Draining lymph nodes often enlarge.

Complications

Secondary bacterial infection may be severe enough to make the child listless and feverish.

Differential diagnosis

All patients with recurrent impetigo or crusted eczema on their scalps should be carefully examined for the presence of nits.

Investigations

None are usually required.

Treatment

The finding of living moving lice means that the infestation is current and active, and needs treatment. Empty egg cases signify only that there has been an infestation in the past, but suggest the need for periodic re-inspection.

Dimeticone is a non-neurotoxic agent that coats the lice and probably suffocates them. It is rubbed into dry hair and scalp and left for 8 hours. This is then repeated 1 week later. Cure rates of 70% or more are reported and it is non-irritant and well tolerated.

Malathion and the synthetic pyrethroid permethrin have traditionally been used, but resistance to these neurotoxic pediculocides has been increasing since the 1990s. Sensitivity of less than 20% is reported in some areas, and resistance to more than one agent is also developing. Unsurprisingly, this has been accompanied by a big rise

Clinical Dermatology, Fifth Edition. Richard B. Weller, Hamish J.A. Hunter and Margaret W. Mann.
© 2015 John Wiley & Sons, Ltd. Published 2015 by John Wiley & Sons, Ltd.

Table 17.1 Arthropods and their effects on the skin.

Type of arthropod	Manifestations
Insects	
Hymenoptera	Bee and wasp stings
	Ant bites
Lepidoptera	Caterpillar dermatitis
Coleoptera	Blisters from cantharidin
Diptera	Mosquito and midge bites
	Myiasis
Aphaniptera	Human and animal fleas
Hemiptera	Bed bugs
Anoplura	Lice infestations
Mites	
Demodex folliculorum	Normal inhabitant of facial hair follicles
Sarcoptes scabei	Human and animal scabies
Food mites	Grain itch, grocer's itch, etc.
Harvest mites	Harvest itch
Feather mites	In pet birds, nests, and sometimes feather pillows
House dust mite	Possible role in atopic eczema
Cheyletiella	Papular urticaria
Ticks	Tick bites. Vector of rickettsial infections and erythema migrans (p. 221)

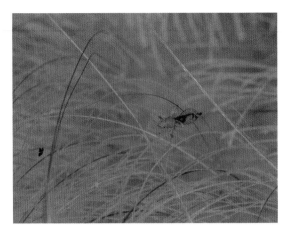

Figure 17.1 This woman had acquired a head louse infection from her grandchild.

in infestation rates. Where resistance is not yet a problem these agents are more effective at killing adult lice and nymphs than eggs and should thus be applied on two occasions, 1 week apart. The second application is needed to kill young nymphs that hatch after the first application, usually 6–10 days after being laid. Lotions should remain on the scalp for at least 12 hours, and are more effective than shampoos.

Wet combing with a fine toothed comb every 3 days for 14 days is an alternative to the treatments mentioned above. The technique relies on physical removal of lice and eggs and is more effective than treatment with neurotoxic agents if carried out thoroughly. Shampoo or conditioner acts as a lubricant and helps with combing, but occasionally matting is so severe that the hair has to be clipped short. A systemic antibiotic may be needed to deal with severe secondary infection. Pillow cases, towels, hats and scarves should be laundered or dry cleaned. Other members of the family and school mates should be checked.

Systemic ivermectin therapy is reserved for infestations resisting the treatments listed above.

Body lice

Body lice have diverged genetically from head lice. This probably occurred between 85 000 and 170 000 years ago, and marks the time at which anatomically modern humans started wearing clothes.

Cause

Body louse infestations are now uncommon except in the unhygienic and socially deprived. Epidemics also occur in times of social disruption, such as civil war or in refugee camps. Morphologically, the body louse looks just like the head louse, but lays its eggs in the seams of clothing in contact with the skin. Transmission is via infested bedding or clothing.

Presentation and course

Self-neglect is usually obvious; against this background there is severe and widespread itching, especially on the trunk. The bites themselves are soon obscured by excoriations and crusts of dried blood or serum. In chronic untreated cases ('vagabond's disease'), the skin becomes generally thickened, eczematized and pigmented; lymphadenopathy is common. Body lice can act as vectors for the organisms causing epidemic typhus, relapsing fever and trench fever.

Differential diagnosis

In scabies, characteristic burrows are seen (p. 253). Other causes of chronic itchy erythroderma include eczema and lymphomas, but these are ruled out by the finding of lice and nits.

Investigations

Clothing should be examined for the presence of eggs in the inner seams.

Treatment

First and foremost treat the infested clothing and bedding. Lice and their eggs can be killed by high temperature laundering, by dry cleaning and by tumble-drying. Less competent patients will need help here. Once this has been achieved, 5% permethrin cream rinse or 1% lindane lotion (United States only; Formulary 1, p. 405) may be used on the patient's skin.

Pubic lice

Cause

Pubic lice (crabs) are broader than scalp and body lice, and their second and third pairs of legs are well adapted to cling on to hair. They are usually spread by sexual contact, and most commonly infest young adults.

Presentation

Severe itching in the pubic area is followed by eczematization and secondary infection. Among the excoriations will be seen small blue–grey macules of altered blood at the site of bites. The shiny translucent nits are less obvious than those of head lice (Figure 17.2). Pubic lice spread most extensively in hairy males and may even affect the eyelashes.

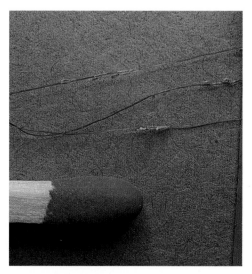

Figure 17.2 Pediculosis pubis. Numerous eggs (nits) can be seen on the plucked pubic hairs.

Differential diagnosis

Eczema of the pubic area gives similar symptoms but lice and nits are not seen.

Investigations

The possibility of coexisting sexually transmitted diseases should be kept in mind.

Treatment

Carbaryl, permethrin and malathion are all effective treatments. Aqueous solutions are less irritant than alcoholic ones. They should be applied for 12 hours or overnight – and not just to the pubic area, but to all surfaces of the body, including the perianal area, limbs, scalp, neck, ears and face (especially the eyebrows and the beard, if present). Treatment should be repeated after 1 week, and infected sexual partners should also be treated. Shaving the area is not necessary.

Infestation of the eyelashes is particularly hard to treat, as this area is so sensitive that the mechanical removal of lice and eggs can be painful. Applying a thick layer of petrolatum twice a day for 2 weeks has been recommended. Aqueous malathion is effective for eyelash infestations but does not have a product licence for this purpose.

Patients should avoid close bodily contact until they and their partners have been treated and completed their follow-up.

Insect bites

Insects inject venoms to kill prey and defend themselves. These stings cause painful inflammatory reactions soon after the attack. Insects also inject chemicals as they feed, usually to anticoagulate the blood. These chemicals and some toxins may cause purpuric and allergic reactions characterized by itching papules or wheals.

Different people may react differently depending upon the type of immunological reaction. Nothing happens after the first bite because there has been no previous exposure and hence no chance for induction of an immune response. With continued biting over time, many individuals develop a cell-mediated immune response that produces itchy red bumps 1–4 days after bites. These last for up to 2 weeks. Others develop immediate IgE-mediated reactions that cause wheals within minutes after a bite and that can cause anaphylaxis. Some develop both types. In this situation, a wheal may appear within a few minutes and then disappear, to be followed hours later by a firm itchy persistent papule, often with a central

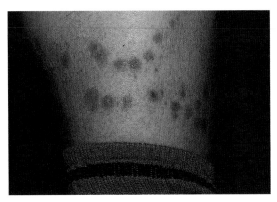

Figure 17.3 Florid insect bites on the leg. Note the tendency of the lesions to lie in lines and groups.

haemorrhagic punctum. Bullous reactions are common on the legs of children.

The diagnosis of insect bites is usually obvious; when it is not, the term papular urticaria is sometimes used.

Papular urticaria

Cause
This term, with its hint that the condition is a variant of ordinary urticaria, is a misnomer. Papular urticaria is nothing more than an excessive, possibly allergic, reaction to insect bites. The source of the bites may be simple garden pests but more often is a parasite on a domestic pet. Often the source cannot be traced.

Presentation
Lesions are usually most common on the arms or legs. They consist of groups or lines of small itchy excoriated smooth pink papules (Figure 17.3) of a uniform size that may become bullous and infected. Some clear to leave small scars or pigmented macules.

Course
An affected child will usually 'grow out' of the problem in a few years, even if the source of the bites is not dealt with. Individual lesions last for 1–2 weeks and recur in distinct crops, especially in the summer – hence the lay term 'heat bumps'. The lesions will disappear with any change of environment, for example by going on holiday. Surprisingly, often only one member of a family is affected, perhaps because the others have developed immunological tolerance after repeated bites.

Complications
Itching leads to much discomfort and loss of sleep. Impetiginization is common.

Differential diagnosis
The grouped excoriated papules of papular urticaria are quite different from the skin changes of scabies, in which burrows are the diagnostic feature. Atopic prurigo may be more difficult to distinguish but here there is usually a family history of atopy and frankly eczematous plaques in a typical distribution.

Investigations
The parents should be encouraged to act as detectives in their own environment, but some resist the idea that the lesions are caused by bites, asking why the other family members are not affected. This attitude is often supported by veterinarians who, after a superficial look at infested animals, pronounce them clear. In such cases the animal should be brushed vigorously while standing on a polythene sheet. Enough dandruff-like material can then be obtained to send to a reliable veterinary laboratory. Often the cause is a *Cheyletiella* mite infestation.

Treatment
Local treatment with a topical corticosteroid or calamine lotion, and the regular use of insect repellents, may be of some help but the ultimate solution is to trace the source of the bites or await spontaneous remission.

Infested animals should be treated by a veterinarian, and insecticidal powders should be used for soft furnishings in the home. Sometimes professional exterminators are needed, but even measures such as these can meet with little success.

Bed bugs (Hemiptera)
Bed bugs are once again prevalent in hotels, houses and hostels. During the day, bed bugs hide in crevices in walls and furniture; at night they can travel considerable distances to reach a sleeping person. Burning wheals, turning into firm papules, occur in groups wherever the crawling bugs have easy access to the skin – the face, neck and hands being the most common sites. Often bites appear in groups of three recalling the bug's breakfast, lunch and dinner. Treatment should be based on the application of insecticides to walls and furniture where the bugs hide.

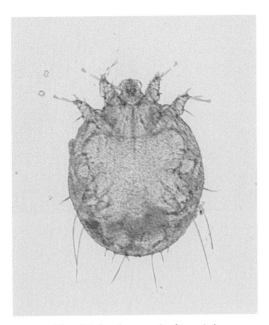

Figure 17.4 The adult female acarus (scabies mite).

Myiasis

The larvae of several species of fly develop only if deposited in living flesh; humans are one of several possible hosts. The skin lesions look like boils, but movement may be detected within them. The diagnosis is proved by incising the nodule and extracting the larva.

Scabies

Cause

Scabies is caused by the mite *Sarcoptes scabiei* var. *hominis* (Figure 17.4). Adult mites are 0.3–0.4 mm long and therefore just visible, although hard to see except through a lens. It is now well established that the mites are transferred from person to person by close bodily contact and not via inanimate objects.

Once on the skin, fertilized female mites can move over the surface at up to 2 cm a minute, but can burrow through the stratum corneum at only about 2 mm/day. They produce two or three oval eggs each day, which turn into sexually mature mites in 2–3 weeks. The number of adult mites varies from case to case – from less than 10 in a clean adult to many more in an unwashed child. The generalized eruption of scabies, and its itchiness, are thought to be caused by a sensitization to the mites or their products.

Epidemiology

Scabies is endemic in many developing countries, and high levels of prevalence go with poverty, overcrowding and poor hygiene. In other populations, scabies rises and falls cyclically, peaking every 15–25 years. The idea of 'herd immunity' has been put forward to explain this, spread being most easy when a new generation of susceptible individuals has arisen. Scabies is most common in the autumn and winter.

Presentation

For 4–6 weeks after a first infestation there may be no itching, but thereafter it dominates the picture, often being particularly bad at night and affecting several people. In contrast, in a second attack of scabies, itching starts within a day or two, because these victims already have immunity to produce the itchy allergic reactions.

The most dramatic part of the eruption – excoriated, eczematized or urticarial papules – is usually on the trunk, and mark feeding spots where the mites were a day or two ago. Do not search for the mite here. Do not search for a moving mite either; they are too small to see. Look instead for burrows where female mites lay their eggs (Figure 17.5).

Most burrows lie on the sides of the fingers, finger webs, sides of the hand and on the flexural aspects of the wrists. Other favourite sites include the elbows, ankles and feet

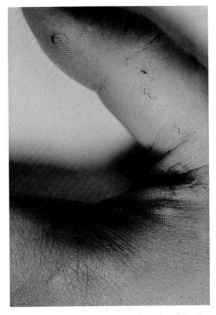

Figure 17.5 Typical burrows seen on the side of the thumb.

(especially in infants; Figure 17.6), nipples and genitals (Figure 17.7). Only in infancy does scabies affect the face. Burrows are easily missed grey–white slightly scaly tortuous lines of up to 1 cm in length. The acarus may be seen through a lens as a small dark dot at the most recent least scaly end of the burrow. With experience it can be removed for microscopic confirmation (p. 38). On the genitals, burrows are associated with erythematous rubbery nodules (Figure 17.8).

Course

Scabies persists indefinitely unless treated. In the chronic stage, the number of mites may be small and diagnosis is correspondingly difficult. Relapses after apparently

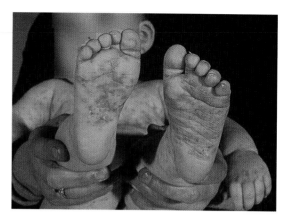

Figure 17.6 The characteristic plantar lesions of scabies in infancy.

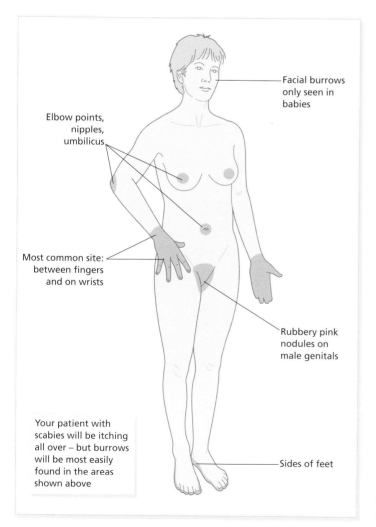

Facial burrows only seen in babies

Elbow points, nipples, umbilicus

Most common site: between fingers and on wrists

Rubbery pink nodules on male genitals

Your patient with scabies will be itching all over – but burrows will be most easily found in the areas shown above

Sides of feet

Figure 17.7 Common sites of burrows in scabies.

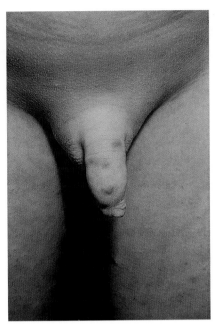

Figure 17.8 Unmistakable rubbery nodules on the penis, diagnostic of scabies.

adequate treatment are common and can be put down to re-infestation from undetected and untreated contacts.

Complications
• Secondary infection, with pustulation, is common (Figure 17.9). Rarely, glomerulonephritis follows this.
• Repeated applications of scabicides can cause skin irritation and eczema.
• Persistent itchy red nodules may remain on the genitals or armpits of children for some months after adequate treatment.

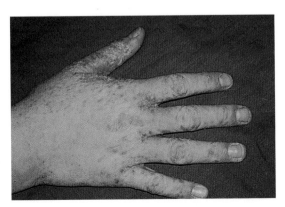

Figure 17.9 Scabies with bacterial superinfection.

• Venereal disease may be acquired at the same time as scabies.
• Crusted (Norwegian) scabies, which may not be itchy, is a widespread crusted eruption in which vast numbers of mites are found. It affects people whose immune system cannot control the infestation, usually due to HIV or immunosuppressive drugs. Such patients can be the unsuspected source of epidemics of ordinary scabies, for example in nursing homes.

Differential diagnosis
Only scabies shows characteristic burrows. Animal scabies from pets induces an itchy rash in humans but this lacks burrows. The lesions of papular urticaria (p. 252) are excoriated papules, in groups, mainly on the legs. Late-onset atopic eczema (p. 87), cholinergic urticaria (p. 100), lichen planus (p. 69), neurotic excoriations (p. 338) and dermatitis herpetiformis (p. 119) have their own distinctive features.

Investigations
With practice an acarus can be picked neatly with a needle from the end of its burrow and identified microscopically; failing this, eggs and mites can be seen microscopically in burrow scrapings mounted in potassium hydroxide (p. 38) or mineral oil. Some find dermatoscopy (p. 36) a quick and reliable way to find the mite.

Treatment
Treatment should be started if the diagnosis seems likely on clinical grounds, even if the presence of mites cannot be confirmed microscopically. Do not treat just the patient: treat all members of the family and sexual contacts too, whether they are itching or not (Figure 17.10).
• Use an effective scabicide (Formulary 1, p. 405). In the United Kingdom, the preferred treatment is with permethrin, with malathion as the second choice. Topical treatment plus ivermectin (on a named patient basis in the United Kingdom), in a single dose of 200 µg/kg by mouth, is effective for Norwegian scabies and scabies that does not respond to topical measures alone.
• A convenient way to apply scabicides to the skin is with a 5-cm (2 inch) paintbrush. The number of applications recommended varies from dermatologist to dermatologist. There is no doubt that some preparations, such as malathion, disappear quickly from the skin, leaving it vulnerable to any mites hatching out from eggs that have survived. A second application, a week after the first, is then essential. With permethrin, this may be less important. Another good reason for recommending a second

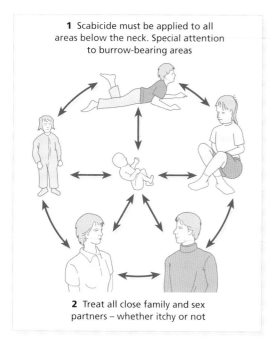

1 Scabicide must be applied to all areas below the neck. Special attention to burrow-bearing areas

2 Treat all close family and sex partners – whether itchy or not

Figure 17.10 The treatment of scabies.

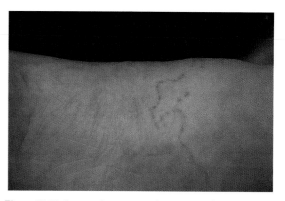

Figure 17.11 Larva migrans – a red serpiginous line on the instep.

• Ordinary laundering deals satisfactorily with clothing and sheets. Mites die in clothing unworn for 1 week.

Parasitic worms

A textbook of tropical medicine should be consulted for more details on this subject.

Larva migrans (creeping eruption)

The larvae of hookworms that go through their full life cycle only in cats or dogs can penetrate human skin when it is in contact with soil or sand contaminated by the faeces of these animals. Larva migrans is most frequently found in the tropics and subtropics, and is the most common parasitic infection of the skin seen in travellers, typically returning from beach holidays in the Caribbean, Central America or Africa. It is now also being acquired in the United Kingdom. The larvae move under the skin creating tortuous red itchy lines (Figure 17.11) that advance at the rate of a few millimetres a day. As man is a dead end host for the larvae they do eventually die, but this can be speeded up by either local treatment with a single oral dose of ivermectin or 1 week of daily albendazole.

Onchocerciasis

This is endemic in much of Central America and Africa where it is an important cause of blindness. The buffalo gnat (*Simulium* species) carries the filarial worm to humans. Infested humans become itchy with an excoriated papular eruption. Later the skin may thicken and become hyper- or hypopigmented. Dermal nodules are found, mainly near bony prominences, and contain both mature worms and microfilariae. It is the latter that invade the eye, leading to blindness. The diagnosis is confirmed

application is that it will cover areas left out during an inefficient first application.

• Most now recommend that the treatment should be applied to the scalp, neck, face and ears as well as to the rest of the skin. Areas that must be included are the genitals, soles of the feet, gluteal fold and the skin under the free edge of the nails. The scabicide should be reapplied if the hands are washed. A hot bath before treatment is no longer recommended.

• Residual itching may last for several days, or even a few weeks, but this does not need further applications of the scabicide. Rely instead on calamine lotion or crotamiton.

• For babies, toddlers and children up to 2 years old we advise special care with treatment. Permethrin is licensed for infants over the age of 2 months, although needs to be used with caution. For many years 6% precipitated sulfur in petrolatum has been used in children without adverse effects. In any case aqueous preparations are best for children as alcoholic ones can sting.

• Permethrin is probably safe in pregnancy and in nursing mothers as little is absorbed, and any that is absorbed is rapidly detoxified and eliminated.

• Have a printed sheet (see *Further reading* at the end of this chapter) to give to the patient and go through it with them – scabies victims are notoriously confused.

by detecting active microfilariae in skin snips teased out in saline and examined microscopically. Rapid serum antibody tests for *Onchocerca volvulus* using cards or fluorescent assays have recently been developed and may replace skin snips. Ivermectin is the treatment of choice. A single dose produces a prolonged reduction of microfilarial levels, and should be repeated every 6–12 months until the adult worms die out. *Onchocerca volvulus* plays host to the endosymbiotic bacterium *Wolbachia*. Targetting this with a 6-week course of doxycycline also appears to slowly kill adult worms.

Filariasis

This is endemic throughout much of the tropics. The adult filarial worms, usually *Wucheria bancrofti*, inhabit the lymphatics where they excite an inflammatory reaction with episodes of lymphangitis and fever, gradually leading to lymphatic obstruction and lymphoedema, usually of the legs or scrotum. Such swellings can be massive (elephantiasis). There is an eosinophilia and microfilariae are found in the peripheral blood, mainly at night; their vector from human to human is the mosquito, in which the larvae mature. Diethylcarbamazine or ivermectin is the treatment of choice.

Other worm infestations

• Threadworm (pinworm) infestation in children can cause severe anal and vulval pruritus. The small worms are seen best at night-time when the itch is worst. Treatment is with a single dose of mebendazole 100 mg, or piperazine.
• Swimmer's itch, in tropical and lake waters, may be caused by the penetration through the skin of the cercariae of schistosomes of human and non-human origin. These cause itching red papule on exposed areas, especially the legs. The skin should be towelled off immediately after swimming to prevent the schistosomes penetrating the skin as it dries.
• The larval stages of the pork tapeworm (cysticercosis) can present as multiple firm nodules in the skin.
• Larger fluctuant cysts may be caused by hydatid disease.

Learning points

1 Always look for signs of head lice before attributing enlarged cervical lymph nodes to anything more sinister.
2 Paravenereal diseases hunt in packs. Does your patient with scabies also have pubic lice, genital mollusca or something even worse?
3 Look for mites in the burrows, where they are laying their eggs, not in the widespread itchy red papular lesions.
4 Never forget to treat the contacts – itchy or not – as if you do not, they will reinfect your patient and waste everybody's time.
5 Remember to look for head lice in children presenting with cervical adenopathy.
6 Do not think that cutaneous larva migrans is a tropical disease. Recent reports document cases acquired in the United Kingdom.

Further reading

Guidelines for scabies have been prepared by the Association of Genitourinary Medicine and are available at http://www.bashh.org/documents/27/27.pdf (accessed 28 June 2014).
A patient information leaflet on scabies is available through the British Association of Dermatologists at www.bad.org.uk (accessed 28 June 2014).

Currie BJ, McCarthy JS. (2010) Permethrin and ivermectin for scabies. *New England Journal of Medicine* **362**, 717–725.
Taylor MJ, Hoerauf A, Bockarie M. (2010) Lymphatic filariasis and onchocerciasis. *Lancet* **376**, 1175–1185.
Tebruegge M, Pantazidou A, Curtis N. (2011) What's bugging you? An update on the treatment of head lice infestation. *Archives of Disease in Childhood: Education and Practice Edition* **96**, 2–8.
Toups MA, Kitchen A, Light JE, Reed DL. (2011) Origin of clothing lice indicates early clothing use by anatomically modern humans in Africa. *Molecular Biology and Evolution* **28**, 29–32.

18 Skin Reactions to Light

Ultraviolet radiation (UVR) has a mixture of beneficial and harmful effects. Our species, *Homo sapiens,* arose in Africa probably around 200 000 years ago. In contrast to our primate cousins, we have lost our covering of fur. In combination with the high volumes of sweat we can produce, this enables us to lose heat effectively, and originally we found our ecological niche as a long distance hunter, able to track our prey until heat and exhaustion fatally weakened it. With this loss of fur, however, has come the need to cope with the effects of the sun directly striking our epidermis. In the last 80 000 years we have scattered from our ancestral African homeland to populate the globe. The range of environments in which we have settled, from the tropics to the polar regions, and Himalayan heights to below sea level, has further altered our exposure to sunlight and imposed powerful evolutionary pressures on our skin. The most obvious effect of this has been in the range of pigmentation we show. This has been caused by two opposing evolutionary pressures. On the one hand we need pale enough skin to synthesise vitamin D, and, on the other, our skin needs enough eumelanin to protect from carcinogenesis and neural tube defect-inducing folate destruction. Recent large-scale population movements have led to high rates of skin cancer in white Australians, and high rates of rickets in immigrants from the Indian subcontinent to Scotland.

The UVR spectrum is divided into three parts (Figure 18.1), each having different effects on the skin, although UVC does not penetrate the ozone layer of the atmosphere and is therefore currently irrelevant to skin disease. Virtually all of the UVB is absorbed in the epidermis, whereas some 30% of UVA reaches the dermis. The B wavelengths (UVB: 290–320 nm) cause sunburn and are effectively screened out by window glass. The A spectrum (UVA) is longwave ultraviolet light, from 320 nm to the most violet colour perceptible to the eye (about 400 nm). It ages and tans the skin. The differences between the wavelengths can be recorded conveniently in the form of action spectra, which show how effective each is at producing different biological effects, such as clearing psoriasis or causing erythema. UVR is non-ionizing, but changes the skin by reacting with endogenous light-absorbing chemicals (chromophores), which include DNA, RNA, urocanic acid and melanin.

The variation in consitutive skin pigmentation and response to UVR is conventionally divided into six types (Table 18.1). These skin types require different degrees of protection against the sun.

Beneficial effects of sunlight

A considerable body of epidemiological data suggest beneficial health effects of sunlight but the interpretation of these data can be contentious. Rickets is a disease of poor diet or inadequate sun exposure resulting in low vitamin D levels and correction of either of these factors is therapeutic. The case for the benefits of vitamin D in other conditions is less clear-cut. Observational studies show that subjects with high levels of circulating vitamin D are less likely to have cardiovascular disease, hypertension, type 2 diabetes or multiple sclerosis than those with low levels. Correlation should not be confused with causation, however, and the results of intervention studies in which vitamin D supplementation has been given have been disappointing. Ill health may lead to reduced sun exposure and thus low vitamin D levels (reverse causation), or vitamin D levels might be acting as a marker for sunlight exposure, which is beneficial via a different mechanism (confounding). A newly identified alternative mechanism is mediated by the vasodilator nitric oxide. The skin contains large stores of nitrate and nitrite, which are converted by sunlight to the nitric oxide

Clinical Dermatology, Fifth Edition. Richard B. Weller, Hamish J.A. Hunter and Margaret W. Mann.
© 2015 John Wiley & Sons, Ltd. Published 2015 by John Wiley & Sons, Ltd.

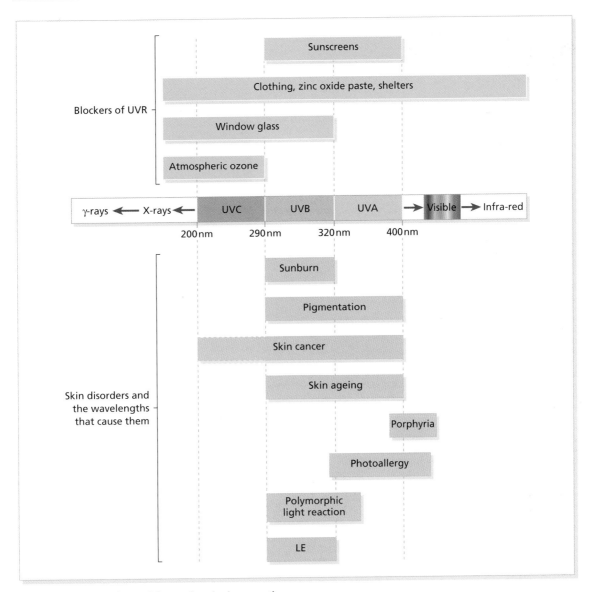

Figure 18.1 Skin disorders and the wavelengths that cause them.

from where it enters the circulation and lowers blood pressure. Other mechanisms may also exist.

Clinically, UVR is helpful in the treatment of diseases such as psoriasis and eczema, but at the same time use of tanning lamps, particularly by young people, increases the risk of developing melanoma and non-melanoma skin cancers. Excess UV exposure also leads to photoageing, and may cause or worsen several skin disorders (Figure 18.2).

Sunburn

Cause

UVB penetrates the epidermis and superficial dermis, stimulating the production and release of prostaglandins, leukotrienes, histamine, interleukin 1 (IL-1) and tumour necrosis factor α (TNF-α). These cause pain and stimulate the production of the inducible nitric oxide synthase (iNOS) enzyme. This generates very high local

Table 18.1 Skin types classified by their reactions to
ultraviolet radiation (UVR).

Type	Definition	Description
I	Always burns but never tans	Pale skin, red hair, freckles
II	Usually burns, sometimes tans	Fair skin
III	May burn, usually tans	Darker skin
IV	Rarely burns, always tans	Mediterranean
V	Moderate constitutional pigmentation	Latin American, Middle Eastern
VI	Marked constitutional pigmentation	Black

concentrations of nitric oxide which causes the characteristic dermal vasodilatation and redness.

Presentation and course

Skin exposed to too much UVB smarts and becomes red several hours later. Severe sunburn is painful and may blister. The redness is maximal after 1 day, contemporaneously with peak levels of the iNOS enzyme, and then settles over the next 2–3 days, leaving sheet-like desquamation (Figure 18.3), diffuse pigmentation (a 'tan') and, sometimes, discrete lentigines.

Differential diagnosis

Phototoxic reactions caused by drugs are like an exaggerated sunburn.

Investigations

None are required.

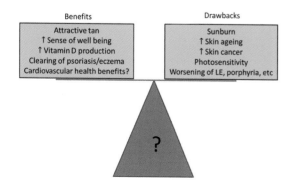

Figure 18.2 The balance between the benefits and drawbacks of sun exposure.

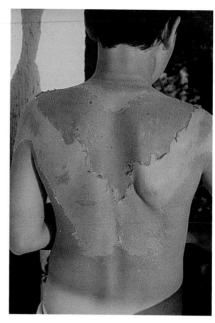

Figure 18.3 Peeling after acute sunburn. This doctor's son should have known better.

Treatment

The treatment is symptomatic. Baths may be cooling and oily shake lotions (e.g. oily calamine lotion) or creams are comforting. Potent topical corticosteroids (Formulary 1, p. 401) help if used early and briefly. Oral aspirin (a prostaglandin synthesis inhibitor) relieves the pain.

Phototoxicity

Basic photochemical laws require a drug to absorb UVR to cause such a reaction. Most drugs listed in Table 18.2 absorb UVA as well as UVB, and so window glass, protective against sunburn, does not protect against most phototoxic drug reactions.

Presentation and course

Tenderness and redness occur only in areas exposed both to sufficient drug and to sufficient UVR (Figure 18.4). The signs and symptoms are those of sunburn. The skin may later develop a deep tan.

Cause

These reactions are not immunological. Everyone exposed to enough of the drug, and to enough UVR, will develop the reaction. Some drugs that can cause

Table 18.2 Drugs commonly causing photosensitivity.

Amiodarone
Chlorpromazine
Doxycycline
Nalidixic acid
Naproxen
Piroxicam
Phenothiazines
Psoralens
Sulfonamides
Tetracyclines
Thiazides
Topical NSAIDs
    Etofenamate
    Ketoprofen
Topical UV absorbers
    Octocrylene
    Benzophenone-3
Voriconazole

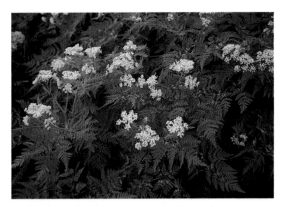

Figure 18.5 Cow parsley contains psoralens and is a common cause of photodermatitis.

phototoxic reactions are listed in Table 18.2. In addition, contact with psoralens in plants (Figure 18.5) can cause a localized phototoxic dermatitis (phytophotodermatitis; Figure 18.6). These areas burn and may blister, leaving pigmentation in linear streaks and bizarre patterns.

Differential diagnosis

Photoallergic reactions are difficult to distinguish; the more so as the same drugs can often cause both photoallergic and phototoxic reactions. The main differences between phototoxicity and photoallergy are shown in Table 18.3.

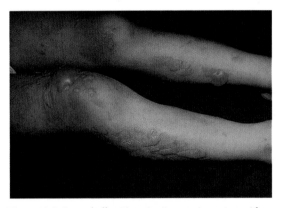

Figure 18.6 Severe bullous eruption in areas in contact with giant hogweed (contains psoralens) and then exposed to sunlight (phytophotodermatitis).

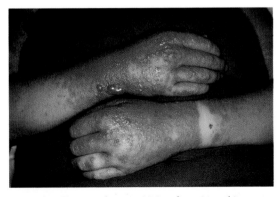

Figure 18.4 Extreme photosensitivity of a patient taking griseofulvin. Note sparing of the area covered by the watch strap and ring.

Table 18.3 Features distinguishing phototoxicity from photoallergy.

Phototoxicity	Photoallergy
Erythematous and smooth (may blister)	Eczematous and rough (may weep)
Immediate onset	Delayed onset (when immunity develops; may not occur on first exposure)
Hurts	Itches
Photopatch testing negative	Photopatch testing positive
Lasts 3–5 days	Lasts 3–14 days

Investigations

None are usually required. In difficult cases, phototesting can be carried out in special centres. The action spectrum (the wavelengths that cause the reaction) may incriminate a particular drug.

Treatment

This is the same as for sunburn. Drugs should be stopped if further exposure to ultraviolet light is likely.

Photoallergy

Drugs, topical or systemic, and chemicals on the skin, can interact with UVR and cause immunological reactions.

Cause

UVR converts an immunologically inactive form of a drug into an antigenic molecule. An immunological reaction, analogous to allergic contact dermatitis (p. 84), is induced if the antigen remains in the skin or is formed there on subsequent exposure to the drug and UVR. Many of the same drugs that cause phototoxic reactions can also cause photoallergic ones. Organic UV absorbers in sunscreens and non-steroidal anti-inflammatory drugs are the most common topical agents to lead to photoallergic reactions.

Presentation

Photoallergy is often similar to phototoxicity. The areas exposed to UVR become inflamed, but the reaction usually becomes eczematous, appears later and lasts longer. The eruption will be on exposed areas such as the hands, the V of the neck, the nose, the chin and the forehead. There is also a tendency to spare the upper lip under the nose, the eyelids and the submental region (Figure 18.7). Often, the eruption does not occur on the first exposure to ultraviolet, but only after a second or further exposures. A lag phase of one or more weeks is needed to induce an immune response.

Course

The original lesions are red patches, plaques, vesicles or bullae, which usually become eczematous. They tend to resolve when either the drug or the exposure to UVR is stopped, but this may take several weeks.

Complications

Some drugs, such as the sulfonamides, can cause a persistent light reaction (see *Chronic actinic dermatitis*).

Investigations

Photopatch testing by an expert can confirm the diagnosis. The chemical is applied for 24 hours and the skin is then irradiated with UVA. An acute photoallergic contact dermatitis is then elicited. A control patch, not irradiated, rules out ordinary allergic contact dermatitis.

Treatment

The drug should be stopped and the patient protected from further ultraviolet exposure (avoidance, clothing and sunscreens). Potent topical corticosteroids or a short course of a systemic corticosteroid will hasten resolution and provide symptomatic relief.

Chronic actinic dermatitis (actinic reticuloid)

Some patients with a photoallergic reaction never get over it and go on developing sun-induced eczematous areas long after the drug has been stopped.

Cause

This is not clear but as most patients have positive patch or photopatch tests, contact allergy presumably plays a part.

Presentation

This is the same as a photoallergic reaction to a drug. The patient goes on to develop a chronic dermatitis, with thick plaques on sun-exposed areas.

Course

These patients may be exquisitely sensitive to UVR. They are usually middle-aged or elderly men who react after the slightest exposure, even through window glass or from fluorescent lights. Affected individuals also are/or become allergic to a range of contact allergens, especially oleoresins in some plants (e.g. chrysanthemums).

Complications

None, but the persistent severe pruritic eruption can lead to depression and even suicide.

Differential diagnosis

Airborne allergic contact dermatitis may be confused, but does not require sunlight. Sometimes the diagnosis is difficult as exposure both to sunlight and to the airborne allergen occurs only out of doors. Airborne allergic contact dermatitis also affects sites that sunlight is less likely to reach, such as eyelids and under the chin

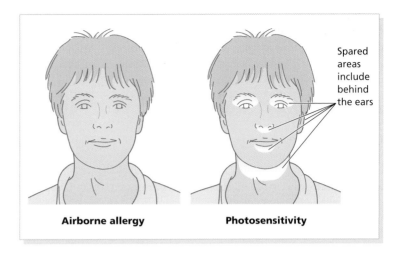

Spared areas include behind the ears

Airborne allergy   **Photosensitivity**

Figure 18.7 Features distinguishing airborne allergy from photosensitivity.

(Figure 18.7). A continuing drug photoallergy, a polymorphic light eruption (see *Polymorphic light reaction*) or eczema as a result of some other cause must also be considered.

Histology shows a dense lymphocytic infiltrate and sometimes atypical activated lymphocytes suggestive of a lymphoma, but the disorder seldom becomes malignant.

Investigations

Persistent light reaction can be confirmed experimentally by exposing uninvolved skin to UVA or UVB. Patch tests and photopatch tests help to distinguish between photoallergy and airborne allergic contact dermatitis, and the action spectrum may point to a certain drug. This sort of testing is difficult, and should be carried out only in specialist centres.

Treatment

Usually cared for by specialists, these patients need extreme measures to protect their skin from UVR. These include protective clothing and frequent applications of combined UVA and UVB blocking agents (Formulary 1, p. 400). Patients must protect themselves from UVR coming through windows or from fluorescent lights. Some can only go out at night. As even the most potent topical steroids are often ineffective, systemic steroids or immunosuppressants (e.g. azathioprine) may be needed for long periods.

Polymorphic light eruption

This is the most frequent cause of a so-called 'sun allergy'.

Cause

It is speculated that UVR causes a natural skin constituent to change into an allergen, to which inadequately suppressed immunological response is made. Mechanisms are similar to those in drug photoallergy. Some people seem genetically predisposed, because other family members may have the problem too.

Presentation

Small itchy red papules, papulovesicles or eczematous plaques arise from 2 hours to 5 days, most commonly at 24 hours, after exposure to UVR. The eruption is itchy and usually confined to sun-exposed areas (Figure 18.8), remembering that some UVR passes through thin clothing. Not all exposed skin develops disease so there are papules and plaques rather than generalized redness.

Course

The disorder tends to recur each spring after UVR exposure. Tanning protects some patients so that if the initial

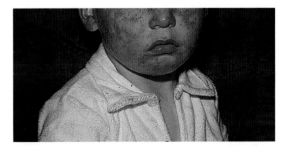

Figure 18.8 Polymorphic light eruption: eczematous plaques on the face of a sad freckly boy. Persists throughout the summer but fades in the winter.

exposures are limited, few or no symptoms occur later. Such patients can still enjoy sun exposure and outdoor activities. Others are so sensitive, or their skin pigments so poorly, that fresh exposures continue to induce reactions throughout the summer. These patients require photoprotection, and must limit their sun exposure and outdoor activities. The rash disappears during the winter.

Differential diagnosis

Phototoxic reactions, photoallergic reactions, miliaria rubra, chronic actinic dermatitis, ordinary eczemas, allergic reactions to sunscreens and airborne allergic contact dermatitis should be considered.

Investigations

It may be possible to reproduce the dermatitis by testing non-sun-exposed skin with UVB and UVA.

Treatment

If normal tanning does not confer protection, sunscreens (Formulary 1, p. 400) should be used. Protective clothing, such as wide-brimmed hats, long-sleeved shirts and long trousers, is helpful. In some patients, a 4-week PUVA course (p. 62) in the late spring can create enough tan to confer protection for the rest of the season. Moderately potent topical steroids (Formulary 1, p. 401) usually improve the eruption. A tapering course of systemic steroids may tide people over during severe or early spring outbreaks. Hydroxychloroquine (Formulary 2, p. 424) may be effective when used over the sunny season.

Actinic prurigo

This is probably a persistent form of polymorphic light eruption. Papules, crusts and excoriations arise on sun-exposed areas and sometimes also on other sites. Lesions may persist through the winter. It is common among North American Indians and may resemble excoriated acne, bites, eczema, erythropoetic protoporphyria or neurotic excoriations. There is a strong association between actinic prurigo and the HLA DRB1*0407 genotype, suggesting that altered antigen presentation plays a part in the development of the disease.

Solar urticaria

This is discussed in Chapter 8. Wheals occur on the sun-exposed areas, within minutes. Some patients are react-

ing to UVB, others to UVA, and still others to visible light. Some patients have erythropoietic protoporphyria (p. 316) and this should be considered particularly if solar urticaria starts in infancy.

Learning points

If the skin reacts badly to light through glass then:
1 Sunscreens are usually ineffective.
2 Think of drugs or porphyria.

Actinic keratoses

These are discussed in Chapter 20.

Actinic cheilitis

This is discussed in Chapter 13 and see Figure 27.17.

Lupus erythematosus

Many patients with lupus erythematosus (p. 126) become worse after exposure to UVR, especially to UVB. This is particularly true of the subacute cutaneous variant associated with antibodies to SS-A and SS-B. They should be warned about this, and protect themselves from the sun (avoidance, clothing and sunscreens).

Carcinomas

The sun's rays can cause basal cell carcinomas, squamous cell carcinomas and malignant melanomas. These are discussed in Chapter 20. People with more than five episodes of sunburn double their risk of developing a melanoma.

Exacerbated diseases

UVR is useful in the treatment of many skin diseases, but it can also make some worse (Table 18.4).

Porphyria cutanea tarda

This is described in Chapter 21.

Table 18.4 The effect of sunlight on some skin diseases.

Helps	Worsens
Atopic eczema	Darier's disease
Cutaneous T-cell lymphoma	Herpes simplex
Parapsoriasis	Lupus erythematosus
Pityriasis lichenoides	Pellagra
Pityriasis rosea	Photoallergy/toxicity
Pruritus of renal failure, liver disease	Porphyrias (excluding acute intermittent)
AIDS	Xeroderma pigmentosum
Psoriasis	

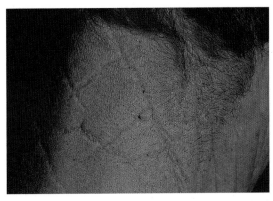

Figure 18.10 Solar elastosis is a sign of photoageing.

Cutaneous ageing

The trouble with old skin is the way it looks rather than the way it behaves. Skin chronically damaged by UVR during childhood thereafter looks old. This 'photoageing' effect causes the skin to become thin on the extremities, so that it bruises (Bateman's purpura) and tears easily (Figure 18.9). The elastic fibres become clumped and amorphous, leading clinically to a yellow pebbly look called actinic elastosis (Figure 18.10). Chronic exposure to sunlight, or to UVR in tanning parlours, also causes lentigines, freckles, roughness and, of course, skin cancers. The bronzed young skins of today will become the wrinkled spotted rough prune-like ones of tomorrow. About 25% of our lifetime dose of sun exposure occurs in childhood.

Wrinkles occur when the dermis loses its elastic recoil, failing to snap back properly into shape. UVR damages elastic tissue and hastens this process. Although cosmetic procedures can smooth wrinkles out, there is no way to reverse the damage fully; however, tretinoin cream (Formulary 1, p. 405) seems to help some patients. Use of lasers, peels, radiotherapy and intense pulsed light have advocates, particulary for reducing redness, telangiectases and lentigines. Surgical 'face lifts' remove redundant skin and pull the rest tighter (see Chapter 27). Fillers can be injected into deep wrinkles. Prevention (reducing exposure to UVR) is better than any 'cure', and is especially important in sunny climates (Table 18.5).

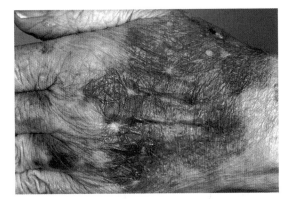

Figure 18.9 Thin skin on the back of the hand. The whitish areas are stellate pseudoscars, the skin having never been broken. The pseudoscars follow the dispersion of senile (Batemen's) purpura.

Table 18.5 Tips to avoid skin damage for those living in a sunny climate.

1 Apply sunscreen daily to all exposed parts – rain or shine, reapply after 20 minutes.
2 Reapply sunscreen often when outdoors.
3 Do not skimp. SPF calculations are based on 2 mg/cm^2 coverage. Most people underuse.
4 Use a sunscreen with a protective factor (SPF) of at least 15, preferably 30.
5 Choose a sunscreen that screens out both UVA and UVB.
6 Wear wide-brimmed hats.
7 Wear dense weave clothing. If you can see through it, it is not protective.
8 Target outdoor activities for early morning or late afternoon.
9 Seek the shade.
10 Avoid tanning salons.
11 Do not sunbathe.
12 Wear cosmetics, including lipstick.
13 Help your children to protect themselves.

Skin ages even in sun-protected areas, but much more slowly. Compare the buttock skin with skin on the face, forearms or back to be convinced. The dermis thins, skin collagen falls by about 1% per year throughout adult life and becomes more stable (less elastic). Fibroblasts become sparser in the dermis, accounting for reduced collagen synthesis and slower wound healing.

> **Learning point**
>
> If your family or patients have type I or II skin tell them that it is never too late to protect themselves from excessive sun exposure. You might be one of the few able to persuade them to think of the future.

Further reading

Berneburg M, Plettenberg H, Krutmann J. (2000) Photoaging of human skin. *Photodermatology, Photoimmunology and Photomedicine* **16**, 239–244.

Das S, Lloyd JJ, Walshaw D, Farr PM. (2004) Provocation testing in polymorphic light eruption using fluorescent ultraviolet (UV) A and UVB lamps. *British Journal of Dermatology* **15**, 1066–1070.

Drucker AM, Rosen CF. (2011) Drug-induced photosensitivity culprit drugs, management and prevention. *Drug Safety* **34**, 821–837.

European Multicentre Photopatch Test Study (EMCPPTS) Taskforce. (2012) A European multicentre photopatch test study. *British Journal of Dermatology* **166**, 1002–1009.

Feelisch M, Kolb-Bachofen V, Liu D, *et al.* (2010) Is sunlight good for our heart? *European Heart Journal* **31**, 1041–1045.

Ferguson J, Dover J. (2006) *Photodermatology*. Blackwell Publishing, Oxford.

Gonzalez E, Gonzalez S. (1996) Drug photosensitivity, idiopathic photodermatitis, and sunscreens. *Journal of the American Academy of Dermatology* **35**, 871–875.

Hawk J. (1998) *Photodermatology*. Hodder Arnold, London.

Krutman J, Hönigsmann H, Elmets CA, Bergstresser PR. (2001) *Dermatological Phototherapy and Photodiagnostic Methods*. Springer, Berlin.

Lim HW, Honigsmann H, Hawk J. (2007). *Photodermatology (Basic and Clinical Dermatology)*. Informa Healthcare, New York.

Ling TC, Gibbs NK, Rhodes LE. (2003) Treatment of polymorphic light eruption. *Photodermatology, Photoimmunology and Photomedicine* **19**, 217–227.

Murphy GM. (2004) Investigation of photosensitive disorders. *Photodermatology, Photoimmunology and Photomedicine* **20**, 305–311.

Harvey NC, Cooper C. (2012) Vitamin D: some perspective please. *British Medical Journal* **345**, e4695.

Pittas AG, Chung M, Trikalinos T, *et al.* (2010) Systematic review: vitamin D and cardiometabolic outcomes. *Annals of Internal Medicine* **152**, 307–314.

Poblete-Gutierrez P, Wiederholt T, Merk HF, Frank J. (2006) The porphyrias: clinical presentation, diagnosis and treatment. *European Journal of Dermatology* **16**, 230–240.

Rabe JH, Mamelak AJ, McElguun PJ, *et al.* (2006) Photoaging: mechanisms and repair. *Journal of the American Academy of Dermatology* **55**, 1–19.

19 Disorders of Pigmentation

Normal skin colour

The colour of normal skin comes from a mixture of pigments. Untanned Caucasoid skin is pink, tinted from white by oxyhaemoglobin in the blood within the dermis. Melanin (see *Melanogenesis*) blends with this colour, and may be increased, for example, after a suntan. Melanin is, of course, also responsible for the shades of brown seen not only in Congoid (Negroid) skin, but also in the other races. Various hues are caused by the addition to these pigments of yellow from carotene, found mainly in subcutaneous fat and in the horny layer of the epidermis. There is no natural blue pigment; when blue is seen, it is either because of an optical effect from normal pigment (usually melanin) in the dermis, or the presence of an abnormal pigment. Skin pigmentation (measured by skin reflectance) is darkest near the equator and correlates with latitude and ultraviolet radiation (UVR). Skin colour seems to have evolved as a compromise between being dark enough to block the damage to DNA caused by UVR and photolysis of the essential metabolite, folate, and light enough to allow vitamin D to be synthesized in the skin (p. 12). Melanins protect against UVR damage by absorbing and scattering the rays, and by scavenging free radicals.

Hair colour is determined by the relative amounts of the different types of melanin (see *Melanogenesis*). Eumelanin predominates in black hair and phaeomelanin in red.

Melanogenesis

Melanin is formed from the essential amino acid phenylalanine through a series of enzymatic steps in the liver and skin. Tyrosine, formed in the liver by hydroxylation of the essential amino acid phenylalanine under the influence of phenylalanine hydroxylase, is the substrate for the reactions that occur in melanocytes (Figure 19.1). Melanocytes are the only cells in the epidermis to contain tyrosinase (dopa oxidase), the rate-limiting enzyme in melanogenesis. Phaeomelanins and trichochromes, the pigments in red hair, are synthesized in a similar way, except that cysteine reacts with dopaquinone and is incorporated into the subsequent polymers. Phaeomelanins and eumelanins may intermesh to form mixed melanin polymers.

Eumelanins and phaeomelanins differ from neuromelanins, the pigments found in the substantia nigra and in cells of the chromaffin system (e.g. adrenal medulla, sympathetic ganglia). The latter are derived from tyrosine using a different enzyme, tyrosine hydroxylase, which is not found in melanocytes.

Melanin is made within melanosomes (see Figure 2.6), tiny particles measuring about 0.1×0.7 μm, shaped either like American footballs (eumelanosomes, containing eumelanin) or British soccer balls (phaeomelanosomes, containing phaeomelanin). Eventually, fully melanized melanosomes pass into the dendritic processes of the melanocyte to be injected into neighbouring keratinocytes. Once there, the melanosomes are engulfed in lysosomal packages (melanosome complexes) and distributed throughout the cytoplasm. Such secretory lysosomes are common to various haematopoietic cells and melanocytes. This explains why some genetic disorders of pigmentation (e.g. rare forms of albinism such as the Hermansky–Pudlak and Chediak–Higashi syndromes, p. 271) are linked with abnormal immune function.

All of us, regardless of race or skin colour, have similar density of melanocytes, with one melanocyte supplying melanin to about 30 keratinocyte neighbours. What determine a person's skin colour is the activity of those melanocytes and their interactions with their keratinocyte neighbours. Darker skin individuals have melanocytes that produce more and larger melanosomes. In addition, these melanosomes are more efficiently transferred to keratinocytes and more slowly degraded in the melanosome complexes.

Clinical Dermatology, Fifth Edition. Richard B. Weller, Hamish J.A. Hunter and Margaret W. Mann.
© 2015 John Wiley & Sons, Ltd. Published 2015 by John Wiley & Sons, Ltd.

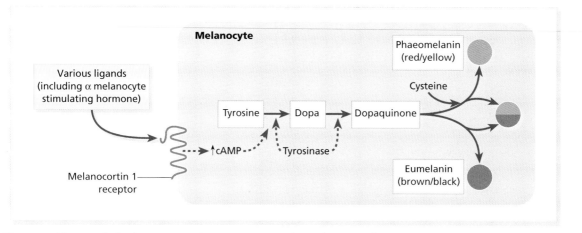

Figure 19.1 The control of melanogenesis. Melanocortin 1 receptor (MC1R) activity is both constitutive and rate limiting when promoting melanogenesis, via cyclic adenosine monophosphate (cAMP) production and tyrosinase stimulation. The MC1R is activated by ligands such as α-melanocyte-stimulating hormone (α-MSH) and other pituitary peptides. In the absence of such ligands or the MC1R itself (knockout animals), and with loss-of-function mutations of the MC1R, phaeomelanin is produced. The precise mechanism by which ultraviolet radiation stimulates melanogenesis remains uncertain.

The control of melanogenesis

Melanogenesis can be increased by several stimuli, the most important of which is UVR. Tanning represents a protective mechanism by our skin against future UV damage and involves two distinct reactions.

1 Immediate pigment darkening (IPD) following exposure to longwave ultraviolet (UVA 320–400 nm). This pigment darkening occurs over minutes to days, dependent on UV dose and constitutive skin colour, and is responsible for the well-known phenomenon of a 'false tan'. It is not caused by melanin synthesis but oxidation of preformed melanin and redistribution of melanin from perinuclear melanosomes to peripheral dendrites.

2 Delayed tanning (DT), the production of *new* pigment occurs some 3–4 days after exposure to medium-wave ultraviolet (UVB: 290–320 nm) and UVA and is maximal at 7 days. UVR results in DNA damage, which leads to the activation of p53. This in turn induces both keratinocytes and melanocytes in the skin to secrete pro-opiomelanocortin. Alpha melanocyte-stimulating hormone (α-MSH), a cleavage product of pro-opiomelanocortin, then binds the melanocortin 1 receptor on melanocytes and signals for the upregulation of microphthalmia transcription factor (MITF). MITF has a central role in melanogenesis by inducing the proliferation of melanocytes, increasing tyrosinase activity and melanosome production, and increasing the transfer of new melanosomes to their surrounding keratinocytes.

A neat control mechanism involving glutathione has been postulated. Reduced glutathione in the epidermis, produced by the action of glutathione reductase on glutathione, inhibits tyrosinase. UVR and some inflammatory skin conditions may induce pigmentation by oxidizing glutathione and so blocking its inhibition of melanogenesis.

Melanocytes are also influenced by MSH peptides from the pituitary and other areas of the brain (Figure 19.1). However, these MSH peptides may play little part in the physiological control of pigmentation. Hypophysectomy will not cause a black skin to lighten and only large doses of adrenocorticotrophic hormone (ACTH), in pathological states (p. 276), will increase skin pigmentation. In the skin, α-MSH also acts as an anti-inflammatory agent by antagonizing the effects of interleukin 1 (IL-1) in inducing IL-2 receptors on lymphocytes (p. 18) and in inducing pyrexia. Oestrogens and progestogens (and possibly testosterone too) may, in some circumstances, stimulate melanogenesis, either directly (by acting on oestrogen and progestogen receptors in the melanocyte) or by increasing the release of MSH peptides from the pituitary.

Genetics and skin pigmentation

Genetic differences determine the pigmentation of the different races (see Chapter 14, p. 197). A black person living in Britain, and a white person living in Africa will remain black and white, respectively. None the less, there is some phenotypic variation in skin colour (e.g. tanning after sun exposure). Red hair is the result of genetic variations in the amino acid sequence of the melanocortin 1 receptor (MC1R; Figure 19.1). Some genodermatoses with abnormal pigmentation are described in Chapter 24.

Abnormal skin colours

These may be caused by an imbalance of the normal pigments mentioned above (e.g. in cyanosis, chloasma and carotenaemia) or by the presence of abnormal pigments (Table 19.1). Sometimes, it is difficult to distinguish between the colours of these pigments (e.g. the gingery brown colour of haemosiderin is readily confused with melanin). Histological stains may be needed to settle the issue. In practice though, apart from tattoos, most pigmentary problems are caused by too much or too little melanin.

Decreased melanin pigmentation

Some conditions in which there is a lack of melanin are listed in Table 19.2. A few of the more important, and the mechanisms involved, are summarized in Figure 19.2. Decreased melanin pigmentation can be caused by the absence of melanocytes (vitiligo) or abnormalities in melanin synthesis (albinism). It is sometimes difficult to distinguish between hypomelanosis (decreased melanin) and amelanosis (complete absence of melanin). Wood's lamp (UVA light) examination can help enhance

Table 19.1 Some abnormal pigments.

Endogenous

Haemoglobin-derived

Methaemoglobin	Blue colour in vessels
Sulphaemoglobin	Cyanosis
Carboxyhaemoglobin	Pink
Bilirubin	Yellow–green
Biliverdin	
Haemosiderin	Brown

Drugs

Gold	Blue–grey (chrysiasis)
Silver	Blue–grey (argyria)
Bismuth	Grey
Mepacrine	Yellow
Clofazamine	Red
Phenothiazines	Slate-grey
Amiodarone	Blue-grey

Diet

Carotene	Orange

Exogenous

Tattoo pigments

Carbon	Blue–black
Coal dust	Blue–black
Cobalt	Blue
Chrome	Green
Cadmium	Yellow
Mercury	Red
Iron	Brown

Local medications

Silver nitrate	Black
Magenta paint	Magenta
Gentian violet	Violet
Eosin	Pink
Potassium permanganate	Brown
Dithranol (anthralin)	Purple
Tar	Brown
Iodine	Yellow

Table 19.2 Some causes of hypopigmentation.

Genetic	Albinism
	Piebaldism
	Phenylketonuria
	Waardenburg's syndrome
	Chediak–Higashi syndrome: autosomal recessive lysosomal defect, pale skin with sparse silvery-grey or blond hair, susceptible to infections
	Tuberous sclerosis (p. 345)
Endocrine	Hypopituitarism
Chemical	Contact with substituted phenols (in rubber industry)
Chloroquine and hydroxychloroquine	
Post-inflammatory	Eczema
	Pityriasis alba
	Psoriasis
	Sarcoidosis
	Lupus erythematosus
	Lichen sclerosus et atrophicus
	Cryotherapy
Infections	Leprosy
	Pityriasis versicolor
	Syphilis, yaws and pinta
Tumours	Halo naevus
	Malignant melanoma
Miscellaneous	Vitiligo
	Idiopathic guttate hypomelanosis

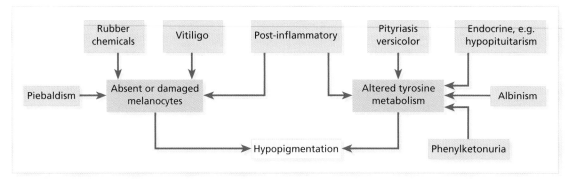

Figure 19.2 The mechanisms involved in some types of hypopigmentation.

the contrast; the greater the loss of epidermal pigment, the more marked the contrast.

Oculocutaneous albinism

Various genetic conditions exist in which there is a defect in the synthesis or packaging of melanin in the melanocyte, or a defective transfer of melanosomes to surrounding keratinocytes (see Chapter 2). In the most common type, little or no melanin is made in the skin and eyes (oculocutaneous albinism) or in the eyes alone (ocular albinism, not discussed further here). The prevalence of albinism of all types ranges from 1 in 20 000 in the United States and United Kingdom to 5% in some communities.

Cause

The hair bulb test (see *Investigations*) separates oculocutaneous albinism into two main types: tyrosinase-negative and tyrosinase-positive. Roughly equal numbers of the two types are found in most communities, both being inherited as autosomal recessive traits. This explains how children with two albino parents can sometimes themselves be normally pigmented, the genes being complementary in the double heterozygote (Figure 19.3).

The tyrosinase gene lies on chromosome 11q14-q21. More than 20 allelic variations have been found there in patients with tyrosinase-negative albinism. The gene for tyrosinase-positive human albinism has been mapped to chromosome 15q11-q13. It probably encodes for an ion channel protein in the melanosome involved in the transport of tyrosine.

Presentation and course

The whole epidermis is white and pigment is also lacking in the hair, iris and retina (Figure 19.3). Albinos have poor sight, photophobia and a rotatory nystagmus. As they grow older tyrosinase-positive albinos gain a

little pigment in their skin, iris and hair. Negroid skin becomes yellow–brown and the hair becomes yellow. Tyrosinine-positive albinos may also develop freckles. Sunburn is common on unprotected skin. As melanocytes are present, albinos have non-pigmented melanocytic naevi and may develop amelanotic malignant melanomas.

Complications

In the tropics these unfortunate individuals develop numerous sun-induced skin cancers even when they are young, confirming the protective role of melanin.

Differential diagnosis

Piebaldism and vitiligo are described below. While patients with albinism have a reduction in melanin content, they have a normal number of melanocytes in their epidermis. This is in contrast to an absence of melanocytes within the affected area of patient with piebaldism and vitiligo.

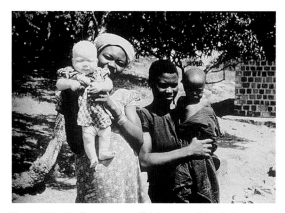

Figure 19.3 Oculocutaneous albinism. An albino baby born to a normally pigmented African family (autosomal recessive inheritance).

Investigations

Prenatal diagnosis of albinism is now possible but may not be justifiable in view of the good prognosis. Nowadays, DNA-based diagnostic screening of amniotic fluid cells or chorionic villi sampling is favoured.

The hair bulb test, in which plucked hairs are incubated in dihydroxyphenylalanine, distinguishes tyrosinase-positive from tyrosinase-negative types.

Treatment

Avoidance of sun exposure, and protection with opaque clothing, wide-brimmed hats and sunscreen creams (Formulary 1, p. 400), are essential and allow albinos in temperate climates to live a relatively normal life. Early diagnosis and treatment of skin tumours is critical.

Other types of albinism

There are several syndromes of albinism. They include the rare autosomal recessive *Hermansky–Pudlak syndrome* (oculocutaneous albinism and platelet storage disease, prolonged bleeding, neutropenia occasionally accompanied by pulmonary fibrosis and granulomatous colitis) and the equally uncommon *Chediak–Higashi syndrome* (oculocutaneous albinism with marked susceptibility to infections, caused by abnormal inclusions in phagocytic leucocytes).

Piebaldism

These patients often have a white forelock of hair and patches of depigmentation lying symmetrically on the limbs, trunk and central part of the face, especially the chin. The condition is present at birth and is inherited as an autosomal dominant trait. The *KIT* proto-oncogene encodes the tyrosine kinase transmembrane cellular receptor on certain stem cells; without this they cannot respond to normal signals for development and migration. Melanocytes are absent from the hypopigmented areas. The depigmentation, often mistaken for vitiligo, may improve with age. There is no effective treatment.

Waardenburg's syndrome includes piebaldism (with a white forelock in 20% of cases), dystopia canthorum (lateral displacement of the inner canthus of each eye), a prominent inner third of the eyebrows, irides of different colour and deafness.

Phenylketonuria

This rare metabolic cause of hypopigmentation has a prevalence of about 1 : 25 000. It is described in Chapter 21 (p. 319).

Hypopituitarism

The skin changes here may alert an astute physician to the diagnosis. The complexion has a pale, yellow tinge; there is thinning or loss of the sexual hair; the skin itself is atrophic. The hypopigmentation is caused by a decreased production of pituitary melanotrophic hormones.

Vitiligo

The word vitiligo comes from the Latin word *vitellus*, which means 'veal' (pale, pink flesh). It is an acquired circumscribed depigmentation, found in all races; its prevalence may be as high as 0.5–1%; its inheritance is polygenic.

Cause and types

There is a complete loss of melanocytes from affected areas. There are two main patterns: a common generalized one and a rare segmental type. *Generalized vitiligo*, including the acrofacial variant, usually starts after the second decade. There is a family history in 30% of patients and this type is most frequent in those with autoimmune diseases such as diabetes, thyroid disorders and pernicious anaemia. It is postulated that, in this type, melanocytes are the target of a cell-mediated autoimmune attack or self-destruct as a result of an inability to remove toxic melanin precursors. *Segmental vitiligo* is restricted to one part of the body, but not necessarily to a dermatome. It occurs earlier in life than generalized vitiligo, and is less likely to be associated with autoimmune diseases. Trauma and sunburn can precipitate both types.

Clinical course

Generalized type. The sharply defined, usually symmetrical (Figure 19.4), white patches are especially common on the backs of the hands, wrists, fronts of knees, neck and around body orifices. The hair of the scalp and beard may depigment too. In Caucasoids, the surrounding skin is sometimes partially depigmented or hyperpigmented (trichrome vitiligo).

The course is unpredictable. Lesions may remain static or spread, sometimes following minor trauma (Köbner phenomenon); occasionally, they repigment spontaneously from the hair follicles.

Segmental type. The individual areas look like the generalized type but their segmental distribution is striking. It responds poorly to most treatments, although spontaneous repigmentation occurs more often in this type than in generalized vitiligo (Figure 19.5).

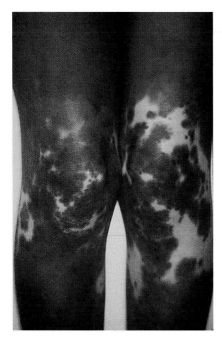

Figure 19.4 Striking patchy vitiligo on the knees.

Differential diagnosis

Contact with depigmenting chemicals, such as hydroquinones and substituted phenols in the rubber industry, should be excluded. Pityriasis versicolor (p. 245) must be considered; its fine scaling and less complete pigment loss separate it from vitiligo. Post-inflammatory depigmentation (p. 273) may look very like vitiligo but is less white and improves spontaneously. The patches of piebald-

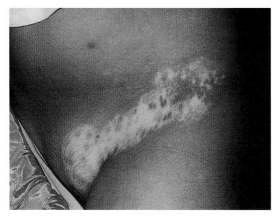

Figure 19.5 Vitiligo: patchy repigmentation is caused by the migration of melanocytes from the depths of the hair follicles.

ism are present at birth. Sometimes, leprosy must be excluded – by sensory testing and a general examination. Other tropical diseases that cause patchy hypopigmentation are leishmaniasis (p. 226), yaws (p. 220) and pinta. Wood's lamp examination can help differentiate between hypopigmentation and depigmentation.

Treatment

The cosmetic disfigurment from vitiligo can be devastating to affected patients. Treatment is often unsatisfactory for those with extensive and long-standing disease. In the white patches pigment cells are only present deep in the hair follicles and treatments mostly try to get melanocytes to divide and migrate into affected skin. Repigmentation is thus often heralded by freckling at follicles within patches. Recent patches may respond to a potent or very potent topical corticosteroid, applied for 1–2 months. After this, the strength should be gradually tapered to a mildly potent steroid for maintenance treatment. Alternatively, calcineurin inhibitors, such as 0.1% tacrolimus ointment (Formulary 1, p. 403), may work, but responses generally seem no better than those to topical corticosteroids. Some patients improve with psoralens (trimethylpsoralen or 8-methoxypsoralen, in a dosage of 0.4–0.6 mg/kg body weight), taken 1–2 hours before graduated exposure to natural sunshine or to artificial UVA (PUVA; p. 62). Narrowband (311 nm) UVB is also effective. Localized irradiation of the skin can also be performed with a 308-nm excimer laser. Therapy is given 2–3 times weekly for at least 6 months; new lesions seem to respond best. Less reliable treatment include antioxidant therapy with *Ginkgo biloba* extract, catalase, and Polypodium leucotomos.

Where pigment is absent in hair follicles or in skin without hair follicles, autologous skin grafts can be performed. The two most common procedures transplant either minigraft implants of 1-mm cylinders or epidermal roofs of suction-raised blisters from unaffected skin. Melanocyte and stem cell transplants, in which single cell suspensions are made from unaffected skin and applied to dermabraded vitiliginous skin, are also being investigated.

Advice about suitable camouflage preparations (Formulary 1, p. 399) to cover unsightly patches should be given. These include staining with dihydroxyacetone self-tanning lotions, or covering with theatrical makeups. Sun avoidance and screening preparations (Formulary 1, p. 400) are needed to avoid sunburn of the affected areas and a heightened contrast between the pale and dark areas. Black patients with extensive vitiligo can be

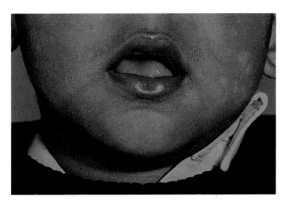

Figure 19.6 Pityriasis alba.

completely and irreversibly depigmented by creams containing the monobenzyl ether of hydroquinone (Formulary 1, p. 399). The social implications must be discussed and carefully considered, and written consent given, before such treatment is undertaken.

Post-inflammatory depigmentation

This may follow eczema, psoriasis, sarcoidosis, lupus erythematosus and, rarely, lichen planus. It may also result from cryotherapy or a burn. In general, the more severe the inflammation, the more likely pigment is to decrease rather than increase in its wake. These problems are most significant in darker skinned individuals. With time, the skin usually repigments. Pityriasis alba is common on the faces of children. The initial lesion is probably a variant of eczema (pinkish with fine scaling), which fades leaving one or more pale, slightly scaly, areas (Figure 19.6). Treatment is to address the underlying inflammatory disorder. Exposure to the sun makes the patches more obvious.

Idiopathic guttate hypomelanosis

Confetti-like asymptomatic 1–5 mm white macules occur amongst the mottled hyperpigmentation of severe sun damage in a condition called idiopathic guttate hypomelanosis.

White hair

Melanocytes in hair bulbs become less active with age and white hair (canities) is a universal sign of ageing (p. 211). Early greying of the hair is seen in the rare premature ageing syndromes, such as Werner's syndrome, and in autoimmune conditions such as pernicious anaemia, thyroid disorders and Addison's disease (p. 276).

Table 19.3 Some causes of hyperpigmentation.

Genetic	Freckles
	Lentigines
	Café au lait macules
	Peutz–Jeghers syndrome
	Xeroderma pigmentosum (see Chapter 21)
	Albright's syndrome: segmental hyperpigmentation, fibrous dysplasia of bones, precocious puberty
Endocrine	Addison's disease
	Cushing's syndrome
	Pregnancy
	Renal failure
Metabolic	Biliary cirrhosis
	Haemochromatosis
	Porphyria (p. 316)
Nutritional	Malabsorption
	Carcinomatosis
	Kwashiorkor
	Pellagra
Drugs	Photosensitizing drugs
	ACTH and synthetic analogues
	Oestrogens and progestogens
	Psoralens
	Arsenic
	Busulfan
	Minocycline
Post-inflammatory	Lichen planus (p. 69)
	Eczema
	Secondary syphilis
	Systemic sclerosis (p. 132)
	Lichen and macular amyloidosis
	Cryotherapy
	Poikiloderma
Tumours	Acanthosis nigricans (p. 311)
	Pigmented naevi (p. 282)
	Malignant melanoma (p. 294)
	Mastocytosis (p. 306)

ACTH, adenocorticotrophic hormone.

Disorders with increased pigmentation (hypermelanosis)

Some of these disorders are listed in Table 19.3. The most common are described here and the mechanisms involved are summarized in Figure 19.7.

Freckles (ephelides)

Freckles are so common that to describe them seems unnecessary. They are seen most often in the red-haired or

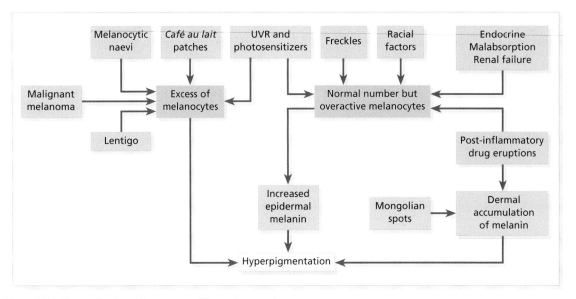

Figure 19.7 The mechanisms of some types of hyperpigmentation.

blond person as sharply demarcated, light brown–ginger macules, usually less than 5 mm in diameter. They multiply and become darker with sun exposure.

Increased melanin is seen in the basal layer of the epidermis without any increase in the number of melanocytes, and without elongation of the rete ridges (Figure 19.8). No treatment is necessary.

Melanotic macule of the lip

This common lesion (Figure 19.9) worries doctors but is benign. Its histology is similar to that of a freckle (Figure 19.8).

Lentigo

Simple and senile lentigines look alike. They are light or dark brown macules, ranging from 1 mm to 1 cm across. Although usually discrete, they may have an irregular outline. Simple lentigines arise most often in childhood as a few scattered lesions, often on areas not exposed to sun, including the mucous membranes. Senile or solar lentigines are common after middle age on the backs of the hands (*age spots* or *liver spots*; Figure 19.10) and on the face (Figure 19.11). In contrast to freckles, lentigines have increased numbers of melanocytes. They should be distinguished from freckles, from junctional melanocytic naevi (p. 283) and from a lentigo maligna (p. 295).

Treatment is usually unnecessary and prevention, by sun avoidance and the use of sunscreens, is the best approach. Cryotherapy has stood the test of time but care must be taken to not cause hypopigmentation. Melanin-specific high energy lasers (e.g. Q-switched ruby laser, 694 nm; Q-switched alexandrite laser, 755 nm; Nd:Yag laser, 1064 nm) and intense pulsed light are extremely effective for treating ugly lesions (p. 379). Topical therapies are also effective for lightening lentigines such as daily application of 0.1% tretinoin cream (Formulary 1, p. 405), 2–4% hydroquinone (Formulary 1, p. 399) or a combination of these with or without a retinoid, alpha-hydroxy acid, or topical corticosteroid (Formulary 1, p. 401).

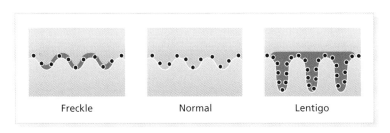

Freckle   Normal   Lentigo

Figure 19.8 Histology of a freckle and a lentigo.

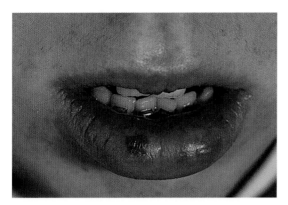

Figure 19.9 Melanotic macule of the lip: slow to evolve and benign, as suggested by its even colour and sharp margin.

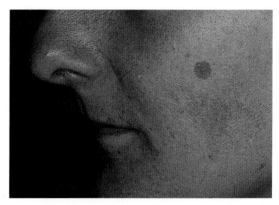

Figure 19.11 A simple lentigo showing a sharp edge and an even distribution of pigment.

Conditions associated with multiple lentigines

Three rare but striking syndromes feature multiple lentigines.

Peutz–Jeghers syndrome

Profuse lentigines are seen on and around the lips in this autosomal dominant condition (Figure 19.12). Scattered lentigines also occur on the buccal mucosa, gums, hard palate, hands and feet. The syndrome is important because of its association with polyposis of the small intestine, which may lead to recurrent intussusception and, rarely, to malignant transformation of the polyps. Ten per cent of affected women have ovarian tumours.

Cronkhite–Canada syndrome

This consists of multiple lentigines on the backs of the hands and a more diffuse pigmentation of the palms and volar aspects of the fingers. It may also associate with gastrointestinal polyposis. Alopecia and nail abnormalities complete the rare but characteristic clinical picture.

Leopard syndrome

This is an acronym for generalized **l**entiginosis associated with cardiac abnormalities demonstrated by **E**CG, **o**cular hypertelorism, **p**ulmonary stenosis, **a**bnormal genitalia, **r**etardation of growth and **d**eafness.

Melasma (chloasma)

Melasma is an acquired symmetrical hypermelanosis occuring on sun-exposed skin, especially the face. The areas of increased pigmentation are well defined and their edges may be scalloped. The condition is much more common in women, affects all races but is most prevalent in dark skinnned individuals with skin types IV–VI (Table 18.1). The hypermelanosis becomes darker after exposure to the sun. The more common

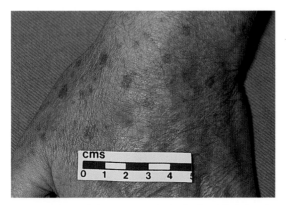

Figure 19.10 Senile lentigines on the back of an elderly hand (*liver spots*). Note accompanying atrophy.

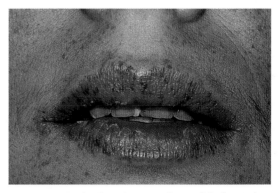

Figure 19.12 Profuse lentigines on and around the lips in the Peutz–Jeghers syndrome.

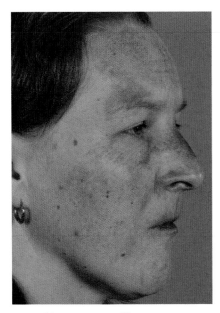

Figure 19.13 Chloasma worsened by sun exposure.

exacerbating factors include sunlight, pregnancy ('the mask of pregnancy'; Figure 19.13) and oestrogens and oral contraceptives. Less reported risk factors include thyroid dysfunction, photosensitizing drugs and cosmetics (see Table 16.2). The placenta may secrete sex hormones that stimulate melanocytes. Recently, over-expression of α-MSH (p. 268) has been demonstrated in lesional skin. Most of the extra melanin lies in the epidermis, but there is some in the dermis too, making treatment difficult.

Treatment

Melasma is challenging to treat, partly because of the presence of melanin at varying depths in the dermis and epidermis. In addition, even minor sun exposure can reactivate the process. Any treatment regimen must include strict sun avoidance, including broad-spectrum sunscreen and hats.

Some find bleaching agents that contain hydroquinone helpful. The optimal effect is achieved with preparations containing 2–5% hydroquinone (Formulary 1, p. 399), applied for 6–10 weeks. After this, maintenance treatment should be with preparations containing no more than 2% hydroquinone. In stubborn cases, the hydroquinone may be combined with a topical steroid and a retinoid for short-term use. Other topical lightening agents include tyrosinase inhibitors such as kojic acid and azelaic acid.

Superficial chemical peels help to remove epidermal melanin and are thus a useful adjunct to topical treatment. Glycolic acid peels are the most efficacious of the peeling agents but require expertise for proper application. Deeper chemical peels and some laser therapy (Q-switched ruby, Q-switched alexandrite, CO_2 and Erb:Yag, p. 379) can worsen melasma and result in dyspigmentation especially for darker skinned individuals. Intense pulsed light may provide modest benefits but should be used with caution. New fractionated lasers show promising results but further studies are needed. Small test sites should be treated and assessed before formal, more widespread, treatment with any modality.

Endocrine hyperpigmentation

Addison's disease

Hyperpigmentation caused by the overproduction of ACTH is often striking. It may be generalized or limited to the skin folds, creases of the palms, scars and the buccal mucosa.

Cushing's syndrome

Increased ACTH production may cause a picture like that of Addison's disease. The hyperpigmentation may become even more marked after adrenalectomy (Nelson's syndrome).

Pregnancy

There is a generalized increase in pigmentation during pregnancy, especially of the nipples and areolae, and of the linea alba. Melasma or chloasma (p. 275) may also occur. The nipples and areolae remain pigmented after parturition.

Chronic renal failure

The hyperpigmentation of chronic renal failure and of patients on haemodialysis is caused by an increase in levels of pituitary melanotrophic peptides, normally cleared by the kidney.

Porphyria

Formed porphyrins, especially uroporphyrins, are produced in excess in cutaneous hepatic porphyria and congenital erythropoietic porphyria (p. 316). These endogenous photosensitizers induce hyperpigmentation on exposed areas; skin fragility, blistering, milia and hypertrichosis are equally important clues to the diagnosis.

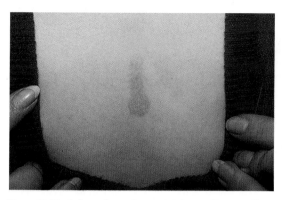

Figure 19.14 A drop of psoralen-containing perfume on the chest photosensitized this pendant-shaped area. It became pigmented after exposure to the sun.

Nutritional hyperpigmentation

Any severe wasting disease, such as malabsorption, AIDS, tuberculosis or cancer, may be accompanied by diffuse hyperpigmentation. Kwashiorkor presents a mixed picture of generalized hypopigmentation and patchy post-inflammatory hyperpigmentation, and in this condition the hair is red–brown or grey.

Chemicals causing hyperpigmentation

Table 18.2 lists drugs that commonly photosensitize. All can cause hyperpigmentation of the exposed skin. Psoralens are used in the photochemotherapy of psoriasis (see Chapter 5) and, more rarely, of vitiligo.

The term *berloque dermatitis* (Figure 19.14) refers to a 'pendant' of hyperpigmentation, often on the side of the neck, where cosmetics have been applied that contain the photosensitizing 5-methoxypsoralen. Cosmetics for men (e.g. pre- and aftershaves) are a thriving source of these.

Arsenic is not used medically nowadays. Once it caused 'raindrop' depigmentation within a diffuse bronzed hyperpigmentation.

Busulfan and bleomycin, used to treat some forms of leukaemia, frequently cause diffuse hyperpigmentation but may also cause brown streaks (flagellate hyperpigmentation). Minocycline can leave blue–black drug deposits in inflamed acne spots on the shins or on the mucosae. They can be removed with Q-switched ruby laser (694 nm) treatment.

Learning points

1 Vitiligo looks ugly and sunburns easily. Treat with cosmetic cover and sunscreens or sun avoidance.
2 Do not promise a cure.

Post-inflammatory hyperpigmentation

This is common after lichen planus (p. 69). It is also a feature of systemic sclerosis (p. 132) and some types of cutaneous amyloidosis, and is often an unwelcome sequela of cryotherapy.

Poikiloderma

Poikiloderma is the name given to a triad of signs: reticulate pigmentation, atrophy and telangiectasia. It is not a disease but a reaction pattern with many causes including X-irradiation, photocontact reactions, and connective tissue and lymphoreticular disorders. Congenital variants (Rothmund–Thomson syndrome, Bloom's syndrome and Cockayne's syndrome) associated with photosensitivity dwarfism and mental retardation also occur. Poikiloderma of Civatte refers to the triad of signs seen on the lateral cheeks and sides of the neck from chronic sun exposure. The submental area is usually spared as it is shaded by the chin.

Learning point

Do not forget that photosensitizing cosmetics can cause facial hyperpigmentation, even in men.

Further reading

Hann S-K, Nordlund JJ. (2000) *Vitiligo.* Blackwell Publishing, Oxford.

Nordlund JJ, Boissy RE, Hearing VJ, *et al.* (2006) *The Pigmentary System*, 2nd edition. Blackwell Publishing, Oxford.

Ortonne JP, Passeron T. (2005) Melanin pigmentary disorders: treatment update. *Dermatology Clinics* **23**, 209–226.

Sheth VM, Pandya AG. (2011) Melasma: a comprehensive update: part II. *Journal of the American Academy of Dermatology* **65**, 699–714.

Taylor SC. (2002) Skin of color: biology, structure, function, and implications for dermatologic disease. *Journal of the American Academy of Dermatology* **46**, S41–62

20 Skin Tumours

This chapter deals both with skin tumours arising from the epidermis and its appendages, and from the dermis (Table 20.1).

Prevention

Many skin tumours (e.g. actinic keratoses, lentigines, keratoacanthomas, basal cell carcinomas, squamous cell carcinomas, malignant melanomas and, arguably, acquired melanocytic naevi) would all become less common if Caucasoids, especially those with a fair skin, protected themselves adequately against sunlight. The education of those living in sunny climates or holidaying in the sun has already reaped great rewards here (Figure 20.1). Successful campaigns have focused on regular self-examination and on reducing sun exposure by avoidance, clothing and sunscreen preparations (Figures 20.2 and 20.3). Public compliance has been encouraged by imaginative slogans like the Australian 'sun smart' and 'slip, slap and slop' (slip on the shirt, slap on the hat and slop on the sunscreen) advice and the American Academy of Dermatology 'ABCs' (away, block, cover up, shade) leaflet.

Tumours of the epidermis and its appendages

Benign

Viral warts

These are discussed in Chapter 13, but are mentioned here for three reasons: first, solitary warts are sometimes misdiagnosed on the face or hands of the elderly; and, secondly, a wart is one of the few benign tumours in humans that is, without doubt, caused by a virus, the human papilloma virus (HPV). Thirdly, some HPVs are prime players in the pathogenesis of malignant tumours. Seventy per cent of transplant patients who have been immunosuppressed for over 5 years have multiple viral warts and there is growing evidence that immunosuppression, certain types of HPV and ultraviolet radiation interact in this setting to cause squamous cell carcinoma (p. 292).

Cutaneous horn

This common horn-shaped excrescence (see Figure 20.25), arising from keratinocytes, may resemble a viral wart clinically. The histology should be checked to distinguish benign and malignant lesions, as both have been known to arise from similar appearing lesions. Excision, or curettage with cautery to the base, is the treatment of choice.

Seborrhoeic keratosis (basal cell papilloma, seborrhoeic wart)

This is a common benign epidermal tumour, unrelated to sebaceous glands, found in older individuals. The term 'senile wart' should be avoided as it offends many patients.

Cause
Usually unexplained but:
• Multiple lesions may be inherited (autosomal dominant);
• Occasionally follow an inflammatory dermatosis; or
• Very rarely, the sudden eruption of hundreds of itchy lesions is associated with an internal neoplasm (Leser–Trélat sign), usually adenocarcinoma of the gastrointestinal tract.

Presentation
Seborrhoeic keratoses usually arise after the age of 50 years, but flat inconspicuous lesions are often visible earlier. They are often multiple (Figures 20.4 and 20.5) but may be single. Lesions are most common on the face and trunk. The sexes are equally affected.

Clinical Dermatology, Fifth Edition. Richard B. Weller, Hamish J.A. Hunter and Margaret W. Mann.
© 2015 John Wiley & Sons, Ltd. Published 2015 by John Wiley & Sons, Ltd.

Table 20.1 Skin tumours.

Derived from	Benign	Premalignant/carcinoma *in situ*	Malignant
Epidermis and appendages	Viral wart	Actinic keratosis	Basal cell carcinoma
	Cutaneous horn		Squamous cell carcinoma
	Seborrhoeic keratosis		Malignant melanoma
	Skin tag		Paget's disease of the nipple
	Linear epidermal naevus		(although, strictly, a breast tumour)
	Melanocytic naevus		
	Sebaceous naevus		
	Epidermal/pilar cyst		
	Milium		
	Chondrodermatitis		
	Nodularis helicis		
Dermis	Haemangioma		Kaposi's sarcoma
	Lymphangioma		Lymphoma
	Glomus tumour		Dermatofibrosarcoma protuberans
	Pyogenic granuloma		Merkel cell carcinoma
	Dermatofibroma		Metastases
	Neurofibroma		
	Neuroma		
	Keloid		
	Lipoma		
	Lymphocytoma cutis		
	Mastocytosis		

Physical signs:
- A distinctive 'stuck-on' appearance due to 'tucked under' shoulders, as chewed chewing gum might appear;
- May be flat, raised, filiform or pedunculated;
- Surface may be smooth or verrucous;
- Colour varies from yellow–white to dark brown–black;
- Surface may have greasy scaling and scattered keratin plugs ('currant bun' appearance); and
- If oval, long axis parallels skin lines.

Clinical course
Lesions may multiply with age but remain benign.

Differential diagnosis
Seborrhoeic keratoses are easily recognized. Occasionally, they can be confused with a pigmented cellular naevus, a pigmented basal cell carcinoma or, most importantly, a malignant melanoma. *Dermatosis papulosa nigra* (Figures 14.3 and 20.6) is a long-winded name for a common variant of seborrhoeic keratoses affecting black adults. Multiple pigmented papules, just raised or filiform, appear on the face and neck but may extend to the trunk. The lesions may be unsightly and catch on jewellery. Histologically they are like seborrhoeic warts. The condition may run in families, being inherited as an autosomal dominant trait.

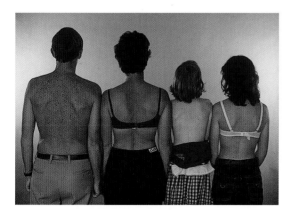

Figure 20.1 This family lived in the tropics. No prizes for guessing which of them avoided the sun.

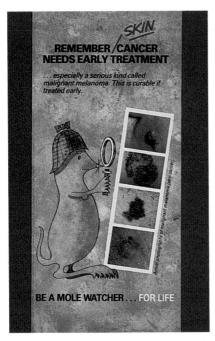

Figure 20.2 An eye-catching and effective way of teaching the public how to look at their moles. A pamphlet produced by the Cancer Research Campaign in the United Kingdom.

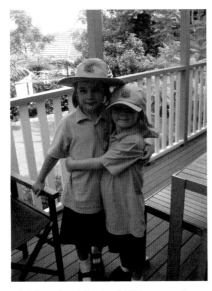

Figure 20.3 These Scottish schoolchildren attending an Australian school were surprised to find that wide-brimmed sun protective hats were a compulsory part of the school uniform. These are fashionable after several clever campaigns, and the 'no hat, no play' rule has become an accepted way of life.

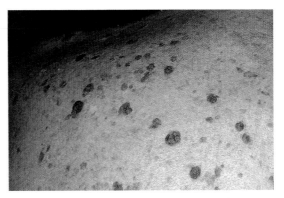

Figure 20.4 Typical multiple seborrhoeic warts on the shoulder. Each individual lesion might look worryingly like a malignant melanoma but, in the numbers seen here, the lesions must be benign.

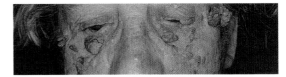

Figure 20.5 Numerous unsightly seborrhoeic warts of the face.

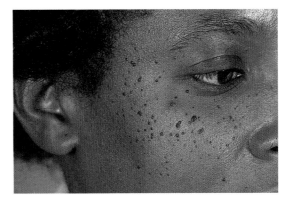

Figure 20.6 Dermatosis papulosa nigra.

Stucco keratoses are another variant of seborrhoeic keratoses and are seen most often around the ankles after the age of 50. They have a similar 'stuck on' appearance to seborrhoeic warts and are small (1–2 mm) white keratotic papules that are easily lifted off the skin with a finger nail, without bleeding.

Investigations

Biopsy is needed only in rare dubious cases. The histology is diagnostic (Figure 20.7): the lesion lies above the

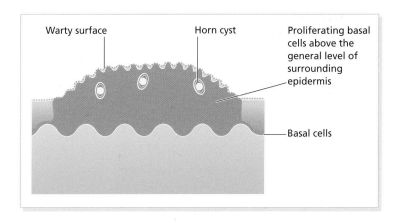

Figure 20.7 Histology of a seborrhoeic keratosis.

general level of the surrounding epidermis and consists of proliferating basal cells and horn cysts. Stucco keratoses have a slightly different histology with loose lamellated hyperkeratosis overlying regular papillomatosis

Treatment

Seborrhoeic keratoses can safely be left alone, but ugly or easily traumatized ones can be removed with a curette under local anaesthetic (this has the advantage of providing histology) or by cryotherapy. If treatment is requested for dermatosis papulosa nigra, gentle electrodessication or snipping of a few trial lesions initially is the best approach. Cryotherapy should be avoided for dermatosis papulosa nigra, as hypo or hyperpigmentation may result.

Learning point

If you cannot tell most seborrhoeic warts from a melanoma you will send too many elderly people unnecessarily to the pigmented lesion clinic.

Skin tags (acrochordon)

These common benign outgrowths of skin affect mainly the middle-aged and elderly.

Cause

This is unknown but the trait is sometimes familial. Skin tags are most common in obese women, and rarely are associated with tuberous sclerosis (p. 345), acanthosis nigricans (p. 311) or acromegaly and diabetes.

Presentation and clinical course

Skin tags are soft skin-coloured or pigmented pedunculated papules commonly found around the neck and within the major flexures (Figure 20.8). They look unsightly and may catch on clothing and jewellery.

Differential diagnosis

The appearance is unmistakable. Tags are rarely confused with small melanocytic naevi.

Treatment

Small lesions can be snipped off with fine scissors, frozen with liquid nitrogen or destroyed with a hyfrecator without local anaesthesia. There is no way of preventing new ones from developing.

Naevi

The term *naevus* refers to a skin lesion that has a localized excess of one or more types of cell in a normal cell site. It is the name used for a cutaneous hamartoma. Histologically, the cells are identical to or closely resemble normal cells. Naevi may be composed mostly of keratinocytes (e.g. in epidermal naevi), melanocytes (e.g. in congenital

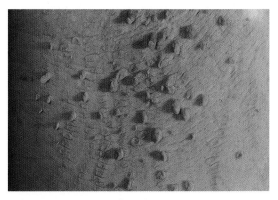

Figure 20.8 Numerous axillary skin tags.

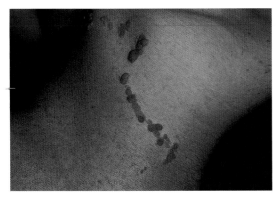

Figure 20.9 Linear warty epidermal naevus.

melanocytic naevi), connective tissue elements (e.g. in connective tissue naevi; p. 346) and a mixture of epithelial and connective tissue elements (e.g. in sebaceous naevi). In this context such naevi are hamartomas or malformations.

Linear epidermal naevus

This lesion is an example of cutaneous mosaicism (p. 343) and so tends to follow Blaschko's lines (Figure 20.9). Keratinocytes in these lines of wart-like growth are genetically different from their normal appearing neighbours. Keratolytics (Formulary 1, p. 401) lessen the roughness of some and small epidermal naevi may be excised. Alternatively, a trial area may be destroyed with a carbon dioxide laser and the subsequent scar assessed before extending treatment (p. 380).

Melanocytic naevi

Melanocytic naevi (moles) are localized benign tumours of melanocytes. Their classification (Table 20.2) is

Table 20.2 Classification of melanocytic naevi.

Congenital melanocytic naevi
Acquired melanocytic naevi
Junctional naevus
Compound naevus
Intradermal naevus
Spitz naevus
Blue naevus
Atypical melanocytic naevus

based on the site of the aggregations of the abnormal melanocytes (Figure 20.10).

Cause and evolution

The cause is unknown. A genetic factor is likely in many families, along with excessive sun exposure during childhood.

With the exception of congenital melanocytic naevi (p. 283), most appear in early childhood, often with a sharp increase in numbers during adolescence and after severe sunburn. Further crops may appear during pregnancy, oestrogen therapy, flare-ups of lupus erythematosus or, rarely, after cytotoxic chemotherapy and immunosuppression. New melanocytic naevi appear less often after the age of 20 years.

Melanocytic naevi in childhood are usually of the 'junctional' type, with proliferating melanocytes in clumps at the dermo-epidermal junction. Later, the melanocytes round off and 'drop' into the dermis. A 'compound' naevus has both dermal and junctional components. With maturation, the junctional component disappears so that the melanocytes in an 'intradermal' naevus are all in the dermis (Figure 20.10).

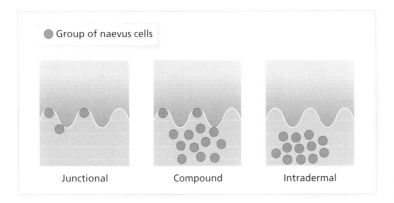

Figure 20.10 Types of acquired melanocytic naevi.

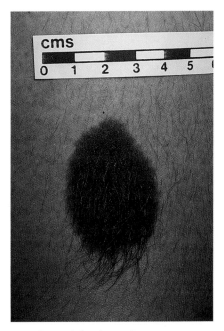

Figure 20.11 Congenital melanocytic naevus.

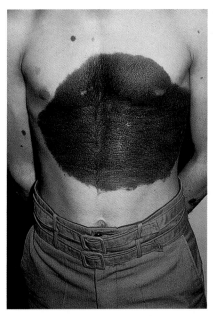

Figure 20.12 A large hairy congenital melanocytic naevus. (Dr Auf Qaba, St John's Hospital, Livingstone. Reproduced with permission of Dr Auf Qaba.)

Presentation

Congenital melanocytic naevi (Figures 20.11 and 20.12). These are present at birth or appear in the neonatal period and are seldom less than 1 cm in diameter. Their colour varies from brown to black or blue–black. With maturity some become protuberant and hairy, with a cerebriform surface. Such lesions can be disfiguring (e.g. a 'bathing trunk' naevus). Congenital melanocytic naevi carry an increased risk of malignant transformation, depending on their size. Giant congenital naevi with a diameter greater than 20 cm have a substantial risk of developing melanoma (lifetime risk up to 5–7%). On the other hand, small-sized congential naevi (less than 1.5 cm) and medium-sized (1.5–20 cm) have a low risk of melanoma. This risk of developing melanoma appears to be maximum in childhood and adolescence. In contrast to common acquired naevi, which are confined to the superfiical dermis, congenital naevi often extend deeply into the subcutaneous fat. The finding of a giant congenital melanocytic naevus in a posterior midline location associated with multiple satellite naevi should prompt a consultation with a neurologist and a magnetic resonance imaging (MRI) scan to rule out neurocutaneous melanosis.

Junctional melanocytic naevi (Figure 20.13). These are roughly circular macules. Their colour ranges from mid

to dark brown and may vary even within a single lesion. Most melanocytic naevi of the palms, soles, mucous membranes and genitals are of this type.

Compound melanocytic naevi (Figure 20.14). These are domed pigmented nodules of up to 1 cm in diameter. They arise from junctional naevi as melanocytes 'drop off' from the epidermis to form collections of cells in the dermis. They may be light or dark brown but their colour is more even than that of junctional naevi. Most are smooth, but larger ones may be cerebriform, or even hyperkeratotic and papillomatous; many bear hairs.

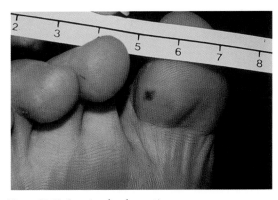

Figure 20.13 Junctional melanocytic naevus.

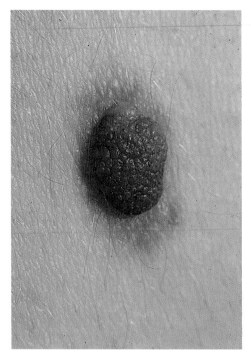

Figure 20.14 Compound melanocytic naevus. No recent change.

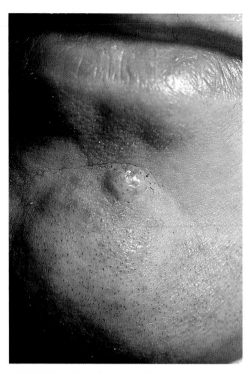

Figure 20.15 Intradermal melanocytic naevus with numerous shaved hairs.

Intradermal melanocytic naevi (Figure 20.15). These look like compound naevi but are less pigmented and often skin-coloured.

Spitz naevi (in the past misleadingly called juvenile melanomas; Figure 20.16). These are seen most often in children. They develop over a month or two as solitary pink or red nodules of up to 1 cm in diameter and are most common on the face and legs. Although benign, they are often excised because of their rapid growth.

Blue naevi (Figure 20.17), So-called because of their striking slate grey–blue colour, blue naevi usually appear in childhood and adolescence, on the limbs, buttocks and lower back. They are usually solitary. Histologically, nests of heavily pigmented melanocytes are found deep in the dermis, which gives the characteristic blue colour as a result of the Tyndall effect.

Mongolian spots (Figure 15.1). Pigment in dermal melanocytes is responsible for these bruise-like greyish areas seen on the lumbosacral area of most Down's syndrome and many Asian and black babies. They usually fade during childhood.

Atypical naevus/mole syndrome (dysplastic naevus syndrome; Figure 20.18). Clinically atypical melanocytic naevi can occur sporadically or run in families as an autosomal dominant trait, with incomplete penetrance, affecting several generations. Some families with atypical naevi are melanoma-prone and in 20% of these mutations in the

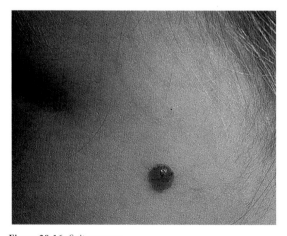

Figure 20.16 Spitz naevus.

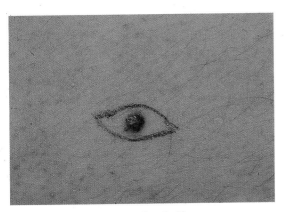

Figure 20.17 The blue ink matches the blue naevus.

cell cycle regulating gene *CDKN2A* on chromosome 9p21 are found. These patients have greater than 50 large irregularly pigmented naevi, commonly on the trunk but some may be present on the scalp. Their edges are irregular and they vary greatly in size – many being over 1 cm in diameter. Some are pinkish and an inflamed halo may surround them. Some have a mamillated surface. Patients with multiple atypical melanocytic or dysplastic naevi with a positive family history of malignant melanoma should be followed up 6-monthly for life. Total body photography can often be helpful to monitor changes in atypical naevi. Melanomas develop in almost all patients with atypical mole syndrome who have both a parent and sibling with the syndrome and a history of melanoma.

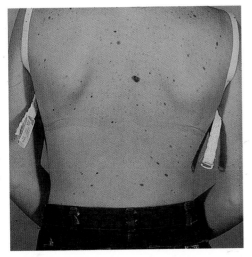

Figure 20.18 Atypical moles in a 12-year-old girl. Note the malignant melanoma lying between the scapulae.

Differential diagnosis of melanocytic naevi

Malignant melanomas. This is the most important part of the differential diagnosis. Melanomas are very rare before puberty, single and more variably pigmented and irregularly shaped (other features are listed below under *Complications*).

Seborrhoeic keratoses. These can cause confusion in adults but have a stuck-on appearance and are warty. Telltale keratin plugs and horny cysts may be seen with the help of a lens or dermatoscope.

Lentigines. These may be found on any part of the skin and mucous membranes. More profuse than junctional naevi, they are usually grey–brown rather than black, and develop more often after adolescence.

Ephelides (freckles). These are tan macules less than 5 mm in diameter. They are confined to sun-exposed areas, being most common in blond or red-haired people.

Haemangiomas. Benign proliferations of blood vessels, including haemangiomas and pyogenic granulomas, may be confused with a vascular Spitz naevus or an amelanotic melanoma. Dermoscopy is most helpful in distinguishing from a naevus or melanoma (Chapter 28).

Histology

Most acquired lesions fit into the scheme given in Figure 20.10: orderly nests of abnormal melanocytes are seen in the junctional region, in the dermis, or in both. However, some types of melanocytic naevi have their own distinguishing features. In congenital naevi the abnormal melanocytes may extend to the subcutaneous fat, and hyperplasia of other skin components (e.g. hair follicles) may be seen. A Spitz naevus has a histology worryingly similar to that of a melanoma. It shows dermal oedema and dilatated capillaries, and is composed of large epithelioid and spindle-shaped melanocytes, some of which may be in mitosis.

In a blue naevus, the abnormal melanocytes are seen in the mid and deep dermis.

The main features of clinically atypical (dysplastic) naevi are lengthening and bridging of rete ridges, and the presence of junctional nests showing melanocytic dysplasia (nuclear pleomorphism and hyperchromatism). Fibrosis of the papillary dermis and a lymphocytic inflammatory response are also seen.

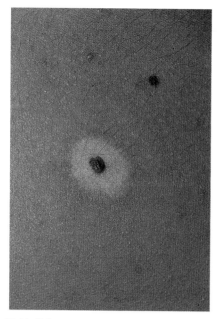

Figure 20.19 Halo naevus.

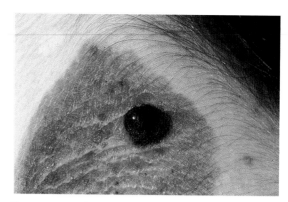

Figure 20.20 Malignant melanoma developing within a congenital melanocytic naevus.

Complications

Inflammation. Pain and swelling are common but are not features of malignant transformation. They are caused by trauma, bacterial folliculitis or a foreign body reaction to hair after shaving or plucking.

Depigmented halo (Figure 20.19). So-called 'halo naevi' are uncommon but benign. There may be vitiligo elsewhere. The naevus in the centre often involutes spontaneously before the halo repigments.

Malignant change. This is extremely rare except in congenital melanocytic naevi, where the risk has been estimated at 0.5–10%, depending on their size (Figure 20.20), and in the atypical naevi of melanoma-prone families. It should be considered if the following changes occur in a melanocytic naevus:

- Enlargement;
- Increased or decreased pigmentation;
- Altered shape;
- Altered contour;
- Inflammation;
- Ulceration;
- Itch; or
- Bleeding.

If **changing** lesions are examined carefully, remembering the 'ABCDE' features of malignant melanoma (Table 20.3), few malignant melanomas will be missed.

Treatment
Excision is needed when:
1 A naevus is unsightly;
2 Malignancy is suspected or is a known risk (e.g. in a large congenital melanocytic naevus); or
3 A naevus is repeatedly inflamed or traumatized.

Learning point

Even if you think it is harmless, do not be afraid to refer a mole that has changed to a dermatologist.

Naevus sebaceus (Figure 20.21)
A flat hairless area at birth, usually in the scalp, these naevi become more yellow and raised at puberty. Secondary benign neoplasms (trichoblastoma, syringocystadenoma papilliferum) can arise over time within a naevus sebaceus. Rarely, malignant transformation into a basal cell carcinoma can occur in adult life.

Table 20.3 The ABCDE of malignant melanoma.

Asymmetry
Border irregularity
Colour variability
Diameter greater than 0.5 cm
Evolution (change)

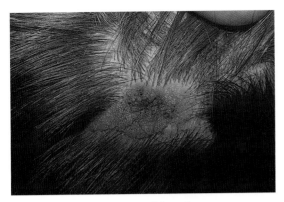

Figure 20.21 Sebaceous naevus of the scalp.

Epidermoid and pilar cysts

Often incorrectly called sebaceous cysts, these are common and can occur on the scalp, face, behind the ears and on the trunk. They often have a central punctum; when they rupture, or are squeezed, foul-smelling cheesy material comes out. Histologically, the lining of a cyst resembles normal epidermis (an epidermoid cyst) or the outer root sheath of the hair follicle (a pilar cyst). Occasionally, an adjacent foreign body reaction is noted. Treatment is by excision, or by incision followed by expression of the contents and removal of the cyst wall. Failure to remove the entire cyst wall may result in recurrence.

Milia

Milia are small subepidermal keratin cysts (Figure 20.22). They are common on the face in all age groups and appear as tiny white millet seed-like papules of 0.5–2 mm in diameter. They are occasionally seen at the site of a previous subepidermal blister (e.g. in epidermolysis bullosa

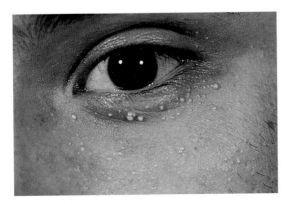

Figure 20.22 Milia.

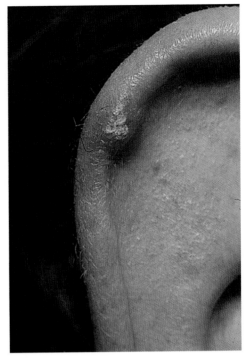

Figure 20.23 Chondrodermatitis nodularis helicis. The inflammation of the underlying cartilage is painful enough to wake up patients repeatedly at night.

and porphyria cutanea tarda). The contents of milia can be picked out with a sterile needle or pointed scalpal blade (No. 11) without local anaesthesia.

Chondrodermatitis nodularis helicis (painful nodule of the ear, ear corn) (Figure 20.23)

This terminological mouthful is, strictly, not a neoplasm, but a chronic inflammation. A painful nodule develops on the helix or antehelix of the ear, most often in men. It looks like a small corn, is tender and prevents sleep if that side of the head touches the pillow. Histologically, a thickened epidermis overlies inflamed cartilage. It may be caused by prolonged excess pressure on the skin overlying the cartilage. A pressure-relieving pillow may help. Wedge resection under local anaesthetic is effective if cryotherapy or intralesional triamcinolone injection fails.

Premalignant tumours

Actinic keratoses

These discrete rough-surfaced lesions crop up on sun-damaged skin. They are best cosidered as premalignant.

Pathologically there is a case for classifying them as squamous cell carcinomas *in situ* but very few progress to invasive squamous cell carcinomas.

Cause
The effects of sun exposure are cumulative. Those with fair complexions living near the equator are most at risk and invariably develop these 'sun warts'. A recent UK survey showed that one-third of men over 70 years had actinic keratoses. Melanin protects, and actinic keratoses are not seen in black skin. Conversely, albinos are especially prone to develop them.

Presentation
They affect the middle-aged and elderly in temperate climates, but younger people in the tropics. The pink or grey rough scaling macules or papules seldom exceed 1 cm in diameter (Figure 20.24). Their rough surface is sometimes better felt than seen.

Complications
Transition to an invasive squamous cell carcinoma, although rare, should be suspected if a lesion enlarges, becomes nodular, ulcerates or bleeds. Luckily, such tumours seldom metastasize. A cutaneous horn is a hard keratotic protrusion based on an actinic keratosis, a squamous cell papilloma or a viral wart (Figure 20.25).

Differential diagnosis
There is usually no difficulty in telling an actinic keratosis from a seborrhoeic wart, a viral wart (p. 227), a keratoacanthoma, an intraepidermal carcinoma or an invasive squamous cell carcinoma.

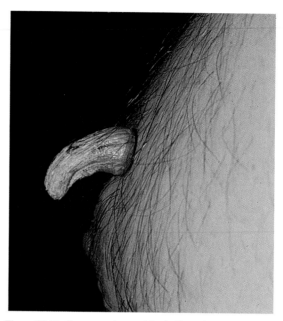

Figure 20.25 Cutaneous horn with a bulbous fleshy base.

Investigations
A biopsy is needed if there is concern over invasive change.

Histology
Alternating zones of hyper- and parakeratosis overlie a thickened or atrophic epidermis. The normal maturation pattern of the epidermis may be lost and occasional pleomorphic keratinocytes may be seen. Solar elastosis is seen in the superficial dermis.

Treatment
Freezing with liquid nitrogen or carbon dioxide snow is simple and effective. Shave removal or curettage is best for large lesions and cutaneous horns. Multiple lesions, including subclinical ones, can be treated with 5-fluorouracil cream (Formulary 1, p. 408) after specialist advice. The cream is applied once or twice daily until there is a marked inflammatory response in the treated area. This takes about 3 weeks and only then should the applications be stopped. Healing is rapid. Most patients dislike the pain and appearance of their faces during treatment but are pleased with their 'new' smooth skin afterwards. Severe discomfort from the treatment may be alleviated by the short-term application of a local steroid. 5-Fluorouracil cream is more effective for keratoses on the face than on the arms. Alternatively, less effective but

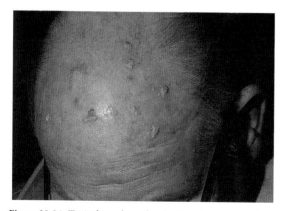

Figure 20.24 Typical rough-surfaced actinic keratoses on the scalp.

causing less inflammation, 5-fluorouracil cream can be applied on just 1–2 days a week for 8 weeks.

Multiple actinic keratoses can also be treated with imiquimod, a modulator of innate immunity (Formulary 1, p. 408). It activates Toll-like receptor 7 causing an immune reaction that destroys abnormal cells. Applied as a cream two to three times weekly for up to 16 weeks, the response is similar to that following 5-fluorouracil, described above. 3% Sodium diclofenac made up in a hyaluronan gel creates less havoc but also lower cure rates. Recently, ingenol mebutate gel was approved in the United States for actinic keratoses as a 2–3 day course. Photodynamic therapy (p. 376), using aminolaevulinic acid hydrochloride followed by blue light, is effective but requires specialist facilities. Lesions that do not respond should be regarded with suspicion, and biopsied.

Malignant epidermal tumours

Basal cell carcinoma (rodent ulcer)

This is the most common form of skin cancer. It crops up most commonly on the faces of the middle-aged or elderly. Neglected lesions can invade and cause significant local destruction but, for practical purposes, never metastasize. Basal cell was first described in 1824 as a rodent ulcer. Most patients often describe a spontaneous non-healing sore that may bleed and scab.

Cause

Prolonged sun exposure is the main factor so these tumours are most common in fair skinned individuals who have lived in sunny areas, high altitudes or near the equator. They may also occur in scars caused by radiation exposure, vaccination or trauma. Photosensitizing pitch, tar and oils can act as cocarcinogens with ultraviolet radiation. Previous treatment with arsenic, once present in many 'tonics', predisposes to multiple basal cell carcinomas, often after a lag of many years.

Multiple basal cell carcinomas are found in the naevoid basal cell carcinoma syndrome (Gorlin's syndrome) where they may be associated with palmoplantar pits, jaw cysts and abnormalities of the skull, vertebrae and ribs. The syndrome is inherited as an autosomal dominant trait and is caused by a mutation of the Patched (PTCH) gene, involved in embryonic tissue growth and organization. Other genetic conditions such as xeroderma pigmentosum, albinism and Bazex syndrome are also associated with the development of multiple basal cell carcinomas.

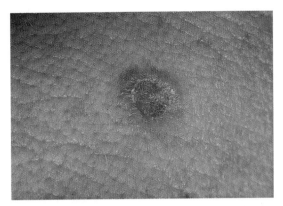

Figure 20.26 Early basal cell carcinoma with rolled opalescent edge and central crusting.

Presentation

Nodular. This is the most common type. An early lesion is a small glistening translucent, sometimes umbilicated, skin-coloured papule that slowly enlarges. Central necrosis, although not invariable, leaves an ulcer with an adherent crust and a rolled pearly edge (Figure 20.26). Coarse telangiectatic vessels often run across the tumour's surface (Figure 20.27). Without treatment such lesions may reach 1–2 cm in diameter in 5–10 years.

Cystic. The lesion is at first like the nodular type, but later cystic changes predominate and the nodule becomes tense and more translucent, with marked telangiectasia.

Morphoeic (cicatricial, sclerosing, infiltrative). These are slowly expanding yellow or white waxy plaques with an ill-defined edge. Ulceration and crusting, followed by fibrosis, are common, and the lesion may

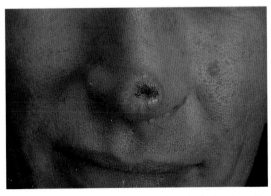

Figure 20.27 Basal cell carcinoma with marked telangiectasia and ulceration.

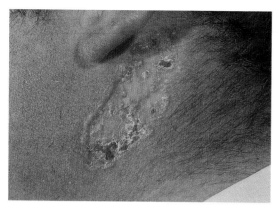

Figure 20.28   Cicatricial basal cell carcinoma.

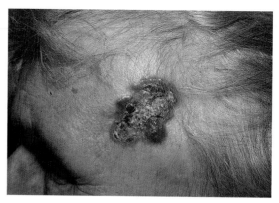

Figure 20.30   A pigmented tumour on the temple. The opalescent rim points to the diagnosis of a basal cell carcinoma.

look like an enlarging scar (Figure 20.28). Histologically, thin strands of tumour infiltrates between collagen fibres, making the clinical margins difficult to distinguish. The actual tumour is often larger than it appears and recurrence is common.

Superficial (multicentric). These arise most often on the trunk. Several lesions may be present, each expanding slowly as a red, pink or brown scaly thin plaque with a fine 'whipcord' edge (Figure 20.29). Such lesions can grow to more than 10 cm in diameter.

Pigmented. Pigment may be present in all types of basal cell carcinoma, causing all or part of the tumour to be brown or have specks of brown or black within it (Figure 20.30).

Clinical course

The slow but relentless growth destroys tissue locally. Untreated, a basal cell carcinoma can invade underlying cartilage or bone (Figure 20.31) or damage important structures such as the tear ducts.

Histology

Small, darkly blue staining basal cells grow in well-defined aggregates which invade the dermis (Figure 20.32). The outer layer of cells is arranged in a palisade. Numerous

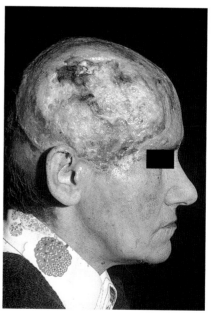

Figure 20.31   A grossly neglected basal cell carcinoma already invading underlying bone.

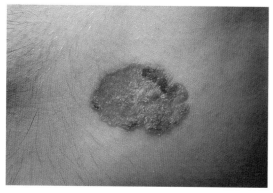

Figure 20.29   Persistent scaly plaque – the whipcord edge gives away the diagnosis of a superficial basal cell carcinoma.

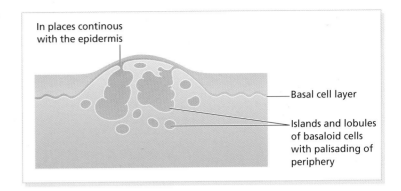

In places continous with the epidermis

Basal cell layer

Islands and lobules of basaloid cells with palisading of periphery

Figure 20.32 Histology of nodular basal cell carcinoma.

mitoses and apoptotic bodies are seen. In the cicatricial type the islands of tumour are surrounded by fibrous tissue.

Differential diagnosis

A nodular basal cell carcinoma may be confused with an intradermal melanocytic naevus, a squamous cell carcinoma, a giant molluscum contagiosum (p. 234), a traumatized benign papule or a keratoacanthoma. Pigmented basal cell carcinomas should be distinguished from seborrhoeic warts and malignant melanomas. A cicatricial basal cell carcinoma may mimic morphoea (p. 135) or a scar. A superficial basal cell carcinoma may be confused with an intraepidermal carcinoma, with psoriasis (see Chapter 5) or with nummular eczema (p. 93).

Treatment

There is no single treatment of choice for all basal cell carcinomas. Treatment should be tailored to the type of tumour, its site and the age and general health of the patient. Surgical wounds closed with sutures generally heal with less apparent scar than those left to heal by secondary intention, and this may be a consideration in the choice of treatment particularly for tumours on the face and keloid-prone areas. Published guidelines are very useful (see *Further reading*). The 5-year cure rate for all types of basal cell carcinoma is over 95% but regular follow-up is advisable to detect local recurrences when they are small and remediable.

In general, excision with 4 mm of surrounding normal skin, is the treatment of choice for discrete nodular and cystic tumours in patients under 60 years. For low risk tumours, this results in complete clearance of over 95%. This can be done by excising an elipse of skin containing the tumour and normal margins. The excised tissue is sent for pathological evaluation to confirm tumour clearance.

Electrodessication and curettage is a common, quick, inexpensive technique used by dermatologists to treat small nodular and superficial tumours. Cure rates exceed 90% for low risk tumours, but specimens cannot be evaluated histologically for margin control.

High risk tumours should be excised by specialist surgeons. Mohs' micrographic surgery is highly effective; it includes careful histological checks in all planes of tissue excised during the operation (p. 371). High risk features include morphoeaform and infiltrative tumours with their ill-defined edges and lesions near vital structures such as the nose, ear, eyelids, eyebrow and temple (the H-zone of the face). Mohs' surgery should also be considered for large tumours (>2 cm), aggressive tumours with perineural or perivascular invasion, recurrent lesions and in patients who are immunosuppressed. The cure rate with Mohs' surgery for primary facial basal cell carcinoma is 98–99% and for recurrent basal cell carcinoma is 96%.

In patients in whom surgery is contraindicated or those with extensive lesions, radiation therapy and medical treatments have also proven effective. Radiotherapy is seldom used now for biopsy-proven lesions in patients under 70 years, because of the high risk of radiodermatitis, scars and induction of new tumours over time. The average cure rate at 5 years with radiotherapy is around 90%. Cryotherapy, imiquimod and photodynamic therapy are sometimes useful for superficial lesions but are associated with high recurrence rates of up to 30%. Sometimes, palliative treatment with curettage and cautery may be preferable to aggressive treatment for elderly patients in poor health; nowadays there is seldom justification for doing nothing.

A new systemic agent, vismodegib, was recently approved for advanced and metastatic disease. It inhibits the Hedgehog signalling pathway, the primary driver of oncogensis in basal cell tumours. While promising, the numerous side effects including dysgeusia, muscle cramps, hair loss and fatigue limit its use.

> **Learning points**
>
> 1 Catch lesions early: small ones are easy to get rid of; larger ones can eat into cartilage or bone.
> 2 Do not sit and watch doubtful lesions near the eye.

Squamous cell carcinoma

This is a common tumour in which malignant keratinocytes show a variable capacity to form keratin. Unlike basal cell carcinomas, larger and invasive squamous cell carcinomas are associated with a significant risk of metastasis, and as such require careful evaluation and aggressive management.

Cause

These tumours often arise in skin damaged by ultraviolet radiation and also by X-rays and infrared rays. The majority of squamous cell skin cancers carry typical ultraviolet-induced mutations in the p53 tumour suppressor gene, emphasizing the significant part ultraviolet radiation plays in the development of this cancer. Other carcinogens include pitch, tar, mineral oils and inorganic arsenic (p. 289). Certain rare genetic disorders, with defective DNA repair mechanisms, such as xeroderma pigmentosum (p. 347), lead to multiple squamous and basal cell carcinomas, and to malignant melanoma. The DNA of some types of HPV (p. 227) can be integrated into the nuclear DNA of keratinocytes and cause malignant transformation. Immunosuppression and ultraviolet radiation predispose to this. Organ transplant recipients are significantly more prone to squamous cell carcinoma rather than basal cell carcinoma due to their immunosuppression. HPV infection and ultraviolet light exposure multiply this risk. These patients are at high risk of dying from their squamous cell carcinomas, and their tumours should thus be treated aggressively. Reduction of their immunosuppressive medication may help reduce future skin cancer development.

Multiple self-healing squamous cell carcinomas are found in the autosomal dominant trait described by Ferguson-Smith. The abnormal gene lies on chromosome 9q.

Clinical presentation and course

Tumours may arise as thickenings in an actinic keratosis or, *de novo*, as small scaling nodules; rapidly grow-

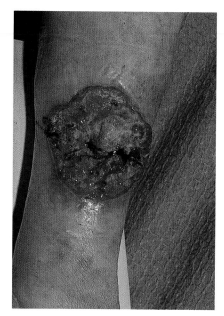

Figure 20.33 Squamous cell carcinoma. Not a venous ulcer – too high up the leg, too raised and no signs of venous insufficiency.

ing anaplastic lesions may start as ulcers with a granulating base and an indurated edge (Figure 20.33). Squamous cell carcinomas are common on the lower lip (see Figure 13.35) and in the mouth. These locations, along with tumours arising in chronic draining sinuses, chronic ulcers, areas of previous X-radiation or thermal injury, or chronic inflammation, are the most likely to metastasize. Tumours arising in non-exposed sites, such as the perineum and sole of foot and on the ear and lip, have a lesser malignant potential but may metastasize. Squamous cell carcinomas arising in sun-exposed areas and in actinic keratoses seldom metastasize except in immunosuppressed patients. Tumours more than 2 cm in diameter are twice as likely to recur and metastasize than smaller tumours. Metastatic potential is also high in tumours greater than 2 mm in depth or invading to the subcutaneous tissue; in poorly differentiated tumours; in tumours with perineural involvement; and in those arising in the immunosuppressed, such as recipients of solid organ transplants and those with lymphoproliferative disorders (e.g. chronic lymphocytic leukemia).

Histology

Keratinocytes disrupt the dermo-epidermal junction and proliferate irregularly into the dermis. Malignant cells

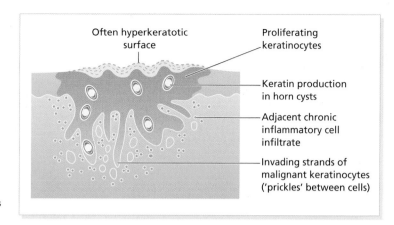

Often hyperkeratotic surface

Proliferating keratinocytes

Keratin production in horn cysts

Adjacent chronic inflammatory cell infiltrate

Invading strands of malignant keratinocytes ('prickles' between cells)

Figure 20.34 The histology of a squamous cell carcinoma.

usually retain the capacity to produce keratin (Figure 20.34).

Treatment

After the diagnosis has been confirmed by biopsy, low risk tumours should be excised with a 5-mm border of normal skin. Wider excision (6 mm or more) or Mohs' micrographic surgery (p. 371) is recommended for high risk tumours. Sometimes, keratin stains are used to help track perineural spread. Sentinal lymph node examination is usually not recommended, but palpation of regional nodes is important in work-up and follow-up. Radiotherapy is effective but should be reserved for the frail and the elderly and as adjuvant therapy following surgical treatment of aggressive squamous cell carcinoma with perineural invasion. Follow-up for up to 5 years is recommended for patients with recurrent disease and for those with high risk tumours.

Other types of squamous cell carcinoma

Intraepidermal squamous cell carcinoma (Bowen's disease, squamous cell carcinoma *in situ*)

Usually single, these slowly expanding pink scaly plaques (Figure 20.35) take years to reach a diameter of a few centimetres. Their border is sharply defined, with reniform projections and notches giving it an amoeboid shape. About 3% progress into an invasive squamous cell carcinoma. The presence of several may be a clue to previous exposure to carcinogens (e.g. excessive sun exposure, arsenic in a tonic when young).

Differential diagnosis

An intraepidermal squamous cell carcinoma is often mistaken for psoriasis (see Chapter 5), discoid eczema (p. 93), superficial basal cell carcinoma (p. 290) or for Paget's disease in the peri-anal region.

Treatment

These lesions are unaffected by local steroids. Small lesions may occasionally be left under observation in the frail and elderly. Cryotherapy or curettage are the treatments of choice for small lesions on a site where healing should be good (e.g. face or trunk); excision is an alternative. Photodynamic therapy (p. 376) is useful for large lesions on a poor healing site (e.g. the lower legs of the elderly). Topical 5-fluorouracil or imiquimod is helpful for multiple lesions (see guidelines in *Further reading*).

Keratoacanthomatous squamous cell carcinoma

These rapidly growing squamous cell tumours do not invade and occasionally resolve spontaneously.

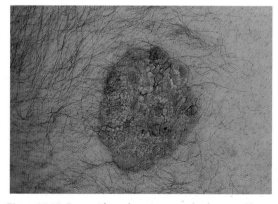

Figure 20.35 Intraepidermal carcinoma: a slowly expanding warty plaque. Note the reniform projections and notches so suggestive of an *in situ* malignancy.

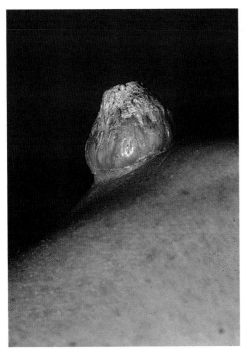

Figure 20.36 Keratoacanthoma with its epidermal shoulders and central plug of keratin.

Cause

Photosensitizing chemicals such as tar and mineral oils can act as cocarcinogens with ultraviolet radiation. They may also follow therapeutic immunosuppression. Patients with multiple keratoacanthoma may have autosomal dominant Ferguson-Smith's syndrome.

Clinical features

They occur mainly on the exposed skin of fair individuals. More than two-thirds are on the face and most of the rest are on the arms. The lesion starts as a pink papule that rapidly enlarges; it may reach a diameter of 1 cm in a month or two. After 5–6 weeks the centre of the nodule forms either a keratinous plug or a crater (Figure 20.36). If left, the lesion may occasionally resolve spontaneously over 6–12 months leaving an ugly depressed scar.

Histology

It is not possible to diagnose a keratoacanthomatous squamous cell carcinoma histologically unless the architecture of the whole lesion can be assessed, including its base (Figure 20.37). A typical lesion is symmetrical and composed of proliferating fronds of epidermis that show mitotic activity but retain a well-differentiated squamous appearance with the production of much 'glassy' keratin. The centre of the cup-shaped mass is filled with keratin, and invasion of the malignant cells into the deeper dermis does not occur.

Treatment

Excision or curettage and cautery are both effective. Occasionally, a further curetting may be needed but this should be performed only once; if this is still ineffective, the lesion must be excised with a narrow margin of surrounding skin.

Malignant melanoma

Malignant melanoma attracts a huge amount of publicity because it is so often lethal but still too many members of the public are unaware of its increasing incidence and dangers.

Incidence

The incidence in the white population in the United Kingdom and United States is doubling every 10 years. In Scotland and northern parts of the United States the incidence is now about 10 per 100 000 per year, with females being affected more often than males. There is a

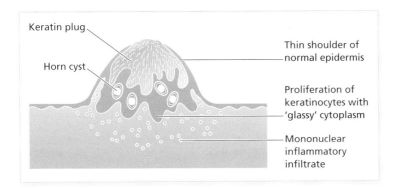

Keratin plug

Horn cyst

Thin shoulder of normal epidermis

Proliferation of keratinocytes with 'glassy' cytoplasm

Mononuclear inflammatory infiltrate

Figure 20.37 Histology of keratoacanthoma.

higher incidence in whites living near the equator than in temperate zones and there the female preponderance is lost. The highest incidence, more than 40 per 100 000 per year, is seen in white people living in Australia and New Zealand. The tumour is rare before puberty but among the most common cancers in those under 40 years. While uncommon in black people, Asians and Orientals, when it does occur in these races it is most often on the palms, soles or mucous membranes.

Cause

Genetic

Susceptibility genes. Approximately 10% of all cutaneous malignant melanoma cases are familial, occuring in families where two or more first-degree relatives have a melanoma. Molecular defects in both tumour suppressor genes and oncogenes have been linked to these melanomas; the one attracting most interest at present lies on chromosome 9p21 and encodes a tumour suppressor gene designated p16, also known as *CDKN2A*. Mutations in *CDKN2A* confer on carriers a risk of melanoma of 20% by the age 40 and 40% by age 60. Other susceptibility genes include *CDK4* and *MC1R*. The more melanomas there are in a single family the more likely they are due to a high risk susceptibility gene. If just two members in a family have a melanoma then they are more likely to be due to low risk susceptibility genes interacting with phenotypic (e.g. red hair and freckles) and environmental factors (e.g. sunlight).

Susceptible phenotypes. Malignant melanomas are most common in white people with blond or red hair, many freckles and a fair skin that tans poorly. Those of Celtic origin are especially susceptible. Melanoma may affect several members of a single family in association with atypical (dysplastic) naevi (p. 284).

Sunlight

Both the incidence and mortality increase with decreasing latitude. Tumours occur most often, but not exclusively, on exposed skin. Episodic exposure of fair skinned individuals to intense sunlight is thought to be the main cause of the steadily increasing incidence of melanoma worldwide. For melanomas, the number of sunburns seems more relevant than cumulative ultraviolet radiation dose.

Pre-existing melanocytic naevi. The risk of developing a malignant melanoma is highest in those with atypical naevi, congenital melanocytic naevi or many banal melanocytic naevi. A pre-existing naevus is seen histologically in about 30% of malignant melanomas.

Prevention and early diagnosis

Every photon of sunlight that hits the skin has a chance to provoke a cancer-causing mutation. So protection of skin from ultraviolet radiation is important. This is best done by avoiding burning exposure of skin to sunlight and tanning booths. Dermatologists joke that the best sunscreen is a house. Tight weave clothing, hats and sunscreens reduce exposure but may provide a false sense of security. Although sunscreens help, avoidance of excessive sun exposure is better. The skin protection factor (SPF) of a sunscreen or sunblock is the ratio of the time it takes to sunburn skin protected by sunscreen divided by the time it takes to sunburn adjacent unprotected skin. The amount of sunscreen applied to get these ratios is the volume of a golf ball. Most sunscreen users apply much less, and apply sunscreen only when outdoor activities are planned. If every photon counts, so sunscreen should be applied to sun exposed skin everyday. When golf, tennis, sailing or other outdoor activity beckons, a sunscreen of SPF 15 or more should be used and reapplied after 20 minutes to add a second coat and to catch missed areas. The sunscreen should be reapplied during the day, especially because it washes off with swimming or sweating. Ideally, sunscreens should be broad spectrum, blocking both UVA and UVB.

Early diagnosis is critical and there is now ample evidence that melanoma publicity campaigns, regular self-examination and the education of primary care physicians have all played their part in reducing the mortality rate from melanoma.

Clinical features

Eighty per cent of invasive melanomas are preceded by a superficial and radial growth phase, shown clinically as the expansion of an irregularly pigmented macule or plaque (Figure 20.38). Most are multicoloured mixtures of black, brown, blue, tan and pink. Their margins are irregular with reniform projections and notches. Malignant cells are at first usually confined to the epidermis and uppermost dermis, but eventually invade more deeply and may metastasize (Figure 20.38).

There are four main types of malignant melanoma.

1 *Lentigo maligna melanoma* occurs on the exposed skin of the elderly. An irregularly pigmented, irregularly shaped macule (a lentigo maligna) may have been enlarging slowly for many years as an *in situ* melanoma before an

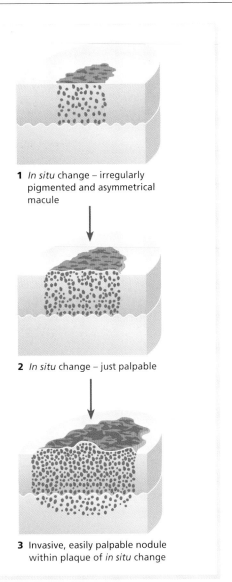

1 *In situ* change – irregularly pigmented and asymmetrical macule

2 *In situ* change – just palpable

3 Invasive, easily palpable nodule within plaque of *in situ* change

Figure 20.38 Radial intraepidermal growth phase of melanoma (1 and 2) precedes vertical and invasive dermal growth phase (3).

invasive nodule (the lentigo maligna melanoma) appears (Figure 20.39).

2 *Superficial spreading melanoma* is the most common type in fair skinned individuals between 30 and 50 years of age. Its radial growth phase shows varied colours and commonly display the classic ABCD signs (Figures 20.40 and 20.41). A nodule coming up within such a plaque signifies deep dermal invasion and a poor prognosis (Table 20.4).

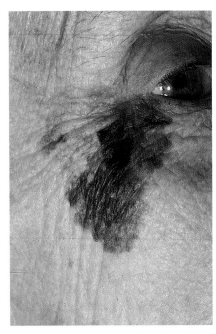

Figure 20.39 This elderly patient, her friends and family doctor, had ignored for too long the slowly spreading macule of a lentigo maligna: now she has a frankly invasive melanoma within it (the darker area).

3 *Acral lentiginous melanoma* occurs on the palms and soles in the elderly and, although rare in Caucasoids, is the most common type in blacks and Asians. The invasive phase is again signalled by a nodule coming up within an irregularly pigmented macule or patch.

4 *Nodular melanoma* (Figure 20.42) appears as a pigmented nodule with no preceding *in situ* phase. It is the most rapidly growing and aggressive type, often found on the legs and truncal areas.

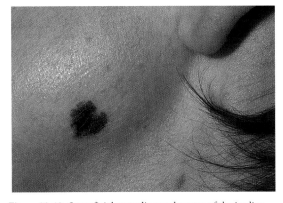

Figure 20.40 Superficial spreading melanoma of the jawline. Small, and still curable at this stage.

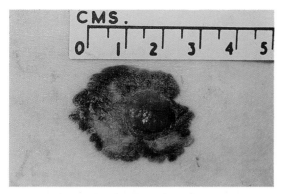

Figure 20.41 This shows the hallmarks of a malignant melanoma with its asymmetry, irregular borders and variations in colour. The pink amelanotic nodule signifies deep dermal invasion.

Melanomas can also be described by their colour, site and degree of spread.
• *Amelanotic melanomas* (Figure 20.43) are rare and occur especially on the soles of the feet. Flecks of pigment can usually be seen with a lens. Diagnosis can be challenging as they can be mistaken for benign skin lesions. Prognosis is the same as for pigmented melanomas.
• *Desmoplastic melanomas* are rare. They are seen most often on the head, neck, palms and soles. They are sometimes amelanotic. This tumour can be locally aggressive with perineural extension, although rarely metastasizes.

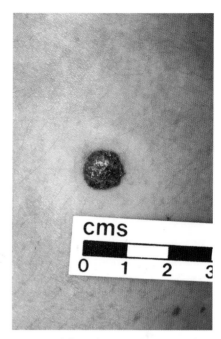

Figure 20.42 A nodular malignant melanoma: just beginning to ulcerate.

• *Subungual melanomas* are painless areas of pigmentation expanding under the nail and on to the nail fold (Hutchinson's sign, Figure 14.6).
• *Metastatic melanoma* has spread to surrounding skin, regional lymph nodes or to other organs. At this stage it can rarely be cured.

Table 20.4 Staging systems for melanoma.

AJCC Stage	TNM Stage		Survival (%)	
			5-year	10-year
0	Tis N0 M0	Melanoma *in situ*	100	100
IA	T1a N0 M0	≤1.0 mm without ulceration or mitoses	97	95
IB	T1b N0 M0	≤1.0 mm + ulceration or mitoses ≥1/mm^2	92	86
	T2a N0 M0	1.01–2.0 mm without ulceration		
IIA	T2b N0 M0	1.01–2.0 mm + ulceration	81	67
	T3a N0 M0	2.01–4 mm without ulceration		
IIB	T3b N0 M0	2.01–4 mm + ulceration	70	57
	T4a N0 M0	>4 mm without ulceration		
IIC	T4b N0 M0	>4 mm + ulceration	53	40
III	Any T N1–3 M0	Any thickness with nodal disease	40–78	24–68
IV	Any T any N M1	Distal metastatic disease	15–20	10–15

AJCC, American Joint Committee on Cancer; TNM, tumour, node, metastasis.

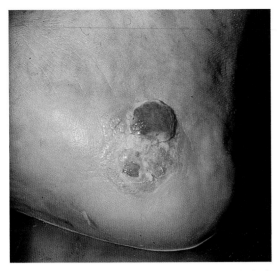

Figure 20.43 An amelanotic malignant melanoma on the heel of an elderly person. Always obtain histology even if you think it is just a pyogenic granuloma or an atypical wart.

Table 20.5 Prognostic indicators in malignant melanoma.

Indicator	Significance
Depth of primary tumour	<0.75 mm, 5-year survival 95%
	0.76–1.5 mm, 5-year survival 85%
	1.51–4.0 mm, 5-year survival 65%
	>4.0 mm, 5-year survival 45%
Sex	Females do better than males
Age	Prognosis worsens after 50 years of age, especially in males
Site	The prognosis is poor for tumours on trunk, upper arms, neck and scalp
Ulceration	Signifies a poor prognosis
Mitosis	Signifies a pooor prognosis
Sentinel node	Prognosis worsens with tumour-positive sentinel node
Clinical stage	Prognosis worsens with advancing stage (Table 20.4)

Staging

The most popular staging systems for melanoma are the TNM classification (Europe) and the American Joint Committee on Cancer (AJCC) system in the United States (Table 20.4). Both have been refined recently to include ulceration and mitosis of the tumour and micrometastases in nodes, but Table 20.4 gives an idea of the broad categories of each classification. The systems provide a useful guide to prognosis (Table 20.5).

Histology

• *Lentigo maligna.* Numerous atypical melanocytes, many in groups, are seen along the basal layer extending downwards in the walls of hair follicles.
• *Lentigo maligna melanoma.* Dermal invasion occurs, with a breach of the basement membrane region. *In situ* changes are seen in the adjacent epidermis.
• *Superficial spreading melanoma* in situ. Large epithelioid melanoma cells permeate the epidermis.
• *Superficial spreading melanoma.* The dermal nodule may be composed of epithelioid cells, spindle cells or naevus-like cells. *In situ* changes are seen in the adjacent epidermis.
• *Acral lentiginous melanoma* in situ. Atypical melanocytes are seen in the base of the epidermis and permeating the mid epidermis.
• *Acral lentiginous melanoma.* Melanoma cells invade the dermis. *In situ* changes are seen in the adjacent epidermis.

• *Nodular melanoma.* The tumour comprises epithelioid, spindle and naevoid cells and there is no *in situ* melanoma in the adjacent epidermis.
• *Desmoplastic melanoma.* Melanoma cells are seen amongst a dense fibrous stroma. The overlying epidermis may show signs of a preceding lentigo maligna or acral lentiginous melanoma *in situ*.

Microstaging

The histology (Figure 20.44) can be used to assess prognosis. Breslow's method is to measure, with an ocular micrometer, the vertical distance from the granular cell layer to the deepest part of the tumour. Clark's method, used less frequently nowadays, is to assess the depth of penetration of the melanoma (Figure 20.45) in relation to the different layers of the dermis. The thicker and more penetrating a lesion, the worse is its prognosis (see *Prognosis*).

Differential diagnosis

This includes a melanocytic naevus, seborrhoeic keratosis, pigmented actinic keratosis, lentigo, pigmented basal cell carcinoma and sclerosing haemangioma; all are discussed in this chapter. A malignant melanoma can also be confused with a subungual or peri-ungual haematoma (see Figure 13.20). A history of trauma helps here, as may paring. 'Talon noir' (Figure 20.46) is a pigmented petechial area on the heel following minor trauma from

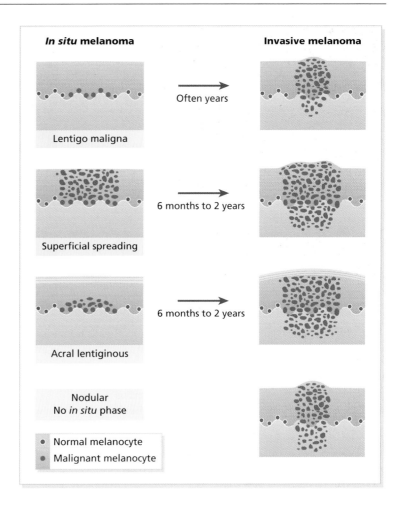

Figure 20.44 Histology of the different types of melanoma.

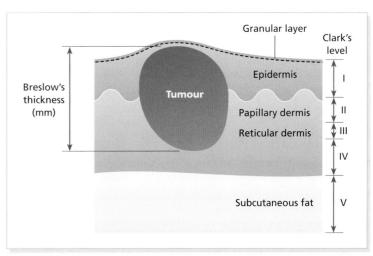

Figure 20.45 Schematic representation of Breslow's and Clark's methods of microstaging malignant melanoma.

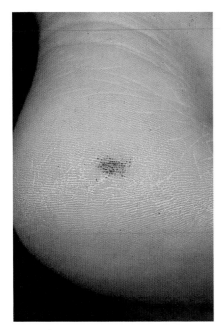

Figure 20.46 Talon noir.

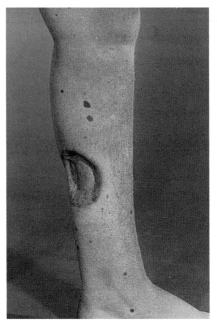

Figure 20.47 Such a wide excision and unsightly graft is no longer acceptable for a thin good-prognosis melanoma. Note the many atypical moles.

ill-fitting training shoes. An amelanotic melanoma is most often confused with a pyogenic granuloma and with a squamous cell carcinoma. Dermatoscopy (Chapter 28), in experienced hands, helps to distinguish the above but doubtful lesions should be removed without delay for histological examination (see *Treatment*).

Prognosis

The prognostic indicators, and their significance, are listed in Table 20.5. They have been established by following up large numbers of patients who have undergone appropriate surgical treatment (see *Treatment*). As a general rule, the prognosis for those patients with non-ulcerated superfical melanomas, less than 1 mm in thickness, is excellent.

Treatment

Surgery. Surgical excision, with minimal delay, is required. An excision biopsy with 1–3 mm of normal skin (or deep saucerization technique down to the subcutaneous fat) is recommended for all suspicious lesions. Shave and punch biopsies are not recommended, but can be done if the lesion is in a cosmetically sensitive site. Punch biopies can lead to a sampling error, and rob the pathologist of the chance to evaluate architecture and

malignant changes elsewhere in the tumour. They do not provoke metastasis. Shave biopsies may not include the deep margin, making it difficult to gauge prognosis, and superficial shave biopsies may be misdiagnosed.

If the histology confirms the diagnosis of malignant melanoma then wider excision, including the wound of the excision biopsy, should be performed as soon as possible. A minimum of 0.5 cm clearance for *in situ* melanomas and 1 cm clearance is required for melanomas ≤1 mm in depth. Intermediate thickness tumours (1–4 mm Breslow depth) should be excised with 1–3 cm margins (Figure 20.47). The maximum clearance is thus 3 cm of normal skin and, depending on the site, primary closure – without grafting – is often possible. There is no convincing evidence that excision margins wider than 3 cm confer any greater survival advantage. Tissue is removed down to, but not including, the deep fascia. The guidelines of the British Association of Dermatologists (see *Further reading*) differ minimally from this simple advice.

If lymph node involvement is suspected clinically then the initial investigation should be with fine needle aspiration. If involvement is confirmed then formal block dissection of the involved group of nodes should be carried out.

The role of sentinel node biopsy in detecting occult nodal metastases remains under investigation. The aim is to carry out elective dissection of the local nodes in positive cases, but avoid this significant procedure when the sentinel node is not involved. Sentinel lymph node biopsy is recommended in patients with thicker melanomas ($\geq$1 mm in depth). It is also recommended in thinner melanomas (0.75–1 mm) with high risk features (ulceration, mitotic rate $\geq$1/mm^2, lymphovascular invasion). The sentinel node, the first and often nearest local node in the lymphatic drainage of the tumour, is detected by a blue dye and a radiolabelled colloid injected intradermally around the tumour before excision. This node is excised and examined histologically for metastases including micrometastases. If metastases are found, the entire lymph node basin is removed. There is little evidence to support elective regional node dissection in the management of sentinel node-negative patients with tumours of intermediate thickness (1.5–4.0 mm). Although sentinel lymph node status is the most important factor in defining prognosis, its therapeutic benefit to overall survival is yet to be determined. Early results of ongoing trials show a positive benefit in 5-year survival rates for patients with positive sentinel lymph nodes who underwent immediate elective lymph node dissection but longer follow-up data are needed.

Adjunctive therapies. Surgery cures most patients with early melanoma, but its effect on survival lessens as the disease advances. The median survival for metastatic disease is 8–9 months and the 3-year overall survival rate is less than 15%. The results of ongoing controlled trials, investigating the role of immunotherapy (e.g. melanoma-specific antigen vacccines, immunotherapy agents and biologic response modifiers) as an adjunct to surgery in patients with poor prognostic melanomas (e.g. TNM stages II and III), are awaited with interest. Adjuvant high dose interferon α-2b and IL-2 have demonstrated comparable response rate, although side effects are difficult to tolerate and patients have a 40–80% chance of relapse and death. Melanoma vaccines, while theoretically promising, have failed to improve overall survival in randomized trials. The discovery of BRAF mutations in melanoma has led to the development of new oncogene directed therapy. BRAF inhibitors block the mitogen-activated protein kinase pathway which is constitutively activated in 80–90% of melanomas. In melanomas with a specific BRAF mutation, vemurafenib, a BRAF inhibitor, shows an improved mean progression-free survival (5.3 months) compared with those treated with dacar-

bazine (1.6 months). One side effect of vemurafenib is the development of multiple keratoacanthomas and squamous cell carcinomas. Recently, immunomodulation with ipilimumab, a monoclonal antibody against cytotoxic T-lymphocyte antigen 4 (CTLA-4), has also shown survival benefits. By binding CTLA-4, ipilimumab enhances T-cell response and activates immune-mediated tumour regression. While these new agents are promising, the long-term effects on survival are uncertain and the high cost of these drugs limit their use outside clinical trials.

Chemotherapy. Although rarely curative, chemotherapy may be palliative in 25% of patients with stage III melanoma. Dacarbazine is often the drug of choice.

Follow-up care. Patients who have had melanoma should be screened for recurrence and for metastases. Recurrence usually appears as a growth or pigmentation at the original site. In transit melanomas are satellite nodules nearby but not connected to the original tumour. The regional nodal basins should be palpated, but studies have shown that chest X-rays, laboratory studies (lactic dehydrogenase, liver function tests), and special scans (CT, positron emission tomography) have an extremely low yield in asymptomatic patients; therefore they are not routinely recommended unless there are suspicious symptoms. Desmoplastic melanomas tend to skip the nodes and metastasize directly to the lungs. Eighty per cent of recurrent or metastatic melanomas occur within 3 years of definitive surgery. Unfortunately, a 5-year melanoma-free follow up is not a guarantee of cure; 5–8% of patients develop late (after 5 years) metastatic melanoma. A second primary melanoma is not unusual, so general examination of the skin is recommended at follow up.

Oral contraceptives and hormone replacement therapy. These are not contraindicated in patients who have had a melanoma. The risk of subsequent pregnancy on the outcome of melanoma is not known.

Learning points

1 Prevention of a malignant melanoma is better than cure. Remember avoidance of sun exposure and 'sun smart' advice to patients.
2 Everyone, and especially those with many moles, should be encouraged to examine their own skin regularly.
3 Take any change in a mole seriously.
4 Do not forget the ABCDE rules when querying a melanoma (Table 20.3).
5 Excise all doubtful lesions and check their histology.

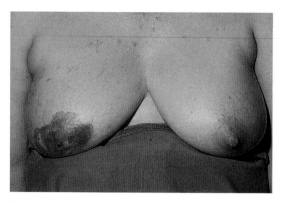

Figure 20.48 Be alert to the possibility of Paget's disease if a red plaque affects only one nipple, and alters its normal architecture.

Table 20.6 Common vascular naevi.

Malformations
Present at birth. Do not involve ('salmon' patch is exception)
1 Capillary ('salmon' patch and 'port-wine' stain)
2 Arterial
3 Venous
4 Combined

Haemangiomas (sometimes called angiomatous naevi)
Usually appear after birth. More common in females, 50–60% on head and neck. Involute by 5–9 years after initial proliferation
1 Superficial (capillary)
2 Deep (cavernous)
3 Mixed

6 If excision biopsy shows that an invasive melanoma is less than 1 mm thick, the only question to be asked is whether it has been excised with a 1-cm clearance in all directions.
7 Support campaigns to educate doctors and the public to recognize melanoma early, in its superficial and curable phase.

Paget's disease of the nipple (apocrine ductal carcinoma) (Figure 20.48)

A well-defined red scaly plaque spreads slowly over and around the nipple. It is caused by the invasion of the epidermis by cells from an underlying intraductal carcinoma of the breast (Paget's cells). The condition is sharply marginated and unilateral, whereas eczemas are usually poorly marginated and affect both nipples. A skin biopsy should be carried out first and if the diagnosis is confirmed mastectomy will be necessary. Extramammary Paget's disease affects other sites bearing apocrine glands and is caused by an underlying ductal carcinoma of these. The perineum is the next most common site after breast.

Tumours of the dermis

Benign

Developmental abnormalities of blood vessels

These are either present at birth or appear soon after. They can be classified clinically (Table 20.6) but there is no good clinicohistological correlation. A capillary malformation is composed of a network of capillaries in the upper and mid dermis. A capillary cavernous haeman-

gioma has multiple ectatic channels of varying calibre distributed throughout the dermis and even the subcutaneous fat.

Malformations

'Salmon' patches ('stork bites')

These common malformations, present in about 50% of all babies, are caused by dilatated capillaries in the superficial dermis. They are dull red, often telangiectatic macules, most commonly on the nape of the neck (*erythema nuchae*), the forehead and the upper eyelids. Nuchal lesions may remain unchanged, but patches in other areas usually disappear within a year.

'Port-wine' stains

These are also present at birth and are caused by dilatated dermal capillaries. They are pale, pink–purple macules and vary from the barely noticeable to the grossly disfiguring. Most occur on the face or trunk. They persist, and in middle age may darken and become studded with angiomatous nodules (Figure 20.49). Occasionally, a port-wine stain of the trigeminal area (Figure 20.50) is associated with a vascular malformation of the leptomeninges on the same side, which may cause epilepsy or hemiparesis (the Sturge–Weber syndrome), or with glaucoma.

Excellent results have been obtained with careful – and time-consuming – treatment with pulsed dye laser (p. 381). Treatment sessions can begin in babies and anaesthesia is not always necessary. Early intervention before 1 year of age may result in better clearance. If a trial patch is satisfactory, 40–50 pulses can be delivered in

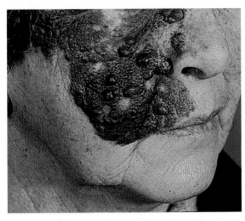

Figure 20.49 Lifelong capillary malformation of the cheek showing no tendency to resolve. Note port-wine appearance of the upper pole, contrasting with the nodular elements elsewhere.

a session and the procedure can be repeated at monthly intervals. Alternatively, some adults become very adept at using cosmetic camouflage (see Figure 1.6).

Combined vascular malformations of the limbs

A large port-wine stain of a limb may be associated with overgrowth of all the soft tissues of that limb with or without bony hypertrophy. There may be underlying venous malformations (Klippel–Trenaunay syndrome), arteriovenous fistulae (Parkes Weber syndrome) or mixed venous–lymphatic malformations.

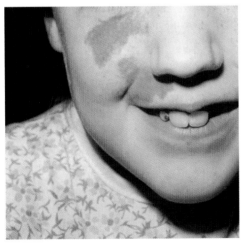

Figure 20.50 Port-wine stain of the right cheek. No neurological problems in this patient.

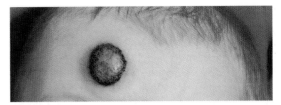

Figure 20.51 Classic strawberry naevus, occurred and enlarged rapidly shortly after birth. (Dr M.J. Tidman, The Royal Infirmary of Edinburgh, Edinburgh, UK. Reproduced with permission of Dr M.J. Tidman.)

Haemangiomas

Capillary cavernous haemangioma (strawberry naevus)

Strawberry naevi appear within a few weeks of birth, and grow for a few months, forming a raised compressible swelling with a bright red surface (Figure 20.51). Spontaneous regression then follows; the surface whitens centrally (Figure 20.52) and regression is complete by the age of 5 years in 50% of children and in 90% by the age of 9 years, leaving only an area of slight atrophy. Bleeding may follow trauma, and ulceration is common in the napkin (diaper) area. Haemangiomas occur in about 10% of infants at age 1 year. They are more common in girls, preterm infants with low birthweight, in infants from multiple gestations and from mothers of advanced maternal age.

Observation and encouragement is the management of choice for the great majority. Serial photographs of the way they clear up in other children help parents to accept this. Large cervicofacial haemangiomas may be associated with other congenital anomalies. Patients with multiple lesions may have visceral involvement. Ophthalmological help should be sought for all growing peri-ocular

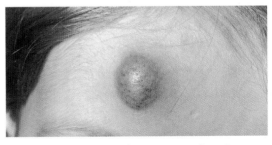

Figure 20.52 The same strawberry naevus as shown in Figure 20.51, showing the whitening of the surface which is a sign of spontaneous remission. (Dr M.J. Tidman, The Royal Infirmary of Edinburgh, Edinburgh, UK. Reproduced with permission of Dr M.J. Tidman.)

haemangiomas to rule out astigmatism and visual deprivation amblyopia. Firm pressure may be needed to stop bleeding. Lesions may ulcerate, bleed repeatedly, interfere with feeding or with vision. In the past, oral and intralesional corticosteroids were used for these complications during the proliferative phase of the haemangioma. Prenisolone at 2–4 mg/kg/day is given in a single dose in the morning and the dosage tapered to zero after 1 month. In 2008 beta-blockers were noted serendipitously to dramatically improve proliferating haemangiomas, and propranolol at a dose of 2–3 mg/kg/day in 2–3 divided doses is now the mainstay of treatment for complicated haemangiomas. Careful monitoring of blood sugar and blood pressure is necessary during the 2–10 month course of treatment. Sometimes, pulsed dye lasers are used for treating large lesions or ulcerated haemangiomas in infancy. Rarely, plastic surgery is necessary for a few large and unsightly haemangiomas that fail to improve spontaneously or to regress with the above measures.

Campbell de Morgan spots (cherry angiomas)

These benign angiomas are common on the trunks of the middle-aged and elderly. They are small bright red papules and of no consequence (Figure 20.53).

Lymphangiomas

The most common type is lymphangioma circumscriptum which appears as a cluster of vesicles resembling frog spawn. If treatment is needed, excision has to be wide and deep as dilatated lymphatic channels and cisterns extend to the subcutaneous tissue.

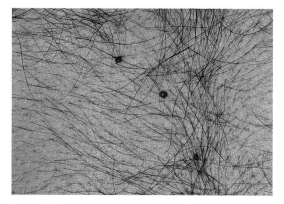

Figure 20.53 Campbell de Morgan spots (cherry angiomas) of the chest.

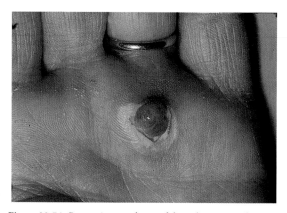

Figure 20.54 Pyogenic granuloma of the palm: soggy after elastoplast dressing and bleeding easily.

Glomus tumours

These are derived from the cells surrounding small arteriovenous shunts. Solitary lesions are painful and most common on the extremities and under the nails. Multiple lesions are seldom painful and may affect other parts of the body. Painful lesions can be removed; others may be left.

Pyogenic granulomas

These badly named lesions are in fact common benign acquired haemangiomas, often seen in children and young adults. They develop at sites of trauma, over the course of a few weeks, as bright red raised, sometimes pedunculated and raspberry-like lesions which bleed easily (Figure 20.54).

The important differential diagnosis is from an amelanotic malignant melanoma and, for this reason, the histology should always be checked. A pyogenic granuloma shows leashes of vessels of varying calibre covered by a thin, often ulcerated, epidermis. Lesions should be removed by curettage under local anaesthetic with cautery to the base. Rarely, this is followed by recurrence or an eruption of satellite lesions around the original site.

Other benign dermal tumours

Dermatofibromas (histiocytomas)

These benign tumours are firm discrete usually solitary dermal nodules (Figure 20.55), often on the extremities of young adults. The lesions have an 'iceberg' effect in that they feel larger than they look. The overlying epidermis is often lightly pigmented and dimples when the nodule is squeezed. Some lesions seem to follow minor trauma or

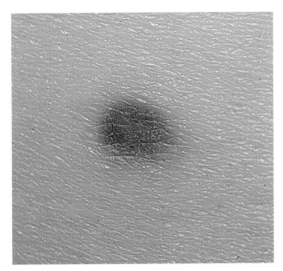

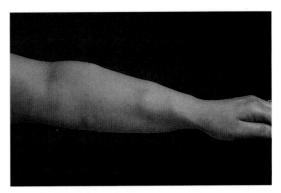

Figure 20.56 Multiple lipomas.

Figure 20.55 A 0.5-cm diameter dermatofibroma. Typically, these lesions feel larger than they look. Its depressed surface became more obvious when the surrounding skin was pinched.

an insect bite. Histologically, the proliferating fibroblasts merge into the sparsely cellular dermis at the margins. A straightforward lesion may be left alone but, if there is any diagnostic doubt, it should be excised.

Neurofibromas

Although solitary tumours occur occasionally, multiple neurofibromas are most common and are usually seen as part of the inherited condition of neurofibromatosis. The clinical features of the tumour are described on p. 344.

Neuroma

This rare benign tumour is usually solitary. It may appear spontaneously but is seen most often as a result of nerve injury at the site of trauma or a surgical wound. There is nothing specific about the appearance of the skin-coloured dermal nodule but the tumour is frequently painful, even with gentle pressure. ENGLAND is a useful acronym for painful tumours (Eccrine spiradenoma, Neuroma, Glomus tumour, Leiomyoma, Angiolipoma, Neurofibroma (rarely) and Dermatofibroma (rarely)).

Keloid

This is an overgrowth of dense fibrous tissue in the skin, arising in response to trauma, however trivial (Figure 14.9). The tendency to develop keloids is genetically inherited. Keloids are common in Negroids and may be familial. Keloid formation is encouraged by infection, for-

eign material and by wounds (including surgical ones), especially those not lying along the lines of least tension or the skin creases. Even in Caucasoids, keloids and hypertrophic scars are seen often enough on the presternal area, the neck, upper back and deltoid region of young adults to make doctors think twice before removing benign lesions there. Silicone sheeting and intralesional steroid injections are helpful but treatment should be given early, preferably for developing lesions.

Lipomas

Lipomas are common benign tumours of mature fat cells in the subcutaneous tissue. There may be one or many (Figure 20.56). Lipomas are rarely a familial trait. They are most common on the proximal parts of the limbs but can occur at any site. They have an irregular lobular shape and a characteristic soft rubbery consistency. They are rarely painful. They need to be removed only if there is doubt about the diagnosis or if they are painful, unsightly or interfere with activities such as sitting back against a chair.

Lymphocytoma cutis

This small dermal nodule is caused by a reactive proliferation of B lymphocytes. The purplish lesions may be single or multiple and/or grouped and are found usually on the face. Some may follow insect bites, scabies nodules and tattoos. If spontaneous regression does not occur, intralesional corticosteroid injection may help.

Mastocytosis (urticaria pigmentosa)

This term describes the various conditions in which the skin, and occasionally other tissues, contains an excess of mast cells. All types are characterized by a tendency for the skin to wheal after being rubbed (Darier's sign). The main types are as follows.

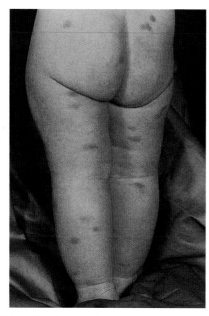

Figure 20.57 Juvenile type of mastocytosis.

• *Mastocytoma*. Usually presents as a solitary pink or brown itchy papule that wheals on rubbing. There are no systemic features.

• *Juvenile mastocytosis*. This is the most common type. Numerous pink or brown papules develop over the trunk and limbs (Figure 20.57). There is no systemic involvement and the condition is often mistaken for multiple melanocytic naevi.

• *Diffuse cutaneous mastocytosis*. This is rare and seen mostly in infants, being characterized by persistent dermographic wheals that appear after minor friction. The skin is diffusely infiltrated with mast cells, producing a thickened appearance like pigskin. The bone marrow, liver and spleen may be involved. Flushing is common. Death from massive histamine release is a real risk. Spontaneous improvement usually occurs.

• *Adult type*. Pink or pink–brown telangiectatic macules appear in early adult life and can spread to cover the whole body. The liver, spleen and bone are involved in up to 20% of cases but systemic features such as headaches, flushing and palpitations are unusual.

Malignant

Kaposi's sarcoma

This malignant tumour of proliferating capillaries and lymphatics may be multifocal. There are four types: classic, endemic, epidemic of HIV and that associated with immunosuppression. Human herpesvirus type 8 (HHV8) has been isolated from, and linked to, all types.

Classic (sporadic) Kaposi's sarcoma is seen most often in elderly Mediterranean and Eastern European men. The tumours are usually on the feet and ankles but may be seen on the hands and on cold parts of the skin (e.g. the ears and nose). Initially, they are dark blue to purple macules progressing to tumours and plaques which ulcerate and fungate. Oedema of the legs may be severe. This form rarely spread to the lymph nodes, mucous membrane or internal organs.

These tumours are very sensitive to radiotherapy, which is the treatment of choice during the early stages. Chemotherapy, with chlorambucil or vinblastine, helps when there is systemic involvement. Life expectancy is 5–9 years.

Endemic African Kaposi's sarcoma is seen primarily in men who are HIV seronegative in Africa. Clinical presentation is similar to the classic form, but endemic Kaposi's sarcoma is more likely to involve the lymph nodes.

Epidemic Kaposi's sarcoma (see Figures 16.32–14.64). Smaller and more subtle (e.g. bruise-like) lesions may occur in an immunodeficient host. This tumour has become well known because of its association with AIDS (p. 235) caused by the human immunodeficiency virus (HIV-1). Lesions of AIDS-related Kaposi's sarcoma can appear anywhere but are most common on the upper trunk and head and neck. The initial bruise-like lesions tend to follow tension lines; they become raised, increasingly pigmented and evolve into nodules and plaques. Lesions frequently arise on the oral mucous membranes. The observation in the early years of the AIDS pandemic that HIV-positive intravenous drug abusers did not develop Kaposi's sarcoma as often as did HIV-positive homosexuals is now explained by the discovery that an infectious agent (HHV8) is an important cause. The prognosis of AIDS patients with Kaposi's sarcoma used to be poor, as the disease usually develops when HIV infected patients have severe immunodeficiency with low CD4 count and increased HIV-1 viral loads. Without antiretroviral therapy, patients with AIDS-related Kaposi's sarcoma develop opportunistic infections and have a life expectancy of around 1 year. The advent of highly active antiretroviral therapy (HAART) has changed this and even multiple lesions of HIV-associated Kaposi's sarcoma usually resolve with this treatment.

Kaposi's sarcoma and immunosuppression. Clinical presentation is similar to the epidemic form. While rare, this form of Kaposi's sarcoma occurs following organ transplantation or immunosuppressive therapy in patients who are at risk for the classic type (e.g. Mediterranean men). An aggressive course with visceral involvement is common. Reduction of immunosuppression may cause regression of the disease.

Learning points

1 Early Kaposi's sarcomas often look trivial but odd in those with immunosuppression. Keep HIV in mind.
2 Turn back 2 pages if you cannot remember which benign nodules are painful.

Lymphomas and leukaemias

The latest (2005) WHO-EORTC classification (see *Further reading*) is too detailed for most non-specialists. These conditions are rare and it is convenient to group skin involvement in them into two broad categories:

1 Disorders that arise in the skin or preferentially involve it:
   - Cutaneous T-cell lymphoma (mycosis fungoides) and its variants: subcutaneous panniculitis-like subcutaneous lymphoma, anaplastic large cell CD30+ lymphoma, granulomatous slack skin, pagetoid reticulosis and folliculotropic mycosis fungoides;
   - Sézary syndrome; and
   - Lymphoma associated with HIV infection.

2 Those arising extracutaneously, but which sometimes involve the skin:
   - Hodgkin's disease;
   - B-cell lymphoma; and
   - Leukaemia.

Cutaneous T-cell lymphoma (CTCL; sometimes called mycosis fungoides)

This lymphoma of skin-associated helper T lymphocytes usually evolves slowly. There are three clinical phases: the patch, plaque and tumour stages, with involvement of lymph nodes and other tissues occurring late in the disease.

The *patch stage* (formerly termed 'premycotic' to denote an early phase of mycosis fungoides) may last for years (see Figure 6.9). Most commonly it consists of scattered, barely palpable, erythematous, slightly pigmented, sharply marginated scaly patches rather like psoriasis or seborrhoeic dermatitis (see *Parapsoriasis*, p. 73). Often they have a bizarre outline (e.g. arciform, or horseshoe-shaped) and, on close inspection, atrophy with surface wrinkling is usually evident. Their distribution is usually asymmetrical. Less commonly, the patch stage can be

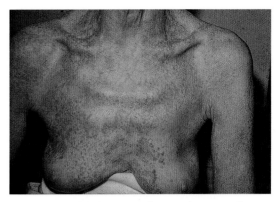

Figure 20.58 Poikiloderma vasculare atrophicans may be a precursor of the tumour stage of cutaneous T-cell lymphoma.

a widespread poikiloderma, with atrophy, pigmentation and telangiectasia (Figure 20.58). As the lymphoma develops, some patches become indurated and palpable: the *plaque stage*. Some then turn into frank tumours which may become large (occasionally like mushrooms, hence the term 'mycosis fungoides') and ulcerate (Figure 20.59). The patch stage of CTCL may be difficult to diagnose clinically, but the plaque and tumour stages are usually characteristic. The first two phases of the disease may occupy 20 years or more, but the tumour stage is often short, with spread and death usually within 3 years.

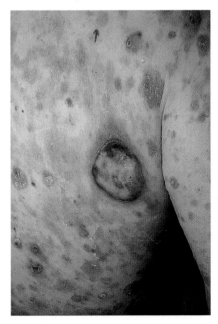

Figure 20.59 An ulcerated tumour of mycosis fungoides against a background of plaques.

Variants

• *Subcutaneous panniculitis-like T cell lymphomas* resemble an ulcerating panniculitis, especially lupus panniculitis profundus (p. 138). Subcutaneous nodules on the trunk and extremities are accompanied by general malaise, fever, chills, and weight loss.

• *Anaplastic large cell CD30+ lymphomas* present as rapidly growing tumours that sometimes regress spontaneously. About 10% have regional lymph node involvement.

• *Granulomatous slack skin* affects young patients. Indurated plaques become atrophic and the skin then becomes pendulous in the affected areas.

• *Pagetoid reticulosis* is seen most often on the acral parts and again affects the young. It appears as a slow-growing psoriasiform or verrucous plaque.

• *Folliculotrophic mycosis fungoides* usually appears as itchy pink scaly plaques with follicular prominence, most commonly on the head and neck. This is followed by alopecia although this may be subtle.

• *Sézary syndrome* is also a CTCL caused by a proliferation of helper T lymphocytes. Generalized skin erythema and oedema is associated with pruritus and lymphadenopathy. Abnormal T lymphocytes, with large convoluted nuclei, are found circulating in the blood (*Sézary cells*).

Histology

The histological hallmarks of plaque stage CTCL are:

• Intraepidermal lymphocytic microabscesses (Pautrier microabscesses);

• A band of lymphoid cells in the upper dermis, infiltrating the epidermis; and

• Atypical lymphocytes.

The histology of the patch stage poses more problems and may differ little from dermatitis. In lymphomas, T cells are clonal with most of the cells in the lesion having the same T-cell receptor. Immunophenotyping and T-cell receptor gene rearrangement studies (p. 18) may sometimes, but not always, be helpful in reaching a definitive diagnosis. Many biopsies, over several years, may be needed to prove that a suspicious rash is indeed an early stage of CTCL. Clinicopathological correlation is essential.

Differential diagnosis

The patch and plaque stages may be mistaken for psoriasis or parapsoriasis (see Chapter 5), seborrhoeic dermatitis (p. 92) or tinea corporis (p. 240). However, they respond poorly to treatment for these disorders; the bizarre shapes of the patches and their asymmetrical distribution often raise suspicion. In the early stages skin scrapings may be needed to exclude tinea. Patients with lymphomatoid papulosis develop papules or small cutaneous nodules of clonal T cells with a worrying malignant histology but a benign clinical course.

Treatment

Moderately potent or potent local steroids, and UVB treatment, may provide prolonged palliation in the patch stage. These patients should be encouraged to moisturize frequently to alleviate their xerosis and pruritus. In the plaque stage, PUVA, oral retinoids and α-interferon are helpful. If lesions become more indurated, electron beam therapy may be used. Topical nitrogen mustard paint and topical retinoids (tazarotene) have also been used with success in both patch and plaque stages. Individual tumours respond well to low-dose radiotherapy. Systemic chemotherapy is disappointing, except for patients with the Sézary syndrome. For them, treatment with extracorporeal photopheresis (irradiationg psoralenized blood with UVA in a machine) or with a targeting monoclonal antibody carrying diphtheria toxin may help destroy circualting malignant cells. Recently, oral histone deacetylase inhibitors have been shown to inhibit gene transcription and show promise in the treatment of CTCL.

Extracutaneous lymphomas

Hodgkin's disease

This is of interest to dermatologists because it may present with severe generalized pruritus (p. 320). Patients with unexplained pruritus must be examined for lymphadenopathy and hepatosplenomegaly. Only rarely does Hodgkin's disease affect the skin directly, as small nodules and ulcers.

Leukaemia

Rarely, the first sign of leukaemia is a leukaemic infiltrate in the skin. Clinically, this shows as plum-coloured plaques or nodules or, less often, a thickening and rugosity of the scalp (cutis verticis gyratum). More often, the rashes associated with leukaemia are non-specific red papules (leukaemids). Other non-specific manifestations include pruritus, herpes zoster, acquired ichthyosis and purpura.

B-cell lymphomas

B-lymphocytic lymphomas presenting with skin lesions are rare. They appear as scattered plum-coloured nodules

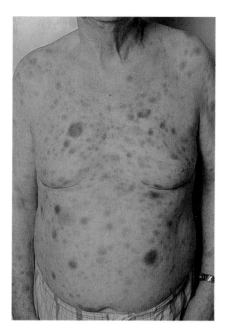

Figure 20.60 Immunopathology showed that these nodules were caused by a B-cell lymphoma. (Dr E.C. Benton. Reproduced with permission of Dr E.C. Benton.)

(Figure 20.60). Histologically, a B-cell lymphoma infiltrates the lower dermis in a nodular or diffuse manner. Immunophenotyping shows a monoclonal expansion of B lymphocytes, all with either lambda or kappa light chains. Treatment is with radiotherapy and systemic chemotherapy.

Other malignant tumours

Dermatofibrosarcoma protuberans

Dermatofibrosarcoma protuberans is a slowly growing malignant tumour of fibroblasts, arising usually on the upper trunk. At first it seems like a dermatofibroma or keloid but, as it slowly expands, it turns into a plaque of red or bluish nodules with an irregular protuberant surface. It seldom metastasizes. It should be removed with extra wide margins, preferably with Mohs micrographic surgery, and even then will sometimes recur.

Merkel cell carcinoma

Merkel cell carcinoma is a rare but aggressive cutaneous tumour from neuroendocrine derived cells. The 2-year survival rate is 50–70%. It presents as a solitary dome-shaped nodule or plaque, most commonly on the head and neck of the elderly and immunosuppressed. It fre-

quently metastasizes to the lymph nodes. In 2008, a new polyomavirus (Merkel cell polyomavirus, MCV) was identified in 80% of Merkel cell carcinomas, suggesting that MCV infection may contribute to the development of this carcinoma. The mainstay of treatment is wide local excision or Mohs' micrographic surgery (p. 371) along with sentinel lymph node biopsy.

Cutaneous metastases

About 3% of patients with internal cancers have cutaneous metastases. They usually arise late and indicate a grave prognosis, but occasionally a solitary cutaneous metastasis is the first sign of the occurrence of a tumour.

The most common cutaneous metastases come from breast cancer. The skin of the breast is also most often involved by the direct extension of a tumour. This may show up as a sharply demarcated and firm area of erythema (carcinoma erysipeloides), firm telangiectatic plaques and papules (carcinoma telangiectoides) or as skin like orange peel (*peau d'orange*) caused by blocked and dilated lymphatics. Carcinoma of the breast may also send metastases to the scalp causing patches of alopecia (Figure 20.61), or to other areas as firm and discrete dermal nodules.

Other common primaries metastasizing to the skin are tumours of the lung, gastrointestinal tract, uterus,

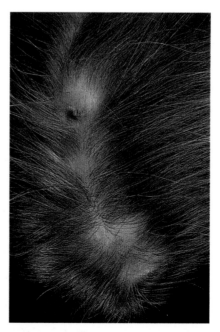

Figure 20.61 Several scalp metastases arising from a breast carcinoma.

prostate and kidney. The most frequent sites for secondary deposits are the umbilicus and the scalp.

Further reading

Cox NH, Eedy DJ, Morton CA. (2007) Guidelines for the management of Bowen's disease. *British Journal of Dermatology* **151**, 11–21.

Kim EJ, Hess S, Richardson SK, *et al.* (2005) Immunopathogenesis and therapy of cutaneous T cell lymphoma. *Journal of Clinical Investigation* **115**, 798–812.

Marsden JR, Newton-Bishop JA. Burrows L, *et al.* (2010) Revised UK guidelines for the management of cutaneous melanoma. *British Journal of Dermatology* **163**, 238–256. Also at www.bad.org.uk (accessed 28 June 2014)

Motley R, Kersey P, Lawrence C. (2002) Multiprofessional guidelines for the management of the patient with primary cutaneous squamous cell carcinoma. *British Journal of Dermatology* **146**, 18–25. Update at http://www.bad.org.uk/library-media%5Cdocuments%5CSCC_2009.pdf (accessed 11 July 2014).

Rigel DS, Friedman R, Dzubow MD, *et al.* (2005) *Cancer of the Skin.* Elsevier-Saunders, Philadelphia.

Telfer NR, Colver GB, Morton CA. (2008) Guidelines for the management of basal cell carcinoma. *British Journal of Dermatology* **159**, 35–48.

Thompson JF, Scolyer RA, Kefford RF. (2005) Cutaneous melanoma. *Lancet* **365**, 687–701.

Ward KA, Lazovich D, Hordinsk MK. (2012) Germline melanoma susceptibility and prognostic genes: a review of the literature. *Journal of the American Academy of Dermatology* **67**, 1055–1067.

Willemze R, Jaffe ES, Burg G, *et al.* (2005) WHO-EORTC classification for cutaneous lymphomas. *Blood* **105**, 3768–3785.

21 The Skin in Systemic Disease

Only selected aspects of this huge subject can be covered here. In the first part of this chapter, the skin changes seen in particular diseases (e.g. sarcoidosis) or groups of diseases (e.g. internal malignancies) are described. The second part covers some individual skin conditions that can be associated with a wide range of internal disorders (e.g. pyoderma gangrenosum).

The skin and internal malignancy

Obvious skin signs can be seen if a tumour invades the skin, or sends metastases to it; but there are other more subtle ways in which tumours can affect the skin. Sometimes they act physiologically, causing, for example, the acne seen with some adrenal tumours, flushing in the carcinoid syndrome, and jaundice with a bile duct carcinoma. These cast-iron associations need no further discussion here. However, the presence of some rare but important conditions should alert the clinician to the possibility of an underlying neoplasm. It should be noted that the onset of these conditions might predate diagnosis of the malignancy. In some instances their natural course closely parallels that of the associated tumour and may provide the first indication of tumour relapse.

1 *Acanthosis nigricans* is a velvety thickening and pigmentation of the major flexures. Setting aside those cases caused by obesity (Figure 21.1), the metabolic syndrome (including type 2 diabetes with insulin resistance), or by drugs such as nicotinic acid used to treat hyperlipidaemia, the chances are high that a malignant tumour is present, usually an adenocarcinoma within the abdominal cavity. Acanthosis nigricans has been reported in association with the sign of Leser–Trélat, a sudden onset of multiple seborrhoeic keratoses or sudden increase in their size and number. This sign is somewhat controversial given that multiple seborrhoeic keratoses are often found in the healthy elderly population.

2 *Erythema gyratum repens* is a shifting pattern of waves of erythema covering the skin surface and looking like the grain on wood. It may precede the onset of bronchial or oesophageal neoplasms.

3 *Acquired hypertrichosis lanuginosa* ('malignant down') is an excessive and widespread growth of fine lanugo hair. It is more common in women, when it is usually associated with colorectal, lung and breast malignancies.

4 *Necrolytic migratory erythema* is a figurate erythema with a moving crusted edge. When present, usually with anaemia, stomatitis, weight loss and diabetes, it signals the presence of a glucagon-secreting tumour of the pancreas.

5 *Bazex syndrome* is a psoriasiform papulosquamous eruption of the fingers and toes, ears and nose, seen with some tumours of the upper respiratory tract.

6 *Dermatomyositis*, other than in childhood (p. 131). About 20% of adult patients have an underlying malignancy. However, this may be a gross under-estimation, with some series quoting figures nearer 50%. The antibody anti-P155 may be helpful in discriminating between idiopathic and malignancy-associated cases. Onset in adulthood should always prompt a thorough search for an underlying malignancy. Pay special attention to the ovaries where tumours may lurk undetected.

7 *Generalized pruritus*. One of its many causes is an internal malignancy, usually a lymphoma (p. 320).

8 *Superficial thrombophlebitis*. The migratory type has traditionally been associated with carcinomas of the pancreas.

9 *Acquired ichthyosis*. This may result from a number of underlying diseases (p. 48. Malignancy should always be excluded, in particular Hodgkin's lymphoma (70–80% of cases) and other haematological neoplasms.

10 *Genetic conditions*. An example is the Muir–Torre syndrome in which sebaceous adenomas are accompanied by surprisingly unaggressive visceral malignancies.

11 *Acute febrile neutrophilic dermatosis* (Sweet's syndrome; Figure 21.2). The classic triad found in association

Clinical Dermatology, Fifth Edition. Richard B. Weller, Hamish J.A. Hunter and Margaret W. Mann.
© 2015 John Wiley & Sons, Ltd. Published 2015 by John Wiley & Sons, Ltd.

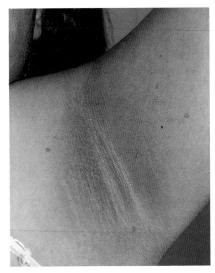

Figure 21.1 Acanthosis nigricans – in this case caused by obesity.

with the red oedematous plaques consists of fever, a raised erythrocyte sedimentation rate (ESR) and a raised blood neutrophil count. Aproximately 20% of cases are associated with an underlying malignancy. The most important internal association is with myeloproliferative disorders.

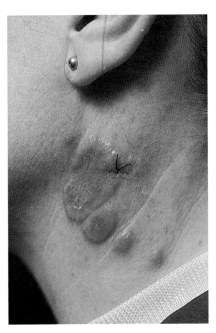

Figure 21.2 Acute febrile neutrophilic dermatosis (Sweet's syndrome).

12 *Paraneoplastic pemphigus* (see Chapter 9). This is similar to pemphigus vulgaris but with extensive and persistent mucosal ulceration. The blisters on the palms and soles can look like erythema multiforme. It is associated with lymphoproliferative malignancies as well as underlying carcinomas.

13 *Others.* Pachydermoperiostosis is a coarsening and thickening of the skin seen in association with severe clubbing. It can be inherited as an autosomal dominant trait or be a result of the standard causes of clubbing, which include conditions such as bronchial carcinoma.

The skin and diabetes mellitus

The following are more common in those with diabetes than in others.

1 *Necrobiosis lipoidica.* Less than 3% of diabetics have necrobiosis, but 11–62% of patients with necrobiosis will have diabetes. Apparently non-diabetic necrobiosis patients should be screened for diabetes as some will have impaired glucose tolerance or diabetes, and some will become diabetic later. The association is with both type 1 (previously termed 'insulin-dependent') and type 2 (previously termed 'non-insulin-dependent') diabetes. The lesions appear as one or more discoloured areas on the fronts of the shins (Figure 21.3). Early plaques are violaceous, but atrophy as the inflammation goes on and are then shiny, atrophic and brown–red or slightly yellow. The underlying blood vessels are easily seen through the atrophic skin and the margin may be erythematous or violet. Minor knocks can lead to slow-healing ulcers; biopsy can do the same.

No treatment is reliably helpful. The atrophy is permanent; the best one can expect from medical treatments is halting of disease progression. The disease is caused by inflammation, yet treatment with topical steroids may add to the atrophy. There is little evidence that good control of the diabetes will help the necrobiosis. A padded dressing should help those whose legs are subjected to trauma. A strong topical corticosteroid applied to the edge of an enlarging lesion may halt its expansion. Varied responses to immunosuppression and photochemotherapy have been reported.

2 *Granuloma annulare.* The cause of granuloma annulare is not known; it now seems that there is no association between the common type and diabetes. An association applies to a few adults with extensive superficial granuloma annulare, characterized by dull red or purple macules. Clinically, the lesions of the common type

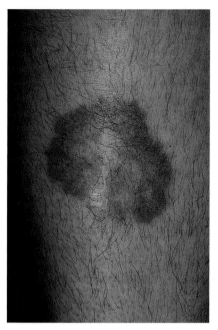

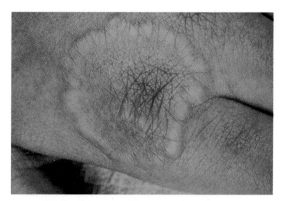

Figure 21.4 Granuloma annulare.

Figure 21.3 Necrobiosis lipoidica: shiny yellowish patch with marked telangiectasia.

of granuloma annulare often lie over the knuckles and are composed of dermal nodules fused into a rough ring shape (Figure 21.4). On the hands the lesions are skin-coloured or slightly pink; elsewhere a purple colour may be seen. Although a biopsy is seldom necessary, the histology shows a diagnostic palisading granuloma, like that of necrobiosis lipoidica. Lesions tend to go away over the course of a year or two. Stubborn ones respond to intralesional triamcinolone injections. Cosmetically disfiguring cases may warrant treatment with psoralen and ultraviolet A (PUVA) treatment.

3 *Diabetic dermopathy.* In about 50% of type I diabetic patients, multiple small (0.5–1 cm in diameter) slightly sunken brownish scars can be found on the limbs, most obviously over the shins. It is thought to be caused by vascular disease and may act as a surrogate marker of systemic complications secondary to diabetes.

4 *Candidal infections* (p. 243).

5 *Staphylococcal infections* (p. 214).

6 *Vitiligo* (p. 271).

7 *Eruptive xanthomas* (p. 318).

8 *Stiff thick skin* (diabetic sclerodactyly or cheiroarthropathy) on the fingers and hands, demonstrated by the 'prayer sign' in which the fingers and palms cannot be opposed properly (Figure 21.5).

9 *Atherosclerosis* with ischaemia or gangrene of feet.
10 *Neuropathic foot ulcers.*

The skin in sarcoidosis

The aetiology of sarcoidosis has yet to be fully elucidated. Current evidence suggests that in genetically susceptible individuals, an infectious or environmental antigen (as yet unknown) stimulates a predominantly Th1 immune-mediated response, resulting in the clinical manifestations discussed below. About one-third of patients with systemic sarcoidosis have skin lesions; it is also possible to have cutaneous sarcoidosis without systemic abnormalities (also known as sarcoid). The most important skin changes are as follows.

1 *Erythema nodosum* (p. 107; and Figure 8.10). This occurs in the early stages of sarcoidosis, especially in young women, and is almost always associated with hilar adenopathy. It is usually associated with transient disease and requires only symptomatic relief.

2 Sarcoidal granulomas in the skin. Histology reveals a 'naked' tubercle comprising foci of macrophages and giant cells without many surrounding lymphocytes. These are seen clinically as:

• *Scar sarcoidosis*: granulomatous lesions arising in long-standing scars should raise suspicions of sarcoidosis.

• *Lupus pernio*: dusky infiltrated plaques appear on the nose and fingers, often in association with sarcoidosis of the upper respiratory tract.

• *Papular, nodular and plaque forms* (Figure 21.6): these brownish-red, violaceous or hypopigmented papules and plaques are indolent although often

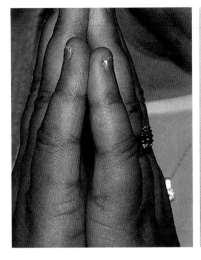 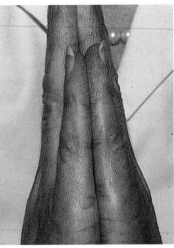

Figure 21.5 Diabetic cheiropathy – the prayer sign. Poor finger apposition in the diabetic hand (on the left) compared with the normal one (on the right).

symptom-free. Sometimes they are annular or psoriasis-like. Lesions vary in number, size and distribution.

Diascopy (see Chapter 3) may be helpful in the diagnosis of cutaneous sarcoid. Pressure with a glass slide over the lesion may reveal the characteristic 'apple jelly nodules' associated with granulomatous disease. Sarcoid is a great imitator of many conditions.

Investigations

Although sarcoid may present solely in the skin it is important to assess the patient for systemic involvement as this may prompt the need for more aggressive therapy. With this in mind, a comprehensive history and examination should be performed. Investigations should include: chest radiograph; routine haematological, biochemical and bone profiles; serum angiotensin-converting enzyme

(ACE) levels; urinalysis; electrocardiogram (ECG); pulmonary function tests (PFTs) and ophthalmological (slit lamp) examination. The results from these will govern the need for further investigation and referral to other specialties.

Treatment

Not all cutaneous sarcoid requires treatment but for extensive disease or disease involving cosmetically sensitive areas intralesional and topical corticosteroids are sometimes helpful. If ineffective then, hydroxychloroquine, cholorquine, minocycline and methotrexate (Formulary 2, p. 426) have been used successfully. Chronic lesions respond poorly to any line of treatment short of systemic steroids, which are usually best avoided if involvement is confined to the skin. For severe disease resistant to systemic corticosteroid therapy, or when it is contraindicated, the anti-TNFα biological agents have shown significant promise.

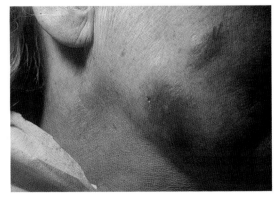

Figure 21.6 Sarcoidosis: plum-coloured plaques on the cheek.

The skin in liver disease

The following are some of the associated abnormalities.

1 *Pruritus.* This is related to obstructive jaundice and may precede it (p. 320).

2 *Pigmentation.* With bile pigments and sometimes melanin (see Chapter 19).

3 *Spider naevi* (Figure 21.7). These are often multiple in chronic liver disease (p. 141).

4 *Palmar erythema* (p. 141).

5 *White nails.* These associate with hypoalbuminaemia.

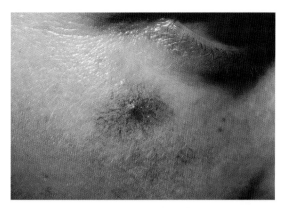

Figure 21.7 Solitary spider naevus showing the central feeding vessel. No underlying liver disease in this case.

6 *Lichen planus* (p. 69) and cryoglobulinaemia (p. 154) with hepatitis C infection.
7 *Polyarteritis nodosa* (p. 110) with hepatitis B infection.
8 *Porphyria cutanea tarda* (p. 316).
9 *Xanthomas.* With primary biliary cirrhosis (p. 318).
10 *Hair loss and generalized asteatotic eczema* may occur in alcoholics with cirrhosis who have become zinc deficient.

The skin in renal disease

The main changes are associated with chronic renal failure are as follow.
1 *Pruritus* and generally dry skin.
2 *Pigmentation.* A yellowish sallow colour and pallor from anaemia.
3 *Half-and-half nail.* The proximal half is white and the distal half is pink or brownish.
4 *Perforating disorders.* Small papules in which collagen or elastic fibres are being extruded through the epidermis.
5 *Pseudoporphyria* (p. 318).
    Some skin changes may be due to the conditions leading to renal disease. For example, leucocytoclastic vasculitis (p. 108), connective tissue disorders (see Chapter 10) and Fabry's disease (p. 320).

Graft versus host disease

Allogeneic haematopoietic stem cell transplantation is now a well-established treatment for several disorders including aplastic anaemia and leukaemia. Recently, bone marrow as a source for stem cells has been replaced by peripheral blood stem cells. Umbilical cord blood grafts are increasingly used. Immunologically competent donor lymphocytes, however, may still cause problems by reacting against host tissues, especially the skin, liver and gut (sites of rapid cell turnover). In an attempt to reduce graft versus host disease (GVHD) the donor graft may have the immunocompetent T cells depleted. However, this increases the chance of graft failure, viral infections, impaired T-cell recovery in the recipient and, most importantly, relapse of the primary condition. GVHD complicates approximately 50% of all allogeneic transplants.

Acute GVHD typically appears within 4 weeks. Fever accompanies malaise and a worsening morbilliform rash, which often starts on the palms and soles and behind the ears. It may progress to a generalized desquamation or even toxic epidermal necrolysis. Histology in the early stage may help to confirm the diagnosis. Typical features include degeneration of basal keratinocytes and/or single cell necrosis of keratinocytes with a surrounding cluster of lymphocytes (*satellite cell necrosis*). Reduced-intensity (non-myeloablative) conditioning regimes prior to graft transplantation reduce the severity of acute GVHD but again increase the risk of relapse of the primary condition. Standard therapy for acute GVHD includes high dose systemic corticosteroids or, if less severe, potent topical corticosteroids or topical tacrolimus.

Chronic GVHD was previously diagnosed if it occurred more than 100 days after transplantation. However, this somewhat arbitrary time has now been revised; the time limit has been dropped and diagnosis is based on clinical features suggestive of chronic GVHD. Skin changes are variable but may be like those of lichen planus (p. 69) or a pigmented scleroderma (p. 132). Contractures and painful skin ulcers may complicate severe cases. The skin changes may be severe enough to need treatment with systemic prednisolone and azathioprine, phototherapy (UVA1, PUVA and possibly narrowband UVB) or ciclosporin (Formulary 2, p. 418). Extracorporeal photophoresis, as used in the treatment of cutaneous T-cell lymphoma (p. 307) is proving efficacious, especially for the cutaneous manifestations of chronic GVHD.

Malabsorption and malnutrition

Some of the most common skin changes are listed in Table 21.1. These conditions should also be borne in mind when confronted with unusual eruptions in alcoholics (relative malnutrition).

Table 21.1 Skin changes in malabsorption and malnutrition.

Condition	Skin changes
Malnutrition	Itching
	Dryness
	Symmetrical pigmentation
	Brittle nails and hair
Protein malnutrition (kwashiorkor)	Dry red-brown hair
	Pigmented 'cracked skin'
Iron deficiency	Pallor
	Itching
	Diffuse hair loss
	Koilonychia
	Smooth tongue
Zinc deficiency	Acrodermatitis enteropathica (dermatiis of hands, feet, peri oral/anal areas)
Vitamin A (retinol) deficiency	Dry skin
	Follicular hyperkeratoses
	Xerophthalmia
Vitamin B_1 (thiamine) deficiency	Beri-beri oedema
Vitamin B_2 (riboflavin) deficiency	Angular stomatitis
	Smooth purple tongue
	Seborrhoeic dermatitis-like eruption
Vitamin B3 (niacin) deficiency	Pellagra with dermatitis, dementia and diarrhoea
	Dermatitis on exposed areas, pigmented
Vitamin B_6 (pyridoxine) deficiency	Ill-defined dermatitis
Vitamin B_7 (biotin) deficiency	Periorofacial macular rash, seborrhoeic dermatitis
	Brittle hair and alopecia
Vitamin C deficiency (scurvy)	Skin haemorrhages especially around follicular keratoses containing coiled hairs
	Bleeding gums
	Oedematous 'woody' swellings of limbs in the elderly

The porphyrias

There are at least eight enzymes in the metabolic pathway that leads to the synthesis of haem. There are also eight different types of porphyria, each being caused by an alteration in the activity of one of these enzymes, and each having its own characteristic pattern of accumulation of porphyrin and porphyrin precursors. Formed porphyrins, but not porphyrin precursors, cause the photosensitivity (to ultraviolet radiation of wavelength 400 nm, which is capable of penetrating through window glass) that is the cardinal feature of the cutaneous porphyrias. Protective clothing and zinc or titanium based 'opaque' sunscreens are required to block skin penetration of this wavelength.

The different types can be separated on clinical grounds, aided by the biochemical investigation of urine, faeces and blood including characteristic emission peaks measured by plasma fluorescence spectroscopy. The genes responsible for all porhyrias have now been characterized. DNA analysis for known mutations in these genes is useful both diagnostically and for the screening of relatives with latent disease. Guidance for genetic testing and enzyme assays can be sought from porphyria reference centres. Historically, porphyrias have been classified by the organs involved; a more useful classification for the clinician is based upon whether the porphyria is confined solely to the skin, is associated with acute attacks and cutaneous signs or only presents with acute attacks. Only six varieties are mentioned here.

Cutaneous porphyrias

Porphyria cutanea tarda (cutaneous hepatic porphyria)

There are two types: a sporadic type (accounting for 75% of cases) and a type inherited as an autosomal dominant trait resulting from mutations in the *UROD* gene (25%). Both are characterized by low hepatic uroporphyrinogen decarboxylase activity. The sporadic type develops when a polygenic predisposition to porphyria cutanea tarda (PCT) is compounded by environmental factors. It is usually seen in men, but rarely in women, who have damaged their livers by drinking too much alcohol but may also occur in women taking oestrogens. It has also been shown that a few cases are caused by iron overload or previous hepatitis C virus or HIV infection. Haemochromatosis gene status should be checked as mutations in the *HFE* genes are over-represented in PCT. Blisters, erosions and milia form on the exposed parts of the face, and on the backs of the hands (Figures 21.8 and 21.9), in response to sunlight or to minor trauma. These areas become scarred and hairy. The urine is pink and fluoresces a bright coral-pink under Wood's light (p. 37) as a result of excessive uroporphyrins (Figure 21.10). Diagnosis is based on a peak plasma fluorescence spectrum of 618–620 nm

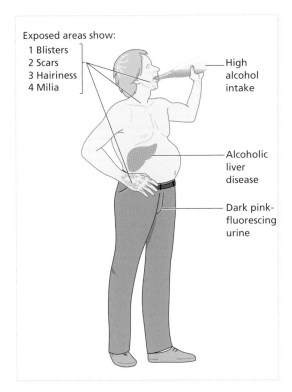

Exposed areas show:
1 Blisters
2 Scars
3 Hairiness
4 Milia

High
alcohol
intake

Alcoholic
liver
disease

Dark pink-
fluorescing
urine

Figure 21.8 Porphyria cutanea tarda.

(differentiating it from variegate porphyria) and over-excretion of urinary and faecal porhyrins; these may normalize after long remissions. Treatment includes avoiding alcohol and oestrogens, but other measures are usually needed too, including iron depletion by regular venesection or very low dose hydroxychloroquine therapy (e.g. 100 mg twice weekly) under specialist supervision. Higher doses cause toxic hepatitis in these patients.

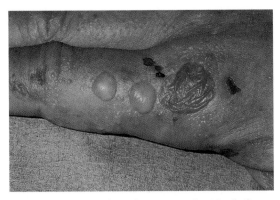

Figure 21.9 Blisters, milia and erosions on the side of a finger.

Congenital erythropoietic porphyria (Günther disease)

This is very rare, caused by mutations in the uropor-phyrinogen III cosynthase gene (*UROS*), and inherited as an autosomal recessive trait. Severe photosensitivity is noted soon after birth, and leads to blistering, scar-ring and mutilation of the exposed parts, which become increasingly hairy. The urine is pink and the teeth are brown, although fluorescing red under Wood's light. A haemolytic anaemia is present. Treatment is unsatisfac-tory but must include protection from, and avoidance of, sunlight. Allogeneic bone-marrow transplantation has been successful in some individuals. The hairy appear-ance, discoloured teeth and the tendency to avoid daylight may have given rise to legends about werewolves.

Erythropoietic protoporphyria (erythrohepatic protoporphyria)

In this more common condition, caused by mutations in the ferrochelatase gene (*FECH*), a less severe but painful photosensitivity develops during infancy. The genetics are complex usually requiring the inheritance of two muta-tions in the *FECH* genes. A burning sensation occurs within minutes of exposure to sunlight. Soon the skin becomes swollen and crusted vesicles may appear, lead-ing to pitted scars. Liver disease and gallstones occur. Protoporphyrin is lypophilic and therefore not excreted in the urine. Diagnosis is based upon raised levels of free protoporphyrin in erythrocytes and a characteristic peak on plasma fluorescence spectroscopy (634 nm). In addition to sun avoidance and the use of sunscreens (For-mulary 1, p. 400), skin-yellowing doses of beta-carotene

Figure 21.10 Porphyria cutanea tarda. Coral-red fluorescence of urine under Wood's light denoting excessive uroporphyrins (chloroform extraction).

may be given orally. A recently recognized X-linked dominant porphyria has a similar clinical presentation to erythropoietic protoporphyria. It results from gain-of-function mutations in the *ALAS2* gene.

Acute and cutaneous porphyria

Variegate porphyria
This disorder, inherited as an autosomal dominant trait, and the result of mutations of the protoporphyrinogen oxidase gene, is particularly common in South Africa. It shares the skin features of PCT and the systemic symptoms and drug provocation of acute intermittent porphyria. A peak at 624–628 nm on plasma fluorescence spectroscopy is diagnostic of variegate porphyria.

Acute porphria

Acute intermittent porphyria
This condition, inherited as an autosomal dominant trait as the result of mutations of the porphobilinogen deaminase gene, is most common in Scandinavia. Skin lesions do not occur. Attacks of abdominal pain, accompanied by neuropsychiatric symptoms and the passage of dark urine, are sometimes triggered by drugs especially barbiturates, griseofulvin, oestrogens and sulfonamides.

'Pseudoporphyria'
This term is used when skin and histological changes like those of cutaneous hepatic porphyria occur without an underlying abnormality of porphyrin metabolism. It has been linked with chronic renal failure and haemodialysis, ultraviolet radiation and sun beds and can be induced by many drugs, notably furosemide, non-steroidal anti-inflammatory drugs, beta-lactam antibiotics and azole antifungals. In the differential diagnosis, be sure to rule out epidermolysis bullosa acquisita (p. 119).

Metabolic disorders

Amyloidosis
Amyloid is a protein that can be derived from several sources, including immunoglobulin light chains and keratins. It is deposited in the tissues in combination with a P component derived from the plasma. Skin changes are prominent in primary systemic amyloidosis, and also in the amyloid associated with multiple myeloma. In contrast, systemic amyloidosis of the type that is secondary to chronic inflammatory disease, such as rheumatoid arthritis or tuberculosis, tends not to affect the skin. Skin

blood vessels infiltrated with amyloid rupture easily, causing 'pinch purpura' to occur after minor trauma. The waxy deposits of amyloid, often most obvious around the eyes, may also be purpuric. More diffuse deposits suggest scleroderma. Distinct from the systemic amyloidoses are localized deposits of amyloid. These are uncommon and usually take the form of macular areas of rippled pigmentation, or of plaques made up of coalescing papules. Both types are itchy.

Mucinoses
The dermis becomes infiltrated with mucin in certain disorders. Skin biopsy specimens readily show the mucin, especially when stained with Giemsa stain.
1 *Myxoedema*. In the puffy hands and face of patients with hypothyroidism.
2 *Pretibial myxoedema*. Pink or flesh-coloured mucinous plaques are seen on the lower shins, together with marked exophthalmos, in some patients with hyperthyroidism. They may also occur after the thyroid abnormality has been treated.
3 *Scleromyxoedema*. A diffuse thickening and papulation of the skin may occur in connection with an immunoglobulin G (IgG) monoclonal paraproteinaemia. In lichen myxoedematosis deposits are more discrete and nodular.
4 *Follicular mucinosis*. In this condition, the infiltrated plaques show a loss of hair. Some cases are associated with a lymphoma.

Xanthomas
Deposits of fatty material in the skin and subcutaneous tissues (xanthomas) may provide the first clue to important disorders of lipid metabolism

Primary hyperlipidaemias are usually genetic. They fall into six groups, classified on the basis of an analysis of fasting blood lipids and electrophoresis of plasma lipoproteins. All, save type I, carry an increased risk of atherosclerosis – in this lies their importance and the need for treatment.

Secondary hyperlipidaemia may be found in a variety of diseases including diabetes, primary biliary cirrhosis, the nephrotic syndrome and hypothyroidism.

The clinical patterns of xanthoma correlate well with the underlying cause. The main patterns and their most common associations are shown in Table 21.2 (Figures 21.11–21.13). Lipid-regulating drugs (e.g. statins and fibrates) not only stop xanthomas from appearing, but also aid their resolution. More importantly, they help

Table 21.2 Xanthomas: clinical appearance and associations.

	Clinical appearance	Types of hyperlipidaemia (Frederickson classification) and Type associated metabolic abnormalities
Xanthelasma palpebrarum (Figure 21.11)	Soft yellowish plaques on the eyelids	None or type II, III or IV
Tuberous xanthomas (Figure 21.12)	Firm yellow papules and nodules, most often on points of knees and elbows	Types II, III and secondary
Tendinous xanthomas	Subcutaneous swellings on fingers or by Achilles tendon	Types II, III and secondary
Eruptive xanthomas	Sudden onset, multiple small yellow papules. Buttocks and shoulders	Types I, IV, V and secondary (usually to diabetes)
Plane xanthomas (Figure 21.13)	Yellow macular areas at any site. Yellow palmar creases	Type III and secondary
Generalized plane xanthomas	Yellow macules lesions over wide areas	Myeloma

reduce the risk of vascular occlusions such as coronary artery disease.

> **Learning point**
>
> Check the blood lipids in all types of xanthoma, including xanthelasma of the eyelids. Abnormalities are remediable with statins and fibrates.

Phenylketonuria

Phenylketonuria is a rare metabolic cause of hypopigmentation. Its prevalence is about 1 in 25 000. It is inherited as an autosomal recessive trait caused by a deficiency of the liver enzyme phenylalanine hydroxylase, which catalyses the hydroxylation of phenylalanine to tyrosine. This leads to the accumulation of phenylalanine, phenylpyruvic acid and their metabolites.

Affected individuals have fair skin and hair. They often develop eczema, usually suggestive of the atopic type, and they may be photosensitive. The accumulation of phenylalanine and its metabolites damages the brain during its phase of rapid development just before and just after birth.

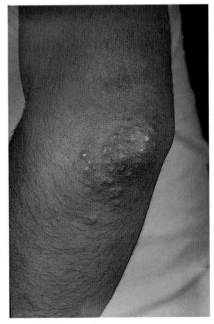

Figure 21.12 Tuberous xanthoma on the points of the elbows – a mixture of nodules and papules.

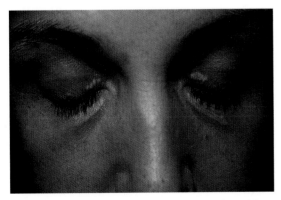

Figure 21.11 Xanthelasma: flat yellow lesions on the eyelids, often with normal blood lipids.

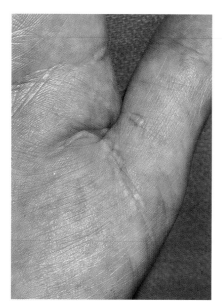

Figure 21.13 Plane xanthoma with yellow palmar creases.

Mental retardation, epilepsy and extrapyramidal manifestations such as athetosis may then occur.

Oculocutaneous albinism (p. 270) can usually be distinguished by its eye signs. The Guthrie test, which detects raised blood phenylalanine levels, is carried out routinely at birth in most developed countries.

A low phenylalanine diet should be started as soon as possible to prevent further neurological damage.

Alkaptonuria

In this rare recessively inherited disorder, based on a homogentisic acid oxidase deficiency, dark urine may be seen in childhood, and in adult life pigment, ranging from grey–blue to brown–black, may be deposited in various places including the ears and sclera (ochronosis). Arthropathy may occur.

Fabry's disease (angiokeratoma corporis diffusum)

A deficiency of the enzyme α-galactosidase A is found in this rare X-linked disorder (chromosome region Xq21.3-22); abnormal amounts of glycolipid are deposited in many tissues as a result. The skin lesions are grouped, almost black, small telangiectatic papules (angiokeratomas) often manifest around the umbilicus and pelvis. Progressive renal failure, cardiovascular disease and stroke occur in adult life. Most patients have gastrointesti-

nal symptoms and attacks of excruciating unexplained pain in their hands. Some female carriers have skin changes, although these are usually less obvious than those of affected males. Recently, treatment with intravenous enzyme replacement has proved beneficial. Similar skin lesions may be seen in lysosomal storage disorders such as fucosidosis.

Generalized pruritus

Pruritus is a symptom with many causes, but not a disease in its own right. Itchy patients fall into two groups: those whose pruritus is caused simply by surface causes (e.g. eczema, lichen planus and scabies), which seldom need much investigation; and the others, who may or may not have an internal cause for their itching. These patients require a detailed physical examination, including a careful search for lymphadenopathy, and investigations including a full blood count, iron status, urea and electrolytes, liver function tests, thyroid function tests and a chest X-ray. The underlying cause for the pruritus may turn out to be one of the following.

1 *Liver disease.* Itching signals biliary obstruction. It is an early symptom of primary biliary cirrhosis. Colestyramine may help cholestatic pruritus, possibly by promoting the elimination of bile salts. Other treatments include naltrexone, rifampicin and ultraviolet B.

2 *Chronic renal failure.* Urea itself seems not to be responsible for this symptom, which plagues about one-third of patients undergoing renal dialysis. UVB phototherapy, naltrexone or administration of oral activated charcoal may help.

3 *Iron deficiency.* Treatment with iron may help the itching.

4 *Polycythaemia.* The itching here is usually triggered by a hot bath; it has a curious pricking quality and lasts about an hour.

5 *Thyroid disease.* Itching and urticaria may occur in hyperthyroidism. The dry skin of hypothyroidism may also be itchy.

6 *Diabetes.* Generalized itching may be a rare presentation of diabetes.

7 *Internal malignancy.* The prevalence of itching in Hodgkin's disease may be as high as 30%. It may be unbearable, yet the skin often looks normal. Pruritus may occur long before other manifestations of the disease. Itching is uncommon in carcinomatosis.

8 *Neurological disease.* Paroxysmal pruritus has been recorded in multiple sclerosis and in neurofibromatosis.

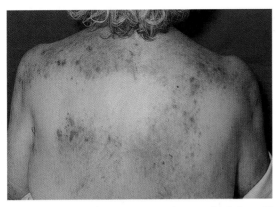

Figure 21.14 An example of the butterfly sign. This lady could not reach her upper back but could scratch her skin everywhere else. In other patients, the spared area is shaped more like a butterfly.

Brain tumours infiltrating the floor of the fourth ventricle may cause a fierce persistent itching of the nostrils.

9 The diffuse sclerotic form of *scleroderma* may start as itching associated with increasing pigmentation and early signs of sclerosis. Itching is usually severe throughout the course of this debilitating disease.

10 The skin of the *elderly* may itch because it is too dry, or because it is being irritated.

11 *Pregnancy* (see Chapter 15).

12 *Drugs.* The history is the most useful indicator here. If the patient takes multiple medications the judicious withdrawal of one at a time may be required to determine the culprit.

The search for a cause has to be tailored to the individual patient, and must start with a thorough history and physical examination. The presence of a 'butterfly sign' (Figure 21.14) sometimes suggests an internal cause for the itching. Unless a treatable cause is found, therapy is symptomatic and consists of sedative antihistamines (Formulary 2, p. 415), skin moisturizers, and the avoidance of rough clothing, over-heating and vasodilatation, including that brought on by alcohol. UVB often helps all kinds of itching, including the itching associated with chronic renal, and liver disease. Local applications include calamine, mixtures containing small amounts of menthol or phenol and topical doxepin (Formulary 1, p. 400).

Learning points

1 Learn how to spell pruritus (not pruritis) but do not accept it as a diagnosis in its own right.

---

2 Ponder underlying causes in those with no primary skin disease.

3 Always consider malignancy if pruritus is unexplained or accompanied by other systemic features such as weight loss, night sweats or lymphadenopathy.

Pyoderma gangrenosum

An inflamed nodule or pustule breaks down centrally to form an expanding painful ulcer with a polycyclic or serpiginous outline, and a characteristic undermined bluish edge (Figure 21.15). The condition is not bacterial in origin but its pathogenesis, presumably immunological, is not fully understood. It may arise in the absence of any underlying disease (50%), or be associated with the following conditions.

1 *Inflammatory bowel disease* (ulcerative colitis and Crohn's disease; Figure 21.16). Of these, 2% of patients develop pyoderma, with peristomal pyoderma being a particular complication in those with abdominal stomas.

2 *Conditions causing polyarthritis*, including rheumatoid arthritis (Figure 21.17).

3 *Haematological malignancies* – particularly of myeloid origin (with a bullous form of pyoderma).

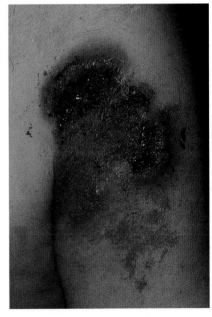

Figure 21.15 Pyoderma gangrenosum: a plum-coloured lesion with a typical cribriform appearance.

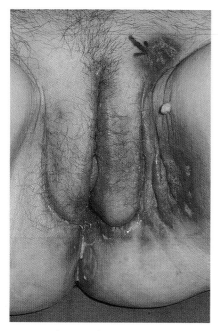

Figure 21.16 Another manifestation of Crohn's disease: grossly oedematous vulva with interconnecting sinuses. Biopsy at the site arrowed showed a granulomatous histology.

Lesions may be single or multiple, and pustular and bullous variants occur. Pyoderma severity does not appear to be related to the activity of inflammatory bowel disease or rheumatoid arthritis when these are the cause. It responds

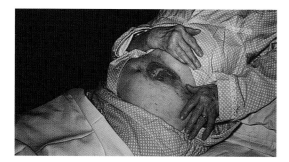

Figure 21.17 This long-standing ulcer was pyoderma gangrenosum secondary to the patient's rheumatoid arthritis. (Dr G.W. Beveridge. Reproduced with permission of Dr G.W. Beveridge.)

to systemic – and in mild cases highly potent topical – corticosteroids, sometimes with adjunctive minocycline. Lesions heal leaving papery scars. Alternative treatments include ciclosporin and the anti-TNF-α agent infliximab. Surgery or skin grafting should be avoided as healing is often poor and may induce pyoderma gangrenosum at the graft donor site. A reduction in pain is usually an early indicator of treatment response.

Further reading

Behm B, Schremi S, Landthaler M, Babilas P. (2012) Skin signs in diabetes mellitus. *Journal of the European Academy of Dermatology and venereology* **26**, 1203–1211.

Braverman IM. (1998) *Skin Signs of Systemic Disease*, 3rd edition. W.B. Saunders, Philadelphia, PA.

Chavan R, El-Azhary R. (2011) Cutaneous graft-versus-host disease: rationales and treatment options. *Dermatologic Therapy* **24**, 219–218.

Chung VQ, Moschella SI, Zembowicz A, Liu V. (2006) Clinical and pathological findings of paraneoplastic dermatoses. *Journal of the American Academy of Dermatology* **54**, 745–762.

Hadi A, Lebowhl M. (2011) Clinical features of pyoderma gangrenosum and current diagnostic trends. *Journal of the American Academy of Dermatology* **64**, 950–954.

Haimovic A, Sanchez M, Judson MA, Prystowsky S. (2012) Sarcoidosis: a comprehensive review and update for the dermatologist. Part I. Cutaneous disease. *Journal of the American Academy of Dermatology* **66**, **699**, e1–e18.

Haimovic A, Sanchez M, Judson MA, Prystowsky S. (2012) Sarcoidosis: a comprehensive review and update for the dermatologist. Part II. Extracutaneous disease. *Journal of the American Academy of Dermatology* **66**, **719**, e1–e10.

Lebwohl M. (2004) *The Skin and Systemic Disease: A Color Atlas and Text*, 2nd edition. Churchill Livingstone, Edinburgh.

Provost TT, Flynn JA. (2001) *Cutaneous Medicine: Cutaneous Manifestations of Systemic Disease*. B.C. Decker, Ontario.

Puy H, Gouya L, Deybach JC. (2010) Porphyrias. *Lancet* **375**, 924–937.

Sánchez NP. (2012) *Atlas of Dermatology in Internal Medicine*. Springer, New York.

Savin JA, Hunter JAA, Hepburn NC. (1997) *Skin Signs in Clinical Medicine: Diagnosis in Colour*. Mosby-Wolfe, London.

Zampetti A, Orteu CH, Antuzzi D, *et al.* (2011) Angiokeratoma: decision-making aid for the diagnosis of Fabry disease. *British Journal of Dermatology* **166**, 712–720.

22 Cosmetic Dermatology

As our population ages, its desire for cosmetic dermatology increases. For the aim of cosmetic dermatology is not to alleviate disease, but to try to make the skin look young again. Perhaps the desire to look young and beautiful seems frivolous, but success has measurable benefits. Studies consistently show that good-looking men and women earn more, are more successful at interviews and have a higher sense of self-worth. In contrast, well-constructed trials and impartial data on the results of cosmetic dermatological procedures are scanty.

In the United Kingdom, with its relatively few dermatologists, hardly any deal only with cosmetic skin problems, but in the United States the proportion is much higher. Dermatologists have been at the forefront of cosmetic procedures. They have made numerous contributions in this field, including the introduction of tumescent anaesthesia, laser physics, hair transplantation and the use of fillers and botulinum toxins. Thus, all dermatologists should know which cosmetic procedures can be performed, and their risks and benefits. This chapter gives an overview of the most common techniques in current use.

Ageing of the skin

Ageing of skin is a mixture of environmental influences and chronological ageing. Exposure to extrinsic factors such as ultraviolet radiation, smoking, poor nutrition and exposure to chemicals result in skin that is more deeply wrinkled, with reduced elasticity, and an epidermis showing solar lentigines, telangiectasia, enlarged pilosebaceous units and keratoses, and scattered pigmentation (see also p. 212). Photoaged skin has reduced levels of the fibrillar collagens, a major structural element in healthy dermis, and a disrupted elastic fibre network. The loss of collagen correlates with the depth and number of wrinkles, and is the result of a combination of reduced procollagen synthesis and increased breakdown by matrix metalloproteinase (MMP) enzymes. Ultraviolet radiation generates free radicals in the dermis and epidermis that alter protein structure directly, as well as initiating signal transduction cascades that activate MMPs. Histologically, the epidermis is thinned, with reduced proliferation and a flattened rete ridge pattern. The Glogau scoring system can be used as a clinical indicator of degree of photoageing (Table 22.1).

Chronological ageing, on the other hand, is largely due to genetics. Intrinsic factors including redistribution of subcutaneous fat, bone remodelling and repeated facial muscular activity contribute to the ageing appearance of the face. The loss of subcutaneous fat in the forehead, temples, malar cheeks and peri-oral area and descent of fat along the jowl and peri-orbital area result in a sagging, sunken appearance. Bone resorption in the inferior orbital rim and mandible further exaggerates the volume loss to the lower face. Finally, repeated muscular contracture around the peri-orbital area give rise to dynamic and static glabellar lines and crow's feet.

In medical dermatology, several different treatments may be needed over time to treat, for example, a psoriatic patient. Similarly in cosmetic dermatology no one technique can reverse all the changes of photoageing, and treatments must be tailored to the individual. The techniques used most commonly are the application of emollients and retinoid creams, facial peels, injection of botulinum toxin and dermal fillers, and laser and light sources. As a general rule, the choice of treatment depends on the depth of the pathological changes. Superficial changes, such as pigmentary ones and early keratoses (Glogau I and II), are best treated with agents acting on the epidermis, such as topical retinoids and shallow facial peels. In contrast, wrinkles caused by dermal changes and underlying volume loss need treatment that reaches the deeper layers of the skin – such as ablative laser therapy or the injection of fillers.

Clinical Dermatology, Fifth Edition. Richard B. Weller, Hamish J.A. Hunter and Margaret W. Mann.
© 2015 John Wiley & Sons, Ltd. Published 2015 by John Wiley & Sons, Ltd.

Table 22.1 Glogau photoageing grade.

Grade	Skin findings
I	No wrinkles
	Mild pigmentary changes
	No keratoses
II	Wrinkles in motion
	Early senile lentigines
	Palpable but invisible keratoses
III	Wrinkles at rest
	Dyschromia and telangiectases
	Visible keratoses
IV	Yellow–grey skin colour
	Prior skin malignancies
	Wrinkled throughout

Cosmeceuticals

The over-the-counter cosmetics industry is worth $160 billion per year worldwide, and in America more is spent on beauty products than on education. However, the definition of what is a cosmetic, as opposed to a medicine, is still confusing. The term 'cosmeceuticals' further confuses consumers, as these topically applied products claim to be a blend of cosmetics and pharmaceuticals, with claims to reduce wrinkles and improve skin tone and texture. In 1938, the American Food and Drug Administration (FDA) defined a cosmetic as anything that can be 'poured, sprinkled or sprayed on, introduced into, or otherwise applied to the human body … for cleansing, beautifying, promoting attractiveness, or altering the appearance without affecting the body's structure or functions'. This has led to confusion in which the cosmetic industry wants to claim rejuvenating properties for its products, but not such dramatic ones that they become classified as medicines, and so are available only with a medical prescription and subject to the review by the FDA. This discourages the open publication of research carried out by the industry, as the absence of effect of their products will not help sales, and the finding of true alterations in the structure of the skin carries the risk having the product classified as a medicine. European regulations are less conservative, and state 'almost every product usually perceived as a cosmetic … does, in some way or another, modify physiological function … the modification has to be more than significant' for the Medicinal Product Directive to apply.

Emollients (p. 397)

Even mildly aged skin looks better after the application of moisturizers. The scaliness of aged skin is due to corneocytes (p. 10) clumping together into lamellae, instead of being shed separately. Emollients help to 'unstick' the corneocytes, and contain two main types of ingredient: occlusives and humectants. Over-the-counter preparations are usually mixtures of these, prepared either as oil-in-water emulsions (creams and lotions) or water-in-oil emulsions (hand creams). Occlusives (such as soft white paraffin or lanolin) are poorly permeable to water, and so reduce trans-epidermal water loss when applied to the skin. Humectants absorb water, generally from the environment, but also from the epidermis. They draw water into the stratum corneum, and the resulting swelling of corneocytes gives an impression of wrinkle reduction, although this is only temporary. Over-the-counter moisturizers advertised as 'anti-wrinkle creams' usually rely on this mechanism. Urea, glycerine and hydroxy acids are all humectants.

Retinoids (p. 405)

Trial data confirm that topical tretinoin improves the appearance of mild to moderate photodamage. Fine and coarse wrinkles, pigmentary changes and keratoses improve as new collagen is formed in the dermis. Skin irritation is common, and both this and the improvement in appearance correlate with the concentration of tretinoin used.

Botulinum toxin

Clostridium botulinum was identified at the end of the nineteenth century as the organism responsible for the potentially fatal disease botulism, in which paralysis of the cranial and autonomic nerves follows the ingestion of its toxin. There are seven serotypes of botulinum toxin, of which A, B and E account for the majority of human disease. The toxins work at the neuromuscular junction, where they produce a chemical denervation by binding irreversibly at the presynaptic junction and blocking the release of acetylcholine. Despite the permanent binding of the toxin, paralysis wears off after several months as collateral axonal sprouts develop, able to release acetylcholine.

Botulinum toxin was first used clinically in the 1980s to correct squints and cervical dystonia, but moved rapidly into cosmetic use when it was found to be effective at reducing wrinkles. Its use is one of the most popular

Table 22.2 Botulinum toxins available in the United Kingdom.

Toxin type	Trade name	Drug name	Manufacturer	UK license for cosmetic use?
Type A	Vistabel (Botox cosmetic)	OnabotulinumtoxinA	Allergan	Yes, 2006
	Azzalure (Dysport)	AbobotulinumtoxinA	Galderma/ Ipsen	Yes, 2009
	Bocouture (Xeomin)	IncobotulinumtoxinA	Merz	Yes, 2010
Type B	Neurobloc (Myobloc)	RimabotulinumtoxinB	Eisai	No

cosmetic procedures because it is easy to administer and starts to work after only a few days.

Types of botulinum toxin

Four types of botulinum toxin are available in the United Kingdom (Table 22.2). Vistabel® (Botox cosmetic® in the United States) is a type A botulinum toxin, licensed to treat glabellar lines, for which it should now be used in place of the identical Botox®. Azzalure® (identical to Dysport®) and Bocouture (identical to Xeomin) are also type A botulinum toxins, while Neurobloc® is a type B toxin. All three type A botulinum toxins contain the same type A toxin molecule consisting of a light chain that promotes its translocation into the presynaptic terminal and a heavy chain that cleaves SNAP-25 (synaptosome-associated protein), inhibiting the release of acetylcholine. They differ in the amount and size of the complexing proteins. Clinical data show similar efficacy and duration of action. All except for Neurobloc are licensed for cosmetic use to treat glabellar frown lines. Type A botulinum toxins do not take effect for several days after injection, and their actions last for 3–4 months. With repeated injections, patients often note the aesthetic improvements last longer than 6 months. Neurobloc® (Myobloc in the United States) has a shorter action of around 6 weeks. Neurobloc is not licensed for cosmetic use and this must be explained to patients. Clinical studies have suggested that Bocouture is bioequivalent to Vistabel or Botox (1 unit Bocouture = 1 unit Botox). The potency of Azzalure is calculated differently, with 1 unit of Botox/Vistabel® being roughly equivalent to 2.5 units of Azzalure®.

Uses of botulinum toxin

Botulinum toxin is primarily used to treat 'dynamic wrinkles' (i.e. wrinkles produced by muscle contraction). The upper part of the face is most amenable to treatment, as wrinkles here are caused by the contraction of specific muscles, such as the frontalis (leading to horizontal wrinkles on the forehead), procerus and corrugator (causing vertical glabellar frown lines) and lateral orbicularis oculi (resulting in crow's feet). While botulinum toxin is only indicated for glabellar lines, experienced physicians have also found other off-labelled uses in treatment of wrinkles of the upper lip, marionette lines, bunny lines from nasal scrunching, mental creases and platysmal bands. These areas should be approached with caution, however, as poor technique may result in difficulty with facial expression and physiological function.

A glabellar frown typically needs injection into each corrugator and the procerus muscle. Five injection sites in a V distribution is often used to eliminate the vertical and horizontal rhytides in the glabellar complex. To avoid lid and brow ptosis, the most lateral injection should be placed slightly medial to the mid-pupillary line and 1 cm superior to the orbital rim. To treat horizontal wrinkles on the forehead, botulinum toxin is injected roughly every 2 cm along the frontalis muscle (Figure 22.1). A more feminine arched brow appearance can be created by raising the lateral injection sites slightly to allow some function of expression in the lateral brow. In men, a horizontal pattern is used to prevent the cockeyed appearance. 'Crow's feet' (peri-ocular rhytides) are treated with injections 1 cm lateral to the lateral canthus.

As botulinum toxin is beneficial for wrinkles caused by muscular contraction, it is not suitable for the 'static wrinkles' associated with photoageing and dermal collagen loss, for which laser and dermal fillers are more effective. It is therefore most commonly used in younger patients. Potential side effects include bruising, ptosis and an asymmetrical or unwanted appearance, but fortunately these go away as the effects of the toxin wear off. Patients should be instructed to avoid massaging the area as diffusion of the botulinum toxin can lead to weakness of muscles adjacent to the injected site. Botulinum toxin is also used to treat hyperhidrosis (p. 167). Contraindication to the use of botulinum toxin include patients with known hypersensitivity to any component of the formulation, those with neuromuscular disorders such as myasthenia gravis,

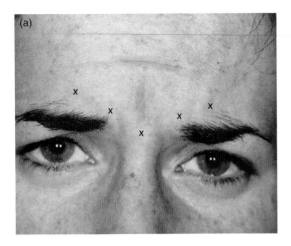

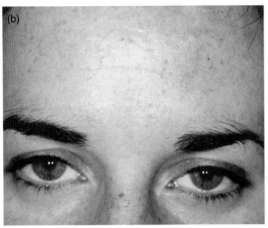

Figure 22.1 Before (a) and after (b) photographs of the effect of botulinum toxin injections on glabella and horizontal forehead frown lines. "X" marks typical injection sites to reduce glabella and forehead rhytids.

pregnant or lactating women and patients on aminoglycoside antibiotics.

Dermal fillers

'Wrinkles at rest' respond poorly to botulinum toxin. The underlying cause here is a loss of elasticity and volume in the dermis and subcutis: and the aim of using dermal fillers is to replace that volume. The ageing face is characterized by loss of volume in the temple, cheeks and perioral area and deep wrinkle lines along the nasolabial folds and corners of the mouth. Dermal fillers can fill in specific furrow lines but also revolumize the sunken, sagging face which results in a more youthful appearance. An ideal filler would be non-inflammatory, non-allergenic, non-carcinogenic, non-migratory, long-lasting and provide a natural appearance. However, no such product exists and there are few trials comparing the different agents.

Fillers are based on naturally derived or synthetic polymers – usually of collagen or hyaluronic acid. Most are injected into the upper or mid-dermis and are useful for wrinkles at rest, acne scars and wrinkles in the lower two-thirds of the face where botulinum toxin is less effective. They are commonly used for the nasolabial folds (Figure 22.2), 'marionette lines' (which radiate from the lateral border of the mouth to the chin), crow's feet and for augmenting the lips.

Collagen fillers
Bovine collagen and its derivatives were the first fillers approved for dermal filling in the United Kingdom and the United States. They are ideal for fine superficial wrinkles such as peri-oral rhytides and are injected intradermally. They have been used for 20 years to augment soft

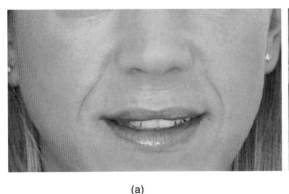

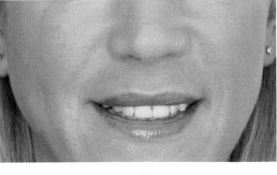

(a)   (b)

Figure 22.2 Before (a) and after (b) photographs showing reduction in nasolabial folds following injection of a hyaluronic acid filler.

tissue, and, with over 1 million subjects treated, have a long safety record. However, because of a decrease in popularity, most of the brands have been voluntarily discontinued.

The first generation collagen fillers were Zyderm and Zyplast, bovine collagens with a relatively short duration of effect in comparison to other dermal fillers. They differ in their concentration of collagen – with lower concentrations being used for the more superficial, finer wrinkles. Products such as Zyplast contain collagen cross-linked with glutaraldehyde: this slows the breakdown of the collagen by host collagenases and lengthens its action to around 4 months. Unmodified collagen (Zyderm) begins to lose its effect after 2–4 months. The major drawback of bovine collagen is the 3% incidence of delayed hypersensitivity reactions. For this reason, two intradermal test injections must be given into the volar forearm, the first at least 6 weeks prior to treatment, followed by a second test at a different site on the forearm 4 weeks later. A positive test is shown by erythema, itching and induration, and precludes the use of bovine collagen.

In recent years, the use of human-derived collagen fillers have surpassed that of bovine collagen because no preliminary skin allergy testing is required prior to treatment. The collagen, either taken from human cadavers, or more commonly produced by human dermal fibroblasts, is cultured in the laboratory (e.g. Cosmoderm/Cosmoplast), eliminating the risk for bovine collagen allergies. Its effects last for around 3 months.

The most recent addition, Evolence, a porcine-based collagen product, was withdrawn in 2009. Because porcine collagen is nearly identical to human collagen, it is less antigenic than bovine collagen and no skin testing is required. It is injected in the mid to deep dermis and lasts 6 months.

Hyaluronic acid fillers

Hyaluronic acid-based products have largely replaced collagen as the filler of choice for several reasons. Unlike bovine collagen, hyaluronic acid is homologous across species, thus delayed hypersensitivity reactions are unusual and preliminary skin testing is not necessary. They tend to last longer (usually 6–12 months) and provide more volume correction than collagen. Finally, the availability of hyaluronidase to dissolve unwanted hyaluronic acid filler also makes it a better alternative than collagen.

Hyaluronic acid is a glycosaminoglycan found naturally in the ground substance of the dermis (p. 16). It is strongly hydrophilic, and so 'plumps up' the dermis by attracting water. In its unmodified state, hyaluronic acid would rapidly be broken down, but chemical modification prevents this. The first hyaluronic acid, Hylaform®, was made from rooster comb. Since then, there have been a growing number of non-animal stabilized hyaluronic acid based products used worldwide, but two main forms are used in Europe: Restylane® and Juvederm®, both synthesized by genetically engineered streptococci. As of 2009, these products are available with the addition of lidocaine for patient comfort during injection. Both product lines have multiple formulations with different particle size and thickness, specifically designed for use in different cosmetic areas. In general, smaller particle sized products are best for superficial wrinkles while larger particle sized products are ideally suited for volumizing deep facial lines.

Calcium hydroxylapatite fillers

Radiesse is a longer lasting dermal filler introduced in the United Kingdom in 2004. It is designed for subdermal correction of deeper lines and volume loss. Radiesse is composed of synthetic calcium hydroxylapatite, which has the same composition as the naturally occurring component of teeth and bone. No skin testing is required as it does not contain any animal-derived components. Foreign body reaction is rare, although nodule formation may occur if the product is injected into the superficial dermis. One should also avoid injecting Radiesse into the lips as nodule and cyst formations are common. The results last on average 12–18 months.

Longer lasting fillers

A number of permanent and semi-permanent fillers are becoming available, intended to provide longer lasting effects. Poly-L-lactic acid (Sculptra®, previously branded as New-Fill®) was introduced in 2000 as a synthetic polymer. It acts differently from hyaluronic acid and collagen, in that it stimulates fibroblasts to produce collagen. Therefore, injection results are not immediate and multiple courses of treatment are required to achieve the optimal effect. Once the desired result is achieved, the results last for 1–3 years. It was initially licensed for the treatment of HIV-related lipoatrophy but is now more widely used as a cosmetic agent in non-HIV patients to treat lines deeper than those that respond to volumetric fillers. Less commonly used permanent fillers include Artecoll®, composed of non-resorbable polymethylmethacrylate (PMMA) microspheres with bovine collagen. Because this product contains bovine collagen, skin testing is required as with previous collagen-based fillers. The benefits of a more permanent effect must be balanced against the higher risk of developing nodules, granulomatous or foreign-body reactions, and biofilm formation. Unfortunately, when these rare side effects develop with more permanent fillers, the consequences are also more likely to be permanent.

As with any medical procedures, all dermal fillers have side effects, but there are no comparative trial data on these. Bovine collagens probably create the most hypersensitivity reactions, but prior skin testing should lessen this risk. Transient but predictable side effects of filler injections include mild ecchymoses, erythema and oedema which usually resolves in 3–7 days. The Tyndall effect, which manifests as a bluish bump under the skin, may occur as a result of superficial placement of hyaluronic acid. Foreign body reactions, granulomas, lumps from maldistribution and infections have been reported for all types of filler. Serious but rare complications include local tissue necrosis and even blindness resulting from vascular compromise, either by compression or occlusion of the vessel.

Autologous fat transfer is used in some centres and has the advantage that it obviates the risk of a foreign body reaction. The patient's own fat is harvested from donor sites such as the buttocks or thighs by gentle aspiration, under local anaesthetic. The aspirate is gently centrifuged down, and fat injected into the area of lipoatrophy. This technique is particularly useful for the peri-orbital and malar areas, and fat can also be frozen and stored for incremental 'touch ups' over time.

Skin resurfacing

Variations in texture, pigmentation and the epidermal lesions of ageing are best treated by resurfacing the skin with chemical peels, dermabrasion or lasers. All three methods create a controlled injury to the superficial layers of the skin to a certain depth to eliminate textural irregularities and promote new collagen.

Chemical peels

Chemical peels are categorized by their depth of action. All rely on the application of a chemical exfoliant, which induces removal or necrosis and inflammation of the epidermis, and sometimes of the dermis too. The release of inflammatory mediators increases new collagen deposition and reduces solar elastosis, resulting in a thicker and smoother appearance of the skin. Superficial peels induce necrosis of part or all of the epidermis; medium depth peels produce destruction of the epidermis and inflammation of the papillary dermis; deep chemical peels create inflammation down to the deep reticular dermis. The depth of the peel depends on the type of chemicals applied and their concentration, the contact time, the mode and number of application, and the thickness and sebaceous gland activity of the patient's skin.

The mainstay of chemical peels are hydroxy acids, classified as α and β hydroxy acids (AHAs and BHAs), depending on the position of the hydroxyl group. Typical AHAs include lactic, glycolic and citric acids, while salicylic acid is the only BHA in clinical use. In the short term, AHAs affect corneocyte cohesiveness in the lower stratum corneum, and in the longer term they thicken the epidermis and papillary dermis, with increased acid mucopolysaccharides and collagen in the dermis. The depth of penetration of AHAs such as glycolic acid is dependent on the time of contact. It must be neutralized with bicarbonate solution which stops the depth of penetration. Salicylic acid has been used as a keratolytic for decades, and enhances the shedding of corneocytes by reducing intercellular stickiness. Salicylic acid peels are particularly useful in treating comedonal acne because salicylic acid is lipid soluble and penetrates better into the sebaceous gland compared to other acids. Its anti-inflammatory effect also results in less erythema and discomfort. Unlike AHAs, salicyclic acid peels do not require neutralization. Resorcinol is a phenol derivative that has keratolytic properties, but is also useful in treating hyperpigmentation.

Most chemical peels rely on a combination of agents. The depth of the peel depends on the agents used, the vehicle in which they are delivered, and the length of time for which they are applied (Table 22.3). Typical of the combination peels is Jessner's solution – a mixture of resorcinol 14%, salicylic acid 14% and lactic acid 14% in ethanol. 'Frosting' due to the precipitation of salicylic acid occurs on treated skin, and can be used as a guide when applying the solution. Single applications of a superficial chemical peel produce only subtle changes, and treatments repeated every few weeks are needed to improve actinic damage, lentigines and melasma. A deeper Jessner's peel can be achieved with multiple applications of solutions on the same day.

Trichloracetic acid (TCA) can be used as a superficial, medium or deep peel. Concentrations of 10–25% are used for superficial peels, whereas TCA 35% is the standard solution for medium depth facial peels. "TCA

Table 22.3 Types of chemical peels and depths of penetration.

Depth of peel	Depth of skin penetration	Types of peels
Very superficial	Strateum corneum/granulosum	TCA 10–25% Jessner's 1–3 layers Glycolic acid 30–50% for 1–2 minutes Salicylic acid Resorcinol 20–30% for 5–10 minutes
Superficial	Basal layer/papillary dermis	TCA 35% Glycolic acid 50–70% for 2–5 minutes Jessner's 4+ layers Resorcinol 40–50% for 30–60 minutes
Medium	Upper reticular dermis	Jessner's + TCA 35% Glycolic acid 70% + TCA 35% TCA 50%
Deep	Mid-reticular dermis	Phenol 88% Baker–Gordon (phenol/septisol/croton oil)

TCA, tricholoroacetic acid.

Cross" technique with high percentage TCA (90–100%) can spot-treat deep ice-pick scars from acne. TCA can be used alone (Figure 22.3), or after preliminary treatment with a superficial peeling agent such as Jessner's peel to achieve a deeper effect. It produces epidermal and dermal necrosis, without serious systemic toxicity, although it may induce post-inflammatory hyperpigmentation in dark skinned subjects, in whom it should not be used.

'Frosting' of the skin occurs shortly after TCA is applied, but is due to the precipitation of denatured proteins in the epidermis. A superficial peel results in minimal streaky frosting with mostly erythema, whereas a deeper peel produces a more powdery white frost with some erythema showing through.

Superficial peels are generally safe, but can cause allergic or irritant contact dermatitis. Salicylate poisoning

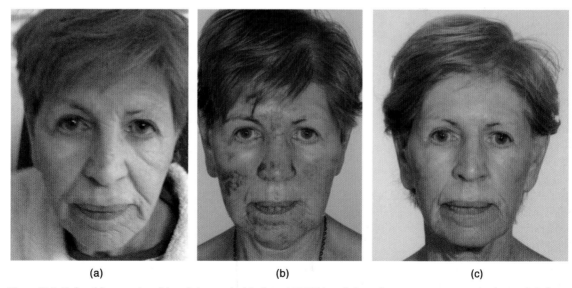

(a)　　　　　　　　　(b)　　　　　　　　　(c)

Figure 22.3 Before (a), seven days (b), and six months (c) after a 25% TCA peel. Once the post-treatment crusting has settled, there is a reduction in peri-oral wrinkles and signs of epidermal photoaging.

has been reported, but only after large areas were treated. Post-inflammatory pigmentation may occur, subjects with darker skins being at greater risk. Medium depth TCA peels inevitably lead to erythema and desquamation of the epidermis, at its worst about a week after treatment. As re-epithelialization is occurring, patients should avoid sun exposure. Prophylactic antiviral medication is often used to prevent the recurrence of a herpes simplex infection in subjects with a history of this.

Deep chemical peels with phenol result in significant postoperative downtime but dramatic results. Commonly used agents include phenol mixed with soap, water, croton oil and olive oil. Proper analgesia, IV hydration, cardiac monitoring and sedation are essential with phenol peels as they are associated with significant discomfort and systemic toxicities. Rare but significant side effects, including hypopigmentation and cardiac arrhythmias, have made most physicians abandon phenol in favour of laser resurfacing.

Dermabrasion

Mechanical resurfacing procedure is a technique for facial rejuvenation. Superficial microdermabrasion can improve pigmentary dyschromias, comedonal acne and superficial rhytides while deeper procedures can correct rhinophyma, deep rhytides, acne scarring and textural irregularities associated with surgical and traumatic scars. Multiple modalities can be used to abrade the skin mechanically including motorized rotary units with wire brush tips or diamond fraise, and even sterile sandpaper. While local anaesthesia is adequate for spot treatment, full-face procedures usually require oral or intramuscular sedation and nerve blocks. Strict adherence to postoperative care including antiviral medications, acetic acid soaks and copious petrolatum ointment application is essential to prevent infection and scarring. As with any skin resurfacing procedures, complications including dyspigmentation, scarring and persistent erythema may occur with deeper procedures.

Laser resurfacing (p. 383)

This is the most effective treatment for deeper changes in the skin such as rhytides and scarring, and also improves epidermal photodamage. Newer laser technology allows the physician to adjust parameters based on patient's skin type and skin problems, making laser resurfacing safer than mechanical and chemical resurfacing. As with all resurfacing modalities, laser resurfacing can induce a partial thickness burn, thus proper training and techniques are required to prevent serious complications.

Ablative laser resurfacing with carbon dioxide (CO_2) and erbium yttrium aluminium garnet (Er:YAG) lasers selectively vaporize the epidermis and papillary dermis, allowing the epidermis to re-epithelialize and new collagen and elastic tissue to be laid down in the upper dermis. The wavelengths of these lasers ($CO_2 = 10\,600$ nm and Er:YAG = 2094 nm) are predominantly absorbed by water in the skin, generating heat and thermal destruction. The millisecond pulse widths of modern CO_2 lasers ensure efficient tissue vaporization and minimizes non-selective thermal damage. The CO_2 laser penetrates deeper than the Er:YAG laser, removing 25–50 μm of tissue with each pass and producing thermal wounding of the dermis. A degree of immediate skin tightening follows, due to denaturation and shrinkage of type I dermal collagen, and dermal remodelling continues for several months afterwards. The shorter wavelength of the Er:YAG laser is absorbed more efficiently by water and penetrates less deeply, usually 15–20 μm each pass, with less collateral thermal injury and collagen contraction. This results in more rapid healing, although often with less clinical improvement. While traditional ablative laser resurfacing procedures produces dramatic results, ablative treatments are limited by their postoperative downtime (1–2 weeks) and side effects including prolonged erythema, pigmentary changes, infections and scarring.

With the recent trend toward more minimally invasive procedures, techniques devised to avoid the morbidity of laser resurfacing include non-ablative treatments and fractional resurfacing. A number of laser sources have been developed in recent years (near-infrared lasers, radiofrequency, intense pulsed light, pulsed dye laser; see Chapter 27), intended to selectively injure the dermis while sparing the epidermis to reduce downtime. While these techniques may improve dyschromia and superficial rhytides, the results were modest at best and required multiple treatments.

In fractional resurfacing, small non-contiguous areas of skin are treated. This allows faster healing to occur from adjacent non-treated tissue and reduces side effects. As only a percentage of the skin surface is treated, the depth of penetration can be increased to trigger deeper thermal damage and tissue repair. Laser parameters such as density and depth can be customized to target specific conditions such as superficial pigmentation or deeper scars. The main drawback of the procedure is that multiple treatments are usually required to produce similar results achieved by conventional laser treatment. Both ablative and non-ablative fractional lasers have relatively short downtime in comparison to traditional ablative laser resurfacing. Non-ablative fractional laser with wavelengths of 1400–1550 nm confines the thermal injury intradermally with preservation of the stratum corneum. This maintains the skin barrier while the columns of microscopic epidermal necrotic debris (MENDs) are extruded through the epidermis. Ablative fractional laser (CO_2 and Er:YAG) on the other hand, creates columns of complete tissue vaporization which induces more collagen remodelling but also more downtime. Studies have shown both ablative and non-ablative fractionated lasers effective in a variety of conditions, including rhytides, acne and traumatic scars, pigmentation and photoageing, with ablative fractionated lasers showing greater improvement in skin laxity and texture abnormalities. Furthermore, these lasers can be used off the face on the neck, chest and extremities with much less risk of scarring than the traditional ablative laser.

Depending on the type of laser used, patients may need topical or general anaesthesia and systemic analgesics. Non-ablative fractionated lasers produce minimal discomfort and most patients only require topical anaesthetic. Skin cooling methods such as ice pack and forced air cooling helps to reduce pain. Ablative lasers are more painful and most patients require nerve blocks and some sort of sedation. Oral antiviral prophylaxis is given before and after the procedure. Postoperatively, patients undergoing non-ablative fractionated laser should expect oedema and erythema for 3–5 days, followed by fine sandpaper desquamation for several more days. Downtime is significantly more with ablative resurfacing. Complete re-epithelialization occurs within 3–7 days for fractionated ablative laser and up to 2 weeks for fully ablative laser. During this time, patients should expect exudation and strict wound care adherence including emollient, acetic acid soaks and wet dressings. Careful patient selection should ensure that only those with realistic expectations, who can tolerate the discomfort of the procedure and will follow the instructions for post-treatment care, are chosen. Preoperative counselling should emphasize that multiple treatments are necessary with fractionated devices to achieve optimal results. Possible side effects include a dissemination of concurrent bacterial or viral infections, pain and pruritus. Long-term complications include hyper- and hypopigmentation, prolonged erythema, scarring and ectropion; these risks are higher with the traditional ablative laser. The concurrent use of oral isotretinoin is an absolute contraindication because of an increased risk of hypertrophic scarring.

Aside from resurfacing, lasers can be used to treat pigmentary lesions in the skin (p. 383), whether due to melanin or unwanted tattoos. Vascular lesions such as haemangioma and telangiectasia can also be treated with a variety of laser modalities (p. 381). The type of laser must be matched to the target chromophore, but as a general rule the best results are obtained when there is a large colour difference between the normal skin and the lesion treated.

Treatment of leg veins (see also p. 153)

Significant contributions have been made by dermatologists in the field of phlebology including advances in sclerotherapy and endovascular vein closure techniques. Many patients present to a dermatologist's office with varicose and telangiectatic leg veins. Their complaints can vary from cosmetic concerns such as unsightly spider veins and pigmentation, to symptoms such as aches, itching, pain from prolong standing, swelling, heaviness, cramps and restless legs. Complications of varicose veins include stasis dermatitis, lower extremity oedema, lipodermatosclerosis, bleeding from a varicose vein, thrombophlebitis and venous ulceration. Thankfully, recent advances have made the treatment of venous disease safer, more effective and with less downtime than ligation and stripping as used previously.

The venous system comprises a network of interconnected veins and one-way valves (p. 147). The pumping actions of the calf muscles propel the blood from the feet back to the heart. Genetics, hormones, age, pregnancy and inactivity are factors that predispose to venous valve failure, which in turn result in the development of varicose veins and spider veins. Long-standing venous insufficiency can result in oedema, skin changes and ulceration. The CEAP (Clinical, Etiologic, Anatomic, Pathophysiologic) classification of chronic venous disorders helps to guide treatment and prognosis (Table 22.4). While class II compression stockings can be very helpful in patients with early venous disease, those with bleeding from a varicosity, inadequate control of skin disease, recurrent superficial thrombophlebitis or progression of ulceration should be referred to a specialist.

As the venous system is interconnected, failure to treat the most proximal point of reflux will likely result in less than optimal outcomes. Thus, while many patients present with unsightly spider and varicose veins, a thorough examination of the venous system must be performed prior to any sclerotherapy or laser treatments. If patients have significant signs or symptoms of venous disease, a venous duplex ultrasound can determine if reflux is present and provide an anatomic map of the venous system to guide treatment. Most often, incompetency is noted in the great or small saphenous vein.

In the last decade, endovascular vein closure and ultrasound guided foam sclerotherapy have rapidly replaced

Table 22.4 Clinical, Etiologic, Anatomic, Pathophysiologic (CEAP) classification of chronic venous disorders.

Clinical	Etiologic	Anatomic	Pathophysiologic
C0: no visible or palpable signs of venous disease	Ec: congenital	As: superficial veins	Pr: reflux
C1: telangiectasia or reticular veins	Ep: primary	Ap: perforator veins	Po: obstruction
C2: varicose veins	Es: secondary	Ad: deep veins	
C3: oedema	(post-thrombotic)		
C4a: haemosiderin pigmentation, eczematous dermatitis			
C4b: lipodermatosclerosis, atrophie blanche			
C5: healed venous ulcer			
C6: active venous ulcer			

ligation and stripping as the treatments of choice for saphenofemoral reflux disease. Both of these procedures can be performed in an outpatient setting, under local anaesthesia, and patients can ambulate immediately after the procedure. In comparison with high ligation and stripping, patients report less pain, fewer complications and a quicker return to work and normal activities. Endovascular closure consists of placing a thin laser fibre or radiofrequency catheter endoluminally inside the great saphenous vein under ultrasound guidance. In most cases, only a small incision is needed to access the vein. Once the fibre is placed, the entire course of the vein is tumesced with local anaesthetic, and the fibre is turned on while withdrawn from just below the saphenofemoral junction to the knee. The laser or radiofrequency device selectively heats the entire section of the treated vein, resulting in contraction and fibrous occlusion.

Foam sclerotherapy is an alternative treatment for treatment of the great saphenous vein (GSV). The GSV is cannulated under ultrasound guidance and injection of the sclerosant foam induces fibrosis of the vein. Foam sclerosant is preferred over liquid sclerosant in the case of large-calibre vessels because the foam displaces the blood inside the vessel. This increases the contact time of the sclerosant thereby enhancing efficacy without having to increase the volume of sclerosant used. Residual varicosities are often treated with a combination of hook phlebectomies (stab avulsions) or foam sclerotherapy.

Sclerotherapy remain the gold standard for treatment of telangiectatic leg veins. A combination of foam sclerosant can be used for larger calibre vessels, and liquid sclerosant for smaller vessels. Commonly used sclerosants include glycerin, sodium tetradecyl sulfate, hypertonic saline and polidocanol. Hypertonic saline can be painful and more likely to cause hyperpigmentation, but is the only agent that does not cause any allergic reactions. Glycerin is best for injecting small vessels. Sodium tetradecyl sulfate and polidocanol are detergent solutions that are the most effective in treating spider veins with the least likelihood of ulceration, hyperpigmentation and pain. These detergent-based solutions have an added advantage in that they can be mixed with air to create foam sclerosant. Patients should be warned that multiple treatments are necessary and temporary hyperpigmentation is common after treatment.

Fat reduction

The ever-expanding field of fat reduction has made it possible to remove stubborn pockets of fat when diet and exercise are not enough. Liposuction is the traditional surgical method of fat reduction in which excess fat is suctioned via cannula for body contouring. The area of interest is first infiltrated with tumescent anaesthesia, consisting of a high volume of diluted solutions of lidocaine and epinephrine. A liposuction cannula connected to a suction device is then used to remove the excess adipose tissue. Newer technology, including ultrasound and laser assisted liposuction devices, are available to facilitate fat removal especially in large volume cases. While these procedures are generally very safe, there is significant recovery time, including pain, oedema and bruising. Most patients need to wear a compression garment for 1–2 weeks after the procedure.

While liposuction remains the gold standard, there has been great interest in recent years in non-surgical methods of fat removal with fewer risks and less downtime. These non-invasive techniques are useful for patients with limited focal deposits of fat. Patients with large volumes of fat are best treated with traditional liposuction. In ultrasound fat reduction, an ultrasound probe is used externally to transmit high-intensity ultrasonic waves to cause lipolysis. Radiofrequency fat reduction utilizes radiofrequency energy to heat deep within the fat cells, thus destroying them. Cryolipolysis disrupts fat by selectively freezing adipocyte cells, which are more sensitive to cold temperature, resulting in their apoptosis and resorption.

Learning points

1 As the demand for cosmetic procedures increases, an understanding of the benefits and pitfalls of cosmetic dermatology will help you steer your patients toward safe and effective procedures.

2 Botulinum toxins are useful for treating dynamic wrinkles produced by muscle contractions. Fillers are more effective for treating static wrinkles, such as those around the cheeks, and nasolabial folds from volume loss.

3 Both fillers and botulinum toxins provide effective reproducible results with minimal downtime.

4 The use of fractionated technology in laser resurfacing has made these procedures safer, more effective and with less downtime.

5 If you suspect someone has complications from venous reflux disease, consider sending them to a vein specialist. Endovascular vein closure and ultrasound guided foam sclerotherapy have largely become the treatments of choice. These outpatient procedures are much more effective without the complications of ligation and stripping.

Further reading

Baumann L. (2002) *Cosmetic Dermatology: Principles and Practice*. McGraw-Hill, New York.

Coleman-Moriarty K. (2004) *Botulinum Toxin in Facial Rejuvenation*. Mosby, Edinburgh.

Fabbrocini G, De Padova MP, Tosti A. (2009) Chemical peels: what's new and what isn't new but still works well. *Facial Plastic Surgery* **25**, 329–36.

Glogau RG. (2012) Fillers: from the past to the future. *Seminars in Cutaneous Medicine and Surgery* **31**, 78–87.

Nesbitt C, Eifell RKG, Coyne P, Badri H, Bhattacharya V, Stansby G. (2011) Endovenous ablation (radiofrequency and laser) and foam sclerotherapy versus conventional surgery for great saphenous vein varices. *Cochrane Database of Systematic Reviews* **10**, CD005624.

Ratner D, Tse Y, Marchell N, *et al.* (1999) Cutaneous laser resurfacing. *Journal of the American Academy of Dermatology* **41**, 365–389.

The Economist (2003) The beauty business. The Economist (22 May). http://www.economist.com/node/1795852 (accessed 3 July 2014).

Saedi N, Jalian HR, Petelin A, Zachary C. (2012) Fractionation: past, present, future. *Seminars in Cutaneous Medicine and Surgery* **31**, 105–109.

Samuel M, Brooke RCC, Hollis S, Griffiths CEM. (2005) Interventions for photodamaged skin. *Cochrane Database of Systematic Reviews* **1**, CD001782.

23 The Skin and the Psyche

Most people accept that there are strong links between the skin and the emotions. Embarrassment causes blushing; anxiety causes cold, sweaty palms; anger causes the face to redden, but only a few skin disorders, such as dermatitis artefacta, have emotional factors as their direct cause. The relationships between the mind and the skin are usually subtle and complex. Nevertheless, patients with skin disorders do have a higher prevalence of psychiatric abnormalities than the general population, although specific personality profiles and disorders can seldom be tied to specific skin diseases. Similarly, it is still not clear how, or even how often, psychological factors trigger, worsen or perpetuate such everyday problems as atopic eczema or psoriasis.

Each school of psychiatry has its own theories on the subject, but their explanations do not satisfy everyone. Do people really damage their skin to satisfy guilt feelings? Does their skin 'weep' because they have themselves suppressed weeping? Until more is known, it may be wise to adopt a simpler and more pragmatic approach, in which interactions between the skin and psyche are divided into two broad groups:

1 Emotional reactions to the presence of skin disease, real or imagined; and

2 The effects of emotions on skin disease (Figure 23.1).

Reactions to skin disease

The presence of disfiguring skin lesions can distort the emotional development of a child: some become withdrawn, others become aggressive, but many adjust well. The range of reactions to skin disease is therefore wide. At one end lies indifference to grossly disfiguring lesions and, at the other, lies an obsession with skin that is quite normal. Between these extremes are reactions ranging from natural anxiety over ugly skin lesions to disproportionate worry over minor blemishes.

A chronic skin disease such as psoriasis can undoubtedly spoil the lives of those affected. It can interfere with work, and with social activities of all sorts including sexual relationships, causing patients to feel like outcasts. Studies have shown that a diagnosis of psoriasis has a negative impact on quality of life equivalent to that of other major medical diseases such as cancer, diabetes and depression. The heavy drinking of so many men with severe psoriasis is one result of these pressures. An experienced dermatologist will be on the lookout for depression and the risk of suicide, as up to 10% of patients with psoriasis have had suicidal thoughts. However, these reactions do not necessarily correlate with the extent and severity of the eruption as judged by an outside observer. Who has the more disabling problem: someone with 50% of his body surface covered in psoriasis, but who largely ignores this and has a happy family life and a productive job, or one with 5% involvement whose social life is ruined by it? The concept of 'body image' is useful here.

Body image

All of us think we know how we look, but our ideas may not tally with those of others. The nose, face, hair and genitals tend to rank high in a person's 'corporeal awareness', and trivial lesions in those areas can generate much anxiety. The facial lesions of acne, for example, can lead to a huge loss of self-esteem, and, for some reason, feelings of shame.

Dermatological delusional disease

Dysmorphophobia

This is the term applied to distortions of the body image. Minor and inconspicuous lesions are magnified in the mind to grotesque proportions.

Clinical Dermatology, Fifth Edition. Richard B. Weller, Hamish J.A. Hunter and Margaret W. Mann.
© 2015 John Wiley & Sons, Ltd. Published 2015 by John Wiley & Sons, Ltd.

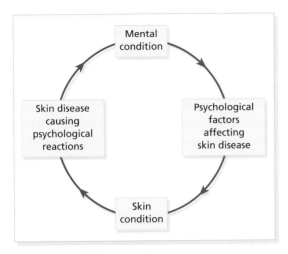

Figure 23.1 Mind–skin interactions.

Dermatological 'non-disease'

This is a form of dysmorphobia. The clinician can find no skin abnormality, but the distress felt by the patient leads to anxiety, depression or even suicide. Such patients are not uncommon. They expect dermatological solutions for complaints such as hair loss, or burning, itching and redness of the face or genitals. The dermatologist, who can see nothing wrong, cannot solve matters and no treatment seems to help. Such patients are reluctant to see a psychiatrist although some may have a monosymptomatic hypochondriacal psychosis.

Other delusions

These patients sustain single hypochondriacal delusions for long periods, in the absence of other recognizable psychiatric disease. They may become eccentric and live in social isolation. Some believe that they have syphilis, AIDS or skin cancer. Others hide in shame from an inapparent body odour. Still other patients have the delusion that their skin is infested with parasites.

Delusional infestation (Figure 23.2)

This term is better than delusions of parasitosis as not all delusions are related to parasites or indeed pathogenic organisms. Parasitophobia implies a fear of becoming infested; patients with delusional infestation are unshakably convinced that they are already infested. No rational argument can convince them that they are not. Many see parasites move on their skin, feel them crawl (formication) or need to dig them out. The pest control agencies that they have called in, and their medical advisers therefore must all be wrong. More recently, patients have begun to describe a condition called Morgellons disease, which involves intense cutaneous dysaesthesia associated with the extrusion of inanimate fibres from the skin surface. This dermatological non-disease has been somewhat perpetuated by ever-increasing internet access and the US media which have attempted to give some credence to its existence; most dermatologists still consider it to be a monosymptomatic hypochondriacal psychosis, a form of delusional infestation. Patients often bring to the clinic samples of extruded fibres or a box of specimens of the 'parasite' at different stages of its supposed life cycle. These must be examined microscopically but usually turn out to be fragments of skin, hair, clothing, haemorrhagic crusts or unclassifiable debris. The skin changes may include gouge marks and scratches, but it is correct to consider these patients separately from those with dermatitis artefacta. Although delusional infestation is the most common psychodermatolological presentation, most dermatologists will see only about two to three cases every 5 years and, due to the nature of the condition, it is likely to be significantly under-reported.

These patients become angry if doubts are cast on their ideas, or if they are referred to a psychiatrist. How could treatment for mental illness possibly be expected to kill parasites? Family members or friends may share their delusions (*folie à deux*) and much tact is needed to secure any cooperation with treatment. Direct confrontations are best avoided; sometimes it may be best simply to treat with psychotropic drugs, explaining that these may be able to help some of the symptoms.

The delusions of a few of these patients are based on an underlying depression or schizophrenia, and of a further few on organic problems such as vitamin deficiency or cerebrovascular disease. Other patients are addicted to alcohol, metamphetamine, cannabis, cocaine or narcotics. These disorders must be treated on their own merits. However, most patients have monosymptomatic hypochondriacal delusions, which can often be suppressed by treatment with drugs, accepting that these will be needed long term. Otherwise, the outlook for resolution is poor. Patients are ideally treated in joint psychodermatology clinics; however. access to these clinics is limited. It is often more practical to seek advice from psychiatric colleagues regarding therapy.

The evidence base for the treatment of delusional infestation is poor but atypical antipsychotics such as risperidone, olanzapine, aripiprazole and amisulpride are gaining favour. Relatively small doses are required when compared with those needed to treat other psychotic

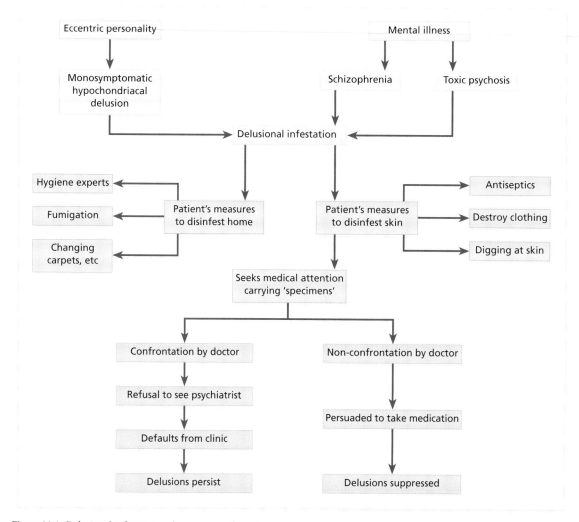

Figure 23.2 Delusional infestation – the sequence of events.

illnesses such as schizophrenia. For example, low dose risperidone (0.5–1 mg/day) may have beneficial effects within 4–6 weeks with treatment required for up to 1 year. Pimozide was traditionally the first line treatment for this condition, but high doses carry cardiac risks. If pimozide is used, an electrocardiogram (ECG) should be performed before starting treatment and the drug should not be given to those with a prolonged Q-T interval or with a history of cardiac dysrhythmia. Fortunately, most patients respond to low doses of 2–4 mg/day. Patients on higher doses need periodic ECG checks. Tardive dyskinesia may develop and persist despite withdrawal of the drug. The skin 'lesions' should not be ignored as these are at the heart of the complaint and effective dressings and treat-

ment of any superadded infection might improve the overall response. Some patients gain insight and relief; others hint that their infestation still persists although this no longer disables them. Many fail to keep their follow-up appointments.

Dermatitis artefacta

Here the skin lesions are caused and kept going by the patient's own actions, but parasites are not held to be to blame. Patients with dermatitis artefacta deny self-trauma but, naturally, if treatment is left to them to carry out, their problems do not improve. Lesions will heal under occlusive dressings, but this does not alter the underlying psychiatric problems, and lesions may recur or crop

Table 23.1 Types of dermatitis artefacta.

Type	Personality
Minor habits (e.g. excoriated acne)	Relatively normal or obsessive
More obvious lesions	Hysterical or neurotic (secondary gain)
Bizarre	Psychotic
Malingering	Criminal

up outside the bandaged areas or after the bandages are removed. Different types of dermatitis artefacta are listed in Table 23.1.

The lesions favour accessible areas, and do not fit with known pathological processes. The diagnosis is often difficult to make, but an experienced clinician will suspect it because there are no primary lesions and because of the bizarre shape or grouping of the lesions, which may be rectilinear or oddly grouped (Figure 23.3). Areas damaged by burning (Figure 23.4), corrosive chemicals (Figure 23.5) or by digging have their own special appearance. Histology varies depending on cause, but many show epidermal necrosis.

More subtle changes are seen in *dermatological pathomimicry*, in which patients reproduce or aggravate their skin disease by deliberate contact with materials to which they know they will react.

Apart from frank malingerers, the patients are often young women with some medical knowledge, perhaps a nurse. Some form of 'secondary gain' from having skin lesions may be obvious. There is often an underlying

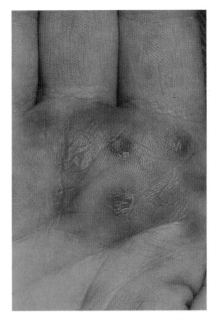

Figure 23.4 A lighted cigarette was responsible for this appearance.

mood or personality disorder. The psychological problems may be superficial and easily resolved, but usually psychiatric help is needed and the artefacts are part of a prolonged psychiatric illness. Suggesting that stress may be increasing 'the reactivity or sensitivity of the skin' may

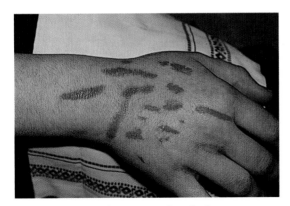

Figure 23.3 Obvious dermatitis artefacta: back your own judgement against the patient's here.

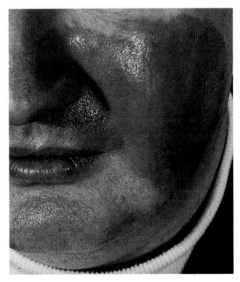

Figure 23.5 Dermatitis artefacta: denials of self-trauma did not convince us that this was caused by any other skin disease.

facilitate referral to psychiatric services. A few patients respond to banal treatments if given the chance to save face. Direct confrontation and accusations are usually best avoided, but the physician must make efforts to help by working to get the patient to psychiatrists and to convince carers that the wounds are self-inflicted. Psychodynamic therapy, low dose antipsychotic medication and selective serotonin reuptake inhibitors such as fluoxetine may be helpful.

Skin-picking syndrome (neurotic excoriations)

Patients with the skin-picking syndrome differ from those with other types of dermatitis artefacta in that they admit to picking and digging at their skin. This habit affects women more often than men and is most active at times of stress. The clinical picture is mixed, with crusted excoriations, peripherally healing irregular ulcers and pale scars, often with a hyperpigmented border, lying mainly on the face, neck, shoulders and arms (Figure 23.6). The syndrome is thought to stem from an inability to ignore the impulse to scratch; subsequent scratching results in a release of tension. There is often a coexistent mood or obsessive–compulsive disorder. The condition may last for years and psychotherapy is seldom successful. Selec-

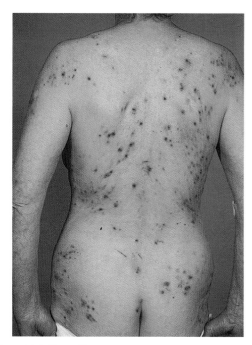

Figure 23.6 Unusually extensive neurotic excoriations.

tive serotonin uptake inhibitors help some patients, especially those with compulsive needs to pick and squeeze skin.

Acne excoriée

Here the self-inflicted damage is based to some extent on the lesions of acne vulgaris, which may in themselves be mild but become disfiguring when dug and squeezed to excess. The patients are usually young girls who may leave themselves with ugly scars. A psychiatric approach is often unhelpful; many patients have insight and recognize their compulsive need to pick at every blemish. A daily ritual of attacking the lesions, helped by a magnifying mirror, may persist for years. Again, selective serotonin uptake inhibitors may help.

Localized neurodermatitis (lichen simplex)

This term refers to areas of itchy eczematization and lichenification, perpetuated by bouts of scratching in response to itching and stress. The condition is not uncommon and can occur on any area of skin. In men, lesions are often on the posterior calves; in women, they favour the nape of the neck where the redness and scaling look rather like psoriasis. Some examples of persistent itching in the anogenital area are caused by lichen simplex there.

Patients with localized neurodermatitis develop scratch responses to minor itch stimuli more readily than controls. Local therapy does not alter the underlying cause, but potent topical or intralesional steroids may ameliorate the symptoms. Occlusive bandaging of suitable areas clears only those lesions that are covered. Capsaicin cream depletes stores of substance P in small sensory cutaneous nerve endings, which can help alleviate the pruritus. Topical antipruritics (Formulary 1, p. 400) provide some relief but this is usually short lived.

Nodular prurigo (Figure 23.7) may be a variant on this theme as manifested in atopic subjects, who scratch and rub remorselessly at their extremely itchy nodules. These patients readily agree that they prefer the pain of excoriations to the itch of their nodules. It is important to exclude underlying causes of generalized pruritus (see Chapter 21). For widespread disease, sedative antihistamines (hydroxyzine), low dose tricyclic antidepressants (amitriptyline or doxepin), gabapentin or pregabalin may be helpful. Phototherapy, both narrowband UVB and PUVA, can provide temporary relief. Under specialist supervision, systemic immunosuppression with

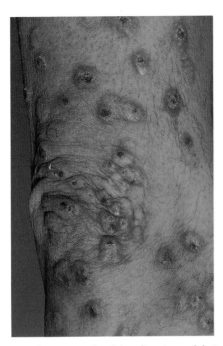

Figure 23.7 The excoriated nodules of prurigo nodularis.

ciclosporin, azathioprine or methotrexate may be considered for more severe cases. These should only be considered if occult malignancy has been ruled out. Recalcitrant disease may respond to thalidomide; its long-term use is often limited by peripheral neuropathy and it must be avoided in women of childbearing age.

Hair-pulling habit

Trichotillomania is too dramatic a word for what is usually only a minor comfort habit in children, ranking alongside nail-biting and lip-licking. Perhaps the term should be dropped in favour of 'hair-pulling habit'. It is usually of little consequence, and children who twist and pull their hair, often as they are going to sleep, seldom have major psychiatric disorders. The habit often goes away most quickly if it is ignored. However, more severe degrees of hair-pulling are sometimes seen in disturbed adolescents and in those with learning difficulties; then the outlook for full regrowth is less good, even with formal psychiatric help.

The diagnosis can usually be made on the history, but some parents do not know what is going on. The bald areas do not show the exclamation-mark hairs of alopecia areata, or the scaling and inflammation of scalp ringworm. The patches are irregular in outline and hair loss is

never complete. Those hairs that remain are bent or broken, and of variable short lengths.

Psychological side effects of dermatological therapy

Several systemic therapies commonly used in the dermatology clinic can impact on the psyche, especially in the elderly (Table 23.2). These reactions are often idiosyncratic but in patients with pre-existing mental health issues careful discussion of the risk versus benefit of treatment should be undertaken. Skin conditions can also be

Table 23.2 Psychological side effects of dermatological medicaments.

Medication	Side effect
Non-sedative antihistamines	Rarely sedation
Sedative antihistamines	Confusion, especially in elderly (use low doses), rarely depression, psychosis
Tetracycline antibiotics	Can cause a lupus-like syndrome with psychosis
Combined oral contraceptive pill	Depression
Retinoids, especially isotretinoin	Depression, cases of suicide linked to isotretinoin use
Tricyclic antidepressants	Sedation, especially in elderly (use low doses), potentially fatal in overdose
Benzodiazepines	Sedation, especially in elderly (use low doses), risk of addiction
Oral corticosteroids	Euphoria, depression and psychosis, confusion common in the elderly
Methotrexate	Mood disturbance
Dapsone	Rarely, psychosis
Antimalarials	Mood disturbance, vivid dreams with hydroxychloroquine, rarely psychosis
Pimozide	Extrapyramidal side effects, tardive dyskinesia
Atypical antipsychotics	Sedation, extrapyramidal side effects (usually mild), tardive dyskinesia

triggered or exacerbated by psychotropic medication, for example the use of lithium in psoriasis.

Dermatoses precipitated or perpetuated by psychosocial stress

Popular candidates for inclusion in this group of diseases are psoriasis, urticaria, atopic eczema, pompholyx, discoid eczema, alopecia areata, lichen simplex and lichen planus. Patient reports of psychosocial stress flaring their skin condition abound but are based on anecdote rather than fact; however, only the most naïve of dermatologists would categorically refute such a relationship. Of late the scientific basis for these effects has begun to emerge. For example, in psoriasis there is now solid evidence that stress not only results from the disease, but can also trigger or exacerbate the condition. The physiological stress response is primarily governed by the hypothalamic–pituitary–adrenal axis and the sympathetic adrenomedullary system, which result in the production of cortisol and catecholamines, respectively. These have a marked influence on nearly all bodily functions including those served by the skin. Recently, an analogous peripheral hypothalamic–pituitary–adrenal axis has been discovered in the skin. This has a similar hierarchical set-up to the central one and possesses all the cellular machinery required for the synthesis of steroids. It is thought that this system may modulate the cutaneous response to stress at a local level. Psychological stress has been shown to impair epidermal barrier function, reduce cutaneous antimicrobial peptide production and delay wound healing, all of which are attributed to the action of cortisol and catecholamines. Whether these are of central or peripheral origin has yet to be confirmed. It is thought that peripheral cutaneous nerves may have a role in the stress-associated triggering and/or flaring of psoriasis. This evidence comes from several sources: untreated chronic plaque psoriasis is frequently symmetrical; psoriatic plaques clear at sites of denervation (following surgery or trauma) and there are increased numbers of nerve fibres in involved skin when compared with uninvolved skin. There is also an increase in the neuropeptide content of plaques, with a concomitant drop in the activity of enzymes that degrade neuropeptides, especially mast cell chymase. In addition, the blood concentrations of certain neuromediators, especially β-endorphin, changes during exacerbations and the hypothalamic–pituitary axis response to social stress appears to differ in psoriatics who feel that stress worsens their disease, compared with

those in whom it does not. Neuropeptides have also been implicated in the pathogenesis of atopic eczema and in its response to psychological stress.

Clearly, the cutaneous stress response varies between individuals; psoriasis patients with increased stress reactivity respond less favourably to treatment. Studies have also shown that reducing the 'psychological burden' of skin disease by employing techniques such as cognitive behavioural therapy lessens the severity of the skin disease and improves the response to standard skin directed therapies.

This area of dermatology is very much in its infancy but there is mounting evidence to support the notion of a 'brain–skin axis'. It is likely that further research will lend weight to anecdotal patient reports of stress flaring their skin conditions, or at least should prompt dermatologists to adopt a more holistic approach when dealing with what may seem at first glance to be a 'skin deep' problem.

Learning points

1 Do not reward a delusion with a treatment for scabies.
2 Direct confrontations with patients with dermatitis artefacta or delusional infestation may make you feel better, but do little for them.
3 Be especially compassionate; having a skin disorder is often stressful and depressing.

Further reading

Anwar W, Murphy N, Powell FC. (2004) Learning the cost of dermatitis artefacta. *Clinical and Experimental Dermatology* **29**, 576–578.

Arck PC, Slominski A, Theoharides TC, Peters EMJ, Paus R. (2006) Neuroimmunology and stress: skin takes center stage. *Journal of Investigative Dermatology* **126**, 1697–1704.

Dewan P, Miller J, Musters C, Taylor RE, Bewley AP. (2011) Delusional infestation with unusual pathogens: a report of three cases. *Clinical and Experimental Dermatology* **36**, 745–748.

Fortune DG, Richards HL, Kirby B, *et al.* (2003) Psychological distress impairs clearance of psoriasis in patients treated with photochemotherapy. *Archives of Dermatology* **139**, 752–756.

Hunter HJA, Griffiths CEM, Kleyn CE. (2013) Does psychosocial stress play a role in the exacerbation of psoriasis? *British Journal of Dermatology* **169**, 965–974.

Koo JY, Do JH, Lee CS. (2000) Psychodermatology. *Journal of the American Academy of Dermatology* **43**, 848–853.

Lawrence-Smith G. (2009) Psychodermatology. *Psychiatry* **8**, 223–227.

Lotti T, Buggiani G, Prignano F. (2008) Prurigo nodularis and lichen simplex chronicus. *Dermatologic Therapy* **21**, 42–46.

Picardi A, Abeni D, Melchi CF, Puddu P, Pasquini P. (2000) Psychiatric morbidity in dermatological outpatients: an issue to be recognized. *British Journal of Dermatology* **143**, 983–991.

Richards HL, Ray DW, Kirby B, *et al.* (2005) Response of the hypothalamic-pituitary-adrenal axis to psychological stress in patients with psoriasis. *British Journal of Dermatology* **153**, 1114–1120.

Robles DT, Olson JM, Combs H, Romm S, Kirby P. (2011) Morgellons disease and delusions of parasitosis. *American Journal of Clinical Dermatology* **12**, 1–6.

Sambhi R, Lepping P. (2009) Psychiatric treatments in dermatology: an update. *Clinical and Experimental Dermatology* **35**, 120–125.

Sandoz A, LoPiccolo M, Kusnir D, Tausk FA. (2008) A clinical paradigm of delusions of parasitosis. *Journal of the American Academy of Dermatology* **59**, 698–704.

Steinhoff M, Bienenstock J, Schemltz M, Maurer M, Wei E, Biro T. (2006) Neurophysiological, neuroimmunological, and neuroendocrine basis for pruritus. *Journal of Investigative Dermatology* **126**, 1705–1718.

Sundström A, Alfredsson L, Sjölin-Forsberg G, Gerdén B, Bergman U, Jokinen J. (2010) Association of suicide attempts with acne and treatment with isotretinoin: retrospective Swedish cohort study. *British Medical Journal* **341**, 1090.

Wong S, Bewley A. (2011) Patients with delusional infestation (delusional parasitosis) often require prolonged treatment as recurrence of symptoms after cessation of treatment is common: an observational study. *British Journal of Dermatology* **165**, 893–896.

24 Other Genetic Disorders

The human genome consists of 23 pairs of chromosomes carrying an estimated 30 000 genes. The pairs of matching chromosomes as seen at colchicine-arrested metaphase are numbered in accordance with their size. A centromere divides each chromosome into a shorter (p) and a longer (q) arm.

Any individual's chromosomal makeup (karyotype) can be expressed as their total number of chromosomes plus their sex chromosome constitution. A normal male therefore is 46XY. A shorthand notation exists for recording other abnormalities such as chromosome translocations and deletions.

The precise location of any gene can be given by naming the chromosome, the arm of the chromosome (p or q), and the numbers of the band and subband of the chromosome, as seen with Giemsa staining, on which it lies. Filaggrin, one of the genes important for atopic eczema, for instance, lies on chromosome 1q21.3, on the long arm of chromosome 1 at band 21, subband 3.

Over the last decade enormous progress has been made in the fields of molecular biology and genetic discovery. Pivotal to these advances was the completion of the Human Genome Project in 2003, which provided a publically available reference template of the human genome. Building on this success, collaborations such as the International HapMap Project mapped common genetic variants (single nucleotide polymorphisms; SNPs) within the genome. Fundamental to these projects was DNA sequencing; initially, using the Sanger sequencing method first described in 1977 but now largely superseded by next generation sequencing (NGS). In the Sanger method one gene is sequenced at a time in contrast to NGS where a DNA sample is fragmented into multiple smaller segments (DNA library), which are sequenced simultaneously (massively parallel sequencing). There are many commercially available NGS platforms which all rely on the same basic steps: DNA extraction; fragmentation in to libraries; amplification; parallel sequencing and imaging; alignment of the sequenced fragments (to a known reference template or de novo alignment) and bioinformatics data analysis. With the advent of NGS, sequencing has become faster, cheaper and universally accessible; a whole genome can now be sequenced in a day. The process can be further streamlined by limiting sequencing to the 1% of the genome that codes for proteins (whole-exome sequencing). However, whole-genome sequencing may be needed to identify non-coding regulatory regions within the introns.

The use of NGS has numerous applications: identification of SNPs; assessment of structural variation within segments of DNA such as deletions, duplications, inversions and translocations (copy number variants or CNVs); and detection of novel mutations. Sequencing panels have also been developed to rapidly identify pathological mutations in single genes or to highlight common mutation hotspots in larger sections of the genome. This more targeted approach further aids in the diagnosis of genetic conditions. Sequencing may also be used in combination with established methods of gene identification.

Linkage analysis. Genes are linked if they lie close together on the same chromosome; they will then be inherited together. The closer together they are, the less is the chance of their being separated by cross-overs, one to six of which, depending on length, occur on each chromosome at meiosis. Each member of an affected family has to be examined both for the presence of the trait to be mapped, and also for a marker, usually a DNA probe, which has already been mapped. If linkage is established then the two loci will be close on the same chromosome. The probability of the results of such a study representing true linkage can be expressed as a logarithm of the odds (Lod) score. A score of three or more suggests that the linkage is likely to be genuine.

Clinical Dermatology, Fifth Edition. Richard B. Weller, Hamish J.A. Hunter and Margaret W. Mann.
© 2015 John Wiley & Sons, Ltd. Published 2015 by John Wiley & Sons, Ltd.

Genome-wide association studies (GWASs). Large populations with a certain phenotype are scanned for the presence of SNPs. These phenotypes are then compared with a reference database to ascertain if any particular SNPs are associated with that particular phenotype. If they are, then sequencing of the section of genome marked by the SNPs may identify disease-causing genes. The technique is especially useful in investigating common conditions with complex modes of inheritance such as psoriasis and eczema.

In situ hybridization. A cloned sequence of DNA, if made single-stranded by heat, will stick to its complementary sequence on a chromosome. Radioactive or fluorescent labelling can be used to indicate its position there.

DNA microarray analysis. This is used to study the expression of multiple genes simultaneously in a given biological tissue. It again relies on the principle of complementary hybridization. Thousands of cDNA or oligonucleotide probes (a specific known DNA sequence) are bonded to a solid surface (glass slide or silicon chip) at a particular site to form a grid; these may be specific to a particular gene or mutation. mRNA is extracted from the tissue under investigation, reverse transcribed into cDNA and labelled with a fluorescent marker. This is then incubated with the microarray and hybridization occurs. The intensity of fluorescence corresponds to the strength of hybridization and hence to the expression of the gene or sequence under investigation. Complex statistical software is used to analyse the results. This technology has been used to identify the over- or under-expression of genes, the frequency of gene mutations and the occurrence of SNPs in many malignant and inflammatory skin conditions. It should be remembered that just because a gene is over- or under-expressed this might not necessarily correspond to its expression at a protein level. Recently, multiple arrays have been combined in high-throughput gene expression profiling platforms. These have enabled the screening of multiple samples at once, dramatically simplifying the screening of larger clinical populations.

Non-Mendelian genetics

Traditional genetics has also been extended by the introduction of several new non-Mendelian concepts of importance in dermatology.

1 *Mosaicism.* A mosaic is a single individual made up of two or more genetically distinct cell lines. The concept is important in several skin disorders including incontinentia pigmenti (p. 348) and segmental neurofibromatosis (p. 345). The mutation of a single cell in a fetus (a post-zygotic mutation) may form a clone of abnormal cells. In the epidermis these often adopt a bizarre pattern of lines and whorls – Blaschko's lines, named after the dermatologist who recorded them in linear epidermal naevi in 1901.

2 *Contiguous gene deletions.* Complex phenotypes occur when several adjacent genes are lost. In this way, for example, X-linked ichthyosis may associate with hypogonadism or anosmia.

3 *Genomic imprinting* means that genes may differ in their effect depending on the parent from which they are inherited. Genes from the father seem especially important in psoriasis, and from the mother in atopy (p. 88).

4 *Uniparental disomy* occurs when both of a pair of genes are derived from the same parent so that an individual lacks either a maternal or a paternal copy. In this way a disorder usually inherited as a recessive trait can arise even though only one parent is a carrier.

5 *Mitochondrial mutations* can cause genodermatoses (e.g. one type of palmoplantar keratoderma). The condition is passed from the mother to both male and female offspring, but affected males do not pass it on to their offspring.

Gene expression may be altered even when the genetic code (DNA sequence) remains unchanged; rarely, these changes may be inherited from one generation to the next. The study of these phenomena is termed epigenetics. There are three broad epigenetic mechanisms: (i) DNA hypermethylation tending to supress gene transcription; (ii) modification of histone proteins (proteins tightly associated with DNA to form chromatin), with acetylation being the most studied usually resulting in activation of genes; (iii) the presence of microRNA genes which themselves do not code for a protein but affect the transcription of other genes. Epigenetic changes are thought to have a role in the pathogenesis of multiple inflammatory and malignant skin conditions.

Two other important genetic concepts are *clinical heterogeneity* (when clinically distinct phenotypes are produced by different mutations within the same gene, such as red hair variants caused by different polymorphisms of the *MC1R* gene) and *genetic heterogeneity* (when the same clinical picture can be produced by mutations in different genes, as in tuberous sclerosis).

Inheritance is important in many of the conditions discussed in other chapters and this has been highlighted in the sections on aetiology. This chapter includes some genetic disorders not covered elsewhere.

Red hair

Red hair is not, of course, a disease but it is the first normal variation in human appearance for which a causative genetic polymorphism was found. The melanocortin-1 receptor (*MC1R*) gene is found at 16q24.3. While at least 30 genetic variants have been described, three in particular are associated with an increased phaeo- (red) to eu- (black) melanin ratio. Individuals homozygous or heterozygous for one or two of these 'red hair alleles' are likely to have pale skin, red hair and poor tanning ability.

The neurofibromatoses

These relatively common disorders affect about 1 in 3500 people and are inherited as an autosomal dominant trait. There are two main types: von Recklinghausen's neurofibromatosis (NF1; which accounts for 85% of all cases) and bilateral acoustic neurofibromatosis (NF2); these are phenotypically and genetically distinct.

NF1

Cause
The *NF1* gene has been localized to chromosome 17q11.2. It is unusually large (300 kb) and many different mutations within it have now been identified. The *NF1* gene is a tumour suppressor gene, the product of which, neurofibromin, interacts with the product of the *RAS* protooncogene. This may explain the susceptibility of NF1 patients to a variety of tumours. The inheritance of NF1 is as an autosomal dominant trait but about half of index cases have no preceding family history. Recently, microRNA expression has been implicated in the control of the *NF1* gene.

Clinical features
The physical signs include the following:
• Six or more café au lait patches (light brown oval macules; Figure 24.1), usually developing in the first year of life.
• Axillary freckling (Figure 24.2) in two-thirds of affected individuals.
• Variable numbers of skin neurofibromas, some small and superficial, others larger and deeper, ranging from flesh-coloured to pink, purple or brown (Figure 24.1). Most are dome-like nodules, but others are irregular raised plaques. Some are firm, some soft and compressible through a deficient dermis ('button-hole' sign); others feel

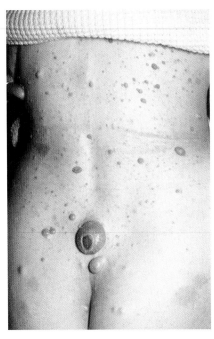

Figure 24.1 Neurofibromatosis: one large but benign neurofibroma has ulcerated over the sacrum. Several café au lait patches are visible.

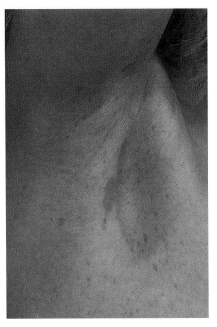

Figure 24.2 Freckling of the axilla and a café au lait patch – both markers of neurofibromatosis.

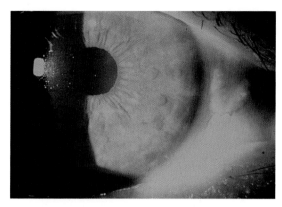

Figure 24.3 Lisch nodules: best seen with a slit-lamp.

'knotty' or 'wormy'. Neurofibromas may not appear until puberty and become larger and more numerous with age.
• Small circular pigmented hamartomas of the iris (Lisch nodules; Figure 24.3) appear in early childhood.

Nearly all NF1 patients meet the National Institutes of Health (NIH) criteria for diagnosis (Table 24.1) by the age of 8 years, and all do so by 20 years. The usual order of appearance of the clinical features is café au lait macules, axillary freckling, Lisch nodules and neurofibromas.

Diagnosis

The café au lait marks, axillary freckling and Lisch nodules should be looked for, as they appear before the skin neurofibromas. A segmental form of NF1 is caused by a post-zygotic mutation, a form of genetic mosaicism. Isolated neurofibromas are not uncommon in individuals without neurofibromatosis and are of little consequence unless they are painful. Genetic testing is now available; it is especially useful in borderline cases where diagnostic uncertainty exists, for example a young individual with a

Table 24.1 National institute for health diagnostic criteria for neurofibromatosis type 1 (NF1).

Two or more criteria are required for a diagnosis of NF1:
• Six or more café au lait macules (>5 mm in children or >15 mm in adults)
• Two or more cutaneous or subcutaneous neurofibromas or one plexiform neurofibroma
• Axillary or groin freckling
• Optic pathway glioma
• Two or more Lisch nodules
• Bony dysplasia
• First-degree relative with NF1

single diagnostic criterion. It may also have a role in prenatal diagnosis.

Complications

A neurofibroma will occasionally change into a neurofibrosarcoma. Other associated features include kyphoscoliosis, learning impairment, epilepsy, renal artery stenosis and an association with phaeochromocytoma. Forme fruste variants occur (e.g. segmental neurofibromatosis).

Management

Ugly or painful lesions, and any suspected of undergoing malignant change, should be surgically removed. Several medical therapies are currently under evaluation but to date none have been approved. The chance of a child of an affected adult developing the disorder is 1 in 2 – parents should be advised about this. Those who are affected should be kept under review and have their blood pressure checked regularly.

NF2

Cause

The inheritance of *NF2* is also autosomal dominant. Mapping to chromosome 22q11.21 followed the observation of changes in chromosome 22 in meningiomas as these tumours may be seen in *NF2*. This gene also normally functions as a tumour-suppressor gene, the product of which is known as Merlin.

Clinical features

• Bilateral acoustic neuromas.
• Few, if any, cutaneous manifestations.
• No Lisch nodules.
• Other tumours of the central nervous system may occur, especially meningiomas and gliomas.

Management

All NF2 patients and their families should have access to genetic testing as presymptomatic diagnosis improves clinical management. Clinical screening for at-risk family members can start at birth.

Tuberous sclerosis

This uncommon condition, with a prevalence of about 1 in 12 000 in children under 10 years, is inherited as an autosomal dominant trait, with variable expressivity even within the same family; thought to be a consequence of mosaicism. Fertility is reduced, so transmission through more than two generations is rare.

Cause

Inactivating mutations at two different loci can, independently, cause clinically identical tuberous sclerosis. Both genes are tumour suppressors. The product of one (*TSC1* on chromosome *9q34*) is hamartin; that encoded by the other (*TSC2* on *16p13.3*) is tuberin. Hamartin and tuberin form a complex, and this may explain why changes in the production of either cause a similar disease phenotype. Familial cases are equally likely to result from mutations in the *TSC1* or *TSC2* genes. In contrast to this, sporadic mutations, which account for two-thirds of all cases, are four times more likely to result from changes in the *TSC2* gene. Mutations in the *TSC2* gene tend to cause a more severe spectrum of disease.

Clinical features

The skin changes include the following.
- *Small oval white patches* (ash leaf macules) occur in over 90% of those affected; three or more are required for them to be of significance. These are important, as they may be the only manifestation at birth. Smaller hypopigmented confetti-like macules are a minor feature of the disease.
- *Angiofibromas* (previously known as adenoma sebaceum*)* occur in about 80% of those affected. They develop at puberty as pink or yellowish acne-like papules on the face, often around the nose (Figure 24.4).
- *Forehead fibrous plaques* are yellowish brown in colour and occur in about 20% of affected individuals.
- *Peri-ungual fibromas* occur in about 15% of patients. These develop in adult life as small pink sausage-like lesions emerging from the nail folds. To be suggestive of the diagnosis there should be no history of digital trauma (Figure 24.5).
- *Connective tissue naevi* (shagreen patches) are seen in 50% of patients. Cobblestone, somewhat yellow, plaques often arise in the skin over the base of the spine.

Other features include:
- Epilepsy (in over 90% of patients);
- Mental retardation (in 50% of patients);
- Ocular signs, including retinal phakomas and pigmentary abnormalities (in 50% of patients);
- Gingival fibromas, which may be exacerbated by antiepileptic drug induced gingival hyperplasia;
- Gliomas along the lateral walls of the lateral ventricles (80% of cases) and calcification of the basal ganglia; and
- Renal and heart tumours.

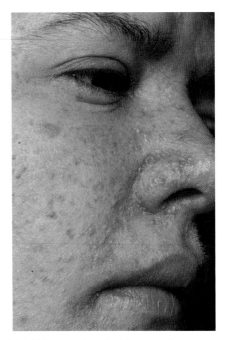

Figure 24.4 Tuberous sclerosis. Adenoma sebaceum, understandably, was referred to the acne clinic.

Diagnosis and differential diagnosis

Any baby with unexplained epilepsy should be examined with a Wood's light (p. 37) to look for ash leaf macules. Skull X-rays and computed tomography scans (Figure 24.6) help to exclude involvement of the central nervous system and kidneys. The differential diagnosis for ash leaf macules includes vitiligo and naevus anaemicus. The lesions of adenoma sebaceum (a misnomer, as

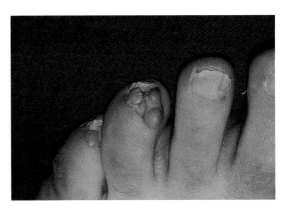

Figure 24.5 The peri-ungual fibromas of tuberous sclerosis are found in adult patients.

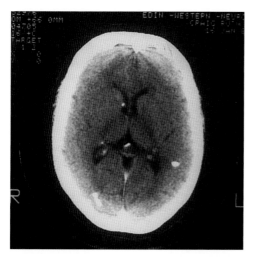

Figure 24.6 Computed tomography scan of a patient with tuberous sclerosis. Modern imaging techniques can sometimes show cortical tubers (white) even when the skin changes are minimal.

histologically they are angiofibromas) may be mistaken for acne. Recently, genetic testing for *TSC1* and *TSC2* mutations has become available; this may be useful in prenatal diagnosis in affected families or when there is diagnostic uncertainty.

Management

Affected families need genetic counselling. Apparently unaffected parents with an affected child will wish to know the chances of further children being affected. Before concluding that an affected child is the result of a new mutation, the parents should be examined with a Wood's light and by an ophthalmologist to help exclude the possibility of genetic transmission from a subtly affected parent. This should be combined with genetic testing of family members.

Facial angiofibromas may improve cosmetically after electrodessication, dermabrasion or destruction by laser, but tend to recur.

Trials of the immunosuppressant rapamycin are ongoing in the treatment of several of the clinical manifestations of tuberous sclerosis. Initial results show some promise.

Xeroderma pigmentosum

Xeroderma pigmentosum is a heterogeneous group of autosomal recessive disorders, characterized by the defec-

tive repair of DNA after its damage by ultraviolet radiation. The condition is rare, affecting about 5 per million in Europe.

Cause

Ultraviolet light damages DNA by producing covalent linkages between adjacent pyrimidines. These distort the double helix and inhibit gene expression. Cells from xeroderma pigmentosum patients lack the ability of normal cells to repair this damage.

DNA repair is a complex process using a large number of genes that encode a variety of interacting products that locate and prepare damaged sites for excision and replacement. It is not surprising therefore that several genetic defects have been shown to lead to a similar clinical picture.

Clinical features

There are many variants but all follow the same pattern.
• The skin is normal at birth.
• Photosensitivity. Some patients, but not all, are exquisitely sensitive to ultraviolet light, developing severe sunburn on minimal exposure.
• Multiple freckles, roughness and keratoses on exposed skin appear between the ages of 6 months and 2 years (Figure 24.7).
• The atrophic facial skin shows telangiectases and small angiomas.
• Many tumours develop on sun-exposed skin: basal cell carcinomas, squamous cell carcinomas, keratoacanthomas and malignant melanomas. Many patients die before the age of 20 years.
• Eye problems are common and include photophobia, conjunctivitis and ectropion.

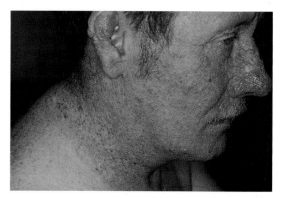

Figure 24.7 Xeroderma pigmentosum: obvious freckling on neck. Scars on nose mark the spots where tumours have been removed.

- The condition may be associated with microcephaly, mental deficiency, dwarfism, deafness and ataxia (De Sanctis–Cacchione syndrome).
- Progressive neurological deficit. Up to one-quarter of patients develop significant neurological decline.

Diagnosis

This becomes evident on clinical grounds, although variants with minor signs may cause difficulty. The DNA repair defect can be detected in a few laboratories after the ultraviolet irradiation of cultured fibroblasts or lymphocytes from the patient.

Treatment

Skin cancers can be prevented by strict avoidance of sunlight, the use of protective clothing, wide-brimmed hats, reflectant sunscreen and dark glasses. Windows can be tinted or fitted with ultraviolet filters at home, school and work. If possible, patients should not go out by day. Early and complete removal of all tumours is essential. Radiotherapy should be avoided. Cutaneous gene therapy may be a possibility in the future. Vitamin D supplementation should not be forgotten in these patients.

Incontinentia pigmenti

This rare condition is inherited as an X-linked dominant disorder. It is usually lethal before birth in males whereas affected females, mosaic as a result of X-inactivation, can survive. The bizarre patterning of the skin is caused by this random X-inactivation (lyonization). The lines of affected and normal skin represent clones of cells in which either the abnormal or normal X chromosome is active. The majority of cases result from a deletion in the nuclear factor-κB modulator gene (*NEMO*); mapped to Xq28. It is a component of a signalling pathway (the NF-κB pathway) that controls the expression of several genes responsible for cytokines.

Clinical features

Skin changes are usually present at birth but may sometimes develop over the first few days of life. There are four stages in their evolution.
1 *Vesicular*. Linear groups of blisters occur more on the limbs than trunk.
2 *Warty*. After a few weeks the blisters dry up and the predominant lesions are papules with a verrucous hyperkeratotic surface.

3 *Pigmented*. A whorled or 'splashed' macular pigmentation, ranging from slate-grey to brown, replaces the warty lesions. Its bizarre patterning follows Blaschko lines and is a strong diagnostic pointer.
4 *Hypopigmented*. Wave-like, hypopigmented, hairless, anhidrotic or atrophic streaks develop, most commonly on the posterior aspects of the calves.

Occasionally, the vesicular and warty stages occur *in utero*; warty or pigmented lesions may therefore be the first signs of the condition.

Associated abnormalities are common. Between 10 and 30% of affected individuals have defects of their central nervous system, most commonly mental retardation, epilepsy or microcephaly. Skull and palatal abnormalities may also be found. Delayed dentition, and even a total absence of teeth, are recognized features. The incisors may be cone- or peg-shaped. Ocular defects occur in one-third of patients, the most common being strabismus, cataract and optic atrophy.

Differential diagnosis

Diagnosis is usually made in infancy when bullous lesions predominate so the differential diagnosis includes bullous impetigo (p. 215), candidiasis (p. 243) and the rarer linear immunoglobulin A (IgA) bullous disease of childhood (p. 119) and epidermolysis bullosa (p. 122).

Investigations

The diagnosis is usually clinical. Genetic testing for deletions in the *NEMO* gene is possible when there is diagnostic uncertainty. There is frequently an eosinophilia in the blood. Biopsy of an intact blister reveals an intraepidermal vesicle filled with eosinophils.

Management

This is symptomatic and includes measures to combat bacterial and candidal infection during the vesicular phase. Family counselling should be available.

Ehlers–Danlos syndrome

This heterogeneous group of conditions has a worldwide prevalence of between 1 in 10 000 and 1 in 20 000 live births. Currently, there are six major subtypes. The classic and hypermobility subtypes account for 90% of cases; the vascular subtype for less than 10% and the remaining cases are attributed to much rarer variants.

Cause

All subtypes of the Ehlers–Danlos syndrome are based on abnormalities in the formation or modification of collagen (types I, III and V) and the extracellular matrix, but are not necessarily a result of mutations in the collagen genes themselves. Established defects include mutations in the collagen V, alpha-1 and alpha-2 genes (classical subtype) and collagen III, alpha-1 gene (vascular subtype). Less common subtypes result from mutations in collagen I, alpha-1 and alpha-2 genes and genes coding for the lysyl hydroxylase and procollagen N-peptidase enzymes.

Clinical features

- Soft hyperelastic skin.
- Hyperextensibility of the joints.
- Fragility of skin and blood vessels.
- Easy bruising.
- Curious ('cigarette paper') scars.
  Sometimes these changes are so mild that the condition is not recognized.

Complications

These depend on the type: subluxation of joints; varicose veins in early life; an increased liability to develop hernias; kyphoscoliosis; and intraocular complications. Individuals may be born prematurely as a result of the early rupture of fragile fetal membranes. The vascular subtype is potentially the most dangerous. It may present as an emergency in adulthood with arterial dissection, pneumothorax or visceral rupture. The delay in diagnosis of this form may be explained by the relatively milder skin hyperextensibility than is seen in other subtypes.

Diagnosis and treatment

The diagnosis is made on the clinical features and family history. The frequent skin lacerations and prominent scars may suggest childhood non-accidental injury. The diagnosis and type can sometimes be confirmed by enzyme studies on isolated fibroblasts. There is no effective treatment but genetic counselling is needed.

Pseudoxanthoma elasticum

This is the classic inherited connective tissue disorder characterized by aberrant mineralization of the elastic structures in the body – most obviously in the skin, blood vessels and eyes. Patients usually present in adolescence with skin signs. Type I is associated with systemic manifestations whereas type II is much rarer with signs confined to the skin.

Cause

It is a metabolic disorder, inherited as an autosomal recessive condition, resulting from mutations in two different genes. The *ABCC6* gene, a member of the ABC transporters superfamily is located on chromosome 16 at 16p13.1 and encodes a transmembrane transporter protein. It is not known exactly how mutations in this gene cause the disease but it is thought that they may prevent the release of circulating 'antimineralization' factors from the liver. The other gene implicated is *GGCX*, located on chromosome 2 at 2p12 and encodes the enzyme gammaglutamyl carboxylase. It is thought to be important in preventing aberrant calcium and phosphate deposition in normal tissue.

Pathology

The elastic fibres in the mid-dermis become swollen and fragmented with progressive aberrant deposition of calcium and phosphate within their substance. The elastic tissue of blood vessels and of the retina may also be affected.

Clinical features

The skin of the neck and axillae, and occasionally of other body folds, is loose and wrinkled. Groups of small yellow papules give these areas a 'plucked chicken' appearance (Figure 24.8). Breaks in the retina show as angioid streaks, which are grey, poorly defined areas radiating from the optic nerve head. Arterial involvement may lead to peripheral, coronary or cerebral arterial insufficiency.

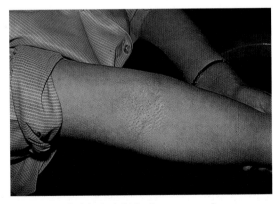

Figure 24.8 The 'plucked chicken' appearance of pseudoxanthoma in the antecubital fossa.

Complications

The most important are hypertension, recurrent gut haemorrhages, ischaemic heart disease and cerebral haemorrhage. Pregnancy is always accompanied by striae and there is an increased risk of miscarriage.

Diagnosis and treatment

The diagnosis is made clinically and confirmed by the histology. Molecular testing for certain mutations is possible. Currently, there is no effective treatment. Blood pressure should be carefully monitored and controlled.

> **Learning point**
>
> In all genodermatoses, the decision to have children, or not, must lie with the family concerned. Make sure they have all of the facts before them.

Further reading

Boyd KP, Korf BR, Theos A. (2009) Neurofibromatosis type 1. *Journal of the American Academy of Dermatology* **61**, 1–14.

DiGiovanna JJ, Kraemer KH. (2012) Shining a light on xeroderma pigmentosum. *Journal of Investigative Dermatology* **132**, 785–796.

Fernandes NF, Schwartz RA. (2008) A "hyperextensive" review of Ehlers–Danlos syndrome. *Cutis* **82**, 242–248.

Grada A, Weinbrecht K. (2013) Next-generation sequencing: methodology and application. *Journal of Investigative Dermatology* **133**, e11.

Gutmann DH, Aylsworth A, Carey JC, et al. (1997) The diagnostic evaluation and multidisciplinary management of neurofibromatosis 1 and neurofibromatosis 2. *Journal of the American Medical Association* **278**, 51–57.

Hadj-Rabia S, Rimell A, Smahi A, et al. (2011) Clinical and histological features of incontinentia pigmenti in adults with nuclear factor-κB essential modulator gene mutations. *Journal of the American Academy of Dermatology* **64**, 508–515.

Huson SM. (2006) The neurofibromatosis: more than just a medical curiosity. *Journal of the Royal College of Physicians Edinburgh* **36**, 44–50.

Irvine MD, McLean WHI. (2003) The molecular genetics of the genodermatoses: progress to date and future directions. *British Journal of Dermatology* **148**, 1–13.

Kimball AB, Grant RA, Wang F, et al. (2012) Beyond the blot: cutting edge tools for genomics, proteomics and metabolomics analyses and previous successes. *British Journal of Dermatology* **166** (Suppl. 2), 1–8.

Kwon EM, Basel D, Siegel D, et al. (2013) A review of next-generation genetic testing for the dermatologist. *Paediatric Dermatology* **30**, 401–408.

Murphy MJ. (2011) Introduction to molecular diagnostics in dermatology and dermatopathology. In Murphy MJ (ed). *Molecular Diagnostics in Dermatology and Dermatopathology: Current Clinical Pathology.* Humana Press, New York: 1–12.

Online Mendelian Inheritance in Man (OMIM) website. http://www.ncbi.nlm.nih.gov/omim/ (accessed 3 July 2014).

Phan TA, Wargon O, Turner AM. (2005) Incontinentia pigmenti case series: clinical spectrum of incontinentia pigmenti in 53 female patients and their relatives. *Clinical and Experimental Dermatology* **30**, 474–480.

Qiaoli L, Jiang Q, Pfendner E, et al. (2009) Pseudoxanthoma elasticum: clinical phenotypes, molecular genetics and putative pathomechanisms. *Experimental Dermatology* **18**, 1–11.

Rees JL. (2000) Genetics, past and present, and the rise of systems dermatology. *British Journal of Dermatology* **143**, 41–46.

Schwartz RA, Fernandez G, Kotulska K, et al. (2007) Tuberous sclerosis complex: advances in diagnosis, genetics and management. *Journal of the American Academy of Dermatology* **57**, 189–202.

Spitz JL. (2004) *Genodermatoses: A Clinical Guide to Genetic Skin Disorders*, 2nd edition. Lippincott Williams & Wilkins, Philadelphia.

25   Drug Eruptions

Almost any drug can cause a cutaneous reaction, and many inflammatory skin conditions can be caused or exacerbated by drugs. A drug reaction can reasonably be included in the differential diagnosis of most skin diseases.

Mechanisms

These are many and various (Table 25.1), being related both to the properties of the drug in question and to a variety of host factors. Drug trials have traditionally studied average population responses to drugs, but the increasing ease with which genetic differences between individuals can be measured offers the promise of personalized medicine. Genetically predicted variations in response – both beneficial and adverse – to a drug will be used to guide the right dose and type of drug for individual patients (pharmacogenetics). For example, drug-induced lupus erythematosus occurs more commonly among 'slow acetylators' who take hydralazine. However, not all adverse drug reactions have a genetic basis; the excess of drug eruptions seen in the elderly may reflect drug interactions associated with their high medication intake.

Non-allergic drug reactions

Not all drug reactions are based on allergy. Some are a result of overdosage, others to the accumulation of drugs or to unwanted pharmacological effects (e.g. stretch marks from systemic steroids; Figure 25.1). Other reactions are idiosyncratic (an odd reaction peculiar to one individual) or a result of alterations of ecological balance (see below).

Cutaneous reactions can be expected from the very nature of some drugs. These are normal but unwanted responses. Patients show them when a drug is given in a high dose, or even in a therapeutic dose. For example, mouth ulcers may occur as a result of the cytotoxicity of methotrexate. Silver-based preparations, given for prolonged periods, can lead to a slate-grey colour of the skin (argyria). Acute vaginal candidiasis occurs when antibiotics remove the normal resident bacteria from the female genital tract and so foster colonization by yeasts. Dapsone or rifampicin, given to patients with lepromatous leprosy, may cause erythema nodosum leprosum as the immune response to the bacillus is re-established.

Non-allergic reactions are often predictable. They affect many, or even all, patients taking the drug at a sufficient dosage for a sufficient time. Careful studies before marketing should indicate the types of reaction that can be anticipated.

Allergic drug reactions

Allergic drug reactions are less predictable. They occur in only a minority of patients receiving a drug and can do so even with low doses. Allergic reactions are not a normal biological effect of the drug and usually appear after the latent period required for induction of an immune response. Chemically related drugs may cross-react.

The majority of allergic drug reactions are caused by type IV cell-mediated immune reactions (p. 25), which can present in a number of forms, most commonly a maculopapular eruption or morbilliform erythema. Rarer allergic reactions include bullae, erythroderma, pruritus, toxic epidermal necrolysis (TEN), acute generalized exanthematous pustulosis (AGEP) and the drug rash with eosinophilia and systemic signs (DRESS) syndrome. Helper CD4+ T cells occur more frequently in the more common morbilliform eruptions, while cytotoxic CD8+ T cells predominate in blistering eruptions (TEN, Stevens–Johnson syndrome) and fixed drug eruptions. Other types of drug reaction include urticaria and angioedema, generally resulting from IgE-mediated type I hypersensitivity reactions, and vasculitis generally caused by type III immune complex-mediated reactions (p. 25).

Clinical Dermatology, Fifth Edition. Richard B. Weller, Hamish J.A. Hunter and Margaret W. Mann.
© 2015 John Wiley & Sons, Ltd. Published 2015 by John Wiley & Sons, Ltd.

Table 25.1 Some mechanisms involved in drug reactions.

Pharmacological
    Caused by overdosage or failure to excrete or metabolize
    Cumulative effects
    Altered skin ecology
Allergic
    IgE-mediated
    Cytotoxic
    Immune complex-mediated
    Cell-mediated
Idiosyncratic
Exacerbation of pre-existing skin conditions

Table 25.2 The six vital questions to be asked when a drug eruption is suspected.

1 Can you exclude a simple dermatosis (such as scabies or psoriasis) and the known skin manifestations of an underlying disorder (e.g. systemic lupus erythematosus)?
2 Does the rash itself suggest a drug eruption (e.g. urticaria, erythema multiforme)?
3 Does a past history of drug reactions correlate with current prescriptions?
4 Was any drug introduced a few days or weeks before the eruption appeared?
5 Which of the current drugs most commonly cause drug eruptions (e.g. penicillins, sulfonamides, thiazides, allopurinol, phenylbutazone)?
6 Does the eruption fit with a well-recognized pattern caused by one of the current drugs (e.g. an acneiform rash from lithium)?

The factors that lead to particular clinical patterns of cutaneous adverse drug reactions remain largely unexplained.

Presentation

Some drugs and the reactions they can cause

Experience helps here, together with a knowledge of the reactions most likely to be caused by individual drugs, and also of the most common causes of the various reaction patterns. Any unusual rash, especially if polymorphic (variation in appearance of rash), should be suspected of being a drug reaction, and approached along the lines listed in Table 25.2.

Antibiotics

Penicillins and sulfonamides are among the drugs most commonly causing allergic reactions. These are often morbilliform (Figure 25.2), but urticaria, erythema multiforme and fixed eruptions are common too. Viral infections are often associated with exanthems, and many rashes are incorrectly blamed on an antibiotic when, in fact, the virus was responsible. Most patients with infectious mononucleosis develop a morbilliform rash if ampicillin is administered. Penicillin is a common cause of severe anaphylactic reactions, which can be life-threatening. Minocycline can accumulate in the tissues and produce a brown or grey colour in the mucosa, sun-exposed areas or at sites of inflammation, as in the lesions of acne. Minocycline can rarely cause the hypersensitivity syndrome reaction, hepatitis, worsen lupus erythematosus or elicit a transient lupus-like syndrome.

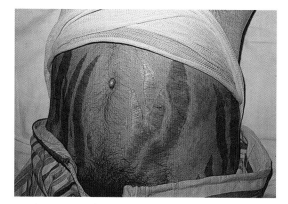

Figure 25.1 Gross striae caused by systemic steroids.

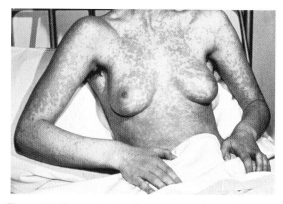

Figure 25.2 Symmetrical erythematous maculopapular rash as a result of ampicillin.

Trimethoprim, now regularly used as a second-line antibiotic for the treatment of acne, can cause an idiosyncratic eruption between days 7 and 14 of therapy; the rash is usually maculopapular or morbilliform in appearance but TEN has been reported.

Penicillamine

Like penicillin itself, penicillamine can cause morbilliform eruptions or urticaria, but the drug has also been incriminated as a cause of haemorrhagic bullae at sites of trauma, of the extrusion of elastic tissue through the skin, and of pemphigus.

Oral contraceptives

Reactions to these are less common now that their hormonal content is small. The hair fall that may follow stopping the drug is like that seen after pregnancy (telogen effluvium; p. 178). Chloasma, hirsutism, erythema nodosum, acne and photosensitivity may also occur.

Gold

This frequently causes rashes. Its side effects range from pruritus to morbilliform eruptions, to curious papulosquamous eruptions such as pityriasis rosea or lichen planus. Erythroderma, erythema nodosum, hair fall and stomatitis may also be provoked by gold.

Steroids

Cutaneous side effects from systemic steroids include a ruddy face, cutaneous atrophy, striae (Figure 25.1), hirsutism, an acneiform eruption and a susceptibility to cutaneous infections, which may be atypical.

Anticonvulsants

Skin reactions to phenytoin, carbamazepine, lamotrigine and phenobarbitol are common and include erythematous, morbilliform, urticarial and purpuric rashes. TEN, erythema multiforme, exfoliative dermatitis, DRESS and a lupus erythematosus-like syndrome are fortunately rarer. About 1% of patients taking lamotrigine develop Stevens–Johnson syndrome or TEN. A phenytoin-induced pseudolymphoma syndrome has also been described in which fever and arthralgia are accompanied by generalized lymphadenopathy and hepatosplenomegaly and, sometimes, some of the above skin signs. Long-term treatment with phenytoin may cause gingival hyperplasia (Figure 25.3) and coarsening of the features as a result of fibroblast proliferation.

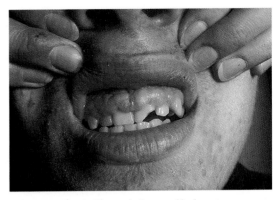

Figure 25.3 Gingival hyperplasia caused by long-term phenytoin treatment.

Highly active antiretroviral drugs

Long-term highly active antiretroviral treatment (HAART) has commonly been associated with lipodystrophy, producing a gaunt facies with sunken cheeks. Interactions between highly active antiretroviral drugs and antituberculous drugs are common.

Biological agents

The antitumour necrosis factor α therapies (etanercept, infliximab and adalimumab) are used extensively in the treatment of severe psoriasis and have all been associated with a lupus erythematosus-like cutaneous reaction. This may be associated with positive autoantibodies but rarely presents with systemic involvement. It usually settles on withdrawal of the drug. Cetuximab and erlotinib are monoclonal antibodies to epidermal growth factor receptors (EGFR) used to treat bowel and lung cancers. These antineoplastic antibodies and their cousins commonly cause a distinctive widespread eruption with follicular pustules that resembles acne. This is because sweat and hair follicle cells express EGFR and the drug causes changes in these structures leading to follicular eruptions. Other side effects are xerosis, fissures of the palms and soles, altered hair growth and paronychia. Many experts feel this is dose-related and not allergic as they may be able to reinstitute the drug at lower dosage, after 1–2 weeks, without recurrence.

Some common reaction patterns and drugs that can cause them

Toxic (reactive) erythema

This vague term describes the most common type of drug eruption, looking sometimes like measles or scarlet fever, and sometimes showing prominent urticarial

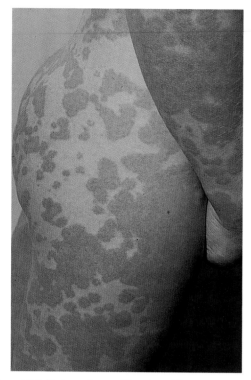

Figure 25.4 Toxic erythema with urticarial features.

(Figure 25.4) or erythema multiforme-like elements. Itching and fever may accompany the rash. Culprits include antibiotics (especially ampicillin), sulfonamides and related compounds (diuretics and hypoglycaemics), barbiturates, phenylbutazone and para-aminosalicylate (PAS).

Urticaria (see Chapter 8)
Many drugs may cause this but salicylates are the most common, followed by angiotensin-converting enzyme (ACE) inhibitors, non-steroidal anti-inflammatory drugs (NSAIDs) and opiates which often work non-immunologically as histamine releasers. Antibiotics are also common culprits. Insect repellents and nitrogen mustards can cause urticaria on contact. Urticaria may be part of a severe and generalized reaction (anaphylaxis) which includes bronchospasm and collapse (Figure 25.5).

Allergic vasculitis (see Chapter 8)
The clinical changes range from urticarial papules, through palpable purpura to necrotic ulcers. Erythema nodosum may occur. Sulfonamides, beta-lactam antibiotics, diuretics, NSAIDs, phenytoin and oral contracep-

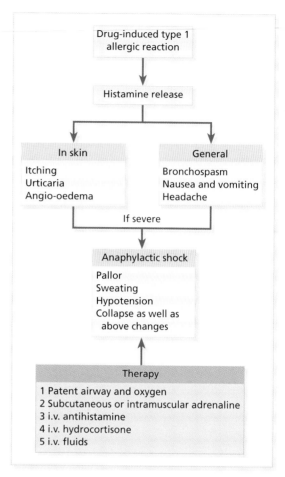

Figure 25.5 The cause, clinical features and treatment of anaphylaxis.

tives are among the possible causes. These disorders are caused by circulating immune complexes of drug and antibody (type III reaction; p. 25). Fever, gut and joint inflammations may be present (serum sickness). Nephropathy is usually mild here, if present at all.

Erythema multiforme (see Chapter 8)
Target-like lesions appear mainly on the extensor aspects of the limbs, and bullae may form. In the Stevens–Johnson syndrome, patients are often ill and the mucous membranes are severely affected. Sulfonamides, barbiturates, lamotrigine and phenylbutazone are known offenders.

Ulceration
Rarely, non-healing ulcers may be attributed to a drug eruption. Nicorandil has been associated with mucosal

(oral, genital, peri-anal and peri-stomal) and leg ulceration. Long-term hydroxycarbamide, commonly used in the treatment of myeloproliferative disorders, can cause painful leg ulceration. Ulceration usually improves following drug withdrawal.

Purpura

The clinical features are seldom distinctive apart from the itchy brown petechial rash on dependent areas that is characteristic of carbromal reactions. Thrombocytopenia and coagulation defects should be excluded (see Chapter 11). Thiazides, sulfonamides, phenylbutazone, sulfonylureas, barbiturates, quinine and anticoagulants are among the drugs causing purpura.

Bullous eruptions

Some of the reactions noted above can become bullous (e.g. Stevens–Johnson syndrome). Bullae may also develop at pressure sites in drug-induced coma. Vancomycin, lithium, diclofenac, captopril, furosemide and amiodarone are associated with development of linear IgA bullous disease (p. 119). Granulocyte–macrophage colony-stimulating factor can induce an eosinophilia and unmask a dormant bullous pemphigoid or epidermolysis bullosa acquisita. Like porphyia cutanea tarda, pseudoporphyria makes photoexposed skin fragile, prone to blisters and causes scarring, but porphyin studies are normal. Suspect NSAIDs, furosemide, retinoids or tetracyclines.

Eczema

This is not a common pattern and occurs mainly when patients sensitized by topical applications are given the drug systemically. Penicillin, sulfonamides, neomycin, phenothiazines and local anaesthetics should be considered. Retinoids may exacerbate pre-existing eczema.

Exfoliative erythroderma

The entire skin surface becomes red and scaly. This can be caused by drugs (particularly phenylbutazone, PAS, isoniazid, vancomycin and gold), but can also be caused by widespread psoriasis, lymphomas and eczema.

Fixed drug eruptions

Round, erythematous or purple, and sometimes bullous plaques recur at the same site each time the drug is taken (Figure 25.6). Pigmentation persists between acute episodes. The glans penis seems to be a favoured site. The causes of fixed drug eruptions in any country follow the local patterns of drug usage there, but these change

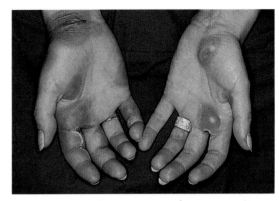

Figure 25.6 Fixed drug eruption – an unusually severe bullous reaction.

as old drugs drop out of use and are replaced by new ones with an unknown potential for causing this type of reaction. For example, in the United Kingdom, three of the four most common causes of fixed drug eruptions in 1970 (barbiturates, phenolphthalein and oxyphenbutazone) are no longer common causes. Paracetamol is currently the most common offender in the United Kingdom; trimethoprim-sulfa leads the list in the United States. NSAIDs (including aspirin), antibiotics, systemic antifungal agents and psychotropic drugs lie high on the list of other possible offenders.

Acneiform eruptions

Lithium, iodides, bromides, oral contraceptives, androgens or glucocorticosteroids, antituberculosis and anticonvulsant therapy may cause an acneiform rash (see Chapter 12) as may the monoclonal antibody drugs targeting EGFRs (see *Biological agents*). Always be suspicious of the illicit use of anabolic steroids in muscle-bound men with severe acne.

Lichenoid eruptions

These resemble lichen planus (see Chapter 6), but not always very closely as mouth lesions are uncommon and as scaling and eczematous elements may be seen. Consider antimalarials, NSAIDs, gold, phenothiazines and PAS.

Toxic epidermal necrolysis (p. 121)

In adults, this 'scalded skin' appearance is often drug-induced (e.g. sulfonamides, cephalosporins, quinolones, barbiturates, phenylbutazone, oxyphenbutazone, phenytoin, oxicams, carbamazepine, lamotrigine or penicillin).

Symmetrical drug-related intertriginous and flexural exanthema (SDRIFE)

As its name suggests, this drug eruption presents with sharply demarcated erythema of the gluteal and/or flexural areas. This newer acronym has superseded the previously used 'baboon syndrome'. It occurs hours to 2 days following drug exposure, is not associated with systemic symptoms and laboratory investigations are normal. The culprit drug is usually a beta-lactam antibiotic, commonly amoxicillin.

Acute generalized exanthematous pustulosis (AGEP) (Figure 25.7)

This disorder suggests acute pustular psoriasis, with a dramatic generalized eruption of red plaques studded with tiny sterile non-follicular pustules. Patients have fever and leucocytosis. Antibiotics, terbinafine, hydroxychloroquine and diltiazem are the most common drugs to induce AGEP, which usually develops within hours, lasts for a few days and then spontaneously resolves on withdrawal of the drug. Treatment is supportive and complications are unusual.

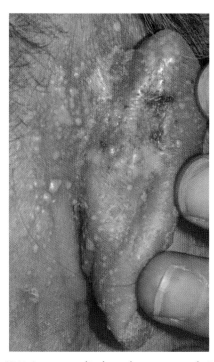

Figure 25.7 Acute generalized exanthematous pustulosis precipitated by amoxicillin.

Drug rash with eosinophilia and systemic signs (DRESS) syndrome

This syndrome includes the triad of fever, rash (from morbilliform to exfoliative dermatitis) and internal organ involvement (hepatitis, pneumonitis, nephritis and haematological abnormalities). An eosinophilia and lymphadenopathy also commonly occur. It characteristically develops 3–8 weeks after starting the causative drug. The most common culprits are anticonvulsants (particularly phenytoin, phenobarbital and carbamazepine), minocycline, allopurinol and sulfonamides.

Nephrogenic systemic fibrosis

This is a rare condition presenting in patients with end stage renal failure following exposure to gandolinium-based contrast media used to enhance magnetic resonance imaging (MRI) scans. It results in systemic fibrosis with cutaneous manifestations akin to scleromyxoedema (p. 132).

Hair loss

This is a predictable side effect of acitretin and cytotoxic agents, an unpredictable response to some anticoagulants and sometimes seen with antithyroid drugs. Diffuse hair loss may occur during, or just after, the use of an oral contraceptive.

Hypertrichosis

This is a dose-dependent effect of diazoxide, minoxidil and ciclosporin.

Pigmentation (p. 267)

Chloasma (p. 275) may follow an oral contraceptive plus sun exposure. Large doses of phenothiazines or amiodarone impart a blue–grey colour to exposed areas (Figure 25.8); heavy metals can cause a generalized browning; clofazimine makes the skin red; mepacrine turns the skin yellow; and minocycline turns areas of leg skin a curious greenish-grey colour that suggests a bruise.

Photosensitivity

This is dealt with in Chapter 18. Always exclude the common drug causes (thiazides, tetracyclines, phenothiazines, sulfonamides or psoralens).

Xerosis

The skin can become rough and scaly in patients receiving oral retinoids, nicotinic acid or lithium.

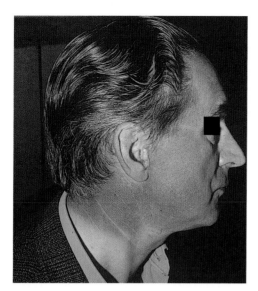

Figure 25.8 Note sparing of skin creases and area shielded by spectacle frames in this patient with photorelated hyperpigmentation from a phenothiazine drug.

Exacerbation of pre-existing skin conditions

Psoriasis and acne are good examples of this. Psoriasis may be made worse by giving β-blockers, antimalarials, terbinafine or lithium. Glucocorticoids, progesterone, androgens, anticonvulsants, bromides, iodides and lithium may exacerbate acne.

Course

The different types of reaction vary so much that a brief summary is not possible. If an allergic reaction occurs during the first course of treatment, it characteristically begins late, often about the ninth day, or even after the drug has been stopped. In such cases, it has taken that lag time to induce an immune reaction. In previously exposed patients the common morbilliform allergic reaction starts 2–3 days after the administration of the drug. The speed with which a drug eruption clears depends on the type of reaction and the rapidity with which the drug is eliminated.

Differential diagnosis

The differential diagnosis ranges over the whole subject of dermatology depending on which disease is mimicked.

For instance, toxic erythema reactions can look very like measles. The general rule is never to forget the possibility of a drug eruption when an atypical rash is seen. Six vital questions should be asked (Table 25.2).

Treatment

The first approach is to withdraw the suspected drug, accepting that several drugs may need to be stopped at the same time. This is not always easy as sometimes a drug is necessary and there is no alternative available. At other times the patient may be taking many drugs and it is difficult to know which one to stop. The decision to stop or continue a drug depends upon the nature of the drug, the necessity of using the drug for treatment, the availability of chemically unrelated alternatives, the severity of the reaction, its potential reversibility and the probability that the drug is actually causing the reaction.

Assessment depends upon clinical detective work (Table 25.2). Judgements must be based on probabilities and common sense. Every effort must be made to correlate the onset of the rash with prescription records. Often, but not always, the latest drug to be introduced is the most likely culprit. Prick tests and *in vitro* tests for allergy are still too unreliable to be of value. Re-administration, as a diagnostic test, is usually unwise except when no suitable alternative drug exists.

Skin biopsy can be helpful in excluding inflammatory conditions but the histopathological features of a drug eruption are often non-specific. However, the presence of necrotic keratinocytes, abundant eosinophils and a degree of interface change may point towards an iatrogenic cause.

Non-specific therapy depends upon the type of eruption. In urticaria, antihistamines are helpful. In some reactions, topical or systemic corticosteroids can be used, and applications of calamine lotion may be soothing. Plasmapheresis and dialysis can be considered in certain life-threatening situations.

Anaphylactic reactions require special treatment (Figure 25.5) to ensure that the airway is not compromised (e.g. oxygen, assisted respiration or even emergency tracheostomy). Epinephrine 1 : 1000, 0.5 mL (adult) or 0.3 mL (child aged 6–12 years) should be injected intramuscularly into the anterolateral mid thigh and repeated every 5 minutes if no improvement. Intravenous access should be established and a fluid challenge given (0.9% isotonic saline): 500–1000 mL in adults, 20 mL/kg in children. H1-antihistamines are used as a second-line agent and may reduce histamine mediated vasodilatation and bronchoconstriction: slow intravenous (over 1 minute) or intramuscular injection of chlorphenamine maleate (10 mg – adult, 5 mg – child aged 6–12 years). Although the action of intravenous hydrocortisone is delayed for several hours it should be given to prevent further deterioration in severely affected patients (200 mg – adults, 100 mg child aged 6–12 years). Patients should be observed for 6 hours after their condition is stable, as late deterioration may occur. On discharge, patients should be warned about the risk of early recurrence. If an anaphylactic reaction is anticipated, patients should be taught how to self-administer intramuscular adrenaline using an automated device, and may be given a salbutamol inhaler to use at the first sign of the reaction. Upon discharge, all patients should be referred to a specialist allergy clinic for further investigation of their anaphylaxis.

To re-emphasize, the most important treatment is to stop the responsible drug. Desensitization, seldom advisable or practical, may rarely be carried out when therapy with the incriminated drug is essential and when there is no suitable alternative (e.g. with some anticonvulsants, antituberculous and antileprotic drugs). An expert, usually a physician with considerable experience of the drug concerned, should supervise desensitization.

Learning points

1 This whole chapter is a warning against polypharmacy. Do your patients really need all the drugs they are taking?
2 Consider the possiblity of a drug reaction when a rash appears suddenly.
3 Watch out for eruptions from new drugs.
4 Avoid provocation tests unless there are very strong indications for them.
5 Fever, lymphadenopathy, internal organ involvement suggest a potentially severe drug reaction, especially if the skin is red, swollen, blistered, purpuric or shedding.

Further reading

Bachot N, Roujeau JC (2003) Differential diagnosis of severe cutaneous drug reactions. *American Journal of Clinical Dermatology* **4**, 561–572.

Gerson D, Sriganeshan V, Alexis JB. (2008) Cutaneous drug eruptions: a 5-year experience. *Journal of the American Academy of Dermatology* **59**, 995–999.

Greenberger PA. (2006) Drug allergy. *Journal of Allergy and Clinical Immunology* **117** (2 Suppl Mini-Primer), S464–470.

Gupta A, Shamseddin MK, Khaira A. (2011) Pathomechanisms of nephrogenic systemic fibrosis: new insights. *Clinical and Experimantal Dermatology* **36**, 763–768.

Häusermann P, Harr TH, Bircher AJ. (2004) Baboon syndrome resulting from systemic drugs: is there strife between SDRIFE and allergic contact dermatitis syndrome? *Contact Dermatitis* **51**, 297–310.

Heinzerling LM, Tomsitz D, Anliker MD. (2012) Is drug allergy less prevalent than previously assumed? A 5-year analysis. *British Journal of Dermatology* **166**, 107–114.

Katz HI. (2000) *Guide to adverse treatment interactions for skin, hair, and nail disorders.* Novartis Pharmaceuticals.

Knowles S, Shear NH. (2009) Clinical risk management of Stevens–Johnson syndrome/toxic epidermal necrolysis spectrum. *Dermatologic Therapy* **22**, 441–451.

Knowles S, Shapiro L, Shear NH. (1999) Drug eruptions in children. *Advances in Dermatology* **14**, 399–415.

Litt JZ. (2007) *Drug Eruption Reference Manual*, 13th ednition. Informa Healthcare, London.

Resuscitation Council (UK). Anaphylaxis algorithm. http://www.resus.org.uk/pages/anaalgo.pdf (accessed 4 July 2014).

Roujeau JC. (2005) Clinical heterogeneity of drug hypersensitivity. *Toxicology* **209**, 123–129.

Sidoroff A, Dunant A, Viboud C, *et al.* (2007) Risk factors for acute generalized exanthematous pustulosis (AGEP): results of a multinational case–control study (EuroSCAR). *British Journal of Dermatology* **157**, 989–996.

Simons FER. (2013) Anaphylaxis the acute episode and beyond. *British Medical Journal* **346**, F602.

Wakelin SH, Maibach HI. (2004) *Handbook of Systemic Drug Treatment in Dermatology.* Manson Publishing, London.

26 Medical Treatment

An accurate diagnosis, based on a proper history and examination (see Chapter 3), must come before a rational line of treatment can be chosen, and even when a firm diagnosis has been reached, each patient must be treated as an individual. For some, no treatment may even be the best treatment, especially when the disorder is cosmetic or if the treatment would be worse than the condition itself. A patient with minimal vitiligo, for example, may be helped more by careful explanation, reassurance and camouflage than by an extended course of enthusiastic treatment producing only marginal improvement.

If a diagnosis cannot be reached, the doctor has to decide whether a specialist opinion is needed, or whether it is best to observe the rash, perhaps treating it for a while with a bland application. In either case, the indiscriminate use of topical corticosteroids or other medications, in the absence of a working diagnosis, often confuses the picture and may render the future diagnosis more difficult.

However, provided the steps described in Chapter 3 are followed, a firm diagnosis can usually be made, and a sensible course of treatment can be planned but even then the results are often better when patients understand their disease and the reasons behind their treatment. The cause and nature of their disease should be explained to patients carefully, in language they are familiar with, and they must be told what can realistically be expected of their treatment. False optimism or undue pessimism, by patients or doctors, leads only to an unsound relationship. Too often patients become discontented, not because they do not know the correct diagnosis but because they have not been told enough about its cause or prognosis. Even worse, they may have little idea of how to use their treatment and what to expect of it; poor compliance often follows poor instruction. If the treatment is complex, instruction sheets are helpful; they reinforce the spoken word and answer unasked questions. A useful source of regularly updated information sheets on different dermatological conditions and their treatment is provided by the British Association of Dermatologists (http://www.bad.org.uk/site/792/default.aspx).

The principal steps in diagnosis and management:
- History;
- Examination;
- Investigations;
- Diagnosis;
- Explanation of the condition, its cause and prognosis;
- Choice of treatment and instructions about it;
- Discussion of expectations; and
- Follow up, if necessary.

Therapeutic options

Some of the treatments used in dermatology are listed in Table 26.1.

Topical and systemic therapy

The great advantage of topical therapy is that the drugs are delivered straight to where they are needed, at an optimum concentration for the target organ. Systemic side effects from absorption are less than those expected from the same drug given systemically. With topical treatment, vital organs such as the marrow, liver and kidneys are exposed to lower drug concentrations than is the skin. However, topical treatment is often messy, time-consuming and incomplete, whereas systemic treatment is clean and quick and its effect is uniform over the entire skin surface. Cost must also be considered.

Some drugs can only be used topically (e.g. permethrin for scabies and mupirocin for bacterial infections), while others only work systemically (e.g. azathioprine for pemphigus and methotrexate for psoriasis).

When a choice exists, and both possibilities are equally effective, then local treatment is usually to be preferred.

Clinical Dermatology, Fifth Edition. Richard B. Weller, Hamish J.A. Hunter and Margaret W. Mann.
© 2015 John Wiley & Sons, Ltd. Published 2015 by John Wiley & Sons, Ltd.

Table 26.1 Therapeutic options in dermatology.

Drugs	Topical
	Systemic
Physical	Surgical
	excision
	curettage
	Intralesional injection
	Electrodessication
	Cryotherapy
	Radiotherapy
	Phototherapy
	Laser therapy

Most cases of mild pityriasis versicolor, for example, respond to topical antifungals alone so systemic itraconazole is not the treatment of first choice.

Topical treatment

Percutaneous absorption

A drug (the *active ingredient*) used on the skin must be dissolved or suspended in a vehicle (base). The choice of the drug and of the vehicle are both important and depend on the diagnosis and the state of the skin. For a drug to be effective topically, it must pass the barrier to diffusion presented by the horny layer (see Chapter 2). This requires the drug to be transferred from its vehicle to the horny layer, from which it will diffuse through the epidermis into the papillary dermis. Passage through the horny layer is the rate-limiting step.

The transfer of a drug from its vehicle to the horny layer depends on its relative solubility in each (measured as the *partition coefficient*). Movement across the horny layer depends both upon the concentration gradient and on restricting forces (its *diffusion constant*). In general, non-polar substances penetrate more rapidly than polar ones. Low molecular weight drugs penetrate the epidermis better than high molecular weight ones. A rise in skin temperature and in hydration, both achieved by covering a treated area with polyethylene occlusion, encourages penetration.

Some areas of skin present less of a barrier than do others. Two extreme examples are palmar skin, with its impermeable thick horny layer, and scrotal skin, which is thin and highly permeable. The skin of the face is more permeable than the skin of the body. Body fold skin is more permeable than nearby unoccluded skin. In humans, absorption through the hair follicles and sweat ducts is of little significance and the amount of hair on the treated site is no guide to its permeability.

In many skin diseases, the horny layer becomes abnormal and loses some of its barrier function. For example, the abnormal nucleated (parakeratotic) horny layers of psoriasis and chronic eczema, although thicker than normal, have lost much of their protective qualities. Water loss is increased and therapeutic agents penetrate more readily. Similarly, breakdown of the horny layer by chemicals (e.g. soaps and detergents) and by physical injury will allow drugs to penetrate more easily. Conversely, as the skin heals, the barrier function of the horny layer returns and drug absorption diminishes. In summary, the penetration of a drug through the skin depends on the following factors:

- Molecular weight;
- Concentration;
- Base;
- Partition coefficient;
- Diffusion constant;
- Thickness of the horny layer;
- State, including hydration, of the horny layer; and
- Temperature.

Active ingredients

These include corticosteroids, tar, dithranol, antibiotics, antifungal and antiviral agents, benzoyl peroxide, retinoic acid and many others (Formulary 1). The choice depends on the action required, and prescribers should know how each works. Topical corticosteroids are the mainstay of much local dermatological therapy and their pharmacology is summarized in Table 26.2 (Figures 26.1 and 26.2).

Vehicles (bases)

Most vehicles are a mixture of powders, water and greases (usually obtained from petroleum), to which emulsifiers, stabilizers and preservatives are often added. Figure 26.3 shows that blending these bases together produces preparations that retain the characteristics of each of their components.

A vehicle should maximize the delivery of topical drugs but may also have useful properties in its own right. A base of petrolatum decreases water loss. Used carelessly, vehicles may do harm. A tincture (containing alcohol) may dry out the skin and injure it. Suggested indications are shown in Table 26.3. The choice of vehicle depends upon the action desired, availability, messiness, ease of application and cost.

Table 26.2 The pharmacology of topical corticosteroid applications.

Active constituents	Include hydrocortisone and synthetic halogenated derivatives Halogenation increases activity
Bases	Available as solutions, lotions, creams, ointments, sprays, mousses foams, masks and tapes
Penetration	Readily penetrate via the horny layer and appendages Form a reservoir in the horny layer Polyethylene occlusion and high concentrations increase penetration
Metabolism	Some minor metabolism in epidermis and dermis (e.g. hydrocortisone converts to cortisone and other metabolites) Leave skin via dermal vascular plexus and enter general metabolic pool of steroids Further metabolism in liver
Excretion	As sulfate esters and glucuronides
Actions	Anti-inflammatory 1 Vasoconstrict 2 Decrease permeability of dermal vessels 3 Decrease phagocytic migration and activity 4 Decrease fibrin formation 5 Decrease kinin formation 6 Inhibit phospholipase A_2 activity and decrease products of arachidonic acid metabolism 7 Depress fibroblastic activity 8 Stabilize lysosomal membranes 9 Immunosuppressive 10 Antigen–antibody interaction unaffected but inflammatory consequences lessened by above mechanisms and by inhibiting cytokines (e.g. IFN-γ, GM-CSF, IL-1, IL-2, IL-3 and TNF-α) 11 Lympholytic 12 Decrease epidermal proliferation
Side effects	1 Thinning of epidermis 2 Thinning of dermis 3 Telangiectasia and striae (caused by 1 and 2; Figures 26.1 and 26.2) 4 Bruising (caused by 2 and vessel wall fragility) 5 Hirsutism 6 Folliculitis and acneiform eruptions 7 May worsen or disguise infections (bacterial, viral and fungal) 8 Systemic absorption (rare but may be important in infants, when applied in large quantities under polyethylene pants) 9 Tachyphylaxis – lessening of clinical effect with the same preparation 10 Rebound – worsening, sometimes dramatic on withdrawing treatment
Uses	Eczema, psoriasis in some instances (facial, flexural and palms/soles) Many non-infective, inflammatory dermatoses

GM-CSF, granulocyte–macrophage colony-stimulating factor; IL, interleukin; INF-γ, γ-interferon; TNF, tumour necrosis factor.

Individual vehicles

Dusting powders are used in the folds to lessen friction between opposing surfaces. They may repel water (e.g. talc) or absorb it (e.g. starch); zinc oxide powder has an absorptive power midway between these extremes. Powders ought not be used in moist areas where they tend to cake and abrade.

Watery lotions evaporate and cool inflamed areas. This effect is hastened by adding an alcohol, but both glycerol and arachis oil slow evaporation and retain skin moisture. Substances that precipitate protein (astringents; e.g. silver nitrate) lessen exudation.

Shake lotions are watery lotions to which powder has been added so that the area for evaporation is increased.

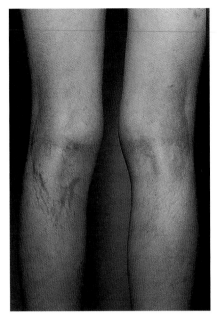

Figure 26.1 Stretch marks behind the knee caused by the topical corticosteroid treatment of atopic eczema.

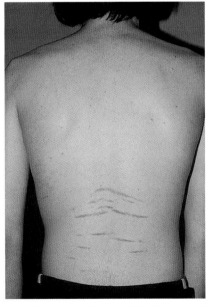

Figure 26.2 Often attributed to Cushing's disease or to local corticosteroid therapy, but stretch marks across the back are common in normal fast-growing teenagers.

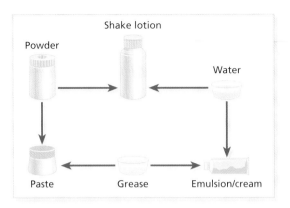

Figure 26.3 The derivation of vehicles.

These lotions dry wet weeping skin. When water has evaporated from the skin, the powder particles clump together and may become abrasive. This is less likely if an oil such as glycerol has been added.

Creams are used for their cooling, moisturizing and emollient effects. They are either oil-in-water emulsions (e.g. aqueous cream, United Kingdom; acid mantle cream, United States) or water-in-oil emulsions (e.g. oily cream, United Kingdom; cold cream, United States). Emulsifying agents are added to increase the surface area of the dispersed phase and that of any therapeutic agent in it.

Ointments are used for their occlusive and emollient properties. They allow the skin to remain supple by preventing the evaporation of water from the horny layer. There are three main types:
1 Those that are water-soluble (macrogols, polyethylene glycols);
2 Those that emulsify with water (e.g. hydrophilic petrolatum); and
3 Those that repel water (mineral oils, and animal and vegetable fats).

Gels may be hydrophilic or hydrophobic. They are especially suitable for scalp applications (because they are less greasy than ointments), treating individual lesions such as insect bites (because they dry on the skin quickly and do not need to be rubbed in) and for use in patients who dislike greasy preparations.

Pastes are used for their protective and emollient properties and usually are made of powder added to a mineral oil or grease, such as petrolatum. The powder lessens the oil's occlusive effect.

Variations on these themes have led to the numerous topical preparations available today. Rather than use them all, and risk confusion, doctors should limit their choice

Table 26.3 Vehicles and their properties.

Base	Used on	Effect	Points of note
Dusting powders	Flexures (may be slightly moist)	Lessen friction	If too wet clump and irritate
Alcohol-based application (tinctures)	Scalp hair	Clean vehicle for corticosteroid applications	Cosmetically elegant, do not matt hair May sting raw areas
Watery and shake lotions	Acutely inflamed skin(wet and oozing)	Drying, soothing and cooling	Tedious to apply Frequent changes (lessened by polyethylene occlusion) Powder in shake lotions may clump
Creams	Both moist and dry skin	Cooling, emollient and moisturizing	Short shelf life Fungal and bacterial growth in base Sensitivities to preservatives and emulsifying agents
Ointments	Dry and scaly skin	Occlusive and emollient	Messy to apply, soil clothing Removed with an oil
Pastes	Dry, lichenified and scaly skin	Protective and emollient	Messy and tedious to apply (bandages needed) Most protective if applied properly
Sprays	Weeping acutely inflamed skin Scalp	Drying, non-occlusive	Vehicle evaporates rapidly No need to touch skin to treat it
Gels	Face and scalp	Vehicle for corticosteroids, salicylic acid and tretinoin	May sting when applied to inflamed skin. Can be covered by makeup
Mousse	Scalp	Clean vehicle for corticosteroid application	Does not matt the hair

to one or two from each category. Table 26.3 summarizes the properties and uses of some common preparations.

Preservatives

Water-in-oil emulsions, such as ointments, require no preservatives. However, many creams are oil-in-water emulsions that permit contaminating organisms to spread in the continuous watery phase. These preparations therefore, as well as lotions and gels, incorporate preservatives. Those in common use include the parahydroxybenzoic acid esters (parabens), chlorocresol, sorbic acid and propylene glycol. Some puzzling reactions to topical preparations are based on allergy to the preservatives they contain.

Methods of application

Ointments and creams are usually applied sparingly twice daily, but the frequency of their application will depend on many factors including the nature, severity and duration of the rash, the sites involved, convenience, the prepara-

tion (some new local corticosteroids need only be applied once daily; Formulary 1, p. 401) and, most important, on common sense. In extensive eruptions, a tubular gauze cover keeps clothes clean and hampers scratching (see Figure 7.18).

Three techniques of application are more specialized: immersion therapy by bathing, wet dressings (compresses) and occlusive therapy.

Bathing

Once-daily bathing helps to remove crusts, scales and medications. After soaking for about 10 minutes, the skin should be rubbed gently with a sponge, flannel or soft cloth; cleaning may be made easier by soaps, oils or colloidal oatmeal.

Medicated baths are occasionally helpful. The most common ingredients added to the bath water are bath oils, antiseptics and solutions of coal tar.

Besides cleaning, the most important function of a bath is hydration. The skin absorbs water and this can be held in the skin for some time if an occlusive ointment is applied immediately after getting out of the bath.

Older patients may need help to get into a bath and should be warned about falling if the bath contains an oil or another slippery substance.

Wet dressings (compresses)

These are used to clean the skin or to deliver a topical medication. They are especially helpful for weeping, crusting and purulent conditions such as eczema, and are described more fully on p. 82. Five or six layers of soft cloth (e.g. cotton gauze) are soaked in the solution to be used; this may be tap water, saline, an astringent or an antiseptic solution, and the compress is then applied to the skin. Open dressings allow the water to evaporate and the skin to cool. They should be changed frequently (e.g. every 15 minutes for 1 hour).

Closed dressings are covered with a plastic (usually polyethylene) sheet; they do not dry out so quickly and are usually changed twice daily. They are especially helpful for debriding adherent crusts and for draining exudative and purulent ulcers.

Occlusive therapy

Sometimes, steroid-sensitive dermatoses will respond to a steroid only when it is applied under a plastic sheet to encourage penetration. This technique is best reserved for the short-term treatment of stubborn localized rashes. The drawback of this treatment is that the side effects of topical steroid treatment (Table 26.2) are highly likely to occur. The most important is systemic absorption if a large surface area of skin, relative to body weight, is treated (e.g. when steroids are applied under the polyethylene pants of infants).

Monitoring local treatment

One common fault is to underestimate the amount required. The guidelines given in Table 26.4 and Figure 26.4 are not precise and are based on twice daily applications. Lotions go further than creams, which go further than ointments and pastes. Inevitably, there will be differences in the quantity of topical preparations needed for the various diseases that affect different age groups. For example, an adult with widespread eczema will need at least 500 g of emollient per week, wheras an adolescent with acne might need only 30 g of a topical gel per month.

Pump dispensers for some topical corticosteroids allow measured amounts to be applied but have not proved popular. Alternatively, the use of *fingertip units* (Figure 26.5)

Table 26.4 Minimum amount of cream (g) required for twice-daily application for 1 week.

Age	Whole body	Trunk	Both arms and legs
6 months	60	25	35
4 years	80	35	45
8 years	130	55	75
12 years	185	75	110
Adult (70-kg male)	250	100	150

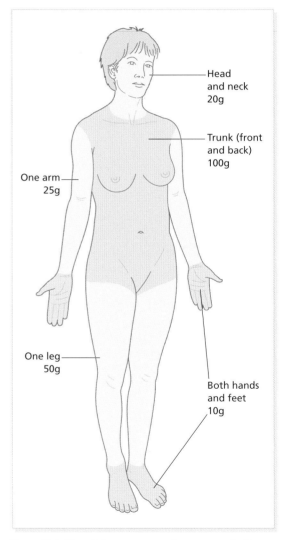

Figure 26.4 The minimum amount of a cream required in 1 week by an adult applying it twice daily.

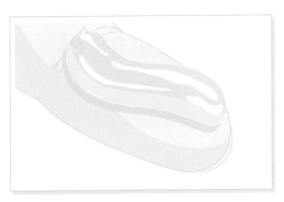

Figure 26.5 A fingertip measures about 0.5 g ointment.

can increase the accuracy of prescribing. As a guide, one fingertip unit in an adult male from a standard nozzle provides 0.5 g ointment.

> **Learning points**
>
> 1 One correct diagnosis is worth a hundred therapeutic trials.
> 2 The doctor who fails to have a placebo effect on patients should become a pathologist or anaesthetist.
> 3 Disease thrives on pessimism.

Systemic therapy

Systemic treatment is needed if a skin condition is associated with systemic disease, or if the medicament of choice is inactive topically (e.g. methotrexate and griseofulvin). The principles of systemic therapy in dermatology are no different from those in other branches of medicine: some drugs act specifically, others non-specifically. For example, antihistamines (H1 blockers) act specifically in urticaria, and non-specifically, by a sedative effect, on the most common skin symptom – itch.

Systemic disease coexists with skin disease in several ways (see Chapter 21). Sometimes, a systemic disease such as systemic lupus erythematosus may cause a rash; at other times, a skin disease causes a systemic upset. Examples of this are the depression that occurs in some patients affected with severe rashes, and high-output cardiac failure, which may occur in exfoliative dermatitis from the shunting of blood through the skin. A systemic upset caused by skin disease can be treated with drugs designed for such problems while the skin is being treated in other ways.

> **Learning points**
>
> 1 You know how much digoxin your patients are taking, but do you know how much of a topical corticosteroid they are applying? Keep a check on this.
> 2 In some patients, drugs produce only side effects.

Further reading

Arndt KA. (1995) *Manual of Dermatologic Therapeutics*, 5th edition. Little Brown, Boston, MA.

Greaves MW, Gatti S. (1999) The use of glucocorticoids in dermatology. *Journal of Dermatological Treatment* **10**, 83–91.

Lebwohl MG, Heymann WR, Berth-Jones J, Coulson I. (2006) *Treatment of Skin Disease*, 2nd edition. Comprehensive Therapeutic Strategies. Mosby, Edinburgh.

Shah VP, Behl CR, Flynn GL, Higuchi WI, Schaefer H. (1993) Principles and criteria in the development and optimization of topical therapeutic products. *Skin Pharmacology* **6**, 72–80.

Shelley WB, Shelley ED. (2001) *Advanced Dermatologic Therapy 11*. W.B. Saunders, Philadelphia.

Wakelin SH. (2002) *Handbook of Systemic Drug Treatment in Dermatology*. Manson Publishing, London.

27 Physical Forms of Treatment

The skin can be treated in many ways, including surgery, freezing, burning, ultraviolet radiation and lasers. Some broad principles are discussed here.

Surgery

As our population ages, and becomes more concerned about appearances, requests for skin surgery are becoming more common. The distinction between traditional dermatological surgery and cosmetic surgery is blurring. There are few over the age of 50 years who do not have a benign tumour (see Chapter 20) that they consider unsightly and wish to have removed. There are also many who are unhappy with a skin damaged by cumulative sun exposure (p. 265), or concerned about medically trivial abnormalities on their face. To term the treatment of all these as 'cosmetic' seems harsh. Health care systems cannot cover the cost of treating all such problems, but family doctors and dermatologists should be able to discuss with their patients any recent developments in phototherapy, laser treatment and specialized surgery that might help them. For example, doctors should be able to explain that diode lasers can remove unwanted hair permanently without visible scarring, and the pros and cons of such treatment, as well as supplying the names of specialists.

Preparation

No surgery is minor. Always mark the site prior to the procedure to reduce error. Use an aseptic technique, if possible in a designated room with appropriate facilities. There are few exceptions but these include bedside biopsies on unconscious patients and those too ill to move. Most biopsies can be performed with clean gloves and isopropyl alcohol prep to the skin (Figure 27.1). Excisions and Mohs' reconstruction should be performed with additional antiseptic prep (chlorhexidine or povidone-iodine solution) and sterile gloves (Figure 27.2). Pre-packed sterile packs of instruments and swabs have made these procedures much easier. Local anaesthesia is usually adequate for skin biopsies, excisions, Mohs' surgery and reconstruction. Most dermatologists use 1 or 2% lidocaine. The addition of adrenaline (epinephrine) constricts local blood vessels to prolong the anaesthetic effect and reduce bleeding (Formulary 2, p. 425).

Antibiotic prophylaxis

Antibiotic prophylaxis is effective in reducing bacteraemia during major surgery, but it probably does not prevent endocarditis or haematogenous total joint infection after simple skin surgery. Routine dermatological surgery (including biopsies, curettage and simple excisions) performed on clean intact skin carry a very low risk of wound infection (1–4%). Because of the low risk of bacteraemia in the setting of skin surgery, British guidelines (see *Further reading*) suggest that antibiotic prophylaxis for endocarditis is not recommended for routine dermatological surgery even in the presence of a pre-existing heart lesion (e.g. prosthetic valves, history of bacterial endocarditis, congenital cardiac malformation, hypertrophic cardiomyopathy, valvular dysfunction and mitral valve prolapse with regurgitation). Similarly, routine antibiotic prophylaxis is not necessary even in patients at high risk (those within the first 2 years of a joint replacement). However, in locations where the risk of wound infection increases to 5–15%, such as eroded or ulcerated skin, respiratory or buccal mucosa, groin and lower leg, antibiotic prophylaxis should be considered in patients at high risk of bacterial endocarditis or joint infection.

Protection against blood-borne infections in dermatological surgery

The risk of contracting a blood-borne virus infection from a patient by a needle stick or scalpel injury during

Clinical Dermatology, Fifth Edition. Richard B. Weller, Hamish J.A. Hunter and Margaret W. Mann.
© 2015 John Wiley & Sons, Ltd. Published 2015 by John Wiley & Sons, Ltd.

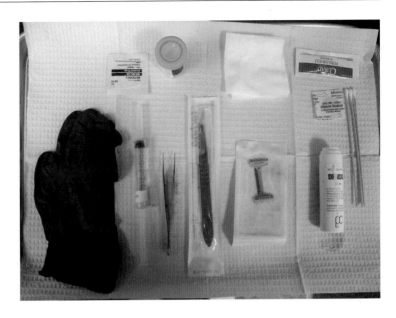

Figure 27.1 An example of a biopsy tray setup with clean gloves.

a surgical procedure is low in the United Kingdom. It varies with the individual virus; it is higher with hepatitis B (HBV) (5–40%) than with hepatitis C (HCV) (3–10%) and HIV (0.2–0.5%). The highest risk of acquiring HIV is following percutaneous injury involving a hollow needle that has been in the vein or artery of an HIV positive patient with a high viral load. The risk of acquiring HIV through mucous membrane exposure is less than 1

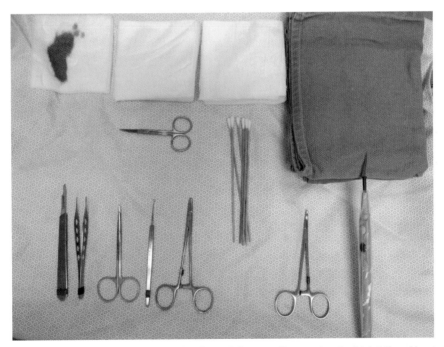

Figure 27.2 Typical excision tray. Hibiclens is positioned at the top left corner (for prepping the skin), followed by sterile gauze and sterile towel (for draping the surgical area). Surgical instruments include forceps, blade and blade holder, suture scissors and undermining scissors, skin hook, needle driver, haemostat and electrocautery.

in 1000 and there is no evidence of risk from blood in contact with intact skin.

These days, any patient can carry an undiagnosed infection, so gloves should be used for all surgical and other procedures where there is risk of contacting blood or body secretions. When operating on a high risk patient the surgeon should wear not only gloves, but also a water-repellent gown, protective headwear, a mask with visor and protective footwear. Other good preventative measures include:

- Good basic hygiene with regular handwashing;
- Cover of existing wounds; and
- Safe procedure for the handling and disposal of needles and blades.

Immunization is currently only effective against HBV infection. All medical staff who come into contact with blood or blood-related products should be immunized against this virus.

Immediate action after a needle and/or scalpel injury.
- Wash off splashes on the skin with soap and running water.
- Encourage bleeding if the skin is already broken. Disinfect the wound using an ample amount of soap and water. If contact with mucous membranes, flush thoroughly with water or saline solution.
- Record the source and nature of the injury.
- Immediately consult the local medical adviser about risk assessment and prophylaxis with antiviral drug(s).
- If the source of the blood is known, the nature and implication of the injury should be explained to the source patient. Efforts should be made to obtain consent from the source patient to sample blood for testing of HBV, HCV and HIV.

Further information can be found in the British Association of Dermatologists' guidelines (see *Further reading*).

Skin biopsy

The indications for biopsy, and the techniques employed, are described in Chapter 3. Briefly, shave or punch techniques can be used to obtain a sample specimen for histopathological examination.

Excision

Excision under local anaesthetic, using an aseptic technique, is a common way of removing small tumours for histopathologic examinatation and surgical cure. First,

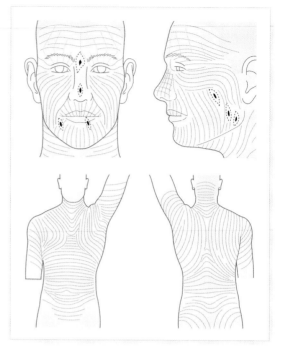

Figure 27.3 Skin wrinkle figures are helpful in deciding the direction of wounds following skin surgery. Those performing dermatological surgery should have ready access to them.

the lesion must be examined carefully and important underlying structures (e.g. the temporal artery) noted. If possible, the incision should run along the line of a skin crease, especially on the face. If necessary, charts or pictures of standard skin creases should be consulted (Figure 27.3). After injection of the local anaesthetic the lesion is excised as an ellipse with a margin of normal skin, the width of which varies with the nature of the lesion and the site (Figure 27.4). Benign lesions can be removed with 1–2 mm margins. Recommended margins for basal cell (BCC) and squamous cell carcionomas (SCC) is usually 4–5 mm and for atypical naevi is 3–4 mm. The length of the fusiform shape should be about 3–4 times the width to minimize redundant cones of tissue or 'dog-ears' at the tips. The scalpel should be held perpendicular to the skin surface and the incision should reach the subcutaneous fat. The ellipse of skin is carefully removed with the help of a skin hook or fine-toothed forceps. Larger wounds, and those where the scar is likely to stretch (e.g. on the back), are undermined carefully to mobilize the tissue and reduce wound tension. It is then closed in a layered fashion – the subcutis and dermis is closed with absorbable sutures (e.g. Dexon) before

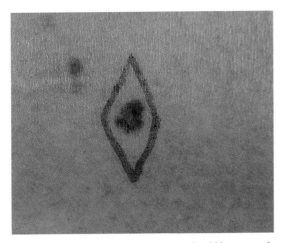

Figure 27.4 Suspicious pigmented lesions should be removed with a 2-mm margin marked out in advance.

apposing the skin edges without tension using non-absorbable interrupted or running sutures such as nylon or Prolene (see *Further reading* for precise techniques of suturing). Stitches are usually removed from the face in 5–7 days and from the trunk and limbs in 10–14 days. Artificial sutures (e.g. Steri-Strip) may be used to take the tension off the wound edges after the stitches have been taken out (Figure 27.5).

Shave excision

Many small lesions are removed by shaving them off at their bases with a scalpel tangential to the skin surface under local anaesthesia. This procedure is suitable only for exophytic tumours that are believed to be benign. Some cells at the base may be left and these, in the case of malignant tumours, could lead to recurrence.

Saucerization excision

This modified shave excision extends into the subcutaneous fat. Instead of tangentially shaving off the growth, it is 'scooped' out, leaving a crater-like wound. The technique is used to remove certain small skin cancers and worrying melanocytic naevi. It tends to leave a more noticeable depressed white scar when compared with a shave excision but the technique provides tissue that allows the dermatopathologist to determine if a tumour is invading and to measure tumour thickness if the lesion is a melanoma. Furthermore, the technique may ensure complete removal more adequately than shave excision.

Cryotherapy

Freezing damages cells by intracellular ice formation. The ensuing thaw compounds this damage by osmotic changes across cell walls and by vascular stasis. The damage is semi-selective in that cellular components are more susceptible to cold injury than stromal ones. There is also some variation in susceptibility between different cells, for example melanocytes are more vulnerable to cold injury than keratinocytes.

Cryotherapy is a most convenient procedure for use in general outpatient and domiciliary practice. Further advantages include its cost effectiveness, its speed and suitability for those who fear surgery, and its lessened chance of transmitting blood-borne infections. These have to be weighed up against its two main disadvantages: short term pain and no histological confirmation of the lesion being treated. Several freezing agents are available. Liquid nitrogen (–196°C) is the most popular and is now used more than carbon dioxide snow ('dry ice', –79°C). It is effective and used often for viral warts, seborrhoeic keratoses, actinic cheilitis, actinic keratoses, simple lentigos and some superficial skin tumours (e.g. intraepidermal carcinoma and lentigo maligna). It is applied either on a cotton bud or with a special spray gun (Figure 27.6). The lesion is frozen until it turns white, with a 1–2 mm halo of freezing around. Two freeze–thaw cycles kill tissue more effectively than one but are usually unnecessary for warts and some keratoses (Figure 27.7). Treatment of BCC with liquid nitrogen cryosurgery requires significantly longer freezing time to reach tissue temperatures of –50 to –60°C. Patients should be warned to expect pain and possible blistering after treatment. Care should be taken when treating warts on fingers as digital nerve damage can follow over-enthusiastic freezing. Standard freeze–thaw times have been established for superficial tumours (see *Further reading*) but temperature probes in and around deep tumours are needed to gauge the degree of freezing for their effective treatment. A crust, including the necrotic tumour, should slough off after about 2 weeks. As melanocytes are very sensitive to cold injury, hypopigmentation at a treated site is common and may be permanent.

Curettage

Curettage under local anaesthetic is also used to treat benign exophytic lesions (e.g. seborrhoeic keratoses;

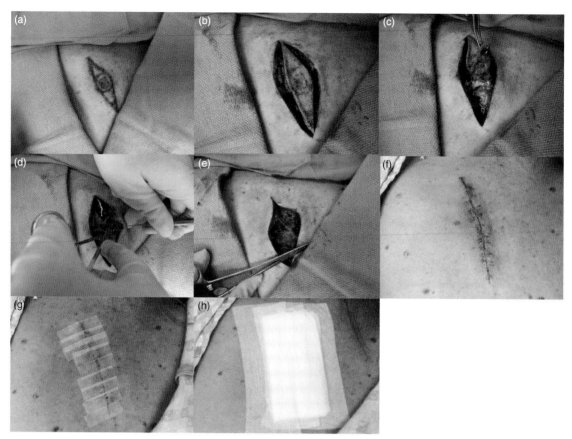

Figure 27.5 Steps for surgical excision of a melanoma in situ. (a) An fusiform shape is marked with 5-mm margins. (b) Incision is carried perpendicular to the skin down to the subcutaneous fat. (c) The tissue specimen is carefully removed with the help of a fine-toothed forceps. (d) Undermining is carried out with a skin hook to minimize trauma to the epidermis. (e) The dermis is closed with absorbable sutures. (f) The epidermis is reapproximated with subcuticular sutures. (g) Steristrips are placed. (h) Pressure dressing is left in place for 24–48 hours.

Figure 27.8) and, combined with electrodesiccation (p. 371), to treat some BCC. Its main advantage over purely destructive treatment such as laser or liquid nitrogen is that histological examination can be carried out on the curettings. As morphology of the tumour is fragmented, the curetting technique does not allow for histological confirmation of tumour clearance and should not be used if there is uncertainty about the primary diagnosis. A sharp curette is used to scrape off the lesion and haemostasis is achieved by local haematinics, by electrocautery or electrodesiccation. The wound heals by secondary intention over 2–3 weeks, with good cosmetic results in most cases.

When a BCC is treated, the curette is scraped firmly and thoroughly along the sides and bottom of the tumour (the surrounding dermis is tougher and more resistant to curettage than the carcinoma) and the bleeding wound bed is then electrodesiccated aggressively. This stops bleeding and destroys a zone of tissue under and around the excised tumour to provide a tumour-free margin. The process is repeated once or twice at the same session to ensure that all of the tumour has been removed or destroyed. Only small BCC outside the skin folds should be treated in this way. The recurrence rates are relatively high for tumours in the nasolabial folds, over the inner canthi and on the nose, glabella and lips. The technique should not ordinarily be used for infiltrative or sclerosing BCC, invasive lesions larger than 1–2 cm, rapidly growing tumours or for those with micronodular features on histology.

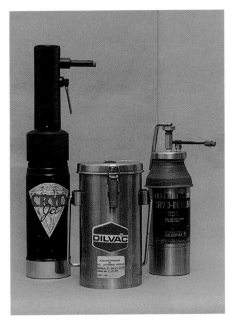

Figure 27.6 Liquid nitrogen can be applied through a spray, or with a cotton wool bud direct from a vacuum flask (centre).

Electrosurgery

This is often combined with curettage, under local anaesthesia, to treat skin tumours. The main types are shown in Figure 27.9.

Microscopically controlled excision (Mohs' micrographic surgery)

This form of surgery for malignant skin tumours is time-consuming and expensive, but allows for greater tissue conservation and the highest cure rate compared with

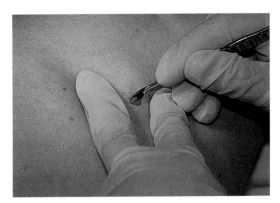

Figure 27.8 Curettage beats excision if a seborrhoeic wart has to be removed. Stretching the skin helps to hold the lesion steady.

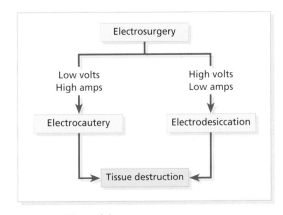

Figure 27.9 Types of electrosurgery.

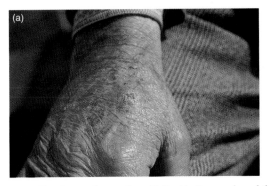
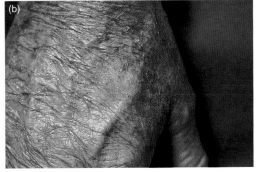

Figure 27.7 Two freeze–thaw cycles with liquid nitrogen cleared this actinic keratosis. (Dr R. Dawber, The Churchill Hospital, Oxford, UK. Reproduced with permission of Dr R. Dawber.)

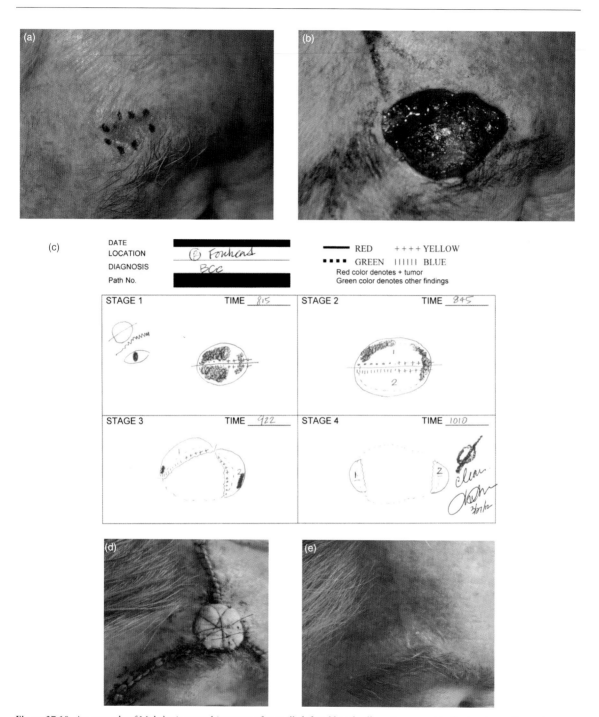

Figure 27.10 An example of Mohs' micrographic surgery for an ill-defined basal cell carcinoma on the forehead near the eyebrow. (a) Initial lesion measured 10 × 8 mm. (b) After four stages of Mohs', the lesion measured 25 × 16 mm. (c) Mohs map showing presence of tumor in red in stage 1–3 with final clearance on stage 4. (d) Reconstruction of the defect with an advancement flap and a skin graft centrally. (e) Final outcome at 6 months.

excision or curettage. Mohs' surgery was pioneered by Dr Frederic E. Mohs in the 1950s. In the United Kingdom, the Mohs surgeon is normally a consultant dermatologist who has undertaken additional fellowship training in Mohs' micrographic surgery, dermatopathology of skin tumours and reconstruction. A surgeon using Mohs' technique functions as both the surgeon and the pathologist, which allows for precise mapping and margin control. First, the tumour is removed with a narrow margin, usually 1–2 mm instead of the usual 4–6 mm required with standard excision. The excised specimen is then marked at the edges, mapped and rapidly frozen for histological processing in horizontal sections. This allows for microscopic examination of 100% of the tissue margin. In contrast, conventional histologic sections requires formalin fixation and takes several days to process. The cross-sectional slices of representative tissue or 'bread loaf' in conventional sections also examines less than 1% of the true margins.

In most cases, each stage of Mohs' surgery requires less than 1 hour to process and the entire procedure is performed under local anaesthetic. If the tumour extends to any margin, further tissue is removed from the appropriate place, based on the markings and mappings, and again checked histologically. This process is repeated until clearance has been proved histologically at all margins. The resulting wound can then be closed directly, reconstructed with a flap, covered with a split skin graft or allowed to heal by secondary intention.

In general, Mohs' surgery is useful to treat skin cancers at high risk of recurrence (Figure 27.10). There are many factors that have an effect on recurrence rate including histological features, location and patient features (Table 27.1). Low risk lesions can be treated with a number of surgical modalities mentioned in this chapter including excisional surgery and electrodessication and currettage (Table 27.2). In addition, patients who cannot undergo surgical treatments (such as the very elderly and those in poor health) may benefit from radiotherapy, topical immunotherapy with imiquimod (Formulary 1, p. 405) and non-surgical therapies.

Flaps and grafts

These can be used to reconstruct a defect left by the wide excision of a tumour (Figure 27.10), or when a tumour is removed from a difficult site (e.g. the eyelid or tip of the nose; see *Further reading* as the techniques are beyond the scope of this book).

Table 27.1 Features associated with high risk of tumour recurrence.

Histological and tumour features	• BCC or SCC with poorly defined edges • BCC or SCC greater than 2 cm • Sclerosing, infiltrative, morphoeic or micronodular BCC (can suggest an enlarging scar clinically) • Basosquamous carcinoma – a tumour with both basal and squamous features • Poorly differentiated SCC • Recurrent BCC or SCC • Perineural invasion or deeply infiltrative lesions • Other malignant tumours such as dermatofibrosarcoma protuberans, microcystic adnexal carcinoma and other rare tumours for margin control
Tumour location	• Tumour overlying an area where excess margins of skin cannot be sacrified to achieve complete removal of the tumour (e.g. near the eye or facial nerve) • Areas with high incidence of recurrence – nose, periocular, ears, scalp and temples, lips • Site of previously injury (e.g. irradiation, chronic ulcer or burns)
Patient features	• Immunosuppression • Genetic disorders such as Gorlin's syndrome

BCC, basal cell carcinoma; SCC, squamous cell carcinoma.

Radiotherapy

Superficial radiation therapy (50–100 kV) can be used to treat biopsy-proven skin cancers in those over 70 years old or who are too frail to tolerate surgery (Figure 27.11). They can also be useful as adjuvant therapy, following incomplete excision of high risk tumours. The usual dose is 3000 cGy, given in fractions over 5–10 days. The scars from radiotherapy worsen with time (Figure 27.12), in contrast to surgical scars which improve. Patients who undergo radiotherapy are also at increased risk of future skin cancer, so this is not an ideal therapy for young patients or those who are prone to skin cancers such as patients with Gorlin's syndrome. Nowadays, radiotherapy is seldom used for inflammatory conditions.

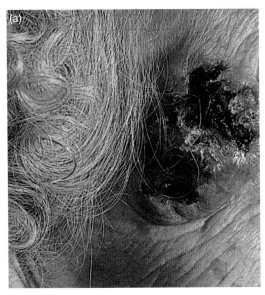
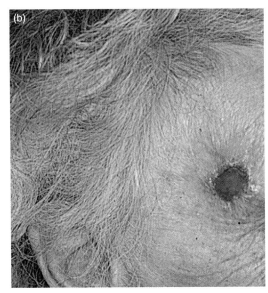

Figure 27.11 (a) A 90-year-old, unfit for surgery, did well with radiotherapy for this massive basal carcinoma. (b) The reaction was healing well after a few weeks.

Phototherapy

Chapter 18 deals mainly with adverse skin reactions to light. On the other side of the coin, the healing power of light has attracted much attention recently, because of technical advances in the manufacture of light sources for phototherapy. Knowledge of a few basic biophysical principles is required in order to understand tissue optics and photobiological reactions.

Visible light is a form of electromagnetic radiation with wavelengths lying between those of the warming infrared and high energy ultraviolet radiation. The ultraviolet spectrum is divided into the ultraviolet C (UVC)

spectrum with wavelengths less than 290 nm, the ultraviolet B (UVB) spectrum of wavelengths between 290 and 320 nm, and ultraviolet A (UVA) with spectrum from 320 nm to the most purple colour the eye can discern as light, roughly 420 nm.

The interaction of light with the skin depends on the amount of photons *reflected, scattered and absorbed. Reflected light* is perceived by the visual system as objects, including the appearances of skin disorders. Penetration of radiation is inversely proportional to its wavelength, so that longer wavelengths such as visible light and infrared radiation penetrate the skin more deeply than shorter wavelength ultraviolet radiation.

Table 27.2 5-year cure rate by treatment modalities for primary basal cell carcinoma (BCC).

Modality	Primary BCC (%)
Mohs' micrographic surgery	99
Surgical excision	90
Currettage and cautery	92
Cryotherapy	92
Radiation therapy	91

Note: Higher cure rates with cyrotherapy and currettage is likely a result of physician selection of smaller lesions for these treatment modalities.

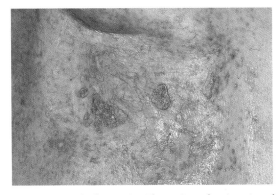

Figure 27.12 Radiodermatitis with scarring, telangiectasia and hyperkeratosis.

Absorption involves the transfer of energy from light to tissue. Photons are absorbed selectively by different chromophores (see Chapter 18) depending on their absorption profile or spectrum. These chromophores in turn determine the extent that light penetrates the skin, as any photon that is absorbed is no longer capable of passing through the skin. With the possible exception of UVB phototherapy (see *Ultraviolet radiation therapy* and p. 62), the specific chromophores for most light-based therapies are known (Table 27.3) and include haemoglobin, water, melanin, tattoo pigments and photosensitizing drugs (e.g. psoralens and photosensitizers used in photodynamic therapy; see *Ultraviolet radiation therapy*). Energy from the photon is transferred to the chromophore either to generate heat to destroy target tissue (as with most lasers and intense pulsed lights) or drive photochemical reactions (as with ultraviolet phototherapy, excimer lasers and photodynamic therapy).

Ultraviolet radiation therapy

Controlled trials have confirmed long-held beliefs that UVB helps some conditions (e.g. chronic plaque psoriasis, see Chapter 5; atopic dermatitis; pityriasis rosea; the pruritus of renal failure; cutaneous T-cell lymphoma; and even pressure sores, see Table 18.4). Open trials show that UVB can improve acne, nummular eczema, neurodermatitis, pityriasis lichenoides chronica, some types of vitiligo, cholinergic urticaria, dermographism and eosinophilic pustular folliculitis. Paradoxically, UVB is effective in 'desensitizing' patients with some photodermatoses, including polymorphic light eruption and solar urticaria. Not surprisingly, these conditions are usually provoked at the beginning of a course, but settle with continuing treatment. It is ironic that the chromophores, and the subsequent biological reactions involved in the most widely used and oldest form of phototherapy, UVB, remain debatable. Candidate chromphores include DNA, RNA, urocanic acid and melanin and the final reaction appears to result in cutaneous immunosuppression. In comparison with oral agents such as prednisone or methotrexate used to treat chronic skin conditions, light therapy has minimal long-term side effects. The major long-term risk being skin carcinogenesis. Proper dosimetry is necessary to prevent sunburn reaction and blistering.

Although broadband UVB (290–320 nm) is still used for selected situations, most ultraviolet radiation (UVR) treatment nowadays falls into two main categories: narrowband (311 nm) UVB therapy and photochemotherapy with PUVA using wavelengths of UVA (p. 62). The advantages of narrowband UVB therapy over PUVA are that:

- There is no need for pre- and post-treatment eye protection;
- It avoids systemic medication; and
- It may be less carcinogenic than PUVA treatment.

PUVA therapy requires the administration of 8-methoxypsoralen (8-MOP), either orally or applied topically, in combination with UVA exposure. The advantages of PUVA therapy are that:

- Treatment is less frequent than with narrowband UVB (twice versus three times weekly);
- It is probably the most effective of all UVR treatments;
- Its carcinogenic risk is known; and
- The rays of UVA penetrate deeper into the skin, and so can affect disorders involving the deeper dermis.

After phototests on the skin or calculations based on the patient's skin type (p. 260) to establish a starting dose, irradiance is increased by small increments, aiming to produce no or minimal erythema after 24 hours (UVB) or 48 hours (PUVA). Close supervision by experienced staff is needed because extreme phototoxicity from an overdose, from sunlight or concomitant use of tanning booths has produced severe burns and even death. A careful record should also be kept of the cumulative UVR dose as the risk of developing skin cancers, including malignant melanoma, may be increased when a patient has received a large cumulative dose. Patients who have had prolonged or repeated UVR courses should be screened for skin cancer at regular (e.g. yearly) intervals after courses.

Recently, the development of excimer laser has made it possible to clear localized stubborn areas of psoriasis and vitiligo. The small 2-cm handpiece allows delivery of high energy 308 nm UVB light to a focused area, thus limiting total body exposure to UVB. Treatment can be time-consuming so is not ideal for treatment of large surface areas,

Sunbeds

Sunbeds, delivering UVA, are used widely throughout the world by those with skin types I–IV (p. 260) to obtain a tan. Some patients assume, often wrongly, that sunbeds also help their skin condition, usually one of those mentioned under *Phototherapy* above. Many sunbed users also believe, again mistakenly, that skin damage is avoided provided their skin does not burn. The potential short-term harmful effects (e.g. sunburn, itch, rashes) of sunbeds are known by many users but

Table 27.3 Wavelength and targets of commonly used dermatological lasers.

Target	Chromophore	Laser	Wavelength	Most suitable for
Vascular lesion	Haemoglobin	KTP	532 nm	• Haemangioma • Facial erythema and telangiectasias
		PDL	585–595 nm	• Haemangioma: treatment of choice • PWS: treatment of choice • Useful for warts, hypertrophic scars, striae, pyogenic granuloma
		Alexandrite	755 nm	• Facial erythema and telangiectasias • Veins >0.4 mm in diameter
		Nd:YAG	1064 nm	• Haemangioma and PWS: thicker lesions • Reticular veins: larger caliper leg veins and ectatic vessels
		IPL	500–1200 nm	• Telangiectasia/poikiloderma
Melanocytic lesions	Melanin	Frequency doubled Q-switched Nd:YAG	532 nm	• Ephelides • Lentigines • Best for light skin types
		Q-switched ruby	694 nm	• Naevi of Ota/Ito: treatment of choice • Ephelides • Lentigines
		Q-switched alexandrite	755 nm	• Naevi of Ota/Ito • Best for light skin types
		Q-switched Nd:YAG	1064 nm	• Naevi of Ota (all skin types) • Best for darker skin type because of its low risk of pigmentary alteration
		IPL	500–1200 nm	• Ephelides • Lentigines
Tattoo	Blue–black ink	Q-switched alexandrite	755 nm	• Best for light skinned individuals • Also helpful for green, red and mauve colours
		Q-switched ruby	694 nm	• Green • Also helpful for blue–black and yellow ink
	Green ink	Frequency doubled Nd:YAG	532 nm	• Red, orange, purple
	Red ink	Pigmented pulse dye	510 nm	• Also helpful for red, orange, purple
	Yellow ink	Ruby	694 nm	
Hair	Melanin in the hair shaft and matrix cells	Alexandrite	755 nm	• Best for dark hair • Best for light skinned individuals
		Diode	800, 810, 930 nm	• Best for dark hair
		Nd:YAG	1064 nm	• Best for dark hair • Best for darker skin types, less risk for pigmentary alteration although less efficacious than shorter wavelengths

IPL, intense pulsed light; KTP, potassium titanyl phosphate; Nd:YAG, neodymium:yttrium-aluminum-garnet; PDL, pulsed dye laser; PWS, port-wine stain.

long-term damage to the skin is either too often under-stated or overlooked:

* Premature ageing of the skin;
* Skin cancer, including melanoma; and
* Increased risk of cataracts.

Based on this evidence most dermatologists strongly discourage the use of sunbeds for cosmetic tanning.

Photodynamic therapy

Photodynamic therapy (PDT) is used for actinic keratoses (p. 287), Bowen's disease (p. 292) and superficial BCC less than 2 mm thick (p. 290). PDT has been increasingly used with variable success for benign conditions including sebaceous gland hyperplasia, acne vulgaris and the rejuvenation of photodamaged skin. Selective tissue destruction is achieved by incorporating the photosensitizer in the target tissue and then activating it with either a laser or non-laser light source. The most common combinations are the naturally occurring porphyrin precursor, 5-aminolaevulinic acid (ALA) or its methyl derivative, methyl aminolaevulinate (MAL), and irradiation with a red or blue light. In one regimen, water-soluble ALA (now commercially available in the United States and Europe) is applied topically, under occlusion, to the target tissue. After 2–4 hours, when the ALA has been selectively absorbed by the tumour and endogenously converted by the haem biosythetic pathway to proptoporphyrin IX (PpIX) (Figure 27.13), the area is exposed to the light for 15–60 minutes. The activated PpIX converts molecular oxygen to cytotoxic singlet oxygen and free radicals, which in turn cause ischaemic necrosis of the target tissue by damaging cell membranes, especially those in the walls of blood vessels. PDT is carried out in an outpatient setting (Figure 27.14) and its potential advantages over standard treatments include:

* Non-invasiveness;
* Ability to treat many lesions at once;
* Rarely causes ulceration and leads to a good cosmetic result;
* Good patient acceptability (although the treatments do hurt and patients must avoid exposure of the photosensitized area to sunlight for 48 hours posttreatment); and
* Usefulness for treating tumours on sites that present surgical difficulty (e.g. the taut skin of the finger; Figure 27.15).

A recent European trial suggests PDT may be helpful as preventative therapy by reducing the number of new premalignant skin lesions in organ transplant recipients.

Laser therapy

Lasers (acronym for light amplification by the stimulated emission of radiation) are high-intensity coherent light sources of a specific wavelength. The choice of a specific laser to treat a specific condition (dyschromia, telangiectasia, rhytides) is based on the theory of selective photothermolysis. The photons are absorbed by a target chromophore (e.g. a tattoo pigment, melanin in hair, oxyhaemoglobin in blood vessels) and, depending on the energy, the duration of the pulse of emission and the thermal relaxation time, cause local, sometimes microscopic, tissue destruction. The mechanisms of action of different lasers are deceptively simple and rely on one of the following tissue reactions:

* *Photothermal:* the laser light is absorbed by the chromophore and converted to heat, resulting in coagulation or vaporization. Continuous wave lasers cause non-selective damage while pulsed lasers cause selective damage.
* *Photomechanical:* laser energy, delivered fast for a few nanoseconds, causes mechanical damage to subcellular organelles containing melanin or exogenous pigment.
* *Photochemical:* the laser light from, for example, excimer and photodynamic therapy lasers triggers a chemical reaction.

Lasers are now being used to treat many skin lesions including port-wine stains, tattoos, epidermal naevi, pigmented lesions, seborrhoeic keratoses, warts and tumours. Technology has advanced rapidly and many types of laser are now available for clinical use. Most treatments can be carried out under topical or local anaesthetic and in an outpatient setting. Cooling the skin surface with chilled probes, cryogen sprays or cold air fans helps to lessen collateral heat damage especially to epidermal melanin in darker patients and to relieve pain. Ocular injury from laser beam exposure can result in permanent blindness, thus adequate eye protection must always be worn by the patient and all personnel in the room.

Lasers of historical interests
The lasers noted below are presented for historical interest. For the most part, they are not frequently used, having been replaced by lasers that are more powerful with less risk of complications.

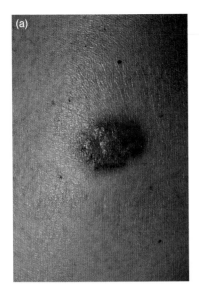

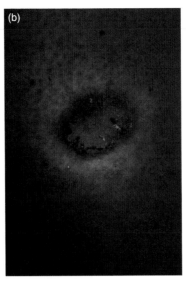

Figure 27.13 A basal cell carcinoma: (a) showing, by fluorescence (b), selective uptake of 5-aminolaevulinic acid (ALA). (The Photobiology Unit, Ninewells Hospital, Dundee, UK.)

Argon laser (488, 514 nm)

The argon laser emits blue–green light with 80% of its emission at 488 and 514 nm, delivered in a continuous beam. This laser was one of the first used to treat vascular and pigmented lesions in the 1970s. While the wavelengths emitted by this laser are well absorbed by haemoglobin, it is associated with a high prevalence of postoperative pigmentary alteration and excess scarring. This is because of its continuous mode which causes nonspecific thermal damage to surrounding tissue. In addition, its shorter wavelength and small spot size (up to

1 mm) results in poor tissue penetration (depth of 1–2 mm) and significant epidermal melanin absorption, increasing the risk for dyspigmentation.

Copper vapour/copper bromide lasers (511, 578 nm)

Copper vapour and copper bromide lasers emit yellow light with wavelengths of 578 and 511 nm and are used for the treatment of vascular and pigmented lesions. This quasi-continuous mode laser delivers 20-nanosecond pulses at a rate of 6000–15 000 pulses per

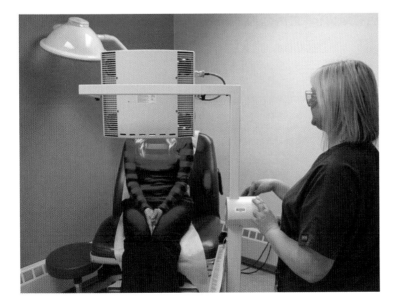

Figure 27.14 Photodynamic therapy of the face with blue light after 2 hours of incubation with ALA. Appropriate safety goggles should be worn by the patient and staff during treatment.

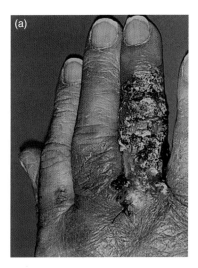 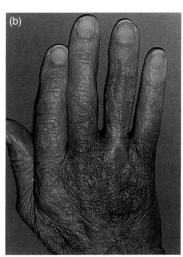

Figure 27.15 (a) Hyperkeratotic Bowen's disease on a finger; (b) treated successfully with photodynamic therapy. This would have been an awkward site for surgery. (The Photobiology Unit, Ninewells Hospital, Dundee, UK.)

second. Similar to the argon laser, these devices have a tendency to produce thermal damage and postoperative pigmentary alteration because of their quasi-continuous mode which exceeds the thermal relaxation time of most vascular and pigment targets. They are best suited for the treatment of large calibre vessels with longer thermal relaxation time, such as cherry angioma and pyogenic granuloma.

Krypton laser (520, 532, 568 nm)

The krypton laser is a quasi-continuous wavelength mode laser that emits green light at 520 and 532 nm and yellow light at 568 nm. The 568-nm krypton laser has been advocated for the treatment of facial telangiectasias. Vessels are traced using a 1-mm, 2-mm or 100-μm handpiece with pulse duration of 0.2–10 seconds until the vessel disappears completely. As with other quasi-continuous wavelength laser systems, multiple treatment sessions at 3- to 4-week intervals are often necessary. The most common adverse effects include erythema, oedema and mild blistering or crusting.

Commonly used lasers in dermatology

Potassium titanyl phosphate crystal laser (532 nm)

The potassium titanyl phosphate (KTP) laser emits a green light at 532 nm, close to the absorption peak of oxy-haemoglobin, making this an ideal laser for vascular targets. Its shorter wavelength also makes it ideal for treating superficial pigmented lesions. The laser is available in a quasi-continuous mode (long pulse) for the treatment of vascular lesions. In addition, the Q-switched mode

delivers a short burst of energy in nanoseconds for treating superficial pigment lesion and red tattoos. Unlike the pulsed dye laser (PDL), KTP lasers do not produce postoperative purpura. This is because of the long pulse duration of the KTP which heats the blood vessel slowly without causing rupture or extravasation of the red blood cell into the interstitial space. Because the 532 nm wavelength is well absorbed by epidermal melanin, there is a higher risk for hyperpigmentation than with the PDL.

Flashlamp-pumped pulsed dye laser (585, 595 nm)

The PDL, which utilizes a rhodamine dye as a laser medium, is the gold standard for the treatment of vascular lesions such as port-wine stains. This laser has also been used for treating telangiectasia, rosacea, haemangiomas, spider angiomas, pyogenic granulomas, hypertrophic scars and warts. Although established hypertrophic scars and keloids can respond to treatment with PDL, it is more effective at prevention of hypertrophy with early treatment of scars in the first few months. Initially available at a wavelength of 577 nm then 585 nm, the newer PDL laser emits 595 nm with an adjustable pulse duration for treatment of larger calibre vessels and a cryogen-cooling device to decrease surrounding tissue injury. By lengthening the wavelength to 585 and 595 nm, the PDL can penetrate and target deeper vessels. The most common adverse effects include transient oedema, erythema and purpura, which may last up to 7 days.

Ruby laser (694 nm)

The ruby laser emits a red 694 nm wavelength useful for treating tattoos with black, blue and green pigment, pigmented lesions and hair removal. The Q-switched mode of this laser allows for the delivery of high energy and short nanosecond pulses to maximize target damage while minimizing surrounding tissue injury. The nanosecond pulse is useful for the treatment of tattoo and pigmented lesions. Compared with the neodymium:yttrium-aluminum-garnet (Nd:YAG), the shorter wavelength of this laser can cause pigmentary alteration and should be used with caution in darker skin types.

Alexandrite laser (755 nm)

The alexandrite laser delivers a wavelength of 755 nm and is available in Q-switched short pulse and normal mode (long pulse). The long-pulsed laser is useful for hair removal. The Q-switched alexandrite laser has excellent absorption by black tattoo pigment and deep pigmentary lesions such as naevus of Ota. It has been shown to be useful in the removal of blue and green ink but with poor results in red ink. Like the Nd:YAG, an average of 5–10 treatment at 1–2 month intervals are required for near complete clearance of black tattoo ink. Hyperpigmentation can occur especially in darker skin types but often clears with hydroquinone and sunscreen. Transient hypopigmentation after 5–7 treatments is common and gradually resolves over 1–12 months. Higher fluences can produce purpura and pinpoint bleeding. Tissue splatter and erosions may occur with the shorter 50-nanosecond pulse width at higher fluence.

Diode lasers (810 nm)

The diode laser emits an 810 nm wavelength which is effective in the removal of dark terminal hairs. Because of its longer wavelength and longer pulse width, it can used safely in darker skin types with less risk of hyperpigmentation than the alexandrite laser.

Neodymium:yttrium-aluminum-garnet laser (1064 nm)

The Nd:YAG laser emits a long wavelength of 1064 nm, which allows for increased dermal penetration (4–6 mm) and decreased melanin absorption, making it an ideal laser for pigmented lesions and tattoos, especially for darker skinned patients. It is useful for hair removal and in the treatment of lentigines, café au lait macules and naevus of Ota. It is available in three modes: continuous mode (millisecond pulse), Q-switched (nanosecond pulse) and frequency doubled. In the continous mode, the Nd:YAG is useful for hair removal. The Q-switched fea-

ture of this laser allows for high peak energies (50 time the laser's power) and short pulse duration (4–7 ns), which is ideal for treatment of tattoos. Compared to the Q-switched ruby laser, the Q-switched Nd:YAG removes blue–black tattoos with less hypopigmentation and skin texture changes. Multiple treatments, sometimes as many as 5–10, are required for lightening of professional tattoos. A unique feature of this laser is the ability to double the frequency and halve the wavelength to 532 nm, allowing it to treat red tattoo ink, with some response with purple and orange ink. The 1064-nm light is passed through a KTP crystal, which converts the wavelength to 532 nm.

This laser is also useful for the treatment of vascular lesions, as both the 1064 and 532-nm wavelengths are well absorbed by oxyhaemglobin. The 1064-nm wavelength can penetrate 4–6 mm into the dermis and is more suitable for thicker vascular lesions. In addition, melanin absorption decreases at longer wavelengths, reducing the risk of post-treatment hyperpigmentation and so is useful for treatment of darker skin types. Continuous wave mode Nd:YAG causes non-specific thermal damage of haemangiomas and increases the risk of scarring, thus it is less ideal for treatment of vascular lesions than the Q-switched pulsed beams. Blistering and purpura are frequently associated with the use of this laser.

Erbium:yttrium-aluminum-garnet laser (2940 nm)

The Er:YAG laser emits an infrared beam at a wavelength of 2940 nm, close to the absorption peak of water. While its absorption coefficient is 16 times that of the CO_2 laser, its penetration depth is only 3 μm compared to CO_2 penetration of 20 μm.

Carbon dioxide laser (10 600 nm)

The carbon dioxide (CO_2) laser emits a 10 600 nm wavelength in either continuous or super-pulse mode which is completely absorbed by water in the epidermis and dermis, limiting its penetration to a depth of 0.1–0.2 mm. Direct tissue vaporization occurs and the skin is ablated at various depths depending on the energy used. It is used for skin resurfacing and treatment of warts, adnexal tumours and skin cancers. Absolute contraindications for laser resurfacing include the use of isotretinoin within the previous year, concurrent bacterial or viral infection and any hint of ectropion. Dark skin (skin types V and V1; p. 260) should be treated with special care as pigmentary irregularities after treatments are common. Cutaneous laser resurfacing is more effective on the face than on the neck and extremities. The CO_2 laser has been used for treatment of tattoos by direct tissue vaporization of the tattoo pigment, although there is a high risk of hypertrophic scarring because of the non-specific tissue necrosis surrounding the tattoo treatment site.

Intense pulsed light therapy (500–1200 nm)

This has become popular recently, partly as a result of its versatility and effective marketing to the public as well as to dermatologists. Intense pulsed light (IPL) sources are not lasers but polychromatic broadband flashlamps that emit non-coherent light within 500–1200 nm portion of the electromagnetic spectrum. Cut-off filters of varying wavelengths are used to filter out shorter wavelengths so that only longer, more deeply penetrating wavelengths are emitted (see Figure 18.2). They produce a photothermal effect. As multiple wavebands are delivered, several chromophores, including haemoglobin and melanin, can be targeted with a single exposure. Rejuvenation of photodamaged skin (lentigines, other pig-

mented lesions, telangiectasia, fine wrinkles and elastosis) may therefore be achieved with one rather than several devices (as would be required with lasers). IPL has been used for hair removal as well. In combination with topical ALA, this laser can be used for photodynamic rejuvenation and treatment of actinic keratoses. The wide variety of wavelengths, pulse duration and delay intervals make this device ideal for a wide range of skin types. Time and trials will define the niche for this treatment.

Lasers for specific indications

Vascular lesions

Vascular birthmarks such as port-wine stains (PWS) can be treated successfully in children as well as in adults, using the flashlamp pulsed dye laser emitting light at 585–595 nm (Figures 27.16 and 27.17). A series of treatment sessions (usually more than 10) are required to improve PWS. PWS with a deeper component benefit from a longer wavelength laser that penetrates deeper

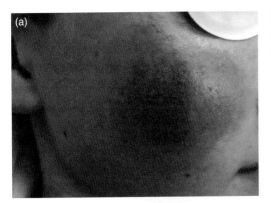
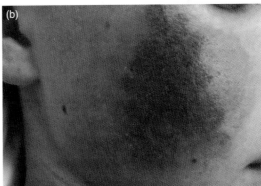
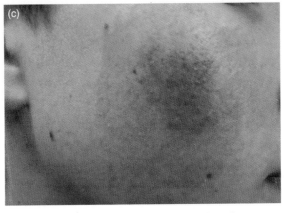

Figure 27.16 An example of a port-wine stain treated with a pulsed-dye laser with resultant purpura: (a) prior to treatment; (b) immediately posttreatment; (c) 1 month posttreatment with improvement in the treated area.

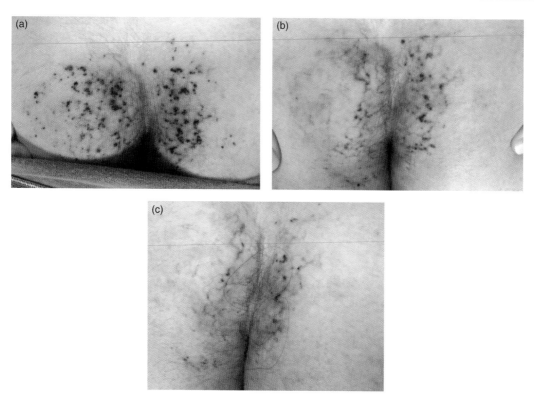

Figure 27.17 Many vascular lesions can be treated with the pulsed-dye laser, including angiokeratoma circumscriptum: (a) pretreatment; (b) after four treatments with significant improvement in the area; (c) after six treatments with near resolution.

such as 1064 nm long-pulsed Nd:YAG. Infantile haemangioma, on the other hand, usually involute with time, thus PDL may not be necessary except in healing ulcerated haemangiomas and treating residual telangiectasia after involution.

PDLs are the treatment of choice for facial erythema and telangiectasia of rosacea with minimal downtime. Most patients experience some post-treatment purpura, although longer pulse duration minimizes this side effect. KTP lasers at 532 nm are also effective at treating fine discrete telangiectatic vessels without purpura as it is better absorbed by haemoglobin, but their shorter wavelength limit their penetration. IPL can be used to treat fine telangiectasia by using the proper cut-off filter; however, more treatments are usually necessary than with PDLs. Also, there is a higher learning curve with KTP lasers as pigmentary damage can occur resulting in blistering and scarring.

Spider veins on the legs can be treated with lasers, although sclerotherapy remains the gold standard for treatment. KTP and PDL are useful for small calibre vessels, in treatment of postsclerotherapy telaniectatic matting and in those patients who are needle phobic. Deeper vessels require treatment with longer wavelengths such as long-pulsed Nd:YAG but these treatments can be painful and labour-intensive, as each vessel must be traced individually. In general, treatment response are poor unless underlying feeding vessels are addressed with sclerotherapy or surgery (p. 331).

Tattoo removal

Tattoos are permanent because the tattoo particles are too large to be phagocytized. Most tattoos can be removed by treatment with a Q-switched laser, the high energy short pulse is preferentially absorbed by the tattoo pigment, causing selective photothermolysis. The fragmented tattoo particles are then phagocytized and removed by the immune system. Four wavelengths are available (ruby 694 nm, alexandrite 755 nm, Nd:YAG 532 and 1064 nm); the choice of laser is dependent on the colour of the tattoo pigment. Recently, a new ultrashort pulsed laser with picosecond duration has shown greater efficacy in

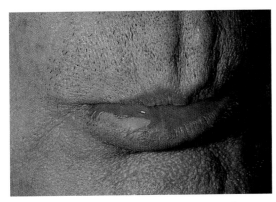

Figure 27.18 Leucoplakia caused by chronic actinic damage – most suitable for laser resurfacing treatment.

tattoo removal. Nevertheless, patients should be warned that multiple (sometimes 8–12) treatments may be necessary and complete removal may not be possible. In patients with an allergic reaction to tattoo ink, the Q-switched laser is not recommended as the fragmentation of the tattoo particles and subsequent phagocytosis may precipitate a systemic allergic reaction.

Pigmented lesions

Benign but unsightly pigmented lesions such as senile lentigines and naevi of Ota can be greatly improved by treatment with long pulsed 532 nm and the Q-switched lasers (ruby 694 nm, alexandrite 755 nm, Nd:YAG 532 and 1064 nm). Other pigmented lesions such as café au lait marks, melasma and Becker's naevi are less resposive to treatment but may be improved. Intense pulsed light is best used for patients with diffuse photodamage with solar lentigines and vascularity.

Hair removal

Unwanted hair can be removed permamently with an alexandrite laser (750 nm), pulsed diode laser (810 nm), with a long-pulsed Nd:YAG laser emitting light at 1064 nm or an IPL system. These lasers preferentially target melanin in the hair follicle. In order to result in permanent hair loss, the heat delivered to the hair follicle must diffuse to damage the follicular stem cells in the hair bulge (which does not contain much melanin). The ideal patient is one with thick dark hair (good melanin target) with fair skin (less collateral damage to the epidermis). Laser hair removal is not effective for blond or white hair given the paucity of melanin. Adequate skin cooling and choice of a longer wavelength lasers are particularly important when treating darker skinned patients.

Laser resurfacing

Rhinophyma, sebaceous gland hyperplasia, seborrhoeic keratoses, syringomas and many of the signs of chronic photodamage (e.g. rhytides, actinic cheilitis, actinic keratoses) can be helped by cutaneous resurfacing using CO_2 lasers emitting a wavelength of 10 600 nm (infrared), with which tissue water is the chromatophore, or a Q-switched Er:YAG laser emitting pulsed waves of 2940 nm in the near infrared, which is absorbed by water 10 times more efficiently than the pulsed CO_2 laser beam (Figures 27.18 and 27.19). Good postoperative care is important, as the patient is left with what is essentially a partial thickness burn which heals by re-epithelialization from the cutaneous appendages. After profuse exudation for 24–48 hours the treated area heals, usually in 5–15 days, but during this time the skin is unsightly. This excessive downtime and risks of scarring and pigmentations

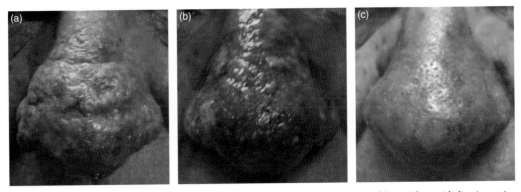

Figure 27.19 Rhinophyma treated with Erb:YAG ablative resurfacing laser: (a) preoperative; (b) partial re-epithelization at 1 week; (c) complete healing at 3 weeks.

have led many to favour other forms of treatment such as fractionated lasers (p. 330) for less severe cases.

If all of the above seems too complicated to the uninitiated then it is clear that laser treatments should be carried out only by fully trained specialists.

Learning points

1 Routine dermatologic surgery performed on clean skin carries a very low risk of infection, therefore antibiotic prophylaxis is rarely necessary.
2 There are numerous techniques for the treatment of malignant skin lesions, including cryosurgery, excision, curettage, electrosurgery, radiotherapy, photodynamic therapy, topical treatment and Mohs' micrographic surgery. Selection of 'best' treatment depends on many factors including the type of tumour, the location, as well as patient factors. One size does not fit all!
3 Advances in laser technology have enabled many skin conditions to be treated with minimal downtime and complications.

Further reading

British Association of Dermatologists (1999) Clinical Guidelines: Antibiotic prophylaxis for endocarditis in dermatological surgery. www.bad.org.uk (accessed 5 July 2014).

British Association of Dermatologists. British Photodermatology Group consensus view on sunbeds for cosmetic tanning. http://www.bad.org.uk/for-the-public/skin-cancer/sunbeds (accessed 15 July 2014).

Dover JS, Arndt KA, Dinehart SM, Fitzpatrick RE, Gonzales E, Guidelines/Outcomes Committee (1999) Guidelines of care for laser surgery. *Journal of the American Academy of Dermatology* **41**, 484–495.

Gold MH, Goldman MP. (2004) 5-aminolevulinic acid photodynamic therapy: where we have been and where we are going. *Dermatologic Surgery* **30**, 1077–1083.

Goldberg MD. (2005) *Lasers and Lights, Vols 1 and 2, Procedures in Cosmetic Dermatology series* (Series editor, Dover JS.) Elsevier Saunders, Philadelphia.

Kuflik EG. (1994) Cryosurgery updated. *Journal of the American Academy of Dermatology* **31**, 925–944.

Lawrence C. (2002) *An Introduction to Dermatological Surgery*, 2nd edition. Elsevier Churchill Livingstone, Edinburgh.

Morison WL. (2005) *Phototherapy and Photochemotherapy of Skin Disease*, 3rd edition. Taylor and Francis Group, Baltimore.

Morton CA, McKenna KE, Rhodes LE. (2008) Guidelines for topical photodynamic therapy: update. *British Journal of Dermatology* **159**, 1275–1266.

Rowe DE, Carroll RJ, Day CL. (1989) Long-term recurrence rates in previously untreated (primary) basal cell carcinoma: implications for patient follow-up. *Journal of Dermatologic Surgery and Oncology* **15**, 315–328.

Telfer NR, Colver GB, Morton CA. (2008) Guidelines for the management of basal cell carcinoma. *British Journal of Dermatology* **159**, 35.

28 Dermoscopy

Dermoscopy, also termed epiluminescence microscopy or skin surface microscopy, has been used since the 1900s by dermatologists as a non-invasive *in vivo* diagnostic technique to aid in early diagnosis of melanoma. Dermoscopy helps to differentiate melanomas from benign naevi and from mimickers such as pigmented basal cell carcinoma, seborrhoeic keratoses or haemorrhages under the skin. A meta-analysis published in 2008 showed that, among dermatologists, dermoscopy increased diagnostic accuracy in pigmented skin lesions (90% diagnosed melanoma correctly versus 74% without dermoscopy), without any difference in specificity. One randomized trial of dermatologists trained in dermoscopy demonstrated a 42% reduction in unnecessary biopsy compared with those using naked eye examination alone. Dermoscopy has also been shown to be increasingly useful in the diagnosis of a variety of other dermatological conditions. It can aid in finding burrows in scabies, locating a splinter, evaluating alopecia and evaluating nail fold capillaries in systemic sclerosis.

A dermascope consists of a hand-held device with magnification (usually 10- to 20-fold) and a light source (Figure 28.1). A digital imaging system can be attached for photographic documentation. A dermascope renders the stratum corneum translucent to allow for the examination of the subsurface morphological details of the skin. It enhances the microstructures in the epidermis, dermo-epidermal junction and papillary dermis, allowing clinicians to identify specific features that correspond to benign and malignant pigmented skin lesions (Table 28.1). Two methods are commonly used to accomplish this: cross-polarized light and contact immersion system. With contact immersion dermoscopy, the dermoscope is placed directly on the skin along with an immersion fluid (mineral oil, ultrasonic gel, alcohol or water) to reduce reflection and refraction of light from the stratum corneum. Alternatively, the use of cross-polarized light eliminates the use of immersion fluid and the need for direct contact with the skin which reducing the risk of cross-contamination between patients. Newer hybrid devices allow for both polarized and contact immersion examination (Figure 28.2).

Dermoscopic evaluation

Dermoscopic evaluation is a two-step process (Figure 28.3). The first step in dermoscopic evaluation is to determine whether a lesion is of melanocytic origin. Melanocytic lesions, basal cell carcinomas, seborrhoeic keratoses, dermatofibromas and vascular lesions have unique dermoscopic features (see Table 28.1; Figure 28.4). In general, melanocytic lesions have pigment network with dots, globules or streaks, and blue–grey pigmentation. If the lesion does not have any of these melanocytic features **and** does not have any features of non-melanocytic lesions listed in Table 28.1, it is considered melanocytic by default. Of note, lesions present on facial, acral and mucosal sites may demonstrate site-specific dermoscopic features; a full discussion of these more complex sites may be found in a dedicated advanced dermoscopy text.

Once a lesion has been categorized as melanocytic, the second step of dermoscopy is to differentiate benign from malignant melanocytic lesions (Table 28.2). Over the last decade, numerous dermoscopic algorithms have been developed to aid in the idenification of melanomas, including pattern analysis, ABCDE rules, 7-point checklist, Menzies method, 4 × 4 × 6 rule and the three-point checklist (Table 28.3). While a thorough discussion of each of these algorithms is beyond the scope of this text, we have listed some general dermscopic features for melanoma that have been emphasized in various

Clinical Dermatology, Fifth Edition. Richard B. Weller, Hamish J.A. Hunter and Margaret W. Mann.
© 2015 John Wiley & Sons, Ltd. Published 2015 by John Wiley & Sons, Ltd.

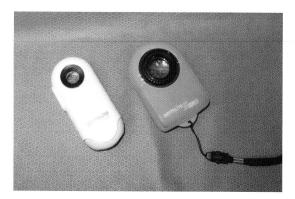

Figure 28.1 Hand-held dermascopes.

algorithms. They can be divided into global features, patterns and local features. Global features of melanoma include asymmetry and mutiple colours (Figure 28.5). Benign lesions tend to show symmetrical dermascopic structures and colour. Patterns refer to types of pigment network, including reticular, globular, homogenous, cobblestone, parallel and starburst. Local features that raise concern for melanoma include irregular dots/globules, streaks, atypical vessels, regression and blue–white veil.

For the newly trained dermoscopy user, the simplified, easy-to-learn three-point checklist is a good screening test. It has proven to be both reproducible and highly sensitive for detecting melanomas, although with lower specificity than the more detailed algorithms listed above. The three-point checklist consists of three criteria: asymmetry, atypical pigment network and blue–white

Table 28.1 Typical dermoscopic features of skin lesions.

Melanocytic lesion	Pigment network
	Dots and globules
	Streaks
	Parallel pattern of pigment (on acral skin)
	Blue–grey pigmentation
	Lack of any specific dermoscopic features
Seborrhoeic keratosis	Milia-like cysts
	Comedo-like openings
	Light-brown fingerprint-like structures
	Fissures/ridges/irregular crypts
Basal cell carcinoma	Absent pigment network
	Arborizing vessels
	Maple leaf-like areas
	Blue–grey ovoid nests/globules
	Spoke wheel areas
	Superficial ulceration
Vascular lesion	Red–blue lacunas
	Red–blue to red–black homogenous areas
Dermatofibroma	Peripheral finely textured pigment network
	Central white area

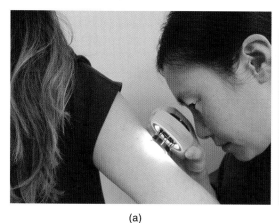

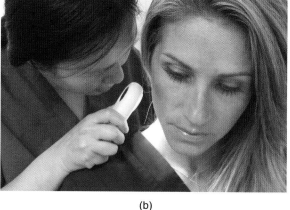

(a)   (b)

Figure 28.2 Physician examining a pigmented lesion using a contact immersion system (a) and cross-polarized light which does not require direct contact (b).

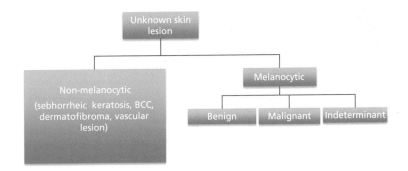

Figure 28.3 Two-step dermoscopic evaluation. BCC, basal cell carcinoma.

structures. Benign lesions may demonstrate any one of these criteria, but lesions with two of three criteria is suspicous for melanoma and should be removed and submitted for pathological review. Lesions with only one colour and one structural pattern are generally benign. Asymmetry of colour or structure in one or two perpendicular axes is concerning for malignancy. Atypical network refers to pigment network with irregular areas of boardened lines or holes. Finally, blue–white structures or blue–while veil consists of any blue or white colour within the lesion (see below). As with most other subjective tools, experience increases diagnostic accuracy.

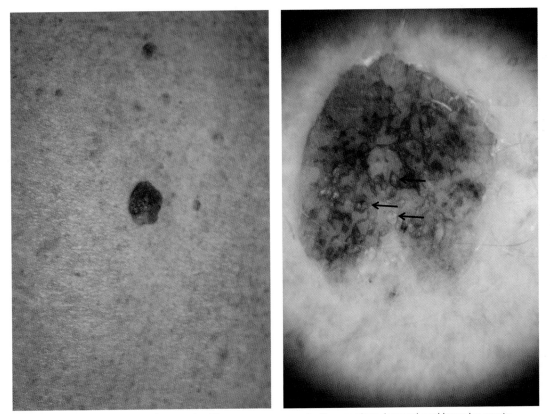

(a) Seborrhoeic keratosis: characterized by numerous comedo-like openings (arrows) and irregular crypts.

Figure 28.4 Typical dermascopic appearance of non-melanocytic lesions. Figures courtesy of Dr. Kelly Nelson, Department of Dermatology, Vanderbilt University, Nashville, Tennessee, USA.

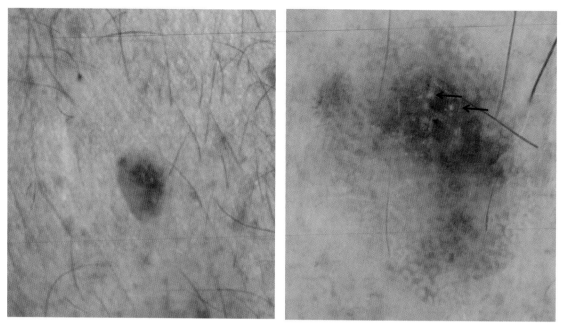

(b) Seborrhoeic keratosis with several milia-like cysts (arrows) and light brown fingerprint-like structures.

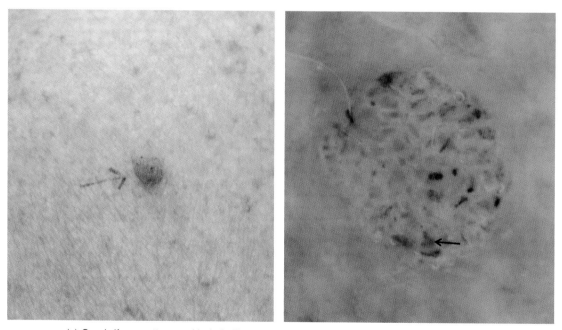

(c) Cerebriform pattern and hairpin-like vessels (black arrow) of a seborrhoeic keratosis.

Figure 28.4 (*Continued*)

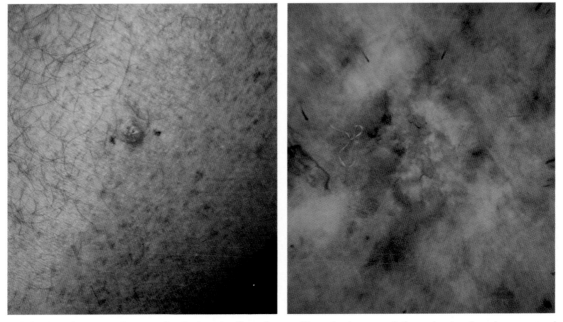

(d) Pigmented basal cell carcinoma. Clinically, this irregularly pigmented lesion is concerning for a melanoma. On dermoscopic examination, one can see features including maple leaf-like structures (black arrows) and arborizing vessels (white arrows) typical of a basal cell carcinoma.

(e) Another dermoscopic example of a basal cell carcinoma. There is absence of pigment network and presence of arborizing vessels in the center of the lesion.

Figure 28.4 *(Continued)*

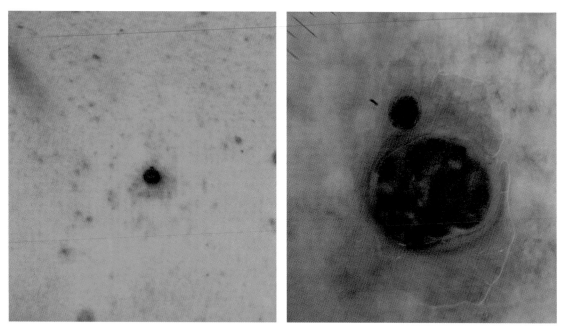

(f) Angioma with classic red lacunae.

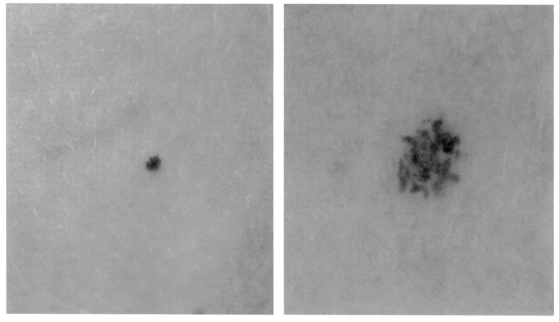

(g) Another example of an angioma with red lacunae.

Figure 28.4 (*Continued*)

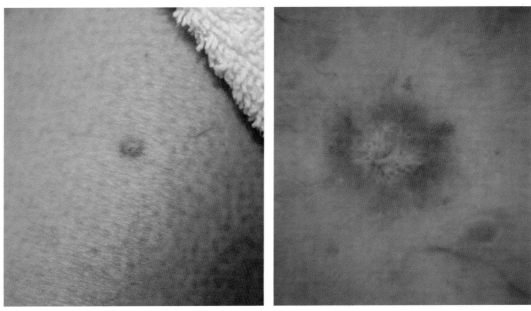

(h) Dermatofibromas are characterized by a central white area with peripheral finely textured pigment network.

Figure 28.4 (*Continued*)

Patterns of pigment network

Reticular pattern

Reticular pattern consists of pigmented 'lines' and hypopigmented 'holes' forming a honeycomb pattern. This grid-like pattern corresponds to the three-dimensional conical structure of the rete ridges. Hypopigmented 'holes' occur at the tips of the dermal papillae where there is relatively less melanin and darker 'lines' are caused by the relative increase in melanin along the base of the papillae or rete ridges.

Most benign naevi have a symmetrical orderly pigment network that fades at the periphery. In contrast, melanomas may demonstrate an atypical pigment network with multiple colours (black, brown and/or grey), with thicker and thinner areas, larger and smaller holes which are irregularly distributed, and abrupt termination of the network at the lesion edges.

Globular pattern

Globules are varying sized round to ovoid structures typically seen in acquired melanocytic naevi in young patients.

Table 28.2 Dermoscopic features suggestive of naevi and melanomas.

Benign naevus	Regular pigment network
	Dots/globules uniform in size and symmetrically distributed (usually centrally located)
	Evenly distributed streaks
Spitz naevus/spindle cell naevus of Reed	Starburst pattern
	Regular streaks at the periphery of lesion
Blue naevus	Homogenous pattern
	Diffuse uniform blue pigment
Melanoma	Atypical pigment network
	Irregular dots/globules (brown globules/black dots)
	Irregular streaks (pseudopods or radial streaming)
	Blue–white veil
	Regression structures
	Atypical vascular pattern

Table 28.3 Common algorithm used to distinguish benign from malignant pigmented lesions.

3-point checklist	• Asymmetry (structure or colour) • Atypical pigment network • Blue–white structures 2 or more points = possible melanoma and needs biopsy		
7-point checklist	Major criteria (2 points each) • Atypical pigment network • Blue–white veil • Atypical vascular pattern Minor criteria (1 point each) • Irregular pigment • Irregular dots/globules • Irregular streaks • Regression structures 3 or more points = possible melanoma and needs biopsy		
		Points	Weight Factor
ABCD Rules	Asymmetry • Complete symmetry • Asymmetry in 1 axis • Asymmetry in 2 axis	0 1 2	1.3
	Border (divided into 8 segments) • 1 point for abrupt cut-off of pigment • 0 point for gradual fade to periphery	0–8	0.1
	Colour (1 point for each) • Black, dark brown, light brown, grey–blue, white and red	1–6	0.5
	Differential structures (1 point for each) • Pigment network, structureless areas, dots, globules, streaks	1–5	0.5
	Total score range 1–8.9 　Score >5.45 = highly suspicious of melanoma and 　　needs biopsy 　Score >4.75 = suspicious, possible dysplastic naevus, 　　needs biopsy 　Score <4.75 = benign		
Menzies method	Negative features: benign • Symmetrical structural pigment pattern • Single colour Positive features: melanoma • Blue–white veil • Multiple brown dots • Pseudopods/radial streaming • Scar-like depigmentation • Peripheral black dots/globules • Multiple colours (5–6) • Multiple blue–grey dots • Broadened network		

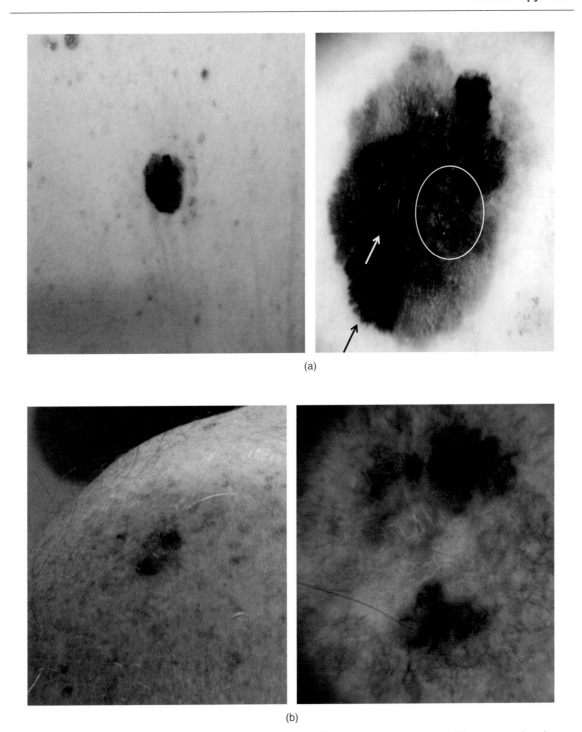

(a)

(b)

Figure 28.5 (a) Melanoma with asymmetry of colour and structure as well as irregular pigment network. There are pseudopods irregularly distributed at one edge of the lesion (black arrows), blue–black structureless area (white arrow) as well as areas of thin and thickened reticular lines. Blue–white veil can be seen at the centre of the lesion (circle). (b) Another example of a melanoma with asymmetry of multiple colours and structure. There are areas of irregular thickened hyperpigmented lines in a reticular pattern at the periphery. Centrally there is a structureless area of regression with scar-like depigmentation. (c) While this lesion is clinically subtle for a melanoma, it has concerning features on dermoscopic examination including multiple colours, asymmetry of structure and multiple peripheral brown and black dots. This lesion was biopsied and histopathology confirmed the diagnosis of melanoma. Figures courtesy of Dr. Kelly Nelson, Department of Dermatology, Vanderbilt University, Nashville, Tennessee, USA.

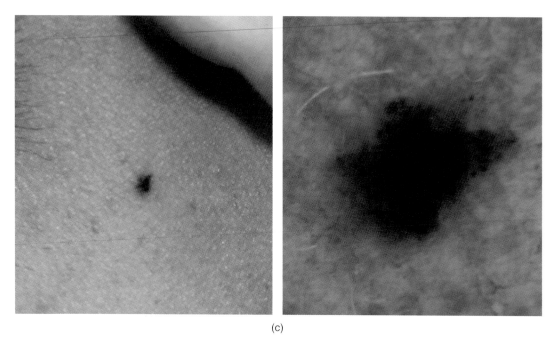

(c)

Figure 28.5 (*Continued*)

Cobblestone pattern

Found in dermal naevi, a cobblestone pattern is similar to a globular pattern but consists of large aggregates of globules or dermal nests of melanocytes arranged in a square or angulated shape that resembles cobblestones.

Homogenous pattern

The homogenous pattern manifests as diffuse areas of colour with an absence of pigment network or structural features and can be seen in blue naevi, seborrhoeic keratoses and benign naevi.

Parallel pattern

The parallel pattern is seen in most melanocytic lesions on acral surfaces. In benign lesions, pigment is generally distributed in a 'parallel furrow' pattern, or along the sulci of the acral skin lines. Variations in the parallel furrow pattern include lattices and fibrillar patterns, in which there is some extension of pigment horizontally on to the ridges. On the other hand, the 'parallel ridge' pattern, in which the pigment is arranged primarily at the base of the papilla, has a high specificity (99%) for melanomas.

Starburst pattern

The starburst pattern is characterized by pigmented streaks in a radial arrangement at the periphery of a pigmented skin lesion and is found in spitzoid melanomas and pigmented spindle cell naevi of Reed.

Multicomponent pattern

The presence of three or more distinctive patterns (reticular, globular and homogenous) is highly correlated with melanoma.

Local features concerning for melanoma

Irregular dots and globules

Dots and globules may occur in both benign naevi and melanomas. In benign lesions, they are uniform in size and regularly distributed centrally, whereas in melanoma they tend to be varied in size and scattered unevenly at the periphery. Dots are small round structures less

Table 28.4 Colour and location of melanin in dermoscopy.

Black	Melanin in the epidermis: stratum corneum or spinous layer
Brown	Melanin in the dermo-epidermal junction
Grey–blue	Melanin in the papillary dermis
Blue	Melanin in the reticular dermis
White	Evidence of fibrosis or regression
Red	Presence of haemoglobin inside vessels

than 0.1 mm in size caused by melanin accumulation, with the colour corresponding to the location of pigment accumulation (Table 28.4). Pigmented structures appear black when located in the stratum corneum, brown in the dermo-epidermal junction and grey–blue in the deep papillary/reticular dermis. Globules are larger than 0.1 mm in size and represent nests of melanocytes.

Irregular streaks

Streaks are brown–black linear structures not clearly part of a pigment network. Symmetrical streaks can be seen in benign naevi while irregular asymmetric streaks are concerning for melanoma. Two types of streak patterns can be seen: radial streaming and pseudopods. Radial streaming refers to radially arranged parallel lines at the periphery of a lesion. Symmetrical and uniform radial streaks are particularly common in pigmented spindle cell naevi (p. 286). Pseudopods are dark finger-like bulbous projections at the periphery of the lesion. Their presence often denotes a melanoma.

Atypical vascular network

Melanomas with neovascularization may result in atypical vascular patterns with dotted, glomerular or bizarre vessels.

Regression

Dermoscopically, regression appears as white scar-like areas, hypopigmented spots or bluish areas. Regression structures may demonstrate a visual continuum with blue–white veil structures. Regression changes are caused by fibrosis, loss of pigmentation and epidermal thinning and may signify a melanoma.

Blue–white veil

Blue–white veil refers to focal areas of indistinct blue–white hazy pigmentation. Histologically, this is caused by excess melanin in a thickened epidermis. This is one of the three criteria used in the three-point checklist and highly suggestive of a melanoma.

Final notes

Just as with learning any new technique, proficiency in dermoscopy requires investment of time and dedication. The learning curve may be shortened by obtaining clinical and dermoscopic images of lesions slated for removal and pathological review. This allows the provider to review the specific dermoscopic features of lesions upon return of the definitive diagnostic pathology report.

There are several limitations of dermoscopy: first, histopathology is still necessary to confirm the diagnosis after a biopsy or excision; secondly, dermatoscopy only allows for examination of the skin up to the level of the papillary dermis, therefore deeper structures in the reticular dermis will not be visualized; thirdly, heavily pigmented areas and small lesions are difficult to examine under dermoscopy, and dermoscopy should not be used as a substitute for a good history and naked eye examination for the diagnosis of pigmented lesions.

Learning points

- Benign lesions tend to show symmetrical dermascopic structures and colour.
- Dermascopic features that raise concern for melanoma include asymmetry in colour and shape, irregular dots/globules, streaks, atypical vessels, regression and blue–white veil.
- The presence of a blue–white veil is highly suggestive of a melanoma.
- Dermoscopy should not be used as a substitute for a good history and naked eye examination for the diagnosis of pigmented lesions.
- If you are ever in doubt, perform a biopsy and confirm the diagnosis with histopathology.
- Dermoscopy can be difficult to master initially. Make an effort to examine every lesion you biopsy. As you get more familiar with the technique, you will improve your diagnostic accuracy and reduce the number of biopsies you perform.

Further reading

Braun RP, Rabinovitz HS, Oliviero M, *et al.* (2005) Dermoscopy of pigmented skin lesions. *Journal of the American Academy of Dermatology* **52**, 109–121.

Hirokawa D, Lee, JB. (2011) Dermatoscopy: an overview of subsurface morphology. *Clinics in Dermatology* **29**, 557–565.

Marghoob AA, Korzenko AJ, Changchien L, Scope A, Braun RP, Rabinovitz H. (2007) The beauty and the beast sign in dermoscopy. *Dermatologic Surgery* **33**, 1388–1391.

Topical Treatments

Our selection has been determined by personal preferences and we accept that we have left out many effective remedies. However, the preparations listed here are those that we use most often. As a result some appear only in the UK column but not in the USA one, and vice versa. To conform with current prescribing recommendations whenever possible we have listed these products under their active ingredients, with their proprietary names in brackets. Up-to-date information can be found at www.bnf.org.uk or www.fda.gov.

There is a limited range of licensed topical products for the treatment of common skin conditions such as eczema and psoriasis. As a result dermatologists may prescribe unlicensed alternatives or 'specials'. These should only be used when a licensed alternative is unavailable. Many of these specials have a proven track record over many years; however, the evidence for their usage is largely empirical. Nonetheless, they have become a trusted and essential part of the dermatological armamentarium. Due to a small potential market and short shelf life they are often considered non-viable for commercial production, which is reflected in their disproportionately high price. In an attempt to rationalize the array of specials, the British Association of Dermatologists has produced an excellent booklet on the most commonly used preparations, their indications and treatment regimes (http://www.bad.org.uk/healthcare-professionals/clinical-standards/specials).

Type of preparation and general comments	UK preparations	USA preparations
Emollients These are used to make dry scaly skin smoother. Most are best applied after a shower or bath. The opposite of dry is wet, not greasy. While greasy formulations make the skin look moister, those containing humectants such as glycerin, urea or lactic acid generally moisturize better. On the face, use moisturizers designed for the face to minimize acne cosmetica	Soft white paraffin BP Emulsifying ointment BP Liquid and White Soft Paraffin Ointment, NPF (liquid paraffin 50%, white soft paraffin 50%) Aqueous cream BP – can be used as a soap substitute Aveeno range Doublebase range Hydromol cream and ointment Epaderm cream and ointment Diprobase cream and ointment E45 range Oilatum range Unguentum M – a useful diluent: contains propylene glycol and sorbic acid, which may sensitize Neutrogena dermatological cream Aquadrate, Balneum, Eucerin Intensive, Hydromol Intensive and Calmurid creams contains urea Dermol range – contains antimicrobials	Petrolatum alba USP Vanicream – devoid of fragrances and many sensitizers Aquaphor – a hydrophilic petrolatum Aveeno cream (Eczema Therapy) Plastibase – a hydrophilic polyglycol Eucerin – hydrophilic petrolatum containing water Curel Moisturel Lubriderm Hydrolatum – petrolatum, methylparaben Carmol range – contains urea humectant Complex 15 facial – phospholipids Lacticare lotion – contains alphahydroxy acid

Clinical Dermatology, Fifth Edition. Richard B. Weller, Hamish J.A. Hunter and Margaret W. Mann.
© 2015 John Wiley & Sons, Ltd. Published 2015 by John Wiley & Sons, Ltd.

Type of preparation and general comments	UK preparations	USA preparations

Bath additives/shower gels
 	
These are a useful way of ensuring application to the whole skin. Most contain emollients which help with dry itchy skin. Others contain tar (see section on psoriasis) or antibacterials. Caution: makes bathtubs slippery
	Balneum range
	Emulsiderm – contains benzalkonium chloride
	Oilatum range
	Aveeno range
	Doublebase range
	Hydromol bath emollient
	Dermol and Oilatum Plus ranges contain
	   antimicrobials
		Mineral oil bath emulsion (Keri
		   Moisture Rich Shower and Bath Oil,
		   Eucerin Bath Therapy)
		Colloidal oatmeal (Aveeno Eczema
		   Therapy Bath Treatment)
		Balneum
		Hydromol Emollient

Shampoos
 	
All contain detergents which help to remove debris and scales; some have added ingredients to combat psoriasis, seborrhoeic eczema and bacterial infections. Most work best if their lather is left on the scalp for 5 minutes before being rinsed off
	Containing tar
	Alphosyl 2 in 1
	Polytar range
	T-Gel
	Capasal – also contains salicylic acid
	
	Others
	Betadine – contains antibacterial povidone
	   iodine
	Ceanel concentrate – contains cetrimide,
	   undecenoic acid
	Selsun – contains selenium sulfide and can be
	   used to treat pityriasis versicolor (p. 245)
	Nizoral – contains ketoconazole and is useful for
	   seborrhoeic dermatitis and pityriasis
	   versicolor
	Meted – contains salicylic acid and sulfur
	Dermax – contains benzalkonium chloride
		Containing tar
		DHS Tar Gel
		Denorex shampoo – tingles on scalp
		Neutrogena T-Gel
		Tarsum Shampoo
		Polytar range
		
		Others
		Selsun contains selenium sulfide and can
		   be used to treat pityriasis versicolor
		   (p. 245)
		Nizoral – contains ketoconazole and is
		   useful for seborrhoeic dermatitis and
		   pityriasis versicolor
		Head and Shoulders, Zincon – contains
		   zinc pyrethione
		Sebulex, Scalpicin, T-sal – contain
		   salicylic and sulfur
		Caprex – contains fluocinonide

Cleansing agents
 	
These are used to remove debris and to combat infection. Some are astringents which precipitate protein and in doing so help to seal the moist surface of a weeping eczema or a stasis ulcer
	Solution of sodium chloride 0.9% (Normasol) –
	   used to clean wounds and ulcers
	Potassium permanganate (Permitabs – one
	   tablet in 4 L water makes a 0.01% solution) –
	   will stain clothing and skin
	Aluminium acetate lotion – use at 0.65% in
	   water – is mildly astringent and used as wet
	   dressing
	Silver nitrate – use at 0.5% in water – is
	   astringent, stains skin brown
	Chlorhexidine acetate 0.05%
	Chlorhexidine gluconate 4% (Hibiscrub)
		Syndets – neutral cleansers generally
		   milder than soap (Dove)
		Chlorhexidine 4% (Hibiclens)
		   concentrate – use diluted to 1 in 100
		   (a 0.04% solution of chlorhexidine in
		   water for skin disinfection)
		Cetaphil gentle skin cleanser (lipid-free)
		Benzalkonium chloride (Ionax line)
		Triclosan (Dial, Lever 2000) –
		   deodorant, antibacterial
		Sulfacetamide/Sulfur (Plexon) – cleanser
		   for rosacea
		Ethyl alcohol gel (non-irritating
		   disinfectant for hand washing)

Type of preparation and general comments	UK preparations	USA preparations
Barrier preparations These are used to protect the skin from irritants and are of value in the napkin (diaper) area and around stomas. Many contain the silicone, dimethicone. The choice of barrier creams for use at work depends upon individual circumstances: recommendations are not given here	Petrolatum Zinc and castor oil ointment BP Dimethicone and benzalkonium chloride (Conotrane) Dimethicone and cetrimide (Siopel)	Petrolatum Zinc oxide ointment Kerodex 51 (water-miscible) Kerodex 71 cream (water-repellent) Bentoquatum (Ivy Block Lotion) protective against toxicodendron (poison ivy allergy) Dermaguard spray Flexible collodion (film) Zinc oxide, lanolin, talc and vitamins A and D (Desitin ointment) Dimethicone (Diaper Guard Ointment) Anusol (zinc oxide plus pramoxine) Bag Balm (contains 8-hydroxyquinoline sulfate)
Depigmenting agents Most contain hydroquinone. The use of agents containing monobenzone causes permanent complete depigmentation	None in BNF but some preparations available without prescription from chemists/cosmetic counters Azelaic acid (Finacea gel 15%, Skinoren cream 20%)	Hydroquinone 2–4% (Ambi Fade Cream (2% HQ), EpiQuin Micro (4% HQ), Glyquin XM (4% HQ, oxybenzone, avobenzone and glycolic acid) Lustra (4% HQ), Lustra-AF (4% HQ, sunscreen) Hydroquinone (4%), tretinoin (0.05%) and fluocinolone acetonide (0.1%) (Tri-Luma) Monobenzene/monobenzyl ether of hydroquinone (Benaquin) (Caution: permanent depigmentation) Azelaic acid (Finacea gel 15%, Azelex cream 20%)
Camouflaging preparations Blemishes that cannot be removed can often be made less obvious by covering. Expert cosmetic advice may be needed to obtain the best colour match	Covermark range Dermablend range Keromask range	Covermark range of products Dermablend Powder Palette (Physician's Formula – Pierre Fabre) in green for correcting red blush of rosacea

Type of preparation and general comments	UK preparations	USA preparations
Sunscreens and sunblocks These help the light-sensitive but are not a substitute for sun avoidance and sensible protective clothing. The sun protection factor (SPF) is a measure of their effectiveness against UVB more than UVA, but those recommended here block UVA also Allergic contact dermatitis from the sunscreen ingredients may be missed and the rash put down to a deterioration of the original photosensitivity	Titanium dioxide (E45 Sun range) Cinnamate, oxybenzone and titanium dioxide (Sunsense Ultra, Roc Sante Soleil, Uvistat range)	Avobenzone, homosalate, oxybenzone (Neutrogena range, Aveeno range, Solbar range) Titanium dioxide, zinc oxide (Blue Lizard, Aveeno Natural Protection, CoTZ, MelaShade, Neutrogena Pure & Free, TiZO3, Vanicream) Helioplex – stabilizes avobenzone and oxybenzone, prolonging duration of protection (Neutrogena Ultra Sheer Dry Touch, Neutrogena Age Shield) Mexoryl SX – contains a photostable UVA-absorbing chemical ecamsule (Anthelios)
Antipruritics Remember that these are of limited value. Try to make a firm diagnosis that will lead to an effective line of treatment	Calamine lotion BP Oily Calamine lotion BP – contains arachis oil Menthol (0.5–2%) or phenol (1.0%) in aqueous cream Crotamiton cream and lotion (Eurax) – also used to treat scabies Doxepin (Xepin cream)	Calamine lotion Crotamiton (Eurax cream and lotion) also used to treat scabies Menthol and camphor (Sarna lotion) contains menthol and camphor Doxepin (Zonalon cream) Pramoxine (Prax, Pramegel, Itch-X) Pramoxine and hydrocortisone (Pramosone, Aveeno Anti-itch cream, Epifoam) Benzocaine (Boil ease ointment, solarcaine) – caution: may sensitize
Antiperspirants Most antiperspirants are deodorants too, but many deodorants (e.g. triclosan) are not antiperspirants	Aluminium chloride hexahydrate 20% (Anhydrol Forte solution or Driclor solution). Botulinum toxin (Botox) injections – for local temporary anhidrosis of axillae or palms Glycopyrronium bromide 0.05% solution by iontophoresis (Robinul) to palmar or plantar skin	Aluminum zirconium tetrachlorhydroxy gly (many drugstore products, e.g. Gillette and Speed stick lines) Aluminum chlorate 20% (Drysol) 12.5% (CertainDri Roll-On), 6.25% (Xerac-AC) Formaldehyde 10% solution (Lazerformaldehyde) – caution: may sensitize Botulinum toxin (Botox) injections – for local temporary anhidrosis of axillae or palms Glycopyrronium bromide 0.05% solution by iontophoresis (Robinul) to palmar or plantar skin

Type of preparation and general comments	UK preparations	USA preparations
Keratolytics These are used to counter an excessive production of keratin. Salicylic acid preparations should be used for limited areas only and not above 6%, as absorption and toxicity may follow their prolonged and extensive application, especially in infants	Salicylic acid, 2–4% in emulsifying ointment or soft white paraffin Zinc and salicylic acid (2%) paste (Lassar's paste). Useful for hyperkeratotic, fissured skin disorders Urea preparations (*see Emollients*) Propylene glycol, 20% in aqueous cream	Salicylic acid (6% Keralyt gel, Salex, Salkera) Salicylic acid, 2–4% in emulsifying ointment or soft white paraffin Urea preparations at high concentrations (Carmol 20%, 40%) Propylene glycol (Epilyt)
Depilatories Over-the-counter depilatories are used to remove unwanted facial hairs and are all irritating. Eflornithine inhibits ornithine decarboxylase in hair follicles	Eflornithine 11.5% (Vaniqa) retards hair regrowth	Sulfides (Magic Shaving Powder) Thioglycollates (Nair line, Neet line) Zip wax, Nair microwave wax – mechanical hair removal Eflornithine hydrochloride cream 13.9% (Vaniqa) retards hair regrowth

Steroids
Our selection here has had to be ruthless as so many brands and mixtures are now on the market
   Conventionally, they are classified according to their potency. Your aim should be to use the least potent preparation that will cope with the skin disorder being treated. Side effects and dangers are listed in Table 26.2, p. 361.
   Nothing stronger than 1% hydrocortisone should be used on the face (except in special circumstances, e.g. discoid lupus erythematosus) or in infancy. Be reluctant to prescribe more than 200 g of a mildly potent, 50 g of a moderately potent or 30 g of a potent preparation per week for any adult for more than 1 month
   Most of the preparations listed are available as lotions, creams, oily creams and ointments; your choice of vehicle will depend upon the condition under treatment (p. 363). Use twice daily except for Cutivate and Elocon, which are just as effective if used once a day
	Mildly potent
	Hydrocortisone 0.5, 1.0, 2.5% preparations
	Fluocinolone acetonide (Synalar cream 1 in 10)
	
	Moderately potent
	Alclometasone dipropionate (Modrasone cream and ointment)
	Betamethasone valerate (Betnovate RD cream and ointment)
	Clobetasone butyrate cream and ointment (Eumovate)
	
	Potent
	Betamethasone valerate (Betnovate range including scalp application, Betacap scalp application, Bettamousse scalp application)
	Fluticasone propionate (Cutivate cream and ointment)
	Mometasone furoate (Elocon range)
	Hydrocortisone butyrate (Locoid range)
	Fluocinolone acetonide (Synalar range)
	
	Very potent
	Clobetasol propionate (Dermovate range, Clarelux foam scalp treatment and Etrivex shampoo)
	Diflucortolone valerate (Nerisone Forte range)
		Mildly potent
		Hydrocortisone 0.5, 1.0, 2.5% (numerous manufacturers)
		Desonide (Desowen, Tridesilon, Desonate)
		Alclometasone (Aclovate)
		Fluocinolone acetonide 0.01% (Synalar, Dermasmoothe)
		
		Moderately potent
		Betamethasone valerate (Valisone, Luxiq Foam)
		Hydrocortisone valerate (Westcort)
		Triamcinolone 0.025%, 0.1% (Kenalog, Aristocort, various manufacturers)
		
		Potent
		Betamethasone dipropionate (Diprosone)
		Mometason Furoate (Elocon)
		Fluticasone propionate (Cutivate)
		Fluocinonide (Lidex)
		Desoximetasone (Topicort range)
		Hydrocotisone butyrate (Locoid range)
		
		Very potent
		Clobetasol propionate (Temovate, Olux Foam, Clobex)
		Halobetasol propionate(Ultravate)
		Betamethasone dipropionate in enhanced vehicle (Diprolene)
		Diflorasone diacetate (Psorcon)

Type of preparation and general comments	UK preparations	USA preparations
Steroid combinations		
With antiseptics	*Potent* Betamethasone valerate and clioquinol cream and ointment Fluocinolone acetonide with clioquinol (Synalar-C cream and ointment)	*Mildly potent* Clioquinol and hydrocortisone (1%) Iodoquinol 1% and hydrocortisone 1% (Vytone cream) Iodoquinol 1% and hydrocortisone 2% (Alcortin cream) Iodoquinol 1.25% and aloe (Aloquin gel)
With antibiotics	*Mildly potent* Hydrocortisone and fusidic acid (Fucidin H cream) Hydrocortisone and oxytetracycline (Terra-Cortril ointment) *Moderately potent and potent* Betamethasone valerate and neomycin (Betnovate-N cream and ointment) Fluocinolone acetonide and neomycin (Synalar-N cream and ointment)	*Mildly potent* Neomycin, bacitracin, hydrocortisone 1% (Corticosporin)
With antifungals	*Mildly potent* Hydrocortisone and clotrimazole (Canesten HC cream) Hydrocortisone and miconazole (Daktacort cream and ointment) *Potent* Betamethasone dipropionate and clotrimazole (Lotriderm cream)	*Very potent* Clotrimazole and betamethasone dipropionate (Lotrisone)
With antibacterials and antifungals	*Mildly potent* Hydrocortisone, chlorhexidine and nystatin (Nystaform HC cream and ointment) Hydrocortisone, benzalkonium, nystatin and dimeticone (a silicone) (Timodine cream) *Moderately potent* Clobetasone butyrate, oxytetracycline and nystatin (Trimovate cream) *Very potent* Clobetasol propionate with neomycin and nystatin cream and ointment	*Moderately potent* Nystatin and triamcinolone (Mycolog II)
With calcipotriol (For psoriasis)	*Potent* Betamethasone dipropionate (Dovobet ointment and gel)	*Potent* Betamethasone dipropionate (Taclonex ointment)
With salicylic acid	*Potent* Betamethasone dipropionate and salicylic acid (Diprosalic ointment – and scalp application)	

Type of preparation and general comments	UK preparations	USA preparations
Preparations for use in the mouth *Useful mouth washes* *Topical analgesics*	Benzydamine hydrochloride solution (Difflam oral rinse) – an analgesic for painful inflammation in the mouth Chlorhexidine gluconate 1% (Corsodyl mouth wash) Hexetidine solution (Oraldene) an antiseptic gargle	Cetylpyridinium (Cepacol antiseptic mouthwash) Listerine antiseptic mouth rinse (contains thymol, eucalyptol, methylsalicylate, menthol) 'All-purpose mouthwash' – different formulations – e.g. compounded as nystatin suspension 100 000 U/mL, 120 mL; diphenhydramine elixir 12.5 mg/5 mL, 480 mL; hydrocortisone powder 240 mg; sodium carboxymethylcellulose 2%, 720 mL 'Magic mouthwash' – different formulations – e.g. compounded as equal parts Maalox (Magnesia and alumina oral suspension) and diphenhydramine elixir 12.5 mg/5 mL) – some also add dexamethasone Mucotrol – slow dissolving wafer, diphenhydramine elixir 12.5 mg/5 mL)
Topical steroids	Betamethasone soluble tablets Hydrocortisone mucoadhesive buccal tablets to be dissolved slowly in mouth near the lesion – usually an aphthous ulcer	Triamcinolone acetonide (Kenalog in orabase) – a paste that adheres to mucous membranes Fluocinonide gel (Lidex gel) Clobetasol gel (Temovate gel)
For yeast infections	Miconazole (Daktarin oral gel) Nystatin (Nystan oral suspension)	Clotrimazole (Mycelex troches) Nystatin oral suspension or pastilles (Nilstat, Mycostatin)
Topical immunomodulators Long-term safety data not yet available, so should not generally be used as first-line agents	Pimecrolimus (Elidel cream 1%). For mild to moderate eczema Tacrolimus (Protopic ointment 0.03%, 0.1%). For moderate to severe eczema	Pimecrolimus (Elidel cream 1%). For mild to moderate eczema Tacrolimus (Protopic ointment 0.03%, 0.1%). For moderate to severe eczema
Preparations for otitis externa Otitis externa, essentially an eczema, is often complicated by bacterial or yeast overgrowth – hence the combinations listed here	Aluminium acetate ear drops 8% – an effective astringent for the weeping phase; best applied on ribbon gauze Hydrocortisone with neomycin and polymyxin (Otosporin drops) Cotrimazole (Canesten solution)	Aluminium acetate ear drops 8% – an effective astringent for the weeping phase; best applied on ribbon gauze Hydrocortisone, neomycin and polymyxin (Corticosporin drops) Ciprofloxacin 0.2% and hydrocortisone 1% (Cipro HC Otic) Acetic acid 2% with or without hydrocortisone (VoSol/VoSol-HC) Tridesilon otic solution

Type of preparation and general comments	UK preparations	USA preparations
Antibacterial preparations The ideal preparation should have high antibacterial activity, low allergenicity and the drug should not be available for systemic use; this combination is hard to find. Some compromises are given here	Mupirocin (Bactroban cream and ointment) Fusidic acid (Fucidin ointment and cream) Polymyxin and Bacitracin (Polyfax ointment) *To eliminate nasal carriage of staphylococci* Mupirocin (Bactroban Nasal ointment) Chlorhexidine and neomycin (Naseptin cream)	Mupirocin (Bactroban 2% ointment, 2% cream) Nitrofurazone (Furacin ointment, cream or solution) Bacitracin Gentamicin (Garamycin ointment) Bacitracin and polymyxin (Polysporin ointment) Silver sulfadiazine 1% cream – various manufacturers Benzoyl peroxide 5–10% (antiseptic) *To eliminate nasal carriage of staphylococci* Mupirocin (Bactroban nasal ointment)
Antifungal preparations In our view, imidazole, terbinafine, butenafine and amorolfine creams have now supplanted their messier, more irritant and less effective rivals (e.g. Whitfield's ointment). They are fungicidal and the fungistatic azoles such as ketoconazole and clotrimazole have the added advantage of combating yeasts as well as dermatophytes Systemic therapy will be needed for tinea of the scalp, of the nails and of widespread or chronic skin infections that prove resistant to topical treatment	Clotrimazole (Canesten cream) Miconazole (Daktarin cream) Ketoconazole (Nizoral cream) Terbinafine (Lamisil cream) Amorolfine (Loceryl nail lacquer) Tioconazole (Trosyl cutaneous solution) – applied locally it may increase the success rate of griseofulvin. Used by itself it may also cure or improve some nails	Clotrimazole (Lotrimin cream, solution and powder, Mycelex) Miconazole (Micatin cream) Econazole (Spectazole cream, Zeasorb-AF Powder) Terbinafine (Lamisil cream) Butenafine (Mentax cream) Ciclopirox (Loprox cream and lotion, Penlac nail lacquer, Ciclodan Kit) Naftifine (Naftin cream) Oxiconazole (Oxistat) Sertaconazole (Ertaczo)
Antiviral preparations Topical products have little part to play in the management of herpes zoster. However, if used early and frequently, they may help with recurrent herpes simplex infections	Aciclovir (Zovirax cream) Penciclovir (Vectavir cream)	Penciclovir (Denavir cream) Aciclovir (Zovirax cream) Docosanol (Abreva cream)
Wart treatments *Palmoplantar warts*	Salicylic acid and lactic acid (Salactol paint or Salatac and Cuplex gel) Salicylic acid (at 26%, Occlusal solution: at 50%, Verrugon ointment) Glutaraldehyde (Glutarol solution) Formaldehyde (Veracur gel)	Salicylic acid (Duofilm, Occlusal-HP) Salicylic acid plasters 40% (Compound W)

Type of preparation and general comments	UK preparations	USA preparations
Anogenital warts Podophyllum should only be used for non-keratinized warts	Imiquimod (Aldara cream) – an immunomodulator (p. 230) Podophyllotoxin (Condyline solution, Warticon cream and solution)	Podophyllin resin, 15% (Podophyllin paint compound – use with care (p. 230) Podophyllin/benzoin (Podocon-25 powder) Podofilox (Condylox gel) Imiquimod (Aldara cream) (p. 230)
Preparations for treatment of scabies (p. 253) Poor results follow inefficient usage rather than ineffective preparations. We prefer permethrin or sulfur in young children, and pregnant and lactating women. Written instructions are helpful (p. 256)	Permethrin (Lyclear Dermal Cream) Malathion (Derbac-M liquid) Benzyl benzoate application (BP). Irritant and less effective than malathion or permethrin. Crotamiton (Eurax cream) for use if itching persists after treatment with more effective scabicides	Permethrin (Elimite cream) Lindane (Kwell lotion) Crotamiton (Eurax cream) for use if itching persists after treatment with more effective scabicides Precipitated sulfur 6% in soft white paraffin
Preparations for treatment of pediculosis (p. 249) Resistance is a growing problem. Lotions left on for a minimum of 12 hours are more effective, although less convenient than shampoos	Malathion (Derbac-M liquid) Permethrin (Lyclear Creme Rinse)	Malathione (Ovide) Permethrin (Nix) Permethrin/piperonyl butoxide (Rid) Benzyl benzoate solution 20–25% Precipitated sulfur 6% in Nivea Oil
Preparations for acne *Active ingredient* Benzoyl peroxide (an antibacterial agent) induces dryness during the first few weeks; this usually settles, even with continued use	Benzoyl peroxide (Panoxyl ranges) Potassium hydroxyquinoline with benzoyl peroxide (Quinoderm range)	Benzoyl peroxide (Panoxyl, Benzac, Desquam-X Oxy, Clearasil range 2.5, 5 and 10%) With sulfur (Sulphoxyl)
Retinoids Potent comedolytic agents, also used to reverse photoageing. May irritate. Must be avoided during pregnancy/lactation	Isotretinoin (Isotrex gel) Isotretinoin and erythromycin (Isotrexin gel) Tretinoin (Retin-A preparations) Adapalene (Differin gel and cream) Adapalene and benzoyl peroxide (Epiduo gel)	Tretinoin (Retin-A preparations) Tretinoin and clindamycin (Ziana, Veltin) Tazarotene (Tazarac gel 0.05 and 0.1%) Adapalene (Differin gel, lotion and cream) Adapalene and benzoyl peroxide (Epiduo gel)
Antibiotics Bacterial resistance is increasing, but can be reduced by concomitant administration of benzoyl peroxide	Clindamycin (Dalacin-T solution or roll-on) Erythromycin (Stiemycin solution) Erythromycin and zinc acetate (Zineryt) Clindamycin and benzoyl peroxide (Duac Once daily gel)	Clindamycin (Cleocin-T solution and gel, Evoclin Foam) Erythromycin 2% solution – various manufacturers Sulfacetamide (Klaron lotion) Clindamycin and benzoyl peroxide (Duac, Benzaclin, Acanya) Erythromycin and benzoyl peroxide (Benzamycin) Sulfur and sulfacetamide (Sulfacet-R, Sumadan)

Type of preparation and general comments	UK preparations	USA preparations
Azelaic acid and salicylic acid	Azelaic acid (Skinoren cream, Finacea gel)	Azelaic acid (Azalex cream, Finacea gel) Salicylic acid (Neutrogena clear pore gel, Clearasil stick, Stridex gel)
Preparations for rosacea	Metronidazole (Metrogel, Rozex cream, Rosiced cream) Azelaic acid (Finacea gel)	Metronidazole gel, lotion, cream (Metrogel, Metrocream, Metrolotion, Noritate) Sulfur and Sulfacetamide (Sulfacet-R) Sulfacetamide (Klaron)
Preparations for psoriasis *Vitamin D derivatives* Calcipotriol (calcipotriene, USA) and tacalcitol. Avoid using in patients with disorders of calcium metabolism	Calcipotriol ointment and scalp solution (Dovonex ointment). Maximum weekly doses: 6–12 years, 50 g; over 12–16 years, 75 g; adults, 100 g. Can be irritant. Avoid on face Calcitriol (Silkis ointment). Maximum daily dose for adults, 30 g. Less irritant than calcipotriol. Can be used on face/flexures. Tacalcitol (Curatoderm ointment and lotion). Maximum daily dose for adults, 10 g. Not recommended for children	Calcipotriene (Dovonex cream, lotion and ointment) Calcitriol (Vectical) Maximum doses same as UK
Steroids Routine long-term treatment with potent or very potent steroids is not recommended. For indications (p. 60)	Calcipotriol with betamethasone diproprionate (Dovobet ointment and gel)	Calcipotriene with betamethasone diproprionate (Taclonex)
Scalp applications	Betamethasone (Betnovate scalp application, Diprosalic scalp lotion – also contains salicylic acid) Fluocinolone (Synalar gel) Dovobet gel Clobetasol propionate (Etrivex shampoo)	Clobetasol (Temovate scalp application, Olux foam) Fluocinonide (Lidex solution) Fluocinonide in peanut oil (Dermasmoothe FS) Betamethasone valerate (Valisone lotion), Luxiq foam)
Dithranol/anthralin Stains normal skin and clothing. May be irritant, therefore start with low concentration (for 30-minute regimen see p. 61)	Micanol range 1% Dithrocream range 0.1, 0.25, 0.5, 1, 2%	Micanol 1% Dithrocreme 0.1, 0.25, 0.5, 1% Dritho-Scalp
Retinoid Contraindicated in pregnancy and during lactation	Tazarotene (Zorac gel)	Tazarotene (Tazorac gel)

Type of preparation and general comments	UK preparations	USA preparations
Tar These clean refined tar preparations are suitable for home use. Messier, although more effective, formulations exist but are best used in treatment centres		
Bath additives	Polytar emollient bath additive Psoriderm bath emulsion	Balnetar liquid
Applications	Exorex lotion Carbo-Dome cream Psoriderm cream	Denorex Psoriasis overnight treatment MG-217 2% ointment
Scalp applications	Polytar liquid Exorex lotion Psoriderm scalp lotion T-Gel shampoo	10% Liquor carbonis detergens in Nivea oil DHS Tar Gel Denorex shampoo Neutrogena T-Gel Tarsum Shampoo Polytar range
Tar – salicylic acid combinations	Sebco scalp ointment Cocois ointment Capasal shampoo	Sebulex, Scalpicin, T-sal
Preparations for venous ulcers Regardless of topical applications, venous ulcers will heal only if local oedema is eliminated. Remember that the surrounding skin is easily sensitized. To choose treatment for an individual ulcer see p. 150		
For cleansing	Saline, potassium permanganate (*see Cleansing agents*) Hydrogen peroxide solution (3%)	Saline, potassium permanganate (*see Cleansing agents*) Hydrogen peroxide solution (3%) Bleach (sodium hypochlorite) 1/4 cup to bathtub of water, or 1 tablespoon per quart for soaking) – may bleach fabrics
Low adherent dressings	Tulle dressings (e.g. Bactigras, contains chlorhexidine; Jelonet, paraffin gauze) Textiles (e.g. Mepitel)	Telfa Vaseline gauze (contains petrolatum)
Enzymes		Enzymes (Elase Ointment – contains fibrinolysin and deoxyribonuclease; Collagenase Santyl ointment – contains collagenase)
Antiseptics	Silver sulfadiazine – active against *Pseudomonas* (Flamazine cream) Cadexomer iodine (Iodosorb powder)	Silver sulfadiazine (Silvadene cream) Nitrofurazone (Nitrofurazone solution) Mupirocin (Bactroban Ointment)

Type of preparation and general comments	UK preparations	USA preparations
Other applications *Medicated bandages* Beware of allergic contact reactions to parabens preservatives which are in most bandages	Zinc paste and ichthammol (Ichthopaste) Zinc oxide (Viscopaste PB7, steripaste)	Zinc oxide Dextranomer (Debrisan) – for absorbing exudates Becaplermin (Regranex) – growth factor
Other dressings	Hydrocolloid (Granuflex, DuoDERM Extra Thin) Calcium alginate (Kaltostat) Hydrogels (Intrasite, Aquaform) Polyurethane foam (Tielle) Vapour-permeable film dressing (Opsite) Activated charcoal with silver (Actisorb silver 200)	Hydrocolloid (Duoderm) Vapour-permeable film dressing (Opsite, Tegaderm) Hydrogel (Vigilon) Calcium alginate Biafin – recruits macrophages
For photodamage *5-Fluorouracil* The treatment of individual lesions in patients with multiple actinic keratoses is tedious or impossible. Lesions on the scalp and face do better than those on the arms and hands	Efudix cream fluorouracil 5% cream containing 5-fluorouracil is useful. It should be applied twice daily for 2–3 weeks. For such cases patients should be warned about the inevitable inflammation and soreness which appears after a few days Actikerall fluorouracil 0.5%, salicylic acid 10%, apply once daily for up to 12 weeks	Efudex cream 2% or 5%) Fluroplex 1% cream Carac 0.5% solution – drug incorporated into microsphere
Imiquimod Enhances the immune response to superficial basal cell carcinomas and actinic keratoses	Imiquimod 5% (Aldara) Applied 5 days per week for 6 weeks. The response is related to the degree of inflammation. When used to treat actinic keratoses, apply three times per week for 4 weeks	Imiquimod 5% (Aldara) Applied 5 days per week for 6 weeks for treatment of superficial basal cell carcinomas. The response is related to the degree of inflammation. When used to treat actinic keratoses, apply two times per week for 16 weeks and wash off after 8 hours
Miscellaneous For actinic keratoses *Diclofenac*	3% Diclofenac sodium in sodium hyaluronate base (Solaraze gel). Applied twice daily for 60–90 days	3% Diclofenac sodium in sodium hyaluronate base (Solaraze). Applied twice daily for 60–90 days
Ingenol mubutate	Picato. For treatment of face and scalp, use 0.015% gel daily for 3 days. For treatment of trunk and extremities, use 0.05% gel daily for 2 days	Picato 0.015% or 0.05%. For treatment of face and scalp, use 0.015% gel daily for 3 days. For treatment of trunk and extremities, use 0.05% gel daily for 2 days

Type of preparation and general comments	UK preparations	USA preparations
Minoxidil May be used as a possible treatment for early male-pattern alopecia. The response is slow, and only a small minority of patients will obtain a dense regrowth even after 12 months. Hair regained will fall out when treatment stops – warn patients about this	Regaine liquid 2 or 5% – only on private prescription	Rogaine 2% solution Rogaine 5% solution for men
Capsaicin A topical pepper that depletes substance P. Useful for the treatment of post-herpetic neuralgia. May itself sting. Apply up to 3–4 times daily after lesions have healed. May take 2–4 weeks to relieve pain	Axsain cream (0.075%), Zacin cream (0.075%)	Zostrix cream (0.025%) Capzasin HP cream (0.075%) Axsain cream (0.075%)
Lidocaine/prilocaine A local anaesthetic for topical use. Applied on skin as a thick layer of cream under an occlusive dressing or on adult genital mucosa with no occlusive dressing. Read manufacturer's instructions for times of application	Lidocaine and prilocaine (EMLA cream)	Lidocaine 4% (LMX 4) Lidocaine 5% (LMX 5) Lindocaine 2.5%/prilocaine 2.5% (EMLA cream)

Systemic Medication

We list here only preparations we use commonly for our patients with skin disease. The doses given are the usual oral doses for adults. We occasionally use some of these drugs for uses not approved by federal regulatory agencies. We have included some, but not all, of the side effects and interactions; these are more fully covered in the *British National Formulary* (BNF) (UK) and *Physician's Desk Reference* (PDR) (USA). Physicians prescribing these drugs should read about them there, in more detail, and specifically check the dosages before treating their patients. If possible, systemic medication should be avoided in pregnant women.

Main dermatological uses and usual adult doses	Adverse effects	Interactions	Other remarks
Antibacterials			
Cefalexin and cefuroxime			
Cephalosporins not inactivated by penicillinase. For Gram-positive and Gram-negative infections resistant to penicillin and erythromycin (Cefalexin 250–500 mg four times daily; Cefuroxine 250 mg twice daily)	Gut upsets Candidiasis Rarely, erythema multiforme or toxic epidermal necrolysis Transient hepatotoxicity Rarely nephrotoxic	Probenecid reduces excretion	0.5–6.5% of penicillin allergic patients will react to this
Ciprofloxacin			
A 4-quinolone used for Gram-negative infections, especially *Pseudomonas*, and Gram-positive infections. First choice for skin infections in the immunosuppressed if the causative organism is not yet known (500 mg twice daily)	Gut upsets Occasionally hepatotoxic and nephrotoxic Haemolysis in those deficient in glucose-6-phosphate dehydrogenase Rarely, associated with tendon damage and rupture	Antacids and dairy products reduce absorption Enhances effects of warfarin and theophylline Inhibits metabolism of duloxetine (antidepressant) May interact with some antipsychotic therapies	Crystalluria if fluid intake is inadequate Care if renal impairment Avoid in pregnancy, breastfeeding, children and epileptics
Co-amoxiclav (Augmentin)			
A broad-spectrum penicillin combined with clavulanic acid; use if organisms resistant to both erythromycin and flucloxacillin. Also for Gram-negative folliculitis (375 mg three times daily)	Gut upsets Candidiasis Rashes, especially in infectious mononucleosis Cholestatic jaundice	As for other penicillins	Use with care in hepatic or renal failure, pregnancy, and breastfeeding Avoid in those allergic to penicillin

Clinical Dermatology, Fifth Edition. Richard B. Weller, Hamish J.A. Hunter and Margaret W. Mann.
© 2015 John Wiley & Sons, Ltd. Published 2015 by John Wiley & Sons, Ltd.

Main dermatological uses and usual adult doses	Adverse effects	Interactions	Other remarks
Erythromycin 1 Acne vulgaris (250–500 mg twice daily) 2 Gram-positive infections, particularly staphylococcal and streptococcal. Useful with penicillin allergy (250–500 mg four times daily)	Gut upsets Rashes Cholestatic hepatitis if treatment prolonged (reversible and most common with estolate salt) Prolongation of QT interval	Increased risk of toxicity if given with theophylline or carbamezapine Potentiates effects of warfarin, ergotamine, ciclosporin, disopyramide, carbamazepine, terfenadine, astemizole, theophylline, cisapride digoxin and other drugs metabolized by CYP3A4	*P. acnes* now widely resistant to erythromycin Avoid estolate in liver disease Care when hepatic dysfunction Excreted in human milk
Flucloxacillin, dicloxacillin and cloxacillin Penicillins used for infections with penicillinase-forming staphylococci (250–500 mg four times daily)	Gut upsets Morbilliform eruptions Arthralgia Anaphylaxis Hepatic jaundice	Probenecid increases blood level Reduces excretion of methotrexate	Accumulate in renal failure Atopics may be at increased risk of hypersensitivity reactions Avoid in those allergic to penicillin
Metronidazole 1 Anaerobic infections (400 mg three times daily) 2 Stubborn rosacea (200 mg twice daily) 3 Trichomoniasis (200 mg three times daily for 7 days)	Gut upsets Metallic taste Candidiasis Ataxia and sensory neuropathy Seizures	Potentiates effects of warfarin, phenytoin and lithium Drugs that induce liver enzymes (e.g. rifampicin, barbiturates, griseofulvin, phenytoin, carbamazepine and smoking) increase destruction of metronidazole in liver and necessitate higher dosage May have disulfiram-like effect with alcohol (headaches, flushing, vomiting, abdominal pain) Co-administration with disulfiram may cause psychotic reactions	Use lower dose in presence of liver disease Neurotoxicity more likely if central nervous system disease Carcinogenic and mutagenic in some non-human models

Main dermatological uses and usual adult doses	Adverse effects	Interactions	Other remarks
Minocycline A tetracycline used for acne and rosacea (50–100 mg daily or twice daily, or 100 mg daily in a modified release preparation)	Gut upsets Dizziness and vertigo Candidiasis Deposition in bones and teeth of fetus and children Deposition in skin and mucous membranes causes blue–grey pigmentation Benign intracranial hypertension Lupus erythematosus-like syndrome with hepatitis	May impair absorption of oral contraceptives May potentiate effect of warfarin Risk for benign intracranial hypertension from tetracyclines may increase with isotretinoin or acitretin	Avoid in pregnancy and in children under 12 years

Tetracycline and oxytetracycline
Acne and rosacea (250–500 mg twice daily)
   Doxycycline (100 mg daily or twice daily) and
   Lymecycline (408 mg daily in acne
   Doxycycline modified release (40 mg daily) in rosacea
	Gut upsets/oesophagitis
	Candidiasis
	Rashes
	Deposition in bones and teeth of fetus and children
	Rare phototoxic reactions
	Benign intracranial hypertension
		Absorption impaired when taken with food, antacids and iron
		Many impair absorption of oral contraceptives
		May potentiate effect of warfarin
		Risk for benign intracranial hypertension from tetracyclines may increase with isotretinoin or acetretin
			Avoid in pregnancy and in children under 12 years
			Should not be used if renal insufficiency

Penicillin V (phenoxymethylpenicillin) **1** For infections with Gram-positive cocci (250–500 mg four times daily) **2** Prophylaxis of erysipelas (250 mg daily)	Gut upsets Morbilliform rashes Urticaria Arthralgia Anaphylaxis	Blood level increased by probenecid Reduces excretion of methotrexate	Accumulates in renal failure Atopics at increased risk of hypersensitivity reactions
Trimethoprim (300 mg twice daily) for use in resistant acne	Gut upsets Rashes Haematopoietic suppression	Hyperkalaemia with ACE inhibitors May enhance anticoagulant effect of coumarins May increase levels of phenytoin and digoxin Increased neprotoxicity if co-administered with ciclosporin	Reduce dose in renal impairment, avoid in pregnancy and breastfeeding

Main dermatological uses and usual adult doses	Adverse effects	Interactions	Other remarks
Dapsone Leprosy, dermatitis herpetiformis, vasculitis, pyoderma gangrenosum (50–150 mg daily)	Haemolytic anaemia Methaemoglobinaemia Headaches Lethargy Hepatitis Peripheral motor neuropathy Exfoliative dermatitis Toxic epidermal necrolysis Agranulocytosis Aplastic anaemia Hypoalbuminaemia Hypersensitivity syndrome	Reduced excretion and increased side effects if given with probenecid	Regular blood checks necessary (weekly for first month, then every 2 weeks until 3 months, then monthly until 6 months and then 6-monthly) Not felt to be teratogenic, but should not be given during pregnancy and lactation if possible. For dermatitis herpetiformis, a gluten-free diet is preferable at these times Avoid in patients with glucose 6-phosphate dehydrogenase deficiency (screen for this, especially in USA)

Antifungals
Terbinafine
Dermatophyte infections when systemic treatment appropriate (as a result of site, severity or extent)
    Usual first-choice systemic antifungal agent. Unlike itraconazole and fluconazole its action does not involve cytochrome P-450 dependent enzymes in the liver
    Dose: 250 mg daily
• Tinea pedis: 2–6 weeks
• Tinea corporis: 4 weeks
• Tinea unguium: 6 weeks to 3 months
	Gut upsets
	Headache
	Rashes – including toxic epidermal necrolysis, subacute cutaneous lupus erythematosus
	Taste disturbance
	Rarely, liver toxicity
		Plasma concentration reduced by rifampicin
		Plasma concentration increased by cimetidine
		Cytochrome 2D6 inhibitor – lowers ciclosporin levels and increases theophylline, tricyclic antidepressant levels
			May exacerbate psoriasis
			Avoid in hepatic and renal impairment and when breastfeeding
			Not for use in pregnancy
			Not yet recommended for children

Griseofulvin Has largely been superseded by newer antifungals Dermatophyte infections of skin, nails and hair. Not for *Candida* or pityriasis versicolor (500 mg microsize daily)	Gut upsets Headaches, rashes, photosensitivity	Induces microsomal liver enzymes (CYP3A4 inducer) and so may increase elimination of drugs such as warfarin and ciclosporin	Not for use in pregnancy, liver failure, porphyria or systemic lupus erythematosus Men should not father children within 6 months of taking it Absorbed better when taken with fatty foods

Main dermatological uses and usual adult doses	Adverse effects	Interactions	Other remarks
Fluconazole **1** Candidiasis *Acute/recurrent vaginal* (single dose of 150 mg) *Mucosal (not vaginal) conditions* (50 mg daily) Oropharyngeal: 7–14 days Oesophagus: 14–30 days *Systemic candidiasis* – see manufacturer's instructions **2** Second-line treatment in some systemic mycoses (e.g. cryptococcal infections) **3** Dermatophyte infections (except of nails) and pityriasis versicolor (50 mg daily for 2–6 weeks)	Gut upsets Rarely rashes Angioedema/anaphylaxis Liver toxicity May be worse in AIDS patients	Hydrochlorothiazide increases plasma concentration Rifampicin reduces plasma concentration Potentiates effects of warfarin, ciclosporin and phenytoin May potentiate effects of sulfonylureas leading to hypoglycaemia May inhibit metabolism of astemizole causing serious dysrhythmias	Avoid in pregnancy Hepatic and renal impairment Use in children only if imperative and no alternative Avoid in children under 1 year and when breastfeeding
Itraconazole **1** Candidiasis *Vulvovaginal* (200 mg twice daily) for 1 day *Oropharyngeal* (100 mg daily) for 15 days **2** Pityriasis versicolor (200 mg daily) for 7 days **3** Dermatophyte infections (100 mg daily) Tinea pedis and manuum for 30 days Tinea corporis for 15 days Tinea of nails – an intermittent regimen can be used (200 mg twice daily for 1 week per month, continued for three or four cycles)	Gut upsets Headache	Antacids reduce absorption Rifampicin and phenytoin reduce plasma concentration May potentiate effects of warfarin May increase plasma levels of digoxin and ciclosporin Inhibits metabolism of astemizole: this may lead to serious dysrhythmias	Avoid in hepatic impairment Avoid in children, in pregnancy and when breastfeeding Prescribe with caution to patients at risk of heart failure
Nystatin **1** Recurrent vulval and perineal candidiasis **2** Persistent gastrointestinal candidiasis in immunosuppressed patients (500 000 units three times daily)	Unpleasant taste Gut upsets		Not absorbed and when given by mouth acts only on mouth and bowel yeasts
Anthelmintics *Albendazole* (400 mg daily for 3 days) *Ivermectin* (12 mg, single dose) **1** Cutaneous larva migrans **2** Filariasis **3** Cutaneous larva currens (*Strongyloides stercoralis*) **4** Scabies resistant to topical therapy			Both drugs available on a named patient basis

Main dermatological uses and usual adult doses	Adverse effects	Interactions	Other remarks
Antivirals *Aciclovir, famciclovir and valaciclovir* (for dosages see specialist literature) Famciclovir and valaciclovir are more reliably absorbed than aciclovir and need be taken only two or three time a day 1 Severe herpes simplex infections – primary or recurrent 2 Severe herpes zoster infections – use may reduce incidence of post-herpetic neuralgia 3 Prophylaxis for recurrent herpes simplex especially in the immunocompromised, to treat eczema herpeticum and to treat chickenpox in the immunocompromised	Generally safe drugs. Rapid gut upsets, transient rise in urea and creatinine in 10% of patients after intravenous use Raised liver enzymes Reversible neurological reactions Decreases in haematological indices	Excretion may be delayed by probenicid Lethargy when intravenous aciclovir given with zidovudine	Adequate hydration of patient should be maintained Risk in pregnancy unknown Reduce dose in renal impairment No effect on virus in latent phase Must be given early in acute infections to have maximum effect
Antiprotozoals Sodium stibogluconate (for specific dosages see specialist literature) 1 Lesions requiring local treatment (100–500 mg intralesional pentavalent antimony every 3–7 days for 1–5 sessions) 2 When systemic treatment required (20 mg/kg pentavalent antimony intramuscularly or intravenously for 10–20 days) 3 Mucocutaneous leishmaniasis (20 mg/kg pentavalent antimony daily intramuscularly or intravenously for 30 days)	Pain on local injection Parenteral administration: Nausea, vomiting, diarrhoea in 2% Cardiac arrhthmias (QTc prolongation) – ECG monitoring advisable during administration. Anaphylaxis. Injection site thrombosis Mucocutaneous disease – oedema around lesions may lead to life-threatening laryngeal/pharyngeal compromise – administer with corticosteroids	Avoid administration with other drugs prolonging QTc interval (e.g. Class III anti-arrhythmics sotalol and amiodarone) Concomitant administration with amphotericin B deoxycholate increases risk of fatal arrhythmias	Trial data on long-term effectiveness of sodium stibogluconate are lacking Monotherapy not advised for treatment of *L. aethiopica*

Antihistamines
All those listed here are H_1-blockers although some dermatologists combine these with H_2-blockers in recalcitrant urticaria

Non-sedative Used for urticaria and type I hypersensitivity reactions			Non-sedative antihistamines should be avoided, or used with caution in pregnancy and lactation

Main dermatological uses and usual adult doses	Adverse effects	Interactions	Other remarks
Loratadine and desloratadine (Loratadine, 10 mg daily; desloratadine, 5 mg daily)		Metabolized by CYP3A4 and to a lesser extent by CYP2D6	Desloratidine to be used with caution in renal impairment
Cetirizine and levocetirizine (Cetirizine, 10 mg daily; levocetirizine, 5 mg daily)	Rarely sedate		Use half the usual dose when renal impairment
Fexofenadine (a metabolite of terfenadine) 60–180 mg daily			
Sedative Urticaria, type I hypersensitivity including intravenous use in anaphylaxis (p. 357). Also used as antipruritic agents in atopic eczema, lichen planus	Sedation (promethazine > trimeprazine (alimemazine) > hydroxyzine > chlorphenamine = diphenhydramine = cyproheptadine) Anticholinergic effects: • dry mouth • blurred vision • urinary retention • tachycardia • glaucoma	Potentiate effect of alcohol and central nervous system depressants Potentiate effect of other anticholinergic drugs	Increased rate of elimination in children Sedation may be useful in an excited itchy patient Warn of risk of drowsiness when driving or operating dangerous machinery
Chlorphenamine (4 mg three or four times daily) *Diphenhydramine* (25–50 mg four times daily) *Hydroxyzine* (25 mg, nocte at first, but up to 100 mg four times daily if needed) *Cyproheptadine* (4 mg four times daily) *Promethazine* (10–20 mg daily to three times daily) *Alimemazine (trimeprazine)* (10 mg two or three times daily)	Consider lower doses in the elderly		Hydroxyzine particularly useful for pruritus

Main dermatological uses and usual adult doses	Adverse effects	Interactions	Other remarks
Antiandrogens			
Cyproterone acetate and ethinylestradiol (UK, Dianette; USA, not available) 1 Acne vulgaris, unresponsive to systemic antibiotics, in women only 2 Idiopathic hirsutism, one tablet (cyproterone acetate 2 mg, ethinylestradiol 35 mg) daily for 21 days, starting on fifth day of menstrual cycle and repeated after a 7-day interval. Treat for 6 months at least	As for combined oral contraceptives	Should not be given with other oral contraceptives	Contraindicated in pregnancy. Cyproterone acetate is an antiandrogen and if given to pregnant women may feminize a male fetus. For women of childbearing age, therefore, it must be given combined with a contraceptive (the ethinylestradiol component) Also contraindicated in liver disease, disorders of lipid metabolism, those with risk factors for venous throboembolic or arterial disease and with past or present endometrial carcinomas Not for use in males or children
Drospirenone and ethinylestadiol (Yasmin)	Hyperkalaemia	NSAIDs and ACE inhibitors increase risk of hyperkalaemia	Contraindicated if abnormal renal or hepatic function Drospirenone is an analogue of spironolactone. Avoid in pregnancy
Spironolactone 25–50 mg daily Used in USA for: 1 Idiopathic hirsutism 2 Acne vulgaris, unresponsive to systemic antibiotics, in women only	Hyperkalaemia	Increases plasma concentration of digoxin	May feminize male fetus Avoid in pregnancy. Causes gynaecomastia. Avoid if renal or hepatic impairment
Finasteride 1 mg daily for male-pattern baldness	Impotence and decreased libido		5α-reductase inhibitor, reduces formation of dihydrotestosterone Not for use by women

Main dermatological uses and usual adult doses	Adverse effects	Interactions	Other remarks
Immunosuppressants			
Azathioprine			
For autoimmune conditions (e.g. systemic lupus erythematosus, pemphigus and bullous pemphigoid) often used to spare dose of systemic steroids (1–2.5 mg/kg daily). We strongly recommend checking thiopurine methyltransferase (TMPT) levels before starting treatment with azathioprine as homozygotes for the low-activity allele have a high risk of bone marrow suppression	Gut upsets Bone marrow suppression, usually leucopenia or thrombocytopenia Hepatotoxicity, pancreatitis Predisposes to infections, including warts and possibly also to skin cancers	Increased toxicity if given with allopurinol	See comment about the need to check for thiopurine methyltransferase levels (in first column) Weekly blood checks are necessary for the first 8 weeks of treatment and thereafter at intervals of not longer than 3 months Reduce dosage if severe renal impairment Avoid in pregnancy Possible increased risk of lymphomas
Ciclosporin (cyclosporine)			
1 Severe psoriasis when conventional treatment is ineffective or inappropriate **2** Short-term (max. 8 weeks) treatment of severe atopic dermatitis when conventional treatment ineffective or inappropriate (2.5 mg/kg daily in two divided doses). See p. 64 for guidance in use	Hepatic and renal impairment Hypertension Gut upset Hypertrichosis Gum hyperplasia Tremor Hyperkalaemia Occasionally facial oedema, fluid retention and convulsions Hypercholestero-laemia Hypomagnesia	(See *BNF* and *PDR* for fuller details) (Use with tacrolimus specifically contraindicated) **1** Drugs that may increase nephrotoxicity • Antibiotics (aminoglycosides, co-trimoxazole) • NSAIDs • Melphalan **2** Drugs that may increase ciclosporin blood level (by cytochrome P-450 inhibition) • Antibiotics (erythromycin, amphotericin B, cephalosporins, doxycycline, aciclovir) • Hormones (corticosteroids, sex hormones) • Diuretics (furosemide thiazides) • Other (warfarin, H_2 antihistamines, calcium channel blockers, ACE inhibitors, grapefruit juice) **3** Drugs that may decrease ciclosporin levels (by cytochrome P-450 induction) • Anticonvulsants (phenytoin, phenobarbital, carbamazepine, sodium valproate) • Antibiotics (isoniazide, rifampicin)	Contraindicated if abnormal renal function, hypertension not under control and concomitant premalignant or malignant conditions Monitor renal function and blood pressure as indicated on p. 64

Main dermatological uses and usual adult doses	Adverse effects	Interactions	Other remarks
Mycofenolate mofetil Used as a second-line immunosuppressive therapy or as an adjunct to corticosteroids for a range of unlicensed indications including severe psoriasis, severe atopic dermatitis, blistering conditions, lupus erythematosus, dermatomyositis, sarcoidosis, necrobiosis lipoidica, cutaneous vasculitis and pyoderma gangrenosum (1–3 g/day in two divided doses)	Taste disturbance, gingival hyperplasia and nausea, vomiting, constipation, diarrhoea and indigestion. Splitting dose into four divided doses may reduce gastrointestinal side effects. Electrolyte abnormalities including hypomagnesaemia, hypocalcaemia, hypophosphataemia and hyper- and hypokalaemia. Hepatic and renal impairment Bone marrow suppression including leucopenia, anaemia, thrombocytopenia, pancytopenia and red cell aplasia which may present with bleeding, easy bruising or increased susceptibility to infection Long-term therapy may predispose to cutaneous malignancy	**1** Absorption reduced by antacids, iron tablets, cholestyramine **2** Bioavailability or plasma concentration possibly reduced by antibacterials: metronidazole, norfloxacin and rifampicin **3** Increases plasma concentrations of antivirals: aciclovir and ganciclovir **4** Reduces absorption of phenytoin **5** May interact with clozapine to increase the risk of agranulocytosis	Full blood count, electrolytes and liver function tests before starting treatment, and then weekly until therapy is stabilized. Thereafter test every 1–3 months Avoid in pregnancy and breastfeeding. Men should use condoms during treatment and for 13 weeks after the last dose Live vaccines should be avoided. Flu vaccines and Pneumovax are recommended
Methotrexate Severe psoriasis unresponsive to local treatment (initially, 2.5 mg test dose and observe for 1 *week*, then 5–20 mg once a week orally or intramuscularly)	Gut upsets Stomatitis Bone marrow depression Liver or kidney dysfunction Pulmonary fibrosis/pneumonitis	Aspirin, probenecid, thiazide diuretics and some NSAIDs delay excretion and increase toxicity Antiepileptics, co-trimoxazole, and pyrimethamine increase antifolate effect Toxicity increased by ciclosporin and acitretin. Co-administration of folate does not antagonize the effect of methotrexate on psoriasis and may confer protective effects (p. 64)	Full blood count and liver function tests before starting treatment, and then weekly until therapy is stabilized. Thereafter test every 2–3 months Avoid in pregnancy Reduce dose if renal or hepatic impairment Folic acid given concomitantly prevents bone marrow depression Reduced fertility in males Traditionally the development of hepatic fibrosis has been detected with a liver biopsy before treatment and periodical biopsies thereafter. Need for liver biopsy is being replaced by serial measurement of serum procollagen III aminopeptide and hepatic fibroscans. Elderly may be more sensitive to the drug

Main dermatological uses and usual adult doses	Adverse effects	Interactions	Other remarks
Corticosteroids *Prednisone and prednisolone* Acute and severe allergic reactions, Acute eczemas, severe erythema multiforme, connective tissue disorders, pemphigus, pemphigoid and vasculitis (5–80 mg daily or on alternate days) Withdrawal should be gradual for patients who have received systemic corticosteroids for more than 3 weeks or those who have taken high doses Gastric and bone protection should be commenced at onset of treatment if long-term therapy is considered	Impaired glucose tolerance Redistribution of fat (centripetal) Muscle wasting, proximal myopathy Osteoporosis and vertebral collapse Aseptic necrosis of head of femur Growth retardation in children Peptic ulceration Euphoria, psychosis or depression Cataract formation Precipitation of glaucoma Increase in blood pressure Sodium and water retention Potassium loss Skin atrophy and capillary fragility Spread of infection Iatrogenic Cushing's syndrome	Liver enzyme inducers CyP3A4 (e.g. phenytoin, griseofulvin; rifampicin) reduce effect of corticosteroids Carbenoxolone and most diuretics increase potassium loss as a result of corticosteroids Corticosteroids reduce effect of many antihypertensive agents and drugs that affect glucose metabolism	**1** Before long-term treatment screen: • Chest X-ray • Blood pressure • Weight • Glycosuria • Electrolytes • Consider the need for a bone density scan • Tuberculin skin test (USA) • Past history of peptic ulcer, cataracts/glaucoma, and affective psychosis **2** During treatment check blood pressure, weight, glycosuria and electrolytes regularly. Patients can carry a steroid treatment card or wear a labelled bracelet. Always bear in mind the possibility of masked infections and perforations **3** Long-term treatment has to be tapered off slowly to avoid adrenal insufficiency **4** Do not use for psoriasis or long-term for atopic eczema **5** Consider the need for adjunctive treatment for prevention of osteoporosis

Main dermatological uses and usual adult doses	Adverse effects	Interactions	Other remarks
Retinoids *Acitretin* Severe psoriasis, resistant to other forms of treatment (may be used with PUVA, p. 63), palmoplantar pustulosis, severe ichthyoses, Darier's disease, pityriasis rubra pilaris (0.2–1.0 mg/kg daily) Acitretin is not recommended for children except under exceptional circumstances	1 *Mucocutaneous* (common). Rough, scaly, dry-appearing skin and mucous membranes Chafing Atrophy of skin and nails Diffuse thinning of scalp and body hair Curly hair Exuberant granulation tissue (especially toe nail folds) Disease flare-up Photosensitivity 2 *Systemic* Teratogenesis Diffuse interstitial skeletal hyperostosis Arthralgia, myalgia and headache Benign intracranial hypertension 3 *Laboratory abnormalities* Haematology: ↓ White blood cells ↑ Erythrocyte sedimentation rate Liver function tests: ↓↑ Bilirubin ↑ AST/ALT ↑ Alkaline phosphatase (abnormal in 20% of patients) Serum lipids: ↑ Cholesterol ↑ Triglycerides ↓ High-density lipoprotein (abnormal in 50% of patients)	Avoid concomitant high doses of vitamin A Possible antagonism to anticoagulant effect of warfarin Increases plasma concentration of methotrexate Increases hepatotoxicity of methotrexate	All women of childbearing age should ideally use two methods of contraception, one of which should be a combined hormonal contraceptive or intrauterine device for 1 month before treatment, during treatment and for at least 3 years after treatment (see specialist literature for details) Patients should sign a consent form indicating that they know about the danger of teratogenicity Should not donate blood during or for 2 years after stopping the treatment (teratogenic risk) Regular screening should be carried out to exclude: 1 Abnormalities of liver function 2 Hyperlipidaemia 3 Disseminated interstitial skeletal hyperostosis Avoid if renal or hepatic impairment

Main dermatological uses and usual adult doses	Adverse effects	Interactions	Other remarks
Isotretinoin (13 cis-retinoic acid) Severe acne vulgaris, unresponsive to systemic antibiotics (0.5–1.0 mg/kg daily for 16 weeks) (p. 162) or to total dose of 120 mg/kg	See *Acitretin* Almost all patients experience chelitis. Other common side effects are aches and pains, epistaxis, dry skin, dry eyes, and occasional change in night vision	See *Acitretin*	Females of childbearing age must take effective contraception for 1 month before treatment is started, during treatment, and for 1 month after treatment is stopped; check pregnancy test(s) before starting treatment and monthly. Maximum 4 weeks' supply of drug to be administered only on receipt of negative pregnancy test. Females should sign a consent form that states the dangers of teratogenicity (see p. 163 for USA recommendations) Before starting a course of isotretinoin, patients and their doctors should know about the risk of the appearance or worsening of depression. The drug should be stopped immediately if there is any concern on this score (p. 163) Avoid in renal or hepatic impairment Blood tests as for acitretin

Alitretinoin (Toctino®)
Severe refractory hand eczema refractory to potent topical steroids
   Adults over 18 years, 30 mg once daily, reduced to 10 mg once daiy if not tolerated. Treat for 12–24 weeks, discontinue if no response after 12 weeks or inadequate response at 24 weeks
	1 *Mucocutaneous* (common)
	   Rough, scaly, dry-appearing skin and mucous membranes
	Chafing
	Alopecia
	2 *Systemic*
	Teratogenesis
	Hyperostosis, ankylosing spondylitis arthralgia and myalgia. Headache and blurred vision
	Benign intracranial hypertension
	Vasculitis
	3 *Laboratory abnormalities*
	Haematology: anaemia
	Deranged thyroid function tests
	↑ Creatine kinase
	Serum lipids:
	↑ Cholesterol
	↑ Triglycerides
		See *Acitretin*	Females of childbearing age must take effective contraception (ideally two methods) for 1 month before treatment is started, during treatment and for 1 month after treatment is stopped; check pregnancy test(s) before starting treatment and monthly. Maximum 4 weeks' supply of drug to be administered only on receipt of negative pregnancy test
			Use with caution if history of depression
			Avoid blood donation during and for 1 month following treatment

Main dermatological uses and usual adult doses	Adverse effects	Interactions	Other remarks
Drugs acting on the central nervous system (CNS)			
Amitriptyline 1 Depression secondary to skin disease 2 Post-herpetic neuralgia (50–100 mg at night; start with 10–25 mg in the elderly)	Sedation, anticholinergic effects, cardiac dysrhythmias Confusion in the elderly Postural hypotension Jaundice Neutropenia May precipitate seizures in epileptics	Potentially lethal CNS stimulation with monoamine oxidase inhibitors Increases effects of other CNS depressants and anticholinergics Metabolism may be inhibited by cimetidine	Avoid in the presence of heart disease or hypertension Use small doses at first to avoid confusion in the elderly Warn about effects on skills such as driving
Doxepin Antidepressant with sedative properties sometimes used for antipruritic effect 10–50 mg at bedtime or twice daily	See *Amitriptyline*	See *Amitriptyline*	Avoid in breastfeeding
Diazepam Anxiety – often associated with skin disease (2–5 mg three times daily)	Sedation Impaired skills (e.g. driving) or ataxia Dependence (withdrawal may lead to sleeplessness, anxiety, tremors)	Potentiates effects of other CNS depressants including alcohol Breakdown inhibited by cimetidine and propranolol Liver enzyme inducers (e.g. phenytoin, griseofulvin, rifampicin) increase elimination	Use for short spells only (to avoid addiction) Avoid in pregnancy and breastfeeding Use with care in presence of liver, kidney or respiratory diseases, and in the elderly

Biological therapies

These are agents that block specific molecular steps in disease pathogenesis. In the UK they are licensed for the treatment of severe psoriasis, which has either failed to respond to standard systemic therapy or for patients who are intolerant of standard systemic therapy. 'Biologics' either target TNF-α or T cells and antigen-presenting cells

Tumour necrosis factor α *(TNF-α) targeting biologics*	Predispose to infection. May reactivate TB. May exacerbate heart failure and demyelinating conditions. Associated with increased risk of malignancies (lymphoma and leukaemia)	Avoid concomitant use with live vaccines Avoid with Anakinra (IL-1 inhibitor)	

Main dermatological uses and usual adult doses	Adverse effects	Interactions	Other remarks
Etanercept (Enbrel®) 1 Psoriasis as above. 2 Psoriatic arthritis 'Subcut' injection. 25 mg, twice weekly, increasing to 50 mg depending on response. Discontinue if inadequate response at 12 weeks	Infections, allergic reactions Injection site reactions Rare lupus syndrome		A recombinant human TNF-α receptor fusion protein, which binds primarily to soluble TNF-α with less affinity for membrane-bound TNF-α Screen for TB pre-treatment Avoid in pregnancy and breastfeeding
Infliximab (Remicade®) 1 Psoriasis as above 2 Psoriatic arthritis IV infusion, 5 mg/kg at weeks 0, 2, 6 and then 8 weekly intervals. Discontinue if inadequate response at 14 weeks	Infections Hypersensitivity reactions, particularly 1 or 2 hours after first or second infusion		A human/mouse chimeric monoclonal IgG antibody to TNF-α. Binds and forms stable complexes with circulating and membrane bound TNF-α Caution in hepatic and renal impairment Contraindicated in patients with moderate or severe heart failure Screen for infections and TB pre-treatment Avoid in pregnancy and breastfeeding
Adalimumab (Humira®) 1 Psoriasis as above 2 Psoriatic arthritis. 'Subcut' injection. Initially 80 mg then 40 mg. Discontinue treatment if no response after 16 weeks	Infections, dizziness, headache, diarrhoea, abdominal pain, stomatitis and mouth ulceration, nausea, increased hepatic enzymes, musculoskeletal pain and fatigue, injection-site reactions		A fully humanized monoclonal IgG antibody to TNF-α. Binds and forms stable complexes with circulating and membrane bound TNF-α Screen for infections and TB pre-treatment Use with caution in patients with a history of mild heart failure, avoid if moderate or severe. Caution in demyelinating conditions (may be exacerbated) and previous malignancy. Monitor for development of skin malignancy. Avoid in pregnancy and breastfeeding

Interleukin-12/interleukin-23 inhibitor

Ustekinumab (Stelara®) 1 Psoriasis as above. 2 Psoriatic arthritis. Subcut' injection. Initially 45 mg then 45 mg at 4 weeks then 45 mg every 12 weeks. If over 100 kg then use 90 mg dose. Discontinue treatment if no response after 16 weeks	Infections, nasopharangitis, diarrhoea, headaches, fatigue, dizzines, myalgia, depression, rarely hypersensitivity reactions Injection site reactions	Discontinue 8 weeks before and until 2 weeks after vaccination with live or live-attenuated vaccines	A fully humanized monoclonal antibody against the shared p40 subunit of interleukin-12 and interleukin-23 that prevents them from binding to the cell surface of T cells Screen for infections and TB pre-treatment Avoid in pregnancy and breastfeeding

Main dermatological uses and usual adult doses	Adverse effects	Interactions	Other remarks

Alefacept
15 mg IM once weekly for 12-week course
  Requires baseline and weekly monitoring of CD4 T-cell counts. Hold dose if <250 cells/μL, DC if count <250 cells/μL for more than 1 month
  TB test before starting
	Injection site reactions, cough, myalgias, nausea	No live vaccines	Not licensed for use in UK. No longer available in the USA
			Fusion protein of human LFA-3 and Fc portion of IgG
			Blocks the interaction of accessory molecules LFA-3 and CD2 needed for T-cell activation
			Monitor for lymphopenia, malignancy, infections, liver enzyme changes and cardiovascular troubles

Rituximab 1 Cutaneous B-cell lymphoma 2 Primary blistering diseases 3 Dermatomyositis 4 Graft versus host disease 5 Cutaneous vasculitis 6 Lupus erythematosus 375 mg/m^2 body surface area, IV infusion weekly for several weeks (regimens vary depending on indication)	Infusion reactions, usually mild, often worse with first infusion, fever, chills, nausea and vomiting. Allergic reactions, rash, pruritus, urticaria, angioedema bronchospasm and dyspnoea. Stevens Johnson syndrome and toxic epidermal necrolysis Severe sepsis, reactivation of hepatitis B, progressive multifocal leukoen-cephalopathy	Avoid concomitant use with cisplatin as risk of renal failure	A human/mouse chimeric monoclonal IgG antibody which binds to CD20 on the surface of normal and malignant B lymphocytes, resulting in cell lysis There are no licensed dermatological indications in the UK or USA Use with caution in patients with cardiovascular disease Avoid in pregnancy and breastfeeding Avoid if concomitant severe active infection
Miscellaneous *Epinephrine injection* Emergency treatment for acute anaphylaxis 0.5 mg (0.5 mL of 1 in 1000 solution given as a slow subcutaneous or, rarely, intramuscular injection. May be repeated after 10 minutes if necessary) An Epipen is a convenient way for patients to carry adrenaline with them for self-injection if needed	Tachycardia Cardiac dysrhythmias Anxiety Tremor Headache Hypertension Hyperglycaemia Hypokalaemia	If given with some β-blockers may lead to severe hypertension	Do not confuse the different strengths Give *slowly*, subcutaneously or intramuscularly, but *not* intravenously, except in cardiac arrest

Main dermatological uses and usual adult doses	Adverse effects	Interactions	Other remarks
Hydroxychloroquine Systemic and discoid lupus erythematosus, polymorphic light eruption: 200–400 mg daily, maintaining level at lowest effective dose. Must not exceed 6.5 mg/kg body weight/day (based on the ideal/lean body weight and not on the actual weight of the patient)	Retinopathy, which may cause permanent blindness Corneal deposits Blue pigmentation Headaches Gut upsets, pruritus and rashes Worsening of psoriasis haemolysis Vivid dreams Cardiac toxicity with overdose Patients with porphyria cutanea tarda may develop acute chemical hepatitis	Should not be taken at the same time as other antimalarial drugs May raise plasma digoxin levels Potential neuromuscular toxicity if taken with gentamycin, kanamycin or tobramycin Bioavailability decreased if given with antacids	In the UK, before treatment, patients should be asked about their visual acuity (not corrected with glasses). If it is impaired, or eye disease is present, assessment by an optometrist is advised and any abnormality should be referred to an ophthalmologist. The visual acuity of each eye should be recorded using a standard reading chart. In the USA, all patients should have a pre-treatment ophthalmological assessment with evaluation of visual fields, and examinations every 6–12 months. In addition, patients can check visual fields and accuity with special charts (Amsler grid) at home Discontinue drug if any change occurs Reduce dose with poor renal or liver function Best avoided in the elderly and children Do not give automatic repeat prescriptions Prefer intermittent short courses to continuous treatment if possible

8-Methoxypsoralen (methoxsalen)
Used usually with UVA as PUVA therapy (p. 62)
    Severe psoriasis, vitiligo, localized pustular psoriasis, cutaneous T-cell lymphoma; rarely, lichen planus, atopic dermatitis
    Tablets: 0.6–0.8 mg/kg body weight taken as a single dose 1–2 hours before exposure to UVA
    Liquid (Ultra Capsules) (USA): 0.3 mg/kg body weight taken 1 hour before exposure to UVA
	Nausea
	Itching
	Photoxicity
	Catracts
	Lentigines
	Ageing changes of skin
	Hyperpigmentation
	Cutaneous neoplasms
		Avoid other photosensitizers (see Chapter 18)	The following should checked before treatment:
			• Skin: examine for premalignant lesions and skin cancer
			• Eyes: check for cataracts. Fundoscopic examination of retina. Visual acuity
			• Blood: full blood count, liver and renal function tests and antinuclear factor test
			• Urine analysis
			Eyes should be protected with appropriate lenses for 24 hours after taking the drug
			Protective goggles must be worn during radiation
			If feasible, shield face and genitalia during treatment
			Patients must protect skin against additional sun exposure after ingestion
			Monitor eyes for development of cataracts
			Try to avoid maintenance treatment, more than 250 treatments and a cumulative dose of more than 1000 joules/cm^2 (skin cancer risk)

Index

Clinical Dermatology, Fifth Edition. Richard B. Weller, Hamish J.A. Hunter and Margaret W. Mann.
© 2015 John Wiley & Sons, Ltd. Published 2015 by John Wiley & Sons, Ltd.

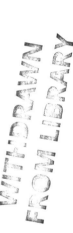
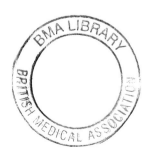